P9-AQI-126

Handbook of Modern Item Response Theory

Wim J. van der Linden
Ronald K. Hambleton
Editors

Handbook of Modern Item Response Theory

With 57 Illustrations

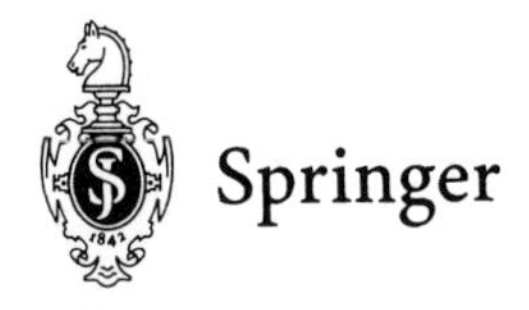
Springer

Wim J. van der Linden
Faculty of Educational Sciences and Technology
University of Twente
7500 AE Enschede
Netherlands

Ronald K. Hambleton
School of Education
University of Massachusetts
Amherst, MA 01003
USA

Library of Congress Cataloging-in-Publication Data

Linden, Wim J. van der
Handbook of modern item response theory / Wim J. van der Linden, Ronald K. Hambleton.
p. cm.
Includes bibliographical references and indexes.
ISBN 0-387-94661-6 (hardcover : alk. paper)
1. Item response theory. 2. Psychometrics. 3. Psychology-- Mathematical models. 4. Rasch, G. (George), 1901-
I. Hambleton, Ronald K. II. Title.
BF176.V56 1996
150′.28′7—dc20 95–49217

Printed on acid-free paper.

Production managed by Terry Kornak; manufacturing supervised by Johanna Tschebull.
Typeset using LaTeX and Springer-Verlag's svsing.sty macro.
Printed and bound by Edwards Brothers Inc., Ann Arbor, MI.
Printed in the United States of America.

9 8 7 6 5 4 3

ISBN 0-387-94661-6 Springer-Verlag New York Berlin Heidelberg

Preface

The central feature of item response theory (IRT) is the specification of a mathematical function relating the probability of an examinee's response on a test item to an underlying ability. Until the 1980s, interest was mainly in response functions for dichotomously-scored items. Nearly all of the research up to that time was focused on the statistical aspects of estimating and testing response functions and making them work in applications to a variety of practical testing problems. Important application of the models were, for example, to the problems of test-score equating, detection of item bias, test assembly, and adaptive testing. In the 1940s and 1950s, the emphasis was on the normal-ogive response function, but for statistical and practical reasons this function was replaced by the logistic response function in the late 1950s. Today, IRT models using logistic response functions dominate the measurement field.

In practice, however, test items often have nominal, partial-credit, graded, or other polytomous response formats. Also, they may have to deal with multidimensional abilities, measure attitudes rather than abilities, or be designed to diagnose underlying cognitive processes. Due to computerization of tests, recording of response latencies has become within reach too, and models to deal with such data are needed. In the 1980s, psychological and educational researchers, therefore, shifted their attention to the development of models dealing with such response formats and types of data. The goal of this *Handbook* is to bring these new developments together in a single volume.

Each chapter in this book contains an up-to-date description of a single IRT model (or family of models) written by the author(s) who originally proposed the model or contributed substantially to its development. Each chapter also provides complete references to the basic literature on the model. Another feature of the book is that all chapters follow the same fixed format (with only a few minor exceptions). They begin with an *Introduction* in which the necessity of the model is historically and practically motivated. In the next section, *Presentation of the Model*, the model is introduced, its mathematical form is described, its parameters are interpreted, and possible generalizations and extensions of it are discussed. The statistical aspects of the model are addressed in the following two sections, *Parameter Estimation* and *Goodness of Fit*. In addition to an explanation of the statistical methods available to estimate the parameters and determine the fit of the model to response data, these sections also contain references to existing software developed for the model. The next section, *Empirical Example*, presents one or more examples based on empirical data. These examples are intended to show how to use the model in a practical application. The final section, *Discussion*, covers possible remaining aspects of the use of the model. All chapters use a common notation for basic quantities such as item responses, ability and attitude variables, and item parameters.

An introductory chapter to the book summarizes the theory available for the original unidimensional normal-ogive and logistic IRT models for items with dichotomously-scored responses. The remaining chapters in the book are presented in six sections:

1. *Models for items with polytomous response formats.* This section contains models for unordered and ordered discrete polytomous response formats.

2. *Models for response time or multiple attempts on items.* Models for tests with a time limit in which response time is recorded and models for tests recording the numbers of successes on replicated trials are presented in this section.

3. *Models for multiple abilities or cognitive components.* Sometimes item responses are produced by more than one ability or by a process with more than one cognitive component. This section of the book presents the models to be used in such cases.

4. *Nonparametric models.* Though models with a parametric form for response functions have dominated the literature, relaxation of these parametric assumptions can often be helpful and lead to some important results. Nonparametric approaches to response functions are brought together in this section.

5. *Models for nonmonotone items.* Models for the analysis of responses to statements in attitude instruments with response functions not monotonically increasing in the underlying variable are given in this section.

6. *Models with special assumptions about the response process.* The final section contains models for mixtures of response processes or ability distributions, conditional dependence between responses, and responses formats designed to allow for partial knowledge of test items.

The book has not only been designed as a comprehensive introduction to modern test theory for practitioners as well as researchers but also as a daily reference by these two groups. In addition, we hope the book may serve as a valuable resource in graduate courses on modern developments in test theory. As its chapters can be read independently, teachers are able to design their own routes through the book to accommodate their course objectives.

The editors appreciate the opportunity to acknowledge the support of the following institutions and persons during the production of this book. The American College Testing, Iowa City, Iowa, provided the first editor with generous hospitality during the first stage of the project. The Department of Educational Measurement and Data Analysis at the University of Twente and the Laboratory of Psychometric and Evaluative Research at the University of Massachusetts created the climate which fostered the work on this *Handbook*. Untiring secretarial support was given by Anita Burchartz-Huls, Colene Feldman, and Peg Louraine. Martin Gilchrist was a helpful source of information at Springer-Verlag throughout the whole project. But most of all, the editors are grateful to the authors of the chapters in this book who believed in the project and were willing to contribute their valuable time.

Wim J. van der Linden — University of Twente
Ronald K. Hambleton — University of Massachusetts at Amherst

Contents

Contributors

Erling B. Andersen
Institute of Statistics, University of Copenhagen, DK-1455 Copenhagen, Denmark

David Andrich
Murdoch University, School of Education, Murdoch Western Australia, 6150, Australia

R. Darrell Bock
University of Chicago, Department of Behavioral Sciences, Chicago, IL 60637, USA

Susan E. Embretson
University of Kansas, Department of Psychology, Lawrence, KS 66045, USA

Gerhard H. Fischer
Institut für Psychologie, Universität Wien, 1010 Wien, Austria

H.H. de Vries
SWOKA, 2515JL, The Hague, The Netherlands

C.A.W. Glas
Department of Educational Measurement and Data Analysis, University of Twente, 7500 AE Enschede, Netherlands

Herbert Hoijtink
University of Gronigen, Department of Statistics and Measurement Theory, 9712 TS Groningen, Netherlands

T.P. Hutchinson
Department of Mathematical Statistics, University of Sydney, Sydney NSW 2006, Australia

Robert J. Jannarone
Electrical & Computer Engineering Department, University of South Carolina, Columbia, SC 29205, USA

Margo G.H. Jansen
Department of Education, University of Groningen, Grote Rozenstraat 38, 9712 TJ Groningen, Netherlands

Henk Kelderman
Department of Industrial and Organizational Psychology, Free University, 1081 BT Amsterdam, Netherlands

Geofferey N. Masters
The Australian Council for Educational Research, Hawthorne, Victoria 3122, Australia

Roderick P. McDonald
Department of Psychology, University of Illinois, Champaign, IL 61820-6990, USA

Robert J. Mokken
Franklinstraat 16-18, 1171 BL Badhoevedorp, Netherlands

Ivo W. Molenaar
University of Gronigen, Department of Statistics and Measurement Theory, 9712 TS Groningen, Netherlands

Eiji Muraki
Educational Testing Service, Princeton, NJ 08541, USA

J.O. Ramsay
Department of Psychology, 1205 Dr. Penfield Avenue, Montreal H3A 1B1 PQ, Canada

Mark D. Reckase
American College Testing, Iowa City, IA 52243, USA

Edward E. Roskam
NICI, Psychologisch Laboratorium, 6500 HE Nijmegen, Netherlands

Jürgen Rost
IPN, D-2300 Kiel 7, Germany

Fumiko Samejima
Psychology Department, University of Tennessee, Knoxville, TN 27996, USA

Elisabeth Seliger
Department of Psychology, University of Vienna, A-1010, Vienna, Austria

Judith A. Spray
American College Testing, Iowa City, IA 52243, USA

Lynne Steinberg
Department of Psychology, Syracuse University, Syracuse, NY 13244-2340, USA

David Thissen
Department of Psychology, University of North Carolina, Chapel Hill, NC 27599-3270, USA

Gerhard Tutz
Technische Universität Berlin, Institut für Quantitative Methoden, 10587 Berlin, Germany

N.D. Verhelst
Cito, 6801 MG Arnhem, Netherlands

Huub Verstralen
Cito, 6801 MG Arnhem, Netherlands

Benjamin D. Wright
Department of Education, University of Chicago, Chicago, IL 60637, USA

Michele F. Zimowski
Department of Behavioral Sciences, University of Chicago, Chicago, IL 60637, USA

Aeilko H. Zwinderman
Department of Medical Statistics, University of Leiden, 2300 RA Leiden, Netherlands

1

Item Response Theory: Brief History, Common Models, and Extensions

Wim J. van der Linden and Ronald K. Hambleton

Long experience with measurement instruments such as thermometers, yardsticks, and speedometers may have left the impression that measurement instruments are physical devices providing measurements that can be read directly off a numerical scale. This impression is certainly not valid for educational and psychological tests. A useful way to view a test is as a series of small experiments in which the tester records a vector of responses by the testee. These responses are not direct measurements, but provide the data from which measurements can be inferred.

Just as in any experiment, the methodological problem of controlling responses for experimental error holds for tests. Experimental error with tests arises from the fact that not only the independent variables but also other variables operational in the experiment, generally known as background, nuisance, or error variables, may have an impact on the responses concerned. Unless adequate control is provided for such variables, valid inferences cannot be made from the experiment.

Literature on experimental design has shown three basic ways of coping with experimental error (Cox, 1958):

(1) matching or standardization;

(2) randomization; and

(3) statistical adjustment.

If conditions in an experiment are matched, subjects operate under the same levels of error or nuisance variables, and effects of these variables cannot explain any differences in experimental outcomes. Although matching is a powerful technique, it does have the disadvantage of restricted generalizability. Experimental results hold only conditionally on the levels of the matching variables that were in force.

Randomization is based on the principle that if error variables cannot be manipulated to create the same effects, random selection of conditions guarantees that these effects can be expected to be the same on average.

Thus, these effects can not have a systematic influence on the responses of the subjects.

Statistical adjustment, on the other hand, is a technique for *post hoc* control, that is, it does not assume any intervention from the experimenter. The technique can be used when matching or randomization is impossible, but the technique does require that the levels of the relevant error variables have been measured during the experiment. The measurements are used to adjust the observed values of the dependent variables for the effects of the error variables.

Adjustment procedures are model-based in the sense that quantitative theory is needed to provide the mathematical equations relating error variables to the dependent variables. In a mature science such as physics, substantive theory may be available to provide these equations. For example, if temperature or air pressure are known to be disturbing variables that vary across experimental conditions and well-confirmed theory is available to predict how these variables affect the dependent variable, then experimental findings can be adjusted to common levels of temperature or pressure afterwards. If no substantive theory is available, however, it may be possible to postulate plausible equations and to estimate their parameters from data on the error and dependent variables. If the estimated equations fit the data, they can be used to provide the adjustment. This direction for analysis is popular in the behavioral sciences, in particular in the form of analysis of covariance (ANCOVA), which postulates linear (regression) equations between error and dependent variables.

Classical Test Theory

Classical test theory fits in with the tradition of experimental control through matching and randomization (van der Linden, 1986). The theory starts from the assumption that systematic effects between responses of examinees are due only to variation in the ability (i.e., true score) of interest. All other potential sources of variation existing in the testing materials, external conditions, or internal to the examinees are assumed either to be constant through rigorous standardization or to have an effect that is nonsystematic or "random by nature."

The classical test theory model, which was put forward by Spearman (1904) but received its final axiomatic form in Novick (1966), decomposes the observed test score into a true score and an error score. Let X_{jg} be the observed-score variable for examinee j on test g, which is assumed to be random across replications of the experiment. The classical model for a fixed examinee j postulates that

$$X_{jg} = \tau_{jg} + E_{jg}, \tag{1}$$

where τ_{jg} is the true score defined as the expected observed score, $\mathcal{E}_{jg}X_{jg}$, and $E_{jg} \equiv X_{jg} - \tau_{jg}$ is the error score. Note that, owing to the definition of the true and error scores, the model does not impose any constraints on X_{jg} and is thus always "true." Also, observe that τ_{jg} is *defined* to cover all systematic information in the experiment, and that it is only a parameter of interest if experimental control of all error variables has been successful. Finally, it is worthwhile to realize that, as in any application of the matching principle, τ_{jg} has only meaning conditionally on the chosen levels of the standardized error variables. The true score is fully determined by the test as designed—not by some Platonic state inside the examinee that exists independent of the test (Lord and Novick, 1968, Sec. 2.8).

If random selection of examinees from a population is a valid assumption, the true score parameter, τ_{jg}, has to be replaced by a random true score variable, T_{j*}. The model in Eq. (1) becomes:

$$X_{j*} = T_{j*} + E_{j*} \tag{2}$$

(Lord and Novick, 1968, Sec. 2.6). It is useful to note that Eq. (2) is also the linear equation of the one-way analysis of variance (ANOVA) model with a random factor. This equivalence points again to the fact that educational and psychological tests can be viewed as regular standardized experiments.

Test-Dependent True Scores

As mentioned earlier, a serious disadvantage of experiments in which matching is used for experimental control is reduction of external validity. Statistical inferences from the data produced by the experiment cannot be generalized beyond the standardized levels of its error or nuisance variables. The same principle holds for standardized tests. True scores on two different tests designed to measure the same ability variable, even if they involve the same standardization of external and internal conditions, are generally unequal. The reason is that each test entails its own set of items and that each item has different properties. From a measurement point of view, *such properties of items are nuisance or error variables that escape standardization.*

The practical consequences of this problem, which has been documented numerous times in the test-theoretic literature [for an early reference, see Loevinger (1947)], are formidable. For example, it is impossible to use different versions of a test in a longitudinal study or on separate administrations without confounding differences between test scores by differences between the properties of the tests.

Statistical Adjustment for Differences Between Test Items

Perhaps the best way to solve the problem of test-dependent scores is through the third method of experimental control listed previously—statistical adjustment. The method of statistical adjustment requires explicit parametrization of the ability of interest as well as the properties of the items, via a model that relates their values to response data collected through the test. If the model holds and the item parameters are known, the model adjusts the data for the properties of items in the test, and, therefore, can be used to produce ability measures that are free of the properties of the items in the test. This idea of statistical adjustment of ability measures for nuisance properties of the items is exactly analogous to the way analysis of covariance (ANCOVA) was introduced to parametrize and subsequently "remove" the effects of covariates in an ANOVA study.

Item Response Theory

Mathematical models to make statistical adjustments in test scores have been developed in item response theory (IRT). The well-known IRT models for dichotomous responses, for instance, adjust response data for such properties of test items as their difficulty, discriminating power, or liability to guessing. These models will be reviewed in this chapter.

The emphasis in this volume, however, it not on IRT models for handling dichotomously scored data, but is on the various extensions and refinements of these original models that have emerged since the publication of Lord and Novick's *Statistical Theories of Mental Test Scores* (1968). The new models have been designed for response data obtained under less rigorous standardization of conditions or admitting open-ended response formats, implying that test scores have to be adjusted for a larger array of nuisance variables. For example, if, in addition to the ability of interest, a nuisance ability has an effect on responses to test items, a second ability parameter may be added to the model to account for its effects. Several examples of such multidimensional IRT models are presented in this volume. Likewise, if responses are made to the individual answer choices of an item (e.g., multiple-choice item), they clearly depend on the properties of the answer choices, which have to be parametrized in addition to other properties of the item. A variety of models for this case, generally known as polytomous IRT models, is also presented in this volume.

The methodological principle underlying all of the models included in this volume is the simple principle of a separate parameter for each factor with a separate effect on the item responses. However, it belongs to the "art of modeling" to design a mathematical structure that reflects the interaction between these factors and at the same time makes the model statistically tractable. Before introducing the models in a formal way, a brief review of common dichotomous IRT models is given in this chapter. These were the first IRT models to be developed, and they have been widely researched and extensively used to solve many practical measurement problems (Hambleton and Swaminathan, 1985; Lord, 1980).

Review of Dichotomous IRT Models

As its name suggests, IRT models the test behavior not at the level of (arbitrarily defined) test scores, but at the item level. The first item format addressed in the history of IRT was the dichotomous format in which responses are scored either as correct or incorrect. If the response by examinee j to item i is denoted by a random variable U_{ij}, it is convenient to code the two possible scores as $U_{ij} = 1$ (correct) and $U_{ij} = 0$ (incorrect). To model the distribution of this variable, or, equivalently, the probability of a correct response, the ability of the examinee is presented by a parameter $\theta \in (-\infty, +\infty)$, and it is assumed in a two-parameter model that the properties of item i that have an effect on the probability of a success are its "difficulty" and "discriminating power," which are represented by parameters $b_i \in (-\infty, +\infty)$ and $a_i \in (0, +\infty)$, respectively. These parameters are simply symbols at this point; their meaning can only be established if the model is further specified.

Since the ability parameter is the *structural parameter* that is of interest and the item parameters are considered *nuisance parameters*, the probability of success on item i is usually presented as $P_i(\theta)$, that is, as a function of θ specific to item i. This function is known as the *item response function* (IRF). Previous names for the same function include *item characteristic curve* (ICC), introduced by Tucker (1946), and *trace line*, introduced by Lazarsfeld (1950). Owing to restrictions in the range of possible probability values, item response functions cannot be linear in θ. Obviously, the function has to be monotonically increasing in θ. The need for a monotonically increasing function with a lower and upper asymptote at 0 and 1, respectively, suggests a choice from the class of cumulative distributions functions (cdf's). This choice was the one immediately made when IRT originated.

Normal-Ogive Model

The first IRT model was the normal-ogive model, which postulated a normal cdf as a response function for the item:

$$P_i(\theta) = \int_{-\infty}^{a_i(\theta - b_i)} \frac{1}{\sqrt{2\pi}} e^{-z^2/z} dz. \tag{3}$$

For a few possible values of the parameters b_i and a_i, Figure 1 displays the shape of a set of normal-ogive response functions. From straightforward analysis of Eq. (3) it is clear that, as demonstrated in Figure 1, the difficulty parameter b_i is the point on the ability scale where an examinee has a probability of success on the item of 0.50, whereas the value of a_i is proportional to the slope of the tangent to the response function at this point. Both formal properties of the model justify the interpretation suggested by the names of the parameters. If b_i increases in value, the response

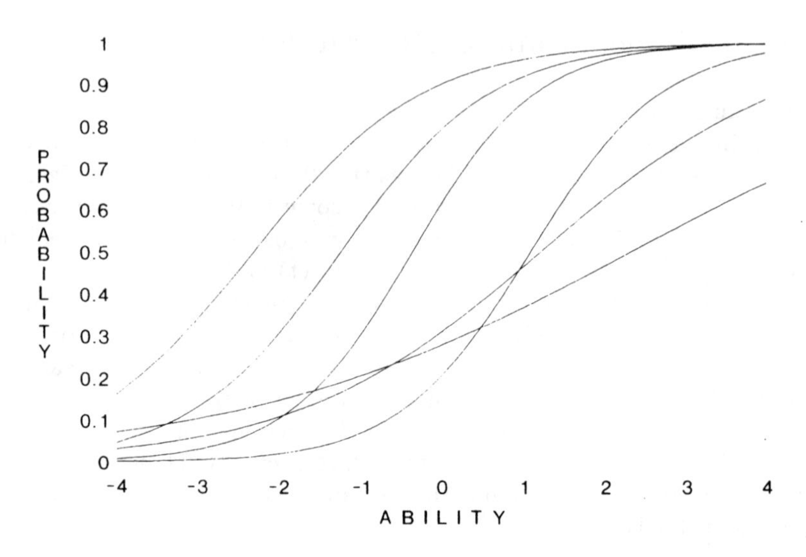

FIGURE 1. Two-parameter normal-ogive response functions.

function moves to the right and a higher ability is needed to produce the same probability of success on the item. Also, the larger the value of a_i, the better the item discriminates between the probabilities of success of examinees with abilities below and above $\theta = b_i$.

Although credit for the normal-ogive model is sometimes given to Lawley (1943), the same basic model had been studied earlier by Ferguson (1942), Mosier (1940, 1941), and Richardson (1936). In fact, the original idea for the model can be traced to Thurstone's use of the normal model in his discriminal dispersions theory of stimulus perception (Thurstone, 1927b). This impact of the psychophysical scaling literature on the early writings of these authors is obvious from their terminology. Researchers in psychophysics study the relation between the physical properties of stimuli and their perception by human subjects. Its main method is to present a stimulus of varying strength, for example, a tone of varying loudness, where the subject's task is to report whether or not he/she was able to detect the stimulus. Since the probability of detection is clearly an increasing function of the physical strength of the stimulus, the normal cdf with the parametrization in Eq. (3) was used as response function. However, in this model, θ stands for the *known* strength of a stimulus and the interest was only in the parameters a_i and b_i, the latter being known as the *limen* of the stimulus—a name also used for the difficulty of the item in the early days of IRT. Mosier (1940, 1941) was quite explicit in his description of the parallels between psychophysics and psychometric modeling. In his 1940 publication he provides a table with the different names used in the two disciplines, which in fact describe common quantities.

Early descriptions of the normal-ogive model as well as of the procedures for its statistical analysis were not always clear. For example, ability θ was not always considered as a latent variable with values to be estimated from the data but taken to be the observed test score. Equation (3) was used as a model for the (nonlinear) regression of item on test scores. Richardson, on the other hand, used the normal-ogive model to scale a dichotomous external success criterion on the observed-score scale of several test forms differing in difficulty. In the same spirit that originated with Binet and Simon (1905), and was reinforced by the widespread use of Thurstone's method of absolute scaling (Thurstone, 1925, 1927a), the ability variable was always assumed to be normally distributed in the population of examinees. The belief in normality was so strong that even if an observed ability distribution did not follow a normal distribution, it was normalized to find the "true" scale on which the model in Eq. (3) was assumed to hold. Also, in accordance with prevailing practice, the ability scale was divided into a set of—typically seven—intervals defined by equal standard-deviation units. The midpoints of the intervals were the discrete ability scores actually used to fit a normal-ogive model.

The first coherent treatment of the normal-ogive model that did not suffer from the above idiosyncrasies was given in Lord (1952). His treatment also included psychometric theory for the bivariate distribution of item and ability scores, the limiting frequency distributions of observed scores on large tests, and the bivariate distribution of observed scores on two tests measuring the same ability variable. All these distributions were derived with the help of the normal-ogive model.

Parameter Estimation. In the 1940s and 1950s, computers were not available and parameter estimation was a laborious job. The main estimation method was borrowed from psychophysics and known as the *constant process.* The method consisted of fitting a weighted regression line through the data points and the empirical probits. [The latter were defined as the inverse transformation of Eq. (3) for empirical proportions of successes on the item.] The weights used in the regression analysis were known as the Müller–Urban weights. Lawley (1943) derived maximum-likelihood (ML) estimators for the item parameters in the normal-ogive model and showed that these were identical to the constant-process estimators upon substitution of empirical probits in the Müller–Urban weights.

Lord and Novick (1968, Secs. 16.8–16.10) presented the following set of equations, derived under the assumption of a normal ability distribution, that relate the parameters b_i and a_i to the classical item-π value and biserial item-test correlation, ρ_i:

$$a_i = \frac{\rho_i}{\sqrt{1 - \rho_1^2}}, \tag{4}$$

$$b_i = \frac{-\gamma_i}{\rho_i}, \tag{5}$$

where γ_i is defined by

$$\gamma_i = \Phi^{-1}(\pi_i) \tag{6}$$

and $\Phi(\cdot)$ is the standard normal distribution function. Although the equations were based on the assumption of the normal-ogive model, plug-in estimates based on these equations have long served as heuristic estimates or as starting values for the maximum likelihood (ML) estimators of the parameters in the logistic model (Urry, 1974).

Goodness of Fit. Formal goodness-of-fit tests were never developed for the normal-ogive model. In the first analyses published, the basic method of checking the model was graphical inspection of plots of predicted and empirical item-test regression functions [see, for example, Ferguson (1942) and Richardson (1936)]. Lord (1952) extended this method to plots of predicted and empirical test-score distributions and used a chi-square test to study the differences between expected and actual item performance at various intervals along the ability continuum.

Rasch or One-Parameter Logistic Model

Rasch began his work in educational and psychological measurement in the late 1940s. In the 1950s he developed two Poisson models for reading tests and a model for intelligence and achievement tests. The latter was called "a structural model for items in a test" by him, but is now generally known as the Rasch model. Formally, the model is a special case of the Birnbaum model to be discussed below. However, because it has unique properties among all known IRT models, it deserves a separate introduction. A full account of the three models is given in Rasch (1960).

Rasch's main motivation for his models was his desire to eliminate references to populations of examinees in analyses of tests (Rasch, 1960, Preface; Chap. 1). Test analysis would only be worthwhile if it were individual-centered, with separate parameters for the items and the examinees. To make his point, Rasch often referred to the work of Skinner, who was also known for his dislike of the use of population-based statistics and always experimented with individual cases. Rasch's point of view marked the transition from population-based classical test theory, with its emphasis on standardization and randomization, to IRT with its probabilistic modeling of the interaction between an individual item and an individual examinee. As will be shown, the existence of sufficient statistics for the item parameters in the Rasch model can be used statistically to adjust ability estimates for the presence of nuisance properties of the items in a special way.

Poisson Model. Only the model for misreadings will be discussed here. The model is based on the assumption of a Poisson distribution for the number of reading errors in a text. This assumption is justified if the reading process is stationary and does not change due to, for example, the examinee becoming tired or fluctuations in the difficulties of the words in the text.

If the text consists of T words and X is the random variable denoting the number of words misread, then the Poisson distribution assumes that

$$P(X = x \mid T) = e^{-\lambda} \frac{\lambda^x}{x!}, \tag{7}$$

where parameter λ is the expected number of misreadings. Equivalently, $\xi \equiv \lambda/T$ is the probability of misreading a single word sampled from the text.

The basic approach followed by Rasch was to further model the basic parameter ξ as a function of parameters describing the ability of the examinee and the difficulty of the text. If θ_j is taken to represent the reading ability of examinee j and δ_t represents the difficulty of text t, then ξ_{it} can be expected to be a parameter decreasing in θ_j and increasing in δ_t. The simple model proposed by Rasch was

$$\xi_{ij} = \frac{\delta_t}{\theta_j}. \tag{8}$$

If the model in Eqs. (7) and (8) is applied to a series of examinees $j = 1, \ldots, N$ reading a series of texts $t = 1, \ldots, T$, it holds that the sum of reading errors in text t across examinees, $X_{t.}$, is a sufficient statistic for δ_t. It is a well-known statistical result that the distribution of X_{tj} given $X_{t.} = x_{t.}$ follows a binomial distribution with a success parameter independent of δ_t. Removing the effect of text difficulty from the data when estimating the ability of an examinee is realized when the inference is based on the conditional likelihood function associated with this binomial.

Rasch Model. The main model for a test with items $i = 1, \ldots, n$ proposed by Rasch departs from the parameter structure defined in Eq. (8). Substituting item difficulty δ_i for text difficulty δ_t, the question can be asked about the simplest model with the parameter structure in Eq. (8). The answer proposed by Rasch was the following transformation:

$$\begin{aligned} P_i(U_{ij} = 1 \mid \theta) &= \frac{\frac{\theta_j}{\delta_i}}{1 + \frac{\theta_j}{\delta_i}} \\ &= \frac{\theta_j}{\theta_j + \delta_i}. \end{aligned} \tag{9}$$

The model, presented in this form, has the simple interpretation of the probability of success being equal to the value of the person parameter relative to the value of the item parameter. Taking the parameters on a logarithmic scale (but maintaining the notation), the model can easily be

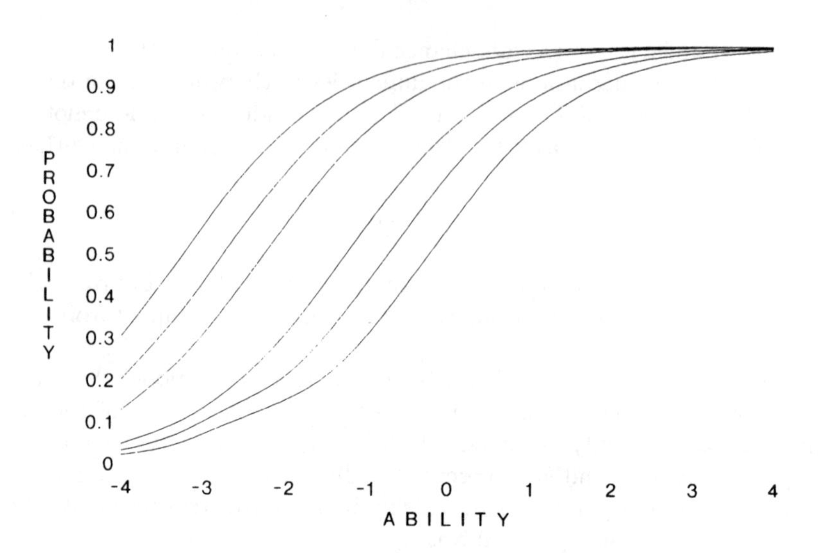

FIGURE 2. One-parameter logistic response functions.

shown to be equivalent to the following form, known as the one-parameter logistic (or 1-PL) model:

$$P(U_{ij} = 1 \mid \theta) = \frac{1}{1 + \exp\{-(\theta - \delta_i)\}}. \tag{10}$$

This representation can be used to show a fundamental property of the Rasch model relative to the two-parameter normal-ogive model, namely, that its IRF's do not intersect. Figure 2 illustrates this property graphically for a few IRF's.

As demonstrated in the next section, the model uses the same form of "item-free" estimation of examinee ability as the Poisson model described above.

Parameter Estimation. Using the representation in Eq. (9), the joint likelihood function associated with the case of N examinees having responded to n items is equal to

$$\begin{aligned} L(\theta, \delta; u) &= \prod_i \prod_j \frac{(\theta_j/\delta_i)^{u_{ij}}}{1 + \theta_j/\delta_i} \\ &= \frac{\prod_i \delta_i^{\,u_{i.}} \prod_j \theta_j^{u_{.j}}}{\prod_i \prod_j (1 + \theta_j/\delta_i)}, \end{aligned} \tag{11}$$

where $\theta \equiv (\theta_1, \ldots, \theta_N)$, $\delta \equiv (\delta_1, \ldots, \delta_n)$, $u \equiv (u_{ij})$, and $u_{i.}$ and $u_{.j}$ are the marginal sums of the data matrix. Since the marginal sums can be shown to be sufficient statistics for the difficulty and item parameters, respectively, it holds for the likelihood function associated with the conditional probability of (U_{ij}) given $U_i = u_i$ that

$$L(\theta; u \mid u_{i.}) = \frac{\prod_j \theta^{u_{j.}}}{\prod_i \gamma_{u_{i.}}}, \tag{12}$$

where the functions $\gamma_{u_{i.}}$ are combinatorial functions of the ability parameters known as elementary symmetric functions (Fischer, 1974, Sec. 13.5).

Three comments on this result should be made. First, the conditional likelihood function contains only the ability parameters. Maximum-likelihood estimates of the ability parameters can thus be obtained from (conditional) likelihood functions free of any item parameter. It is in this sense that sufficient statistics for the item parameters can be used to adjust the data for the difficulty of the items. (Note, however, that these CML estimators are not independent of the item parameters. They have small-sample first moments that may depend on the item parameters, whereas their second moments always depend on these parameters.) The result in Eq. (12) holds for any model in the exponential family, which includes the Rasch model (Lehmann, 1959, Theor. 1.2.1).

Second, the same procedure can be followed to obtain CML estimates for the item parameters. In practice, however, only the item parameters are estimated by CML estimation. These parameters are then considered as known and the examinee parameters are estimated under this assumption by regular maximum likelihood methods.

Third, until recently, the numerical problems involved in dealing with the elementary symmetric functions in the CML equations seemed insurmountable, and applications to tests with more than 60 items were not feasible. The situation has changed favorably since new algorithms with improved efficiency have become available that permit CML estimation of hundreds of parameters (Liou, 1994; Verhelst et al., 1984).

As an alternative to CML estimation, estimates of the item parameters can be found through maximization of the marginal likelihood function, obtained from Eq. (11) by integrating over a common density for the θ's, which is typically taken to be a normal density with parameters μ and σ:

$$L(\delta; u, \mu, \sigma) = \int_{\infty}^{-\infty} L(\delta, \theta; u) f(\theta; \mu, \sigma) d\theta. \tag{13}$$

An efficient way to calculate these marginal maximum-likelihood (MML) estimates is to use an EM algorithm (Thissen, 1982). Marginalization as in Eq. (13) is another way to eliminate the impact of the ability parameters when estimating item parameters.

A variety of other estimation procedures have been studied, including (hierarchical) Bayesian methods (Swaminathan and Gifford, 1982), semi-parametric methods in which the ability density in Eq. (13) is estimated from the data (de Leeuw and Verhelst, 1986; Engelen, 1989), an iterative least-squares method (Verhelst and Molenaar, 1988), and a minimum chi-square method (Fischer, 1974, Sec. 14.8).

Goodness of Fit

Rasch was not particularly interested in formal tests of the goodness of fit of his model. In his 1960 book, in a fashion which was similar to the early work with the normal-ogive model, he only diagnosed the fit of his model using plots of residuals.

The first statistical test for the goodness of fit of the Rasch model was Andersen's (1973) likelihood-ratio test. The test was designed to check whether item parameter estimates in different score groups are equal up to the sampling errors of the estimates. Several other statistical tests have followed. Molenaar (1983) offered a statistic sensitive to differences in discriminating power between items. Van den Wollenberg (1982) introduced the test statistics Q_1 and Q_2, the second of which is sensitive to violations of the assumption of unidimensionality. Large families of possible tests, with power against specific violations of the model, are given in Glas (1988, 1989) and Kelderman (1984).

A controversial aspect of analyzing test items for model fit has always been whether the case of a misfitting item should lead to removal of the item from the test or to a relaxation of the model. In principle, both strategies are possible. Test practice does have a long tradition of item analysis in which items not meeting certain conventional values for the classical difficulty and discrimination parameters are removed from the pool or the test. On the other hand, a relaxation of the Rasch model is available in the form of the two- and three-parameter logistic models, which may better fit problematic items (but need not necessarily do so). The position taken here is that no general recommendation can be made with respect to this choice between a more stringent model with excellent statistical tractability and a more flexible model likely to fit a larger collection of items. Additional factors such as (1) the nature of the misfit, (2) the availability of substitute items, (3) the amount of time available for rewriting items, (4) the availability of a sufficiently large sample to properly estimate item parameters for more general models, and—probably most important—(5) the goal of the testing procedure play a significant role in the handling of items that are not fit by the Rasch model. For example, different decisions about the handling of model misfit are likely to be made in a long-term project developing a psychological test versus an educational assessment project with an item pool that has to cover comprehensively the content of a textbook used by the schools.

Birnbaum's Two- and Three-Parameter Logistic Models

Birnbaum worked on his contributions to IRT in the late 1950s but his work became widely known through the chapters he contributed to Lord and Novick (1968, Chaps. 17–20). Unlike Rasch, Birnbaum's work was not motivated by a desire to develop a different kind of test theory. As a statistician, his main aim was to make the work begun by Lord (1952) on the normal-ogive model statistically feasible. In particular, he provided the statistical theory for ability and item parameter estimation, applied statistical information measures to ability estimation and hypothesis testing with respect to ability values, and proposed a rational approach to test construction.

Birnbaum's main contribution, however, was his suggestion to replace the normal-ogive model in Eq. (3) by the logistic model:

$$P_i(\theta) = \frac{1}{1 + \exp\{-a_i(\theta - b_i)\}}. \tag{14}$$

The motivation for this substitution was the result of Haley (1952) that for a logistic cdf with scale factor 1.7, $L(1.7x)$, and a normal cdf, $N(x)$:

$$|N(x) - L(1.7x)| < 0.01 \qquad \text{for } x \in (-\infty, \infty)$$

[for a slight improvement on this result, see Molenaar (1974)]. At the same time, the logistic function is much more tractable than the normal-ogive function, while the parameters b_i and a_i retain their graphical interpretation shown in Figure 1.

Birnbaum also proposed a third parameter for inclusion in the model to account for the nonzero performance of low-ability examinees on multiple-choice items. This nonzero performance is due to the probability of guessing correct answers to multiple-choice items. The model then takes the form

$$P_i(\theta) = c_i + (1 - c_i)\frac{1}{1 + \exp\{-a_i(\theta - b_i)\}}. \tag{15}$$

Equation (15) follows immediately from the assumption that the examinee either knows the correct response with a probability described by Eq. (14) or guesses with a probability of success equal to the value of c_i. From Figure 3, it is clear that the parameter c_i is the height of the lower asymptote of the response function. In spite of the fact that Eq. (15) no longer defines a logistic function, the model is known as the three-parameter logistic (or 3-PL) model, while the model in Eq. (14) is called the two-parameter logistic (or 2-PL) model. The c-parameter is sometimes referred to as the "guessing parameter," since its function is to account for the test item performance of low-ability examinees.

One of Birnbaum's other contributions to psychometric theory was his introduction of Fisher's measure to describe the information structure of a

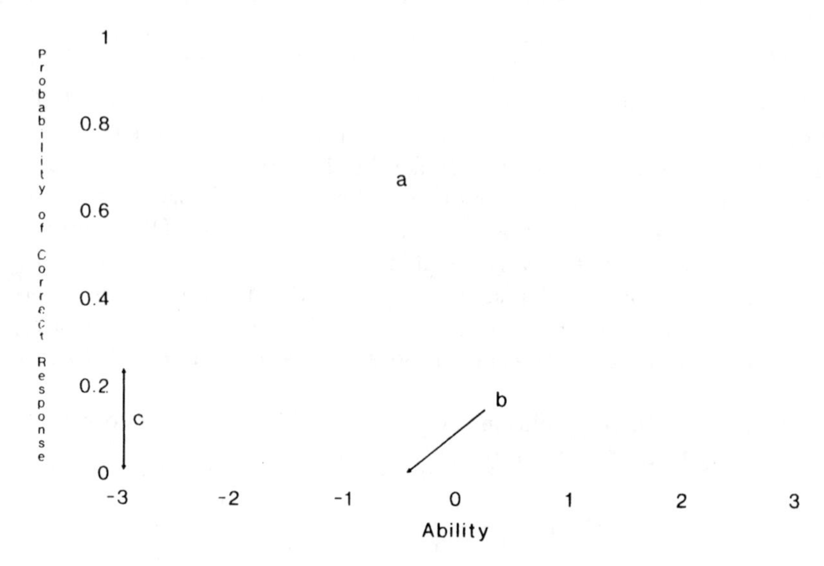

FIGURE 3. Three-parameter logistic response function.

test. For a dichotomous IRT model, Fisher's measure for the information on the unknown ability θ in a test of n items can be written as

$$\begin{aligned} I(\theta) &= \sum_{i=1}^{n} I_i(\theta) \\ &= \sum_{i=1}^{n} \frac{[P_i'(\theta)]^2}{P_i(\theta)[1 - P_i(\theta)]}, \end{aligned} \tag{16}$$

where $I_i(\theta)$ is the information on θ in the response on item i and $P_i'(\theta) \equiv \frac{\partial}{\partial\theta} P_i(\theta)$. One of his suggestions for the use of these information measures was to influence test construction by first setting up a target for the information function of the test and then assembling the test to meet this target using the additivity in Eq. (16).

Birnbaum also derived weights for optimally scoring a test in a two-point classification problem and compared the efficiency of several other scoring formulas for the ability parameter in the model. His strongest statistical contribution no doubt was his application of the theory of maximum likelihood to the estimation of both the ability and the item parameters in the logistic models, which will now be addressed.

Parameters Estimation. Continuing the same notation as before, the likelihood function for the case of N examinees and n items associated with the 2-PL model can be written as

$$L(\theta, a, b; u) = \prod_i \prod_j P_i(\theta_j; a_i, b_i)^{u_{ij}} [1 - P_i(\theta_j; a_i, b_i)]^{1-u_{ij}}. \tag{17}$$

Maximizing the logarithm of the likelihood function results in the following set of estimation equations:

$$\sum_i a_i(u_{ij} - P_i(\theta_j; a_i, b_i)) = 0, \qquad j = 1, \dots, N;$$

$$\sum_j a_i(u_{ij} - P_i(\theta_j; a_i, b_i)) = 0, \qquad i = 1, \dots, n; \tag{18}$$

$$\sum_j (u_{ij} - P_i(\theta_j; a_i, b_i))(\theta_j - b_i) = 0, \qquad i = 1, \dots, n.$$

The technique suggested by Birnbaum was jointly to solve the equations for the values of the unknown parameters in an iterative scheme, which starts with initial values for the ability parameters, solves the equations for the item parameters, fixes the item parameters, and solves the equations for improved estimates of the values of the ability parameters, etc. The solutions obtained by this procedure are known as the joint maximum likelihood (JML) estimates, although the name alternating maximum likelihood (AML) would seem to offer a better description of the procedure.

Problems of convergence and a somewhat unknown statistical status of the JML estimators have led to the popularity of MML estimation for the 2-PL and 3-PL models. The method was introduced by Bock and Lieberman (1970) for the normal-ogive model but immediately adopted as a routine for the logistic model. For a density function $f(\theta)$ describing the ability distribution, the marginal probability of obtaining a response vector $u \equiv (u_1, \dots, u_n)$ on the items in the test is equal to

$$P(u \mid a, b) = \int_{-\infty}^{\infty} \prod_i P_i(\theta; a_i, b_i)^{u_i} [1 - P_i(\theta; a_i, b_i)]^{1-u_i} f(\theta) d\theta. \tag{19}$$

The marginal likelihood function associated with the full data matrix $u \equiv (u_{ij})$ is given by the multinomial kernel

$$L(a, b; u) = \prod_{u=1}^{2^n} \pi_u^{r_u}, \tag{20}$$

where π_u is the probability of the response pattern in Eq. (19), which has frequency r_u in the data matrix. Owing to the large number of possible response vectors, the Bock and Lieberman method was slow and not practical for more than about 10 items. However, Bock and Aitkin (1981) introduce a version of the method in which an EM algorithm is implemented. This version is able to handle realistic numbers of items and has become the popular approach for the estimation of item parameters in the 2-PL and 3-PL model.

It is clear from the likelihood function in Eq. (20), that the ability parameters have been removed. Therefore, MML estimators of the item parameters are estimators that share such properties of regular ML estimators as consistency and asymptotic efficiency (Andersen, 1980, Chap. 2). The assumption of a density for the ability distribution needed to arrive at Eq. (20), for which generally the standard normal density is chosen, is mild. For an extensive description of an application of MML estimation with the EM algorithm to actual test data, see Tsutakawa (1984). For more details on ML estimation in these models, see Baker (1992) and Hambleton and Swaminathan (1985, Chaps. 5 and 7).

A variety of Bayesian approaches to parameter estimation in the 2-PL and 3-PL model have been studied. Relevant references are Mislevy (1986), Swaminathan and Gifford (1985, 1986), and Tsutakawa and Lin (1986).

Ability estimation with known item parameters may produce likelihood functions with multiple modes (Samejima, 1973; Yen et al., 1991). The 3-PL model also suffers from a problem that is known in the context of linear models as multicollinearity. From Fig. 3, it is clear that, for an interval of ability values about the location of the IRF, small changes in the value of the lower asymptote can be compensated for by small changes in the slope of the curve. Therefore, estimates of a_i and c_i are sensitive to minor fluctuations in the responses used to produce these estimates. Unless huge samples of examples or tight priors around the true parameter values are used, the estimates unstable.

Goodness of Fit. Whereas with the Rasch model, a number of sound statistical tests have been produced for addressing fit, the situation for the two- and three-parameter models is quite different. Well-established statistical tests do not exist, and even if they did, questions about the utility of statistical tests in assessing model fit can be raised, especially with large samples. Since no model is likely to fit perfectly a set of test items, given sufficient amounts of data, the assumption of model fit or adequacy, whatever the model, is likely to be rejected. Clearly then, statistical tests should not be used solely to determine the adequacy of model fit. It is quite possible that the departures between test data and predictions from the best fitting model are of no practical consequence but that a statistical test of model fit would reject the null hypothesis of model adequacy. It has been said that failure to reject an IRT model is simply a sign that sample size was too small (McDonald, 1989).

The approach to the assessment of fit with the two- and three-parameter models often involves the collection of a wide variety of evidence about model fit, including statistical tests, and then making an informed judgment about model fit and usefulness of a model with a particular set of data (Hambleton, 1989). This approach often includes fitting multiple models to test data and comparing the results and the practical consequences of any differences. It is common to carry out three types of studies: (1) checks on model assumptions, (2) checks on model parameter invariance, and (3) checks on predictions from the model. The basic idea is to become familiar with the model (and other possible models), the test data, model fit, and the consequences of model misfit, prior to making any decision about the utility of a particular model.

Checks on model assumptions will almost certainly involve investigations of the extent to which the unidimensionality assumption is valid. Common checks might include analysis of (1) the eigenvalues from the matrix of interitem correlations, (2) residuals after fitting a one-factor linear or nonlinear factor analytic model, or (3) IRT item statistics obtained in the total test and in a subset of items from the test that might potentially measure a second ability. For a useful review of approaches to the study of unidimensionality, Hattie (1985) is an excellent resource. Other checks on the test data might consist of a review of item biserial correlations (if variation is substantial, the usefulness of the two- and three-parameter models is increased), test format and difficulty (with multiple-choice items and especially if the items are difficult, a guessing parameter in the model could be helpful), and test speededness (test speededness is a threat to the assumption of unidimensionality).

Checks on model parameter invariance can be carried out. Here, the model of interest is assumed to be true and model parameter estimates are obtained. If the model fit is acceptable, examinee ability estimates ought to be the same (apart from measurement error) from different samples of items within the test (e.g., easy versus hard). Item parameter estimates ought to be about the same (except for sampling errors) from different samples of examinees from the population of examinees for whom the test is intended (e.g., males and females). Checks on the presence of ability and item parameter invariance provide valuable information about model fit (see Hambleton, Swaminathan and Rogers, 1991).

Predictions from the model, assuming it to be true or correct, can also be checked. Analysis of residuals or standardized residuals for items as well as persons is common via the study of residual plots (Hambleton, 1989). Statistical tests of departures in the data from model predictions can be carried out too [e.g., Yen (1981)]. Comparisons of residuals from fitting multiple models is especially helpful in determining the adequacy of model fit. Other studies that might be carried out include the comparison of predicted score distributions with the actual distributions (from several models) and the consequences of model fit (such as the ranking of examinee abilities under different models).

Historical Remark

The above review of IRT followed the history of models for dichotomous responses as they were developed in mental test theory. A potential danger of such treatments is to ignore parallel developments in other disciplines. It was mentioned earlier in the chapter that the first attempts to introduce the normal-ogive model in test theory were motivated by the successful application of the same model in psychophysical scaling. A parallel development is found in the work on models for dose-response curves in bioassay. In this field, the use of the normal-ogive model was popular until the early 1940s when it was replaced by the logistic model. An advocate of this change was Berkson (1944, 1951) who later worked on the statistical refinements of the use of the logistic model (Berkson 1953, 1955). Probably Berkson's work motivated Birnbaum to apply the same model in test theory. Baker (1992), in his book on parameter estimation in IRT, carefully spelled out the various historic links between methods used in bioassay and test theory.

Another main stimulus to work in IRT was Lazarsfeld's work on latent structure analysis. Although the major portion of Lazarsfeld's work was devoted to models for a finite number of latent classes of examinees with different probabilities of responding to items, his earlier work also included models for continuous response functions such as the polynomial, linear, and latent-distance models [for an overview, see Lazarsfeld and Henry (1968)]. Lazarsfeld's most important impact on test theory, however, was methodological. He introduced the terminology to distinguish between latent parameters of interest and manifest data and convinced test theorists that probabilistic models were needed to account for the relation between the two quantities. Lazarsfeld's latent class models have had a larger impact on sociology than on education and psychology. However, some of the modern IRT models in this volume have built the presence of latent classes into IRT models for continuous ability variables, for example, to represent differences between examinees in solution strategies used to solve test items (Kelderman, this volume; Rost, this volume).

Finally, an important link exists between the normal-ogive model and work on factor analysis of dichotomous variables. Both the normal-ogive and the linear factor model dealt with latent quantities, and the question about the relationship between the models has been of concern to several researchers. Lord and Novick (1968, Sec. 16.8) proved that a one-factor model holding for data resulting from a dichotomization of underlying multivariate normal variables is a sufficient condition for the normal-ogive model with normally distributed θ. Equivalence was proved by Takane and de Leeuw (1987), who also addressed extensions to polytomous and pair-comparisons data. Earlier contributions to this domain were provided by Christoffersson (1975) and Muthén (1978).

Historically, factor analysis was developed to deal with problems of multidimensionality in test construction. Given the equivalence between the one-factor and normal-ogive models, it should not come as a surprise that work on problems of multidimensionality in IRT has also been stimulated by factor analysis. An important example is the work by McDonald (1967; this volume).

Introduction to Extensions of Dichotomous IRT

Although some IRT models for tests producing polytomous response data or for tests measuring more than one ability variable were published earlier (Bock, 1972; Rasch, 1961; Samejima, 1969, 1972), the majority of the models in this volume were produced in the 1980s and later. Several authors have provided illuminating reviews of these newer models. Masters and Wright (1984) reviewed extensions of the 1-PL or Rasch model, including the partial credit model, rating scale model, bionomial trials, and Poisson counts model. The main theme in their review was to show that some of these models can be obtained as generalizations or limiting cases of others.

Thissen and Steinberg (1984) reviewed a larger collection of models developed to deal with categorical data and provided a framework for classifying them. They also showed some ingenious reparametrizations through which some of the models could be obtained from others. The same theme was present in a review by Mellenbergh (1994), who showed how, via an adequate choice of a linking function and parameter structure, the majority of the extant models could be obtained from the generalized linear model (GLIM) (McCullagh and Nelder, 1989).

Mellenbergh (1995) classified the polytomous IRT models according to their response format. His main point of view is that both categorical and ordinal response variables can be split into dichotomies that can be combined in different ways to yield the various models. Important principles of combination for ordinal formats are Agresti's (1990, Sec. 9.3) principles of adjacent categories, cumulative probabilities, and continuation ratios. The same notion of underlying dichotomies was present in a review by van Engelenburg (1995), who considered these dichotomous as representations of the cognitive step an examinee needs to take to solve a test item.

The models in this volume are grouped into six different sections. The first section contains eight chapters on models for responses to items with a polytomous format or to open-ended items scored for the degree of completeness of the response. If the distractors of the item play a role in the solution process or the item formulates a problem consisting of different sequential components, the properties of these distractors or components must be parametrized in the model. All of the models in this section are unidimensional logistic models that have been extended to handle polytomous response data, either ordered or unordered. The pioneer in this area of model development is Fumiko Samejima with her graded response model, which could be applied to ordered categorical data. Variations on the graded response model of Samejima are the IRT models presented in the chapters by Andersen, Masters and Wright, Verhelst, Glas, and Vries, Tutz, and Muraki. For unordered categorical data, as might be reflected in the set of answer choices for a test item, the chapter by Bock describes his nominal response model. By scoring the answer choices to an item instead of simply scoring the item response as correct or incorrect, the potential was available for extracting more information about examinee ability. An extension of that model to handle the problem of guessing on multiple-choice items is described by Thissen and Steinberg.

The second section deals with models for items in which response time or numbers of successful attempts are recorded. Response time plays a role in tests with a time limit. Generally, the presence of a time limit requires response speed as a second ability in addition to response accuracy. Tests with a time limit can only be scored satisfactorily if the interaction of the two abilities on the probability of success on the item as well as the response time needed are carefully modeled. Both the chapters by Verhelst, Verstralen and Jansen and Roskam provide models for this interaction. If test items can be considered as parallel, it makes sense to record the number of successes in a fixed number of trials or the number of trials needed to complete a fixed number of successes. The chapter by Spray provides models for these cases that have been proven to be successful for analyzing data from psychomotor tests.

A persistent problem in the history of test theory has been the modeling of examinee performance when multiple abilities are required to complete items in a test. Traditionally, factor analysis was used to analyze the presence of multiple abilities and to reveal the structure of its impact on the responses to items in the test. IRT models for multiple abilities or for a single ability variable needed to solve multiple components or parts in the items are presented in the third section of this volume. This section of the volume contains the descriptions of several multidimensional IRT models. Reckase, McDonald, and Fischer provide parallel developments for the multidimensional logistic, normal-ogive, and linear logistic models, respectively. These are extensions of the corresponding unidimensional versions of the models (although the Reckase chapter extends the polytomous response version of the unidimensional logistic IRT model). Kelderman provides a loglinear version of a multidimensional IRT model for handling polytomous data. A very different type of multidimensional model is represented in the chapter by Zwinderman. Here, multidimensionality is accounted for in the data using a multiple regression model with observed scores used instead of latent variables as the predictors. Two additional models are introduced in Section 3 to provide for a psychological accounting of examinee item performance and items. The unidimensional linear logistic Rasch models of Fischer allow the difficulty parameter to be accounted for by cognitive components. With a better understanding of what makes items difficult, more systematic test construction becomes possible. Embretson's work with multicomponent response models permits a better understanding of examinee performance when item performance involves the completion of many small steps.

The models in Section 4 share the focus on response functions to describe the properties of the items with the other models in this volume. However, rather than defining these functions on a parameter structure to deal with the various factors that influence success on the items, it is the less demanding (nonparametric) shape of the functions that does this job. One of the first to pioneer nonparametric probabilistic models for dichotomous responses was Mokken. His chapter reviews the assumptions underlying his model and provides the statistical theory needed to work with it. The chapter by Molenaar follows the same approach as Mokken's but addresses the case of responses to items with a polytomous format. In the chapter by Ramsay, statistical techniques based on ordinal assumptions are presented to estimate response functions for dichotomous responses nonparametrically. Parametric models for item responses not only have to parametrize completely all factors with an impact on the response process but also must have a realistic functional form. An important distinction in this respect is the one between monotone and nonmonotone response functions. Items in an achievement test should have a monotonically increasing form. The more ability possessed by the examinee, the greater the probability of success. Items or statements in an instrument for the measurement of attitudes or values appear to miss this property. Models for such nonmonotone items are offered in the fifth section of this volume. The chapter by Andrich presents a hyperbolic cosine model to describe the probability of endorsement of statements in an instrument for the measurement of attitudes. The chapter by Hoijtink introduces a model based on the Cauchy density, which can be used as an alternative to Andrich's model.

The final section of this volume contains chapters with models accounting for various special properties of the response process. The multiple-group IRT model of Bock permits, for example, the group rather than the individual to become the unit of analysis. Such a shift may be important in program evaluation studies and educational accountability initiatives and several other applications. Better model parameter estimates is one of the advantages of this line of modeling. A unified treatment of IRT problems involving multiple groups is another. The chapter by Rost offers a description of a discrete mixture model that can be used to describe differences between subpopulations of examinees using different strategies to solve the items. Since these subpopulations are assumed to be latent, there is no need to identify the strategy used by the individual examinees to apply the model. Models to handle local dependencies in the data are provided by Jannarone. As these dependencies can be serious and lead to the rejection of the assumption of unidimensionality in the test data, it is likely these models will become more important in the future. To date, it has been common to simply disregard these dependencies. But it has been shown that failure to attend to these departures can lead to quite negative consequences (Fennessy, 1995). The models presented by Hutchinson allow for the fact that examinees may have partial information about the question asked in a test item. Each of these models is based on the same idea of an underlying continuous variable reflecting how much mismatch an examinee experiences between the question in the stem of the item and a specific alternative.

Future of Item Response Theory

As outlined in the introduction to this chapter, IRT started out as an attempt to adjust test scores for the effects of such nuisance properties of test items as their difficulty, discriminating power, or liability to guessing. Realistic models with parameters for each of these effects were needed. Owing to the success of these models, soon the need was felt to develop models for a larger collection of tests than standard tests with a single ability variable and a dichotomous response format. Such models had to deal, for example, with the presence of nuisance abilities, the role of time limits and speed, the possibility of learning during the test, the impact of properties of item distractors, or different cognitive strategies to solve test items. To date, many such models have been studied—this volume reviews 27 of them. The implicit goal in modern IRT research is to expand the class of models to cover response data from tests with any "natural" format. To realize this goal, deeper insights into response processes and the precise way item properties and human abilities interact are needed.

The important question can be raised whether, in so doing, psychometrics has not entered the domain of mathematical psychology. Indeed, it may seem as if IRT is about to give up its interest in measurement and adopt a new identity as an enthusiastic provider of psychological models for cognitive processes. Some of the families of models presented in this volume do not suggest any interest in estimating ability parameters at all but are presented mainly as vehicles for specifying competing hypotheses regarding, for instance, problem-solving strategies, the composition of skills, or cognitive growth. Pertinent examples are given in the chapters by Embretson, Fischer, Kelderman, and Fischer and Selinger in this volume. Rather than freeing ability measurements from the effects of nuisance variables, the interest of these authors has shifted to the behavior of the nuisance variables themselves. In our opinion, this development should not result in embarrassment but be welcomed as an unexpected bonus from the application of IRT models. Even when the attempt would be to do so, the emergence of this new branch of mathematical psychology would never be able to replace psychometrics as an independent discipline of measurement. The need for measurement models to solve the daily problems in, for instance, selection procedures, licensing, test equating, and monitoring achievement will remain, and improved models to deal with such problems are always welcome. If, in addition, such models also have a spin off to psychological theory, so much the better. They may help to better integrate measurement and substantive research—areas that to date have lived too apart from each other.

Owing to the attempts to make its model applicable under more "natural" conditions, IRT has met several of the technical problems inherent in statistical modeling that more experienced sciences have struggled with for a longer period of time. Large numbers of parameters and a more complicated structure may make a model realistic, but there always is a price to be paid.

First of all, if the number of parameters increases, less data per parameter are available and parameter estimates may show serious instability. The problem usually becomes manifest if estimates for the same parameters vary largely in value between applications. The problem is aggravated if the model has a tradeoff between some of the parameters in their effects on the response probabilities. As already discussed for the 3-PL model, this condition is reminiscent of the problem of multicollinearity in multivariate linear regression, and a prohibitively large amount of data may be needed to realize stable parameter estimates. For more complicated models than the 3-PL, serious versions of the problem can be expected to arise.

Another likely problem with complicated models is lack of identifiability of parameter values. Formally, the problem exists if different sets of parameter values in the model generate the same success probabilities for the examinees on the items. If so, estimation of model parameters cannot result in unique estimates. Practical experience with seemingly simple nonlinear models has taught us that such models often entail vexing identifiability problems. For several of the models in this volume, the issue of nonidentifiability has not been completely addressed yet, and practical criteria necessary and sufficient for identifiability are still lacking.

Even if unique parameters exist, attempts to estimate them may result in ML estimates which are not unique or cases in which no ML estimates exist at all. An example discussed earlier was the 3-PL model with known item parameters which for several data sets has a likelihood function with multiple local modes (Samejima, 1973; Yen et al., 1991). Necessary and sufficient conditions under which data sets produce unique parameter estimates are not yet known for the majority of the models in this volume. A favorable exception is the linear logistic model (LLTM) by Fischer [for the conditions, see Fischer (1983)].

Finally, if unique parameter estimates are known to exist, they may still be hard to calculate. As already mentioned, even a simple model like the Rasch or 1-PL model, numerical complexities had prevented the use of CML estimation for a long time until improved algorithms became available (Liou, 1994; Verhelst et al., 1984). For some of the models in this volume, numerical complexity can only be mastered using a modern technique such as the EM algorithm or one of the recent Monte Carlo methods for finding modes of posterior distributions or likelihood functions [for an introduction, see Tanner (1993)].

An important question, thus, is how far IRT modeling can go without loosing statistical tractability of its models. One obvious strategy is to work within families of distributions, which are known to have favorable properties and are flexible enough to fit empirical data. A well-explored example is the exponential family, which offers favorable minimal sufficient statistics for its parameters (Andersen, 1980). The advantage of these statistics is not so much the fact that they retain all information on the parameters in the sample but have a dimensionality much lower than the original data—a fact that may facilitate computation considerably. However, even within this family, application of advanced numerical procedures to estimate parameters may still be time consuming when applied to models for tests of realistic lengths (for an illustration, see Kelderman, this volume).

It is well known and often stated that models are always based on idealizations and will never completely fit reality. But even if this fact is taken into account, IRT may find that its goal of a realistic model for each possible test design cannot be fully realized because of technical restrictions. When this point will be reached is an issue that depends as much on the creativity of IRT researchers as on future developments in statistical theory and computing. It will be fascinating to follow IRT when models are further extended and refined in the decades to come.

References

Agresti, A. (1990). *Categorical Data Analysis.* New York, NY: Wiley.

Andersen, E.B. (1973). A goodness of fit test for the Rasch model. *Psychometrika* **38**, 123–140.

Andersen, E.B. (1980). *Discrete Statistical Models with Social Science Applications.* Amsterdam, The Netherlands: North-Holland.

Baker, F.B. (1992). *Item Response Theory: Parameter Estimation Techniques.* New York, NY: Marcel Dekker.

Berkson, J.A. (1944). Application of the logistic function to bio-assay. *Journal of the American Statistical Association* **39**, 357–365.

Berkson, J.A. (1951). Why I prefer logits to probits. *Biometrics* **7**, 327–329.

Berkson, J.A. (1953). A statistically precise and relatively simple method of estimating the bioassay with quantal response, based on the logistic function. *Journal of the American Statistical Association* **48**, 565–600.

Berkson, J.A. (1955). Maximum likelihood and minimum chi-square estimates of the logistic function. *Journal of the American Statistical Association* **50**, 120–162.

Binet, A. and Simon, Th.A. (1905). Méthodes nouvelles pour le diagnostic du niveau intellectuel des anormaux. *l'Annéе Psychologie* **11**, 191–336.

Bock, R.D. (1972). Estimating item parameters and latent ability when responses are scored in two or more nominal categories. *Psychometrika* **37**, 29–51.

Bock, R.D. and Aitken, M. (1981). Marginal maximum likelihood estimation of item parameters: An application of an EM algorithm. *Psychometrika* **46**, 443–459.

Bock, R.D. and Lieberman, M. (1970). Fitting a response model for n dichotomously scored items. *Psychometrika* **35**, 179–197.

Christoffersson, A. (1975). Factor analysis of dichotomized variables. *Psychometrika* **40**, 5–32.

Cox, D.R. (1958). *The Planning of Experiments.* New York, NY: Wiley.

de Leeuw, J. and Verhelst, N.D. (1986). Maximum-likelihood estimation in generalized Rasch models. *Journal of Educational Statistics* **11**, 183–196.

Engelen, R.H.J. (1989). *Parameter Estimation in the Logistic Item Response Model.* Unpublished doctoral dissertation, University of Twente, Enschede, The Netherlands.

Fennessy, L.M. (1995). *The Impact of Local Dependencies on Various IRT Outcomes.* Unpublished doctoral dissertation, University of Massachusetts, Amherst.

Ferguson, G.A. (1942). Item selection by the constant process. *Psychometrika* **7**, 19–29.

Fischer, G.H. (1974). *Einführung in die Theorie psychologischer Tests.* Bern, Switzerland: Huber.

Fischer, G.H. (1983). Logistic latent trait models with linear constraints. *Psychometrika* **48**, 3–26.

Glas, C.A.W. (1988). The derivation of some tests for the Rasch model from the multinomial distribution. *Psychometrika* **53**, 525–546.

Glas, C.A.W. (1989). *Contributions to Estimating and Testing Rasch Models.* Unpublished doctoral dissertation, University of Twente, Enschede, The Netherlands.

Haley, D.C. (1952). *Estimation of the Dosage Mortality Relationship When the Dose is Subject to Error* (Technical Report No. 15). Palo Alto, CA: Applied Mathematics and Statistics Laboratory, Stanford University.

Hambleton, R.K. (1989). Principles and selected applications of item response theory. In R.L. Linn (ed.), *Educational Measurement* (3rd ed., pp. 143–200). New York, NY: Macmillan.

Hambleton, R.K. and Swaminathan, H. (1985). *Item Response Theory: Principles and Applications.* Boston: Kluwer Academic Publishers.

Hambleton, R.K., Swaminathan, H., and Rogers, H.J. (1991). *Fundamentals of Item Response Theory.* Newbury Park, CA: Sage.

Hattie, J. (1985). Assessing unidimensionality of tests and items. *Applied Psychological Measurement* **9**, 139–164.

Kelderman, H. (1984). Loglinear Rasch model tests. *Psychometrika* **49**, 223–245.

Lawley, D.N. (1943). On problems connected with item selection and test construction. *Proceedings of the Royal Society of Edinburgh* **61**, 273–287.

Lazarsfeld, P.F. (1950). Chapters 10 and 11 in S.A. Stouffer et al. (eds.), *Studies in Social Psychology in World War II: Vol. 4. Measurement and Prediction.* Princeton, NJ: Princeton University Press.

Lazarsfeld, P.F. and Henry, N.W. (1968). *Latent Structure Analysis.* Boston, MA: Houghton Mifflin.

Lehmann, E.L. (1959). *Testing Statistical Hypotheses.* New York, NY: Wiley.

Liou, M. (1994). More on the computation of higher-order derivatives of the elementary symmetric functions in the Rasch model. *Applied Psychological Measurement* **18**, 53–62.

Loevinger, J. (1947). A systematic approach to the construction and evaluation of tests of ability. *Psychological Monographs* **61** (Serial No. 285).

Lord, F.M. (1952). A theory of test scores. *Psychometric Monographs*, No. 7.

Lord, F.M. (1980). *Applications of Item Response Theory to Practical Testing Problems.* Hillsdale, NJ: Erlbaum.

Lord, F.M. and Novick, M.R. (1968). *Statistical Theories of Mental Test Scores.* Reading, MA: Addison-Wesley.

Masters, G.N. and Wright, B.D. (1984). The essential process in a family of measurement models. *Psychometrika* **49**, 529–544.

McCullagh, P. and Nelder, J.A. (1989). *Generalized Linear Models* (2nd edition). London: Chapman and Hill.

McDonald, R.P. (1967). Nonlinear factor analysis. *Psychometric Monograph*, No. 15.

McDonald, R.P. (1989). Future directions for item response theory. *International Journal of Educational Research* **13**, 205–220.

Mellenbergh, G.J. (1994). Generalized linear item response theory. *Psychological Bulletin* **115**, 300–307.

Mellenbergh, G.J. (1995). Conceptual notes on models for discrete polytomous item responses. *Applied Psychological Measurement* **19**, 91–100.

Mislevy, R.L. (1986). Bayes modal estimation in item response theory. *Psychometrika* **51**, 177–195.

Molenaar, W. (1974). De logistische en de normale kromme [The logistic and the normal curve]. *Nederlands Tijdschrift voor de Psychologie* **29**, 415–420.

Molenaar, W. (1983). Some improved diagnostics for failure in the Rasch model. *Psychometrika* **55**, 75–106.

Mosier, C.I. (1940). Psychophysics and mental test theory: Fundamental postulates and elementary theorems. *Psychological Review* **47**, 355–366.

Mosier, C.I. (1941). Psychophysics and mental test theory. II. The constant process. *Psychological Review* **48**, 235–249.

Muthén, B. (1978). Contributions to factor analysis of dichotomous variables. *Psychometrika* **43**, 551–560.

Novick, M.R. (1966). The axioms and principal results of classical test theory. *Journal of Mathematical Psychology* **3**, 1–18.

Rasch, G. (1960). *Probabilistic Models for Some Intelligence and Attainment Tests.* Copenhagen, Denmark: Danish Institute for Educational Research.

Rasch, G. (1961). On general laws and the meaning of measurement in psychology. *Proceedings of the IV Berkeley Symposium on Mathematical Statistics and Probability* (Vol. 4, pp. 321–333). Berkeley, CA: University of California.

Richardson, M.W. (1936). The relationship between difficulty and the differential validity of a test. *Psychometrika* **1**, 33–49.

Samejima, F. (1969). Estimation of latent ability using a response pattern of graded scores. *Psychometric Monograph*, No. 17.

Samejima, F. (1972). A general model for free-response data. *Psychometric Monograph*, No. 18.

Samejima, F. (1973). A comment on Birnbaum's three-parameter logistic model in the latent trait theory. *Psychometrika* **38**, 221–233.

Spearman, C. (1904). The proof and measurement of association between two things. *American Journal of Psychology* **15**, 72–101.

Swaminathan, H. and Gifford, J.A. (1982). Bayesian estimation in the Rasch model. *Journal of Educational Statistics* **7**, 175–192.

Swaminathan, H. and Gifford, J.A. (1985). Bayesian estimation in the two-parameter logistic model. *Psychometrika* **50**, 349–364.

Swaminathan, H. and Gifford, J.A. (1986). Bayesian estimation in the three-parameter logistic model. *Psychometrika* **51**, 589–601.

Takane, Y. and de Leeuw, J. (1987). On the relationship between item response theory and factor analysis of discretized variables. *Psychometrika* **52**, 393–408.

Tanner, M.A. (1993). *Tools for Statistical Inference: Methods for the Exploration of Posterior Distributions and Likelihood Functions.* New York, NY: Springer-Verlag.

Thissen, D. (1982). Marginal maximum-likelihood estimation for the one-parameter logistic model. *Psychometrika* **47**, 175–186.

Thissen, D. and Steinberg, L. (1984). Taxonomy of item response models. *Psychometrika* **51**, 567–578.

Thurstone, L.L. (1925). A method of scaling psychological and educational tests. *Journal of Educational Psychology* **16**, 433–451.

Thurstone, L.L. (1927a). The unit of measurements in educational scales. *Journal of Educational Psychology* **18**, 505–524.

Thurstone, L.L. (1927b). A law of comparative judgement. *Psychological Review* **34**, 273–286.

Tsutakawa, R.K. (1984). Estimation of two-parameter logistic item response curves. *Journal of Educational Statistics* **9**, 263–276.

Tsutakawa, R.K. and Lin, H.Y. (1986). Bayesian estimation of item response curves. *Psychometrika* **51**, 251–267.

Tucker, L.R. (1946). Maximum validity of a test with equivalent items. *Psychometrika* **11**, 1–13.

Urry, V.W. (1974). Approximations to item parameters of mental test models. *Journal of Educational Measurement* **34**, 253–269.

van Engelenburg, G. (1995). *Step Approach and Polytomous Items* (internal report). Amsterdam, The Netherlands: Department of Methodology, Faculty of Psychology, University of Amsterdam.

van der Linden, W.J. (1986). The changing conception of testing in education and psychology. *Applied Psychological Measurement* **10**, 325–352.

van den Wollenberg, A.L. (1982). Two new test statistics for the Rasch model. *Psychometrika* **47**, 123–139.

Verhelst, N.D., Glas, C.A.W. and van der Sluis, A. (1984). Estimation problems in the Rasch model: The basic symmetric functions. *Computational Statistics Quarterly* **1**, 245–262.

Verhelst, N.D. and Molenaar, W. (1988). Logit-based parameter estimation in the Rasch model. *Statistica Neerlandica* **42**, 273–295.

Yen, W.M. (1981). Using simulation results to choose a latent trait model. *Applied Psychological Measurements* **5**, 245–262.

Yen, W.M., Burket, G.R. and Sykes, R.C. (1991). Nonunique solutions to the likelihood equation for the three-parameter logistic model. *Psychometrika* **56**, 39–54.

Part I. Models for Items with Polytomous Response Formats

Introduction

The first generation of item response models developed in the 1940s and 1950s were intended to be applied to unidimensional test items that were dichotomously scored. Item response functions incorporated one, two, or three parameters and were one of two mathematical forms, normal-ogive or logistic.

Lord (1952) introduced the two-parameter normal-ogive model for analyzing multiple-choice test data. Applications of his model were hampered by the complexities of model parameter estimation and Lord's concern about the failure to handle the problem of guessing in his two-parameter model. A few years later (1957 and 1958), Birnbaum in a series of reports described the more tractable two- and three-parameter logistic models. This important work is most accessible today in Birnbaum (1968).

Although neither Lord nor Birnbaum showed any interest in a one-parameter normal-ogive or logistic parameter model because of their belief that test items needed at least two parameters to be accounted adequately for in an IRT model, one to describe difficulty and the other to describe discriminating power, the one-parameter logistic model is a special case of the models they developed. On the other hand, Rasch (1960) was the first to introduce the one-parameter logistic model (known today as the Rasch model) and this he did from a totally different perspective than Lord or Birnbaum. Lord and Birnbaum were interested in finding models to fit their data. They were statisticians fitting statistical models to data. On the other hand, Rasch, who himself was a statistician, attempted to build psychological models to account for examinee performance on tests. His model was derived from a simple starting point: the odds for success of an examinee on a particular item should depend on the product of the examinee's ability and the easiness of the test item. Basically, the more ability possessed by an examinee and the easier the item, the higher the chances that an examinee would perform successfully. Lower chances of success would be associated with harder items and/or lesser examinee ability. An explicit assumption such as equal item discrimination was never apparent from Rasch's formulation of his one-parameter model.

Although the normal-ogive and logistic models were in the measurement literature for some time, little technical progress was made until the publication of Lord and Novick's (1968) *Statistical Theories of Mental Test Scores.* Shortly thereafter, software began to appear (e.g., LOGIST and BICAL), technical advances were made [see, for example, Bock (1972); Lord, (1974)], and a few applications started to appear. Still, for most of the 1970s, unidimensional IRT models to handle dichotomous data were sufficient, and when the data were polytomous (such as might be obtained from the scoring of essays and performance tasks), it was common to dichotomize the available data prior to analysis. And, the great bulk of the research was focused on parameter estimation, goodness of fit, model robustness and applications of these models. Little if any attention was given to the development of new models.

While important technical and application work was going on with the unidimensional normal and logistic IRT models, other developments started in the late 1960s and became a serious activity of researchers beginning in the early 1980s. Samejima (1969), for example, introduced the very important *graded response model* (Chapter 5) to analyze data from Likert attitude scales and polynomously scored performance tasks such as might arise in the scoring of writing samples. Her model and variations on it were the first of many models developed by her and other scholars to handle ordered polytomous data. The work was stimulated by both the desire to generate and investigate new and potentially interesting models and by an increase in the presence of polytomous data in educational testing.

The *steps model* by Verhelst, Glas, and de Vries (Chapter 7), the (independently developed but formally identical) *sequential model for order responses* of Tutz (Chapter 8), the *generalized partial credit model* of Muraki (Chapter 9), and the *partial credit model* of Masters and Wright (Chapter 6) are variations on Samejima's graded response model intended to model examinee performance on ordered polytomous tasks. How the polytomous data are modeled and the number of parameters in the models are the main differences. Another variation was the *rating scale model* of Andersen (Chapter 4), developed as an extension of the Rasch model to handle polytomous rating scale data that might arise in the assessment of personality. With the increasing use of polytomous rating scales in educational and psychological assessment, these models are going to receive wide use in the future.

All of the IRT models above are intended to be applied to ordered categorical data. The *nominal response model* of Bock (Chapter 2) and a variation on that model by Thissen and Steinberg, *response model for multiple-choice items* (Chapter 3), are intended to be applied to unordered data such as the m choices provided in a multiple-choice test item. The intent is to extract more information about an examinee's ability level from a test item than simply whether or not the examinee answers the item correctly. When there is an empirical ordering of the categories, the nominal response model and the graded response models lead to similar results. A shortcoming of Bock's nominal response model for multiple-choice items is that the model contains only two item parameters. A provision to handle the guessing behavior of examinees is contained in the Thissen–Steinberg model.

References

Birnbaum, A. (1968). Some latent trait models and their use in inferring an examinee's ability. In F.M. Lord and M.R. Novick, *Statistical Theories of Mental Test Scores*, Reading MA: Addison-Wesley.

Bock, R.D. (1972). Estimating item parameters and latent ability when responses are scored in two or more nominal categories. *Psychometrika* **37**, 29–51.

Lord, F.M. (1952). Theory of test scores. *Psychometric Monographs*, No. 7.

Lord, F.M. (1974). Estimation of latent ability and item parameter when there are omitted responses. *Psychometrika* **39**, 247–264.

Rasch, G. (1960). *Probabilistic Models for Some Intelligence and Attainment Tests.* Copenhagen, Denmark: Danish Institute for Educational Research.

Samejima, F. (1969). Estimation of latent ability using a response pattern of graded scores. *Psychometric Monograph*, No. 17.

2
The Nominal Categories Model

R. Darrell Bock

Introduction

The nominal categories model (Bock, 1972), with its various specializations and extensions, comprises a large family of functions suitable for statistical description of individual qualitative behavior in response to identified stimuli. The models specify the probability of a person's response in one of several mutually exclusive and exhaustive categories as a function of stimulus characteristics and person attributes. Bock's nominal model, like Birnbaum's (1968) binary item response model, is an elaboration of a primitive, formal model for choice between two alternatives.

Presentation of the Model

The Choice Model

It is assumed that a person, when presented a choice between alternatives $\mathcal{A}$ and $\mathcal{B}$, will choose $\mathcal{A}$ with probability

$$P_A = \frac{\pi_A}{\pi_A + \pi_B},$$

or choose $\mathcal{B}$ with probability

$$P_B = \frac{\pi_B}{\pi_A + \pi_B},$$

where π_A and π_B are nonnegative quantities attributed to the respective alternatives (Luce, 1959).

In an experiment in which respondents are presented pairs of alternatives chosen from a larger set, it is possible with a suitable set of pairs to estimate efficiently the π-values of the alternatives up to an arbitrary scale factor (Bradley and Terry, 1952). The data for this estimation are the observed frequencies of the choices in a sample of respondents drawn from some population.

For computational convenience in the estimation, it is advantageous to reparametrize the model by setting, say,

$$\pi_A = e^{z_A} \quad \text{and} \quad \pi_B = e^{z_B}.$$

Then,

$$P_A = \frac{e^{z_A}}{e^{z_A} + e^{z_B}} = \frac{1}{1 + e^{-(z_A - z_B)}} = \frac{1}{1 + e^{-z}}, \tag{1}$$

and the model for choice becomes a binary logistic model with logit $z = z_A - z_B$. Similarly,

$$P_B = \frac{e^{z_B}}{e^{z_A} + e^{z_B}} = \frac{e^{-z}}{1 + e^{-z}} = \frac{1}{1 + e^{z}} = 1 - P_A. \tag{2}$$

The advantage of this parametrization is that the logit is unbounded and suitable for linear modeling. The choice model is easily extended to selection among m alternatives by writing

$$P_k = \frac{\pi_k}{\pi_1 + \pi_2 + \cdots + \pi_m}$$

or

$$P_k = \frac{e^{z_k}}{\sum_h^m e^{z_h}}. \tag{3}$$

In Eq. (3), the indeterminacy of scale becomes one of location, and it may be resolved either by setting $\sum_k^m z_k = 0$ or estimating $m - 1$ linearly independent contrasts between the m logits. In this model, the "logit" is the vector

$$z' = [z_1, z_2, \ldots, z_m] \tag{4}$$

in $(m-1)$-dimensional space. In conditions where the respondents' choices may be considered independent trials with constant probabilities, the scalar logit in Eq. (1) may be called a *binomial logit*, and the vector logit in Eq. (4), called a *multinomial logit*. The binomial logit was introduced into statistics by Fisher and Yates (1953), and its values may be read from their table of the transformation of r to z, with $r = 2P - 1$. The multinomial logit was introduced by Bock (1966, 1970, 1975) and independently by Mantel (1966).

Relationship to Thurstone's Choice Models

The logistic choice model approximates closely Thurstone's discriminal-process model based on the normal distribution. According to the latter, a person's perception of the difference between alternatives $\mathcal{A}$ and $\mathcal{B}$ gives rise to a random "discriminal process"

$$y = \mu_A - \mu_B + \varepsilon,$$

where ε is distributed normally with mean 0 and variance σ^2. If the arbitrary unit of scale is set so that $\sigma = 1$, the chances of the person choosing $\mathcal{A}$ is then the probability that $y > 0$, or

$$P_A = \frac{1}{\sqrt{2\pi}} \int_{-(\mu_A - \mu_B)}^{\infty} e^{-t^2/2} dt = \Phi(\mu_A - \mu_B); \tag{5}$$

similarly,

$$P_B = \Phi(\mu_B - \mu_A) = 1 - P_A. \tag{6}$$

This is the basis for Thurstone's (1927) model for comparative judgment. Its connection with the Bradley–Terry–Luce model lies in the close approximation of these probabilities by the logistic probabilities in Eqs. (1) and (2), with error nowhere greater than 0.01, when $z = 1.7(\mu_A - \mu_B)$.

The normal discriminal process model may be extended to the choice of one alternative out of m on the assumption that a person chooses the largest of m multivariate normal processes (Bock, 1956; Bock and Jones, 1968). Suppose the alternatives give rise to an m-vector process with normally distributed means μ_h, standard deviations σ_h, and correlations $\rho_{h\ell}$. Then the differences between the process for alternative k and the remaining processes are $(m-1)$-variate normal with means $\mu_{kh} = \mu_k - \mu_h$, variances $\sigma_{kh}^2 = \sigma_k^2 + \sigma_h^2 - 2\rho_{kh}\sigma_k\sigma_h$, and correlations $\rho_{kh,k\ell} = (\sigma_k^2 - \rho_{kh}\sigma_k\sigma_h - \rho_{k\ell}\sigma_k\sigma_\ell + \rho_{h\ell}\sigma_h\sigma_\ell)/\sigma_{hk}\sigma_{k\ell}$. The probability P_k that alternative k will be the first choice among the m alternatives is the positive orthant of the latter distribution.

In the special case of constant process variances and covariances, $\sigma_{kh} = \rho$ and $\rho_{kh,k\ell} = \frac{1}{2}\rho$, and with the above 1.7 scale adjustment of $\mu_B - \mu_A$, these orthant probabilities are well approximated by the generalized choice model in Eq. (3). In this case, the model is one of the extremal distributions studied by Gumbel (1961), who showed that this distribution has logistic marginals with mean zero and variance $\pi^2/3$. Unlike the multivariate normal distribution, it is not symmetric and is useful only for approximating the positive or negative orthant (McKeon, 1961).

The accuracy of the choice model as an approximation of multivariate normal orthant probabilities has not been studied in general because of the computational difficulty of obtaining the latter for a general Σ when m is large. For $m = 3$, Bock and Jones (1968) gave the comparisons shown in Table 1.

Logit Linear Models

In addition to its IRT applications discussed below, the multinomial logit is widely applied in a logit-linear analysis of contingency tables and estimation of multinomial response relations (Bock, 1975, 1985; Haberman, 1979). It gives the same results as the log-linear model when sample sizes are treated as fixed in these applications (Goodman, 1970).

Table 1. Comparison of the normal and logistic choice models.

Trivariate Normal Distributions

Means			SDs			Correlations		
Var1	Var2	Var3	Var1	Var2	Var3	1,2	1,3	2,3
0.293	0.170	−0.212	0.887	0.979	0.942	0.165	−0.018	0.135
0.587	0.778	0.703	1.081	1.010	1.074	0.196	0.116	0.033
−0.116	0.131	−0.818	1.287	0.755	1.109	0.001	.256	.003
−0.824	−0.831	−0.160	0.992	0.995	1.079	0.638	0.353	0.318

Probability of first choice

Normal			Logistic[1]		
1	2	3	1	2	3
0.429	0.351	0.220	0.430	0.360	0.211
0.280	0.375	0.345	0.289	0.373	0.338
0.381	0.490	0.129	0.361	0.496	0.143
0.191	0.194	0.615	0.210	0.210	0.579

[1]The logistic probabilities were computed using $\pi/\sqrt{3} = 1.8138$ as the scale factor; that is, $z_k = 1.8138\mu_k/\sigma_k$.

A familiar example is the so-called "logit" analysis of binomial response relations (an alternative to probit analysis) in which trend in observed binomial proportions $p_1, p_2, \ldots, p_n$ is modeled by setting

$$z_k = \alpha + \beta x_k, \qquad k = 1, 2, \ldots, n$$

for known values of an independent variable x_k.

The extension of this analysis to multinomial response relations plays a central role in item response models for multiple categories. A typical data structure in multinomial response relations arises from the classification of persons characterized by n levels of the known variable x_k. According to their responses, the persons in level k are classified in m mutually exclusive categories. Their number in category h of level k is r_{kh}, and the total is $N_k = \sum_h^m r_{kh}$.

We assume a method of sampling such that r_{kh} is multinomially distributed with parameters N_k and P_{kh}, where $\sum_h^m P_{kh} = 1$. Assuming N_k given, the purpose of the logit linear analysis of these data is to estimate the P_{kh}, preferably with fewer than $n(m-1)$ free parameters. It is convenient when working with the model to adopt matrix notation and write

$$\underset{n\times m}{Z} = \underset{n\times 2}{X} \cdot \underset{2\times(m-1)}{\Gamma} \cdot \underset{(m-1)\times m}{T}, \tag{7}$$

where: (1) Z contains the multinomial logits corresponding to the response probabilities P_{kh}; (2) the matrix $X = [1, x_k]$ contains a vector of unities and the vector of $n \geq 2$ levels associated with the groups; (3) Γ is a matrix of $2s \geq 2(m-1)$ linearly independent parameters to be estimated; and (4) T is a rank $m-1$ matrix containing coefficients of selected linear functions of the parameters. If the elements in the rows of T are contrasts (i.e., sum to zero), the logits in the rows of Z are constrained to sum to zero.

In the large samples typical of these applications, maximum likelihood estimation has well-known good properties. The likelihood of Γ, given the data, is

$$L(\Gamma) = \prod_{k=1}^{n} \frac{N_k!}{r_{k1}!r_{k2}!\cdots r_{km}!} P_{k1}^{r_{k1}} P_{k2}^{r_{k2}} \cdots P_{km}^{r_{km}} \tag{8}$$

and the gradient vector of the log likelihood is

$$\underset{2s\times 1}{G(\Gamma)} = \frac{\partial \log L}{\partial \operatorname{vec} \Gamma} = \sum_{k}^{n} \underset{s\times 1}{T(r_k - N_k P_k)} \otimes \underset{2\times 1}{\begin{bmatrix} 1 \\ x_k \end{bmatrix}}, \tag{9}$$

where r_k and P_k are, respectively, m-vectors of frequencies and probabilities, $\otimes$ is the Kronecker product $C = A \otimes B = [a_{ij}B]$, and the vec operator stacks the columns of the matrix Γ (Bock, 1975, 1985).

Because logit linear models belong to the exponential family and the parameter space is unbounded, the likelihood surface is everywhere convex and any interior maximum is unique. Any finite solution of the likelihood equations based on Eq. (9) may therefore be obtained from, say, zero starting values by multivariate Newton–Raphson iterations with the Hessian matrix

$$H(\Gamma) = -\sum_{k}^{n} N_k T W_k T' \otimes \begin{bmatrix} 1 \\ x_k \end{bmatrix} [1, x_k]. \tag{10}$$

The elements of the $m \times m$ matrix W_k are $P_{kh}(\delta_{hj} - P_{kj})$, where δ_{hj} is Kronecker's delta (i.e., $\delta_{hj} = 1$ for $j = h$ and $\delta_{hj} = 0$ for $j \neq h$) (Bock, 1975, 1985, p. 524 ff). Boundary solutions at $\pm\infty$ are sometimes encountered with unfavorable data.

The corresponding Fisher information matrix is $I(\Gamma) = -H(\Gamma)$ at the solution point, and $I^{-1}(\Gamma)$ is the large-sample-covariance matrix of the estimator.

The Nominal Categories Model

Item response theoretic applications of logistic models are, from a statistical point of view, extensions of the above fixed-effects logit linear analyses to the mixed-effects setting. Item response models describe a potential population of responses of each person, and the persons themselves are drawn from some specified population. These two stages of sampling introduce corresponding sources of variation—the first arising from random item-by-person interaction and response instability on random occasions—the second, from the attributes of randomly selected persons.

In a typical nominal categories application, each of N persons responds to each of n items, where item i admits responses in m_i mutually exclusive categories. Multiple-choice tests fit this situation, as do short-answer tests when the possible answers to each question are categorized in some way. Assuming that responses to these items depend on a scalar person-attribute θ, we can express the model for the probabilities of a response in category h of item i in terms of the vector logit

$$z_i' = [z_{ih} = a_{ih}\theta + c_{ih}], \qquad h = 1, 2, \ldots, m_i. \tag{11}$$

Let us write the corresponding category response function as

$$P_{ih}(\theta) = e^{z_{ih}} \Big/ \sum_{k}^{m_i} e^{z_{ik}}. \tag{12}$$

The vector logit may be expressed in terms of $2(m_i - 1)$ free parameters as

$$\underset{1\times m_i}{z_i'} = \underset{1\times 2}{[1, \theta]} \cdot \underset{2\times(m_i-1)}{\begin{bmatrix} \alpha_i \\ \gamma_i \end{bmatrix}} \cdot \underset{(m_i-1)\times m_i}{T_i} . \tag{13}$$

In Eq. (13), the original $2m_i$ parameters are replaced by the $2(m_i - 1)$ linear parametric functions

$$\begin{bmatrix} a_i \\ c_i \end{bmatrix} = \begin{bmatrix} \alpha_i \\ \gamma_i \end{bmatrix} T_i.$$

This parametrization of the model is convenient in fitting the model because the elements of α_i and γ_i are unconstrained. The T_i matrix may take various forms depending on the constraints imposed on z_i (see Discussion).

Assuming conditional independence of the responses, the probability of the response pattern $U_\ell = [U_{1\ell}, U_{2\ell}, \ldots, U_{n\ell}]$ as a function of θ is, say,

$$L_\ell(\theta) = P(U_\ell \mid \theta) = \prod_i^n P_{ih}(\theta), \tag{14}$$

where $h = U_{i\ell}$ is the item score designating the category to which the response to item i in pattern ℓ corresponds. There are $S = \prod_i^n m_i$ possible response patterns.

Assuming θ is distributed in the population of persons with density $g(\theta)$, the unconditional probability of pattern ℓ is the integral of Eq. (14) over the θ distribution:

$$\bar{P}_\ell = \int_{-\infty}^{\infty} L_\ell(\theta) g(\theta) d\theta. \tag{15}$$

In other contexts, $L_\ell(\theta)$ is called the *likelihood* of θ, given the pattern U_ℓ, and $\bar{P}_\ell$ is called the *marginal probability* of U_ℓ.

TABLE 2. A Multiple-Choice Item and Its Estimated Parameter Values.

Stem	Alternative	Category (h)	a_h	c_h
"Domicile"	"Residence"	1	0.905	0.126
	"Servant"	2	0.522	−0.206
	"Legal document"	3		
	"Hiding place"	3	−0.469	−0.257
	"Family"	3		
	Omit	4	−0.959	0.336

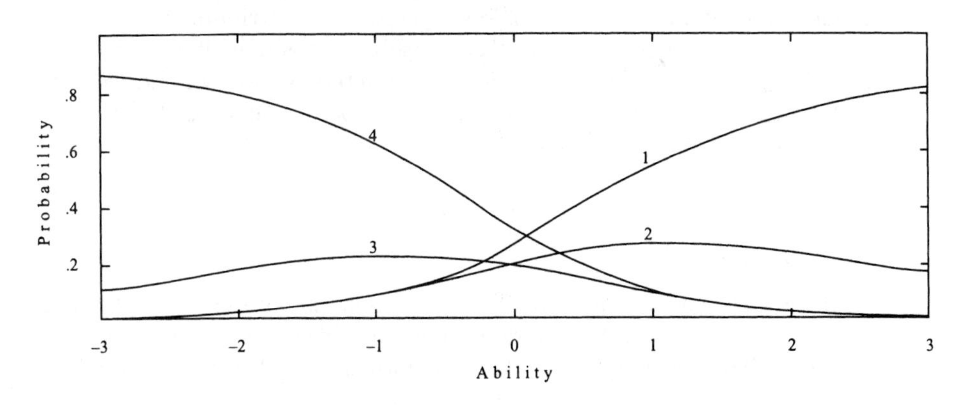

FIGURE 1. Category response functions for the vocabulary item in Table 1.

Figure 1, redrawn from Bock (1972), shows estimated category response functions for the multiple-choice vocabulary item shown in Table 2. The item is from a test administered with the instruction "Do not guess! If you do not know the correct answer, omit the item."

Differentiating the category response functions with respect to θ and equating to zero, Samejima (1972) showed, as Figure 1 suggests, that the function with the smallest a parameter is monotonic decreasing from 1 at $-\infty$, the function with the largest value is monotonic increasing to 1, and those with the intermediate values have unique maxima at finite θ; moreover, functions with the same a values have the same maximum regardless of the value of c.

Samejima (1972) also showed that if the a values are strongly ordered, then the corresponding cumulative category probabilities are strongly ordered, just as in a graded model with strongly ordered thresholds. Conversely, Wainer showed that, if the category response functions are ordered in the sense that the odds of responding to a higher category increase with θ, then the corresponding a values are ordered [see Muraki (1992)]. These results establish that, by an analysis based on the nominal model, one can in general find an ordering of the categories that would justify analysis with a graded model, assuming the empirical ordering is substantively plausible.

Parameter Estimation

As in other applications of item response theory, practical use of the nominal model involves the estimation of one or more parameters of each of a number of items and at least one quantitative attribute, or "ability," of each of a number of persons. For ease of exposition, it is convenient to assume provisionally that the item parameters are known and that the ability, θ, given the response pattern U_j, is to be estimated. For the latter purpose, maximum likelihood, Bayes modal, and Bayes estimation have been proposed.

Maximum Likelihood

Although estimation of θ is not often a large-sample proposition (the number of items is seldom really large), maximum likelihood is widely used in this role.[1] The likelihood takes the same form as Eq. (14), and the gradient

[1] Although maximum likelihood estimation can be adapted to smaller samples by including higher terms in asymptotic expansions (Shenton and Bowman, 1977), this has not yet been attempted for multiple-category IRT models.

of the log likelihood of θ, given the response pattern U_j of person j, is

$$G(\theta) = \frac{\partial \log L_j(\theta)}{\partial \theta} = \sum_i^n a_i' T_i [u_{ij} - P_i(\theta)], \tag{16}$$

where the elements of the m_i-vector u_{ij} are

$$u(h, U_{ij}) = \begin{cases} 1 & \text{if } h = U_{ij} \\ 0 & \text{if } h \neq U_{ij} \end{cases}, \quad h = 1, 2, \ldots, m_i;$$

those of the vector $P_i(\theta)$ are the category response functions $P_{ih}(\theta)$ evaluated at θ.

The corresponding information is

$$I(\theta) = \sum_i^n a_i' W_i(\theta) a_i, \tag{17}$$

where element (k, h) of the matrix $W_i(\theta)$ is $P_{ik}(\theta)[\delta_{kh} - P_{ih}(\theta)]$ as in Eq. (10).

The likelihood surface is in general convex, and the Newton–Raphson iterations,

$$\hat{\theta}^{(t+1)} = \hat{\theta}^{(t)} + G(\hat{\theta}_j^{(t)})/I(\hat{\theta}^{(t)}),$$

will converge to any interior solution from any finite starting values. Boundary solutions at $\theta = \pm\infty$ are possible, however, if the responses to the items are all in the category with the largest a value or all in the category with the smallest a value.

For any finite solution $\hat{\theta}$, the large-sample standard error of the estimator is

$$\text{S.E.}(\hat{\theta}) = I^{-1/2}(\hat{\theta}_j).$$

Bayes Modal

For θ drawn from a proper distribution with a continuous density function $g(\theta)$, the posterior density, given U_j, is

$$p_j(\theta) = L_j(\theta) g(\theta) / \bar{P}_j.$$

The gradient of the log posterior density is

$$G_P(\theta) = \frac{\partial \log L_j(\theta)}{\partial \theta} + \frac{\partial \log g(\theta)}{\partial \theta}, \tag{18}$$

and the posterior information is

$$I_P(\theta) = I(\theta) - \frac{\partial^2 \log g(\theta)}{\partial \theta^2}. \tag{19}$$

When $g(\theta)$ is the normal density function for $N(\mu, \sigma)$, the right-hand terms of Eqs. (18) and (19) are $-(\theta - \mu)/\sigma^2$ and $-\sigma^{-2}$, respectively. In that case, the posterior is strictly convex and all solutions are unique and finite.

The standard error of the Bayes modal estimator, say $\tilde{\theta}$, when n is moderate to large, is

$$\text{S.E.}(\tilde{\theta}) - I_P^{-1/2}(\tilde{\theta}).$$

An index of reliability for the test may then be computed from the population variance σ^2 and the average error variance

$$\bar{\sigma}_e^2 = \int_{-\infty}^{\infty} I_P^{-1}(\theta) g(\theta) d\theta.$$

The marginal test reliability is the intraclass correlation

$$\rho = \frac{\sigma^2 - \bar{\sigma}_e^2}{\sigma^2}.$$

Bayes

The Bayes estimator of θ is the mean of the posterior distribution of θ, given U_j:

$$\bar{\theta} = \int_{-\infty}^{\infty} \theta p_j(\theta) d\theta. \tag{20}$$

The variance of the estimator is

$$\sigma^2_{\theta|U_j} = \int_{-\infty}^{\infty} (\theta - \bar{\theta}_j)^2 p_j(\theta) d(\theta). \tag{21}$$

The square root of the latter serves as a standard error of $\bar{\theta}$. Neither of these estimators depend on large-sample assumptions. They require only that the posterior distribution has finite first and second moments.

The definite integrals in Eqs. (20) and (21) cannot be expressed in closed form in general, but they may be readily evaluated by quadrature. When $g(\theta)$ is normal, Gauss–Hermite quadrature is the method of choice. In other cases, including those where $g(\theta)$ is approximated nonparametrically (e.g., by kernel estimation), the number of nodes can be easily taken large enough to obtain good accuracy with a simple Newton–Cotes formula (Press et al., 1986).

Estimation of the Item Parameters

With the typical large sample sizes of IRT applications, the maximum marginal likelihood method of estimating the parameters of the nominal model is quite satisfactory (Bock and Lieberman, 1970). When the numbers of items and categories are small relative to the sample size, there are computational advantages in sorting and counting the response patterns

U_j. Let r_ℓ be the frequency of pattern ℓ occurring in a sample of N respondents, where $\ell = 1, 2, \ldots, s$ and $s \leq \min(N, S)$. Then the likelihood of the unconstrained parameters, given the data, is

$$L(\alpha, \gamma) = \frac{N!}{r_1! r_2! \cdots r_s!} \bar{P}_1^{r_1} \bar{P}_2^{r_2} \cdots \bar{P}_s^{r_s},$$

where $\bar{P}_\ell$ is the marginal probability given in Eq. (15) of pattern ℓ. The $2(m_i - 1)$ likelihood equations for the parameters of item i are

$$\frac{\partial \log L(\alpha, \gamma)}{\partial \begin{bmatrix} \gamma_i \\ \alpha_i \end{bmatrix}} = \sum_\ell^s \frac{r_\ell}{\bar{P}_\ell} \int_{-\infty}^{\infty} T_i[u_{i\ell} - P_i(\theta)] \otimes \begin{bmatrix} 1 \\ \theta \end{bmatrix} L_\ell(\theta) g(\theta) d\theta = 0.$$

[See Bock (1975, 1989).]

Although it is possible to solve the full system of $2n(m_i - 1)$ likelihood equations by quadrature and Newton–Raphson iterations using the empirical information matrix of Louis (1982) in place of the Hessian matrix, the computational burden quickly becomes prohibitive as the numbers of items and categories increase. An EM solution, however, remains practical (Bock and Aitkin 1981; Dempster et al., 1977). For this solution, one carries out, item by item, successive iterative cycles of computing expected m_i-vectors of response frequencies

$$\bar{r}_{iq} = \sum_{\ell=1}^{s} r_\ell u_{i\ell} L_\ell(X_q) g(X_q) / \bar{P}_\ell, \tag{22}$$

with u as in Eq. (16), and the scalar,

$$\bar{N}_q = \sum_{\ell=1}^{s} r_\ell L_\ell(X_q) g(X_q) / \bar{P}_\ell, \tag{23}$$

at the quadrature nodes X_q, $q = 1, 2, \ldots, Q$. Then the Newton–Raphson solution for the fixed-effects case discussed earlier in this chapter may be applied to obtain provisional estimates for the parameters of item i. The gradient $2(m_i - 1)$-vector is

$$G \begin{bmatrix} \gamma_i \\ \alpha_i \end{bmatrix} = \sum_q^Q T_i \left[\bar{r}_{iq} - \bar{N}_q P_i(X_q)\right] \otimes \begin{bmatrix} 1 \\ X_q \end{bmatrix}, \tag{24}$$

where elements of the m_i-vector $P_i(X_q)$ are the category probabilities for item i at $\theta = X_q$. The Hessian matrix is

$$H \begin{bmatrix} \gamma_i \\ \alpha_i \end{bmatrix} = -\sum_q^Q \bar{N}_q T_i W_i(X_q) T_i' \otimes \begin{bmatrix} 1 \\ X_q \end{bmatrix} [1, X_q], \tag{25}$$

and element (k, h) of $W_i(X_q)$ are $P_{ik}(X_q)[\delta_{kh} - P_{ih}(X_q)]$ as in Eq. (10).

Evaluations of Eqs. (22) and (23) for all items comprise the E-step of the algorithm. The Newton–Raphson iterations, using Eqs. (24) and (25), comprise the M-step. The number of EM cycles required for an acceptable level of convergence may be large—as many as 50 is not unusual. The above estimation procedures are all implemented in the MULTILOG computer program (Thissen, 1991).

Goodness of Fit

When the sample size is large and the number of items and categories relatively small, all of the possible response patterns have a reasonable probability of occurring (e.g., $\bar{P}_\ell > 0.01$). In that case, the expected number of responses among the patterns may be large enough to justify the chi-square approximation of the distribution of the marginal statistic

$$\chi^2_M = \sum_{\ell}^{S} \frac{(r_\ell - N\bar{P}_\ell)^2}{N\bar{P}_\ell} \tag{26}$$

on $(S-1) - 2n(m_i - 1)$ degrees of freedom. This statistic provides a test of fit of the model against the general multinomial alternative.

In smaller samples and large n and m_i, the many patterns with small expectations would make the use of Eq. (26) dubious. For models with differing numbers of independent constraints on the parameters, a test based on the difference between values of χ^2_M could still be valid, however (Haberman, 1977, 1988). The number of degrees of freedom would equal the difference in the number of constraints. Alternatively, the likelihood ratio chi-square,

$$\chi^2_{ML} = \sum_{\ell}^{s} r_\ell \log(\bar{P}_\ell^{(\Omega)} / \bar{P}_\ell^{(\omega)}),$$

where $\bar{P}_\ell^{(\omega)}$ is the marginal probability of pattern ℓ under greater restriction and $\bar{P}_\ell^{(\Omega)}$, the probability under fewer restrictions, would serve the same purpose. These tests are valuable when comparing the specializations and extensions of the nominal model referred to below.

Example

Ratings of responses of 2000 students to three open-ended items of the 1989 Alberta Diploma Examination in human biology provide the data for a small computing example. Originally, the student papers were rated in five categories describing levels of understanding related to the content of each item. For items 1 and 2, the infrequently used category 1 was combined with category 2, and for item 3, a like category 5 was combined with 4. The resulting (relabeled) response patterns, combined and counted, are shown in Table 3.

The EM solution of the MML equations for the item parameters accurate to four decimal places converged in 32 EM cycles. The estimated parameter contrasts between category 1 and each of the remaining categories are shown in Table 4 with their standard errors. The a parameters of the three items are strongly ordered, confirming the item writers' judgmental orderings of the corresponding categories. The likelihood ratio chi-square of 53.7, on 45 degrees of freedom, shows that the goodness of fit of the 18 (free-) parameter nominal model is excellent ($\chi^2/df = 1.2$). When the a parameters are constrained to a common linear function of the category indices 1 through 4, the nominal model becomes equivalent to the partial credit model with 10 free parameters (see Discussion). It fits almost as well as the unconstrained model ($\chi^2/df = 1.3$).

Although the items are few in number, their relatively high discriminating power and well-spaced thresholds enable them to convey useful information about the ability of the examinees. The marginal reliability of the Bayes estimator is 0.60 and the posterior standard deviations are well below the 1.0 standard deviation of the specified population distribution of θ.

Discussion

Thissen and Steinberg (1984) have observed that when Eq. (13) is specialized to

$$z_i' = [1, \theta] \cdot \begin{bmatrix} \alpha & \alpha & \cdots & \alpha \\ \gamma_{i1} & \gamma_{i2} & \cdots & \gamma_{i,m-1} \end{bmatrix} \cdot \begin{bmatrix} 0 & 1 & 1 & \cdots & 1 \\ 0 & 0 & 1 & \cdots & 1 \\ \cdot & \cdot & \cdot & \vdots & \cdot \\ 0 & 0 & 0 & \cdots & 1 \end{bmatrix}, \tag{27}$$

the nominal categories model becomes the Partial Credit Model for ordered categories (Masters, (1982); this volume). [Note that positive α in Eq. (27) satisfies the Samejima–Wainer conditions for strong ordering.] By choice of scale, α may be set equal to 1. In that case, $a_{ik} = k$, $k = 0, 1, \ldots, m_i - 1$, is the so-called "scoring" function of the multiple category Rasch model (Andersen, 1973; this volume). For this model, the crossing points of successive category response curves, which occur at

$$\theta_{ih} = \frac{c_{ih} - c_{i,h-1}}{a_{i,h-1} - a_{ih}}$$

in the nominal model, become $\theta_{ih} = c_{ih} - c_{ih+1} = \gamma_{ih}$.

TABLE 3. Observed and Expected Frequencies of Each Response Pattern; Corresponding Bayes Estimates of Ability and Posterior Standard Deviations (PSD).

	Frequency		Estimate			Frequency		Estimate	
Pattern	Obs.	Exp.	Bayes	PSD	Pattern	Obs.	Exp.	Bayes	PSD
111	50.0	46.5	−1.72	0.68	311	9.0	7.0	−0.96	0.63
112	32.0	37.2	−1.22	0.64	312	12.0	13.3	−0.51	0.60
113	15.0	18.1	−0.95	0.63	313	13.0	10.3	−0.27	0.61
114	10.0	8.7	−0.61	0.61	314	7.0	9.0	0.06	0.62
121	54.0	59.9	−1.39	0.65	321	11.0	16.1	−0.66	0.61
122	80.0	69.9	−0.91	0.63	322	29.0	42.6	−0.23	0.61
123	40.0	41.8	−0.65	0.61	323	37.0	40.2	0.03	0.62
124	24.0	25.9	−0.33	0.61	324	44.0	45.3	0.36	0.62
131	27.0	28.0	−1.07	0.64	331	15.0	13.0	−0.38	0.60
132	52.0	46.7	−0.62	0.61	332	62.0	47.9	0.06	0.62
133	33.0	33.9	−0.37	0.60	333	60.0	55.2	0.32	0.62
134	27.0	26.9	−0.04	0.62	334	88.0	80.8	0.67	0.64
141	4.0	4.0	−0.62	0.61	341	4.0	4.0	0.05	0.62
142	13.0	10.9	−0.20	0.61	342	27.0	24.7	0.51	0.63
143	10.0	10.5	0.06	0.62	343	43.0	38.7	0.78	0.65
144	10.0	12.3	0.40	0.62	344	73.0	85.9	1.17	0.68
211	27.0	20.2	−1.29	0.65	411	4.0	2.5	−0.74	0.61
212	19.0	26.3	−0.82	0.62	412	8.0	6.1	−0.31	0.61
213	11.0	16.6	−0.57	0.60	413	7.0	5.4	−0.06	0.62
214	11.0	11.1	−0.25	0.61	414	9.0	5.7	0.28	0.62
221	30.0	36.0	−0.97	0.63	421	7.0	6.8	−0.46	0.60
222	78.0	66.8	−0.53	0.60	422	21.0	22.9	−0.02	0.62
223	69.0	51.3	−0.28	0.61	423	25.0	24.9	0.24	0.62
224	48.0	43.9	0.05	0.62	424	31.0	33.8	0.58	0.63
231	24.0	23.0	−0.68	0.61	431	8.0	6.4	−0.18	0.61
232	48.0	59.3	−0.25	0.61	432	23.0	30.3	0.27	0.62
233	52.0	55.3	0.01	0.62	433	35.0	40.3	0.54	0.63
234	53.0	61.3	0.34	0.62	434	73.0	71.6	0.90	0.66
241	3.0	5.0	−0.26	0.61	441	4.0	2.5	0.27	0.62
242	21.0	21.3	0.19	0.62	442	21.0	20.0	0.73	0.64
243	20.0	26.8	0.45	0.62	443	36.0	36.6	1.02	0.67
244	54.0	44.0	0.80	0.65	444	105.0	101.2	1.43	0.71

TABLE 4. Estimated Parameter Contrasts and Standard Errors.

	a-parameters						c-parameters				
Item	2–1	SE	3–1	SE	4–1	SE	2–1	SE	3–1	SE	4–1
1	1.00	0.11	1.82	0.14	2.37	0.15	0.67	0.10	.54	0.10	−.01
2	0.77	0.11	1.54	0.14	2.70	0.17	1.45	0.14	1.64	0.14	0.65
3	1.17	0.14	1.85	0.16	2.72	0.17	1.49	0.16	1.51	0.16	1.46

In his Generalized Partial Credit Model, Muraki (1992, this volume) relaxes Eq. (27) by setting $\alpha = \alpha_i$, thus introducing a discriminating parameter into the model. He also employs the device introduced by Andrich (1978) of separating the intercept parameter into a term due to the item and a term due to the category,

$$c_{ih} = b_i + d_h,$$

thus obtaining a rating scale model for items that are rated in a common suite of categories. This device reintroduces the item threshold parameter of binary IRT models.

In a manner similar to the extension of the two-parameter logistic model to three parameters, Samejima (1979) and Thissen and Steinberg (1984) extended the nominal model to allow for effects of guessing on multiple-choice items. Samejima assumed the guessed responses distribute with equal probability over the alternatives, whereas Thissen and Steinberg allowed the position or labeling of the alternatives to affect the distribution of these responses. (In tests balanced for the position of the correct alternative, for example, examinees tend to choose the third of four multiple-choice alternatives slightly more often than the others.)

Thissen and Steinberg's response function for the multiple-choice model appears in this volume. They estimate the d_h under the constraint $\sum_{h=1}^{m_i} d_h = 1$. The exponential with coefficients a_{i0} and c_{i0} in their model represents the latent category of guessed responses to item i, while d_h is the probability that any such response will fall on alternative h.

Most of the above forms of the nominal categories model are also implemented in the MULTILOG program of Thissen (1991). The rating-scale version of the Partial Credit Model is implemented in the PARSCALE program of Muraki and Bock (1991).

References

Andersen, E.B. (1973). Conditional inference for multiple-choice questionnaires. *British Journal of Mathematical and Statistical Psychology* **26**, 31–44.

Andrich, D. (1978). A rating formulation for ordered response categories. *Psychometrika* **43**, 561–573.

Birnbaum, A. (1968). Some latent trait models and their use in inferring an examinee's ability. In F.M. Lord and M.R. Novick (Eds.), *Statistical Theories of Mental Test Scores* (pp. 397–479). Reading, MA: Addison-Wesley.

Bock, R.D. (1956). A generalization of the law of comparative judgment applied to a problem in the prediction of choice (abstract). *American Psychologist* **11**, 442.

Bock, R.D. (1966). *Estimating Multinomial Response Relations* (Research Memorandum No. 5). Chicago: University of Chicago Educational Statistics Laboratory.

Bock, R.D. (1970). Estimating multinomial response relations. In R.C. Bose, I.M. Chakravarti, P.C. Mahalanobis, C.R. Rao, and K.J.C. Smith (Eds.), *Contributions to Statistics and Probability* (pp. 111–132). Chapel Hill, NC: University of North Carolina Press.

Bock, R.D. (1972). Estimating item parameters and latent ability when responses are scored in two or more nominal categories. *Psychometrika* **37**, 29–51.

Bock, R.D. (1975). *Multivariate Statistical Methods in Behavioral Research.* New York: McGraw-Hill.

Bock, R.D. (1985, reprint). *Multivariate Statistical Methods in Behavioral Research.* Chicago: Scientific Software International.

Bock, R.D. (1989). Measurement of human variation: A two-stage model. In R.D. Bock (Ed.), *Multilevel Analysis of Educational Data* (pp. 319–342). New York: Academic Press.

Bock, R.D. and Aitkin, M. (1981). Marginal maximum likelihood estimation of item parameters: Application of an EM algorithm. *Psychometrika* **46**, 443–445.

Bock, R.D. and Jones, L.V. (1968). *The Measurement and Prediction of Judgment and Choice.* San Francisco: Holden-Day.

Bock, R.D. and Lieberman, M. (1970). Fitting a response model for n dichotomously scored items. *Psychometrika* **35**, 179–197.

Bradley, R.A. and Terry, M.E. (1952). Rank analysis of incomplete block designs. I. Method of paired comparisons. *Biometrika* **39**, 324–345.

Dempster, A.P., Laird, N.M. and Rubin, D.B. (1977). Maximum likelihood from incomplete data via the EM algorithm (with discussion). *Journal of the Royal Statistical Society, Series B* **39**, 1–38,

Fisher, R.A. and Yates, F. (1953). *Statistical Tables for Biological, Agricultural and Medical Research* (4th ed.). New York: Hafner.

Goodman, L.A. (1970). The multivariate analysis of qualitative data: Interactions among multiple classifications. *Journal of the American Statistical Association* **65**, 226–256.

Gumbel, E.J. (1961). Bivariate logistic distributions. *Journal of the American Statistical Association* **56**, 335–349.

Haberman, S.J. (1977). Log-linear models and frequency tables with small expected cell counts. *Annals of Statistics* **5**, 1148–1169.

Haberman, S.J. (1979). *Analysis of Qualitative Data, Vol. 2.* Chicago: University of Chicago Press.

Haberman, S.J. (1988). A warning on the use of chi-squared statistics with frequency tables with small expected cell counts. *Journal of the American Statistical Association* **83**, 555–560.

Louis, T.A. (1982). Finding the observed information matrix when using the EM algorithm. *Journal of the Royal Statistical Society, Series B* **44**, 226–233.

Luce, R.D. (1959). *Individual Choice Behavior.* New York: Wiley.

Mantel, N. (1966). Models for complex contingency tables and polychotomous dosage response curves. *Biometrics* **22**, 83–95.

Masters, G.N. (1982). A Rasch model for partial credit scoring. *Psychometrika* **47**, 149–174.

McKeon, J.J. (1961). Measurement procedures based on comparative judgment. Unpublished doctoral dissertation, Department of Psychology, University of North Carolina.

Muraki, E. (1992). A generalized partial credit model: Application of an EM algorithm. *Applied Psychological Measurement* **16**, 159–176.

Muraki, E. and Bock, R.D. (1991). *PARSCALE: Parametric Scaling of Rating Data.* Chicago: Scientific Software International.

Press, W.H., Flannery, B.P., Teukolsky, S.A., and Vetterling, W.T. (1986). *Numerical Recipes.* New York: Cambridge University Press.

Samejima, F. (1972). A general model for free-response data. *Psychometric Monograph*, No. 18.

Samejima, F. (1979). *A New Family of Models for the Multiple Choice Item* (Research Report No. 79-4). Knoxville, TN: Department of Psychology, University of Tennessee.

Shenton, L.R. and Bowman, K.O. (1977). *Maximum Likelihood Estimation in Small Samples.* New York: Macmillan.

Thissen, D. (1991). *MULTILOG User's Guide, Version 6.* Chicago: Scientific Software International.

Thissen, D. and Steinberg, L. (1984). A response model for multiple choice items. *Psychometrika* **49**, 501–519.

Thurstone, L.L. (1927). A law of comparative judgment. *Psychological Review* **34**, 278–286.

3
A Response Model for Multiple-Choice Items

David Thissen and Lynne Steinberg

Introduction

In the mid-1960s, Samejima initiated the development of item response models that involve separate response functions for all of the alternatives in the multiple choice and Likert-type formats. Her work in this area began at the Educational Testing Service and continued during a visit to the L.L. Thurstone Psychometric Laboratory at the University of North Carolina. Both Samejima's (1969; this volume) original model for graded item responses and Bock's (1972; this volume) model for nominal responses were originally intended to produce response functions for all of the alternatives of multiple-choice items. For various reasons, neither model has proved entirely satisfactory for that purpose, although both have been applied in other contexts. Using a combination of ideas suggested by Bock (1972) and Samejima (1968, 1979), a multiple-choice model was developed that produces response functions that fit unidimensional multiple-choice tests better (Thissen and Steinberg, 1984); that model is the subject of this chapter.

Presentation of the Model

To give content to an illustration of the multiple-choice model, consider the mathematics item, shown in Fig. 1, that was administered in 1992 to about a thousand third-grade students as part of an item tryout for the North Carolina End of Grade Testing Program. Calibration of this item, embedded in an 80-item tryout form, gives the response functions shown in Fig. 2. As expected, the response function for the keyed alternative B, increases monotonically, and has approximately the form of the three-parameter logistic curves commonly used for the right–wrong analysis of multiple choice items. The response functions for alternatives A and D, which are fairly obviously incorrect, are monotonically decreasing.

The interesting feature of this analysis involved alternative C, which is

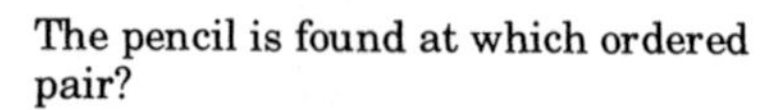
The pencil is found at which ordered pair?

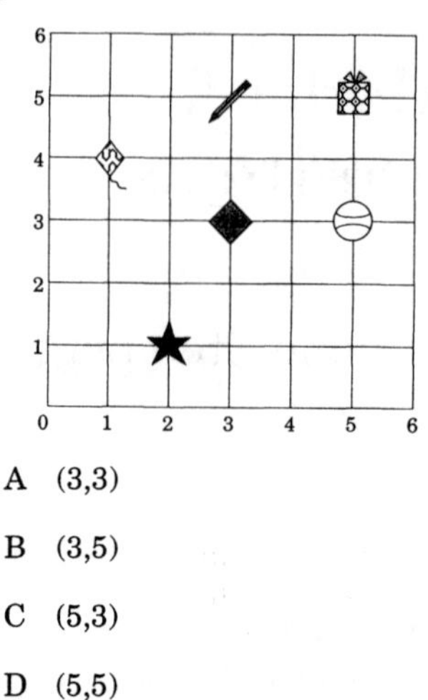

A (3,3)

B (3,5)

C (5,3)

D (5,5)

FIGURE 1. Item 62 from an 80-item tryout form administered to third and fourth grade students as part of the development of the North Carolina End of Grade Testing Program.

a very popular distractor; it was selected by about 27% of the test takers, or about 60% of those who answered incorrectly. Further, the response functions in Figure 2 show that alternative C tended to be selected by examinees of relatively higher proficiency. There is also some interesting anecdotal evidence about this item: When it was used as an illustration of the material to be on the new testing program, a number of classroom teachers complained that the item had two right answers. And when this item was presented informally to some (un-named) psychometricians, they tended to choose alternative C. The problem appears to be that the item-writers assumed that the only acceptable meaning of the phrase "ordered pair" involved the Cartesian coordinate system that is included in the third grade mathematics curriculum; that assumption makes B the keyed alternative. However, in other contexts (e.g., using the row-column rule of matrix algebra and table construction, as in spreadsheets), alternative C is equally the "ordered pair." While it is impossible to tell if any of the third-grade test takers followed such sophisticated rules in responding to this item, it would probably be regarded as more fair, and it would probably be more discriminating, if the context asked for, say, "graphical coordinates," instead of an "ordered pair."

The primary purpose of the multiple choice model is facilitation of graphically-based item analysis; curves like those in Fig. 2 may be very useful for item analysis and test construction. Wainer (1989) has described the use of such graphics in a dynamic item analysis system. Thorough analysis

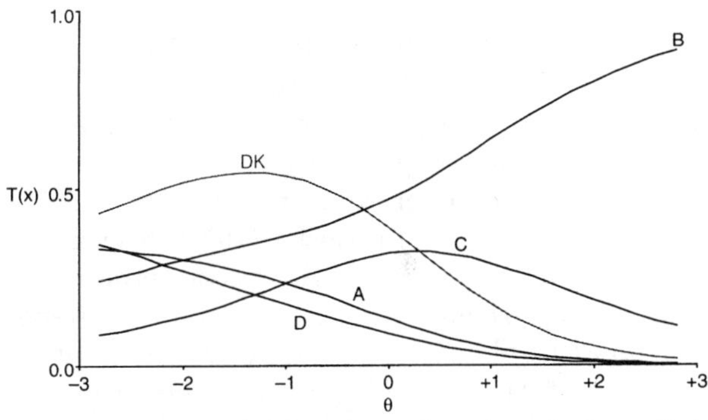

FIGURE 2. Multiple-choice-model response functions for item 62 (shown in Fig. 1), for third grade students.

of the behavior of the alternatives of a multiple-choice item is beyond the convenient reach of the traditional test theory because the relation between proficiency and the probability of most incorrect alternatives is not monotonic. The traditional theory rests on correlations, which summarize only monotonic relationships well. Item response theory need not be concerned with monotonicity, and furthermore, IRT facilitates graphical display of the concepts of interest. Wainer (1989) argues that graphical description of the data for each of the item's alternatives is superior to the numerical summaries of traditional item analysis. The multiple-choice model uses a parametric function as the mechanism for producing graphics such as that shown in Fig. 2; see Ramsay (1991; this volume; Abrahamowicz and Ramsay, 1992) for alternative, less parametric approaches.

Response functions for each category of the item for the multiple choice model are

$$T(u = h) = \frac{\exp[a_h\theta + c_h] + d_h \exp[a_0\theta + c_0]}{\sum_{k=0}^{m} \exp[a_k\theta + c_k]}. \tag{1}$$

The latent variable (*ability* in this volume; also often called *proficiency*) is denoted by θ, and the response functions describe the probability of a response in category h as a function of θ. The observed data are in categories $h = 1, 2, \ldots, m$, where m is the number of multiple-choice alternatives.

Elsewhere in the literature, the response functions are often referred to as *trace lines*; Lazarsfeld (1950, pp. 363ff) introduced that term to describe a curve representing the probability that a respondent selects a particular alternative as a response to an interview question or test item, as a function of the underlying variable that is being measured. That is the reason for the use of the notation T to denote the response functions (trace lines), both as a mnemonic and to emphasize the fact that, while the response function has probabilistic interpretations, it does not describe an observable relative-frequency probability. $T(u = h)$ is a hypothetical type of probability: It can be described as the proportion of a (hypothetical) group of test takers with $\theta = \theta^*$ who select alternative h, or the proportion of (hypothetical) items just like this one (in some sense) for which a particular test taker would select alternative h. It is used to describe these hypothetical probabilities, and the notation P is reserved for later use to describe the model for observable, relative-frequency proportions.

There is no *a priori* ordering of the response categories. The response function model is identical to that for Bock's (1972; this volume) model for nominal responses, with the addition of the second term in the numerator in Eq. (1). Thus, the underlying stochastic model for the response process is identical to that described by Bock (1972; this volume), with the addition of responses in a latent category, referred to as *category 0* or *don't know* (DK). The idea is that the examinees who do not know the correct answer to a multiple-choice item comprise a latent class, and membership in that latent class has a response function that is:

Examinees in the latent DK class give an observed response, by selecting one of the multiple-choice alternatives; the model in Eq. (1) describes this process by adding

$$T(u=0) = \frac{\exp[a_0\theta + c_0]}{\sum_{k=0}^{m} \exp[a_k\theta + c_k]} \tag{2}$$

some proportion (d_h) of the DK responses to the response functions for each of the observed categories. The DK curve is shown in Fig. 2.

The parameters denoted by a reflect the order, as well as discrimination, for the categories (see Thissen et al., 1989). In the nominal model, the category with the largest algebraic value of a has a monotonically increasing response function; generally, that is the keyed alternative. After the addition of the DK curve in Eq. (1), the response function for the keyed response may be nonmonotonic, although it usually approaches 1.0 as θ becomes large. The category with the lowest algebraic value of a has a monotonically decreasing response function; generally, that is DK. (The reader will note that the DK curve in Fig. 2 is not monotonically decreasing; that aspect of the model for this item will be considered below.) Response alternatives associated with intermediate values of a have nonmonotonic response functions. The parameters denoted by c reflect the relative frequency of the selection of each alternative; for alternatives with similar values of a, those with larger values of c are selected more frequently than those with lower values of c.

The parameters a_h and c_h are not identified with respect to location, so these parameters are estimated subject to some linear constraint, most often that $\sum a_h = \sum c_h = 0$; the constraint is most easily imposed using reparametrization (Bock, 1972, 1975, pp. 239–249):

$$\mathbf{a}' = \alpha' \mathbf{T}_{\mathbf{a}},$$

where α contains the unconstrained parameters that are actually estimated. The c_hs are estimated using a similar reparametrization:

$$\mathbf{c}' = \gamma' \mathbf{T}_{\mathbf{c}}.$$

In some contexts, it may be desirable to use other types of contrasts as the rows of the matrix $\mathbf{T}$ [see Thissen (1991)]. The parameters represented by d_h are proportions, representing the proportion of those who don't know who respond in each category on a multiple-choice item. Therefore, the constraint that $\sum d_h = 1$ is required. This constraint may be enforced by estimating d_h such that

$$d_h = \frac{\exp[d_h^*]}{\sum \exp[d_h^*]}$$

and contrasts among the d_h^* are the parameters estimated. Then reparametrization gives

$$\mathbf{d}^{*\prime} = \delta' \mathbf{T}_{\mathbf{d}}.$$

The elements of the vector δ are the parameters estimated.

The use of the parametric model brings with it all of the benefits now associated with IRT: parametric (very smooth) curves for item analysis, information functions for use in test assembly, straightforward computation of scaled scores (but see cautions, below), and likelihood-based procedures for linking scales for different groups, and for testing hypotheses, e.g., about differential item functioning [DIF; see Thissen et al. (1993)]. In addition, the multiple choice model has been used as the generating model in simulation studies of the performance of other IRT systems (Abrahamowicz and Ramsay, 1992; Wainer and Thissen, 1987). However, the use of such a complex parametric model also brings the burden of parameter estimation.

Parameter Estimation

While there are no doubt many conceivable approaches to parameter estimation for the multiple-choice model and closely related IRT models, the only approaches that have been described in the literature are maximum likelihood estimation (that gives the MLEs) and the closely related *maximum a posteriori* (Bayesian) approach, for estimates referred to as MAPs.

Using maximum likelihood estimation, the item parameter estimates maximize the likelihood

$$L = \prod_{\{u\}} P(u)^{r_u}, \tag{3}$$

in which the product is taken over the set $\{u\}$ of all response patterns, $r_{\mathbf{u}}$ is the frequency of response pattern $\mathbf{u}$, and $P(\mathbf{u})$ represents the probability of that response pattern in the data,

$$P(\mathbf{u}) = \int \prod_{i=1}^{n} T_i(u_i \mid \theta)\phi(\theta)d\theta. \tag{4}$$

The population distribution for θ, $\phi(\theta)$, is usually assumed to be $N(0,1)$; given the complexity of the model, it is not clear to what degree aspects of the population distribution might be jointly estimable with the item parameters.

In general, there are no closed-form solutions for the parameter estimates, and so some iterative solution is required. In the context of the normal-ogive and two-parameter logistic models, Bock and Lieberman (1970) described an algorithm for direct maximization of Eq. (3); however, that approach was limited to a small number of items, with many fewer parameters per item than the multiple-choice model.

The direct approach to maximization of Eq. (3) has never been attempted for the multiple-choice model. The reason is that the number of parameters involved is very large: For five-alternative multiple-choice items, each $T_i(u_i \mid \theta)$ in Eq. (4) is a function of 14 parameters (five αs, five γs, and four δs); thus, for a 50-item test, Eq. (3), taken as a function of the item parameters (as it is for likelihood estimation), is a function of 700 parameters. In principle, it might be possible to maximize Eq. (3) directly as a function of those 700 parameters—but no commonly-used approach to likelihood maximization appears promising for this purpose. Derivative-free methods, maximizing Eq. (3) by brute force, would almost certainly flounder in a 700-dimensional parameter space. The Newton–Raphson approach used by Bock and Lieberman (1970) for the simpler IRT models with few items would require the computation of the first and second partial derivatives of the log of Eq. (3) with respect to each of the 700 free parameters—where the item parameters are within the product in Eq. (3) of the integrals of the products in Eq. (4); within that, the parameters are within the response function model [Eq. (1)], as well as the linear transformation used to ensure identifiability. Given the dimensionality of the parameter space, a direct approach to maximization of the likelihood for the multiple-choice model appears unlikely to be manageable. The likelihood in Eq. (3) [using the cell probabilities in Eq. (4)] is stated here only because it is the likelihood that is (indirectly) maximized in practical applications.

Bock and Aitkin (1981) described an indirect approach to the maximization of such IRT likelihoods using a variation of the EM algorithm, and that approach can be generalized to the multiple-choice model (Thissen and Steinberg, 1984). This algorithm is implemented in the computer program Multilog (Thissen, 1991). In broad outline, the iterative procedure involves a repeated sequence of so-called E-steps (for *expectation*) followed by M-steps (for *maximization*) until convergence. The steps are:

E-Step: For each item, using the current estimates of the item parameters and some prespecified list of values of θ, θ_q, compute the expected frequencies of responses for each alternative as

$$r^*_{hq} = \sum_{\{u_i=h\}} \prod_{i=1}^{n} T_i(u_i \mid \theta^*_q)\phi(\theta^*_q),$$

where the sum is taken over all examinees with $u_i = h$.

M-Step: Using some suitable general function maximization technique, for each item maximize

$$\ell^* = \sum_h \sum_q r^*_{hq} \log T_i(u_i \mid \theta^*_q) \tag{5}$$

as a function of α, γ, and δ.

The E-step is completely defined above. The M-step defines a set of loglikelihoods that must be maximized; if no constraints are imposed on the model that involve the parameters of more than one item, there is one loglikelihood per item, involving only the parameters for that item. To reconsider the case of 50 multiple-choice items with five alternatives each, the M-Step involves 50 14-parameter estimation problems, maximizing the loglikelihood in Eq. (5). This can be done using derivative-free methods, or using a Newton–Raphson approach with the derivatives of Eq. (5) given by Thissen and Steinberg (1984, pp. 506–507). If constraints are imposed on the model that involve the parameters of two or more items, then the M-step must be done for the entire set of items over which the constraints have been imposed.

There is no proof of the uniqueness of the parameter estimates for the multiple-choice model (or, to our knowledge, of the parameters of any IRT model outside the so-called Rasch family). This is probably because it is easy to show that the parameter estimates are *not* unique. The obvious demonstration that the parameter estimates that maximize the likelihood are not unique arises from the observation that the goodness of fit remains the same if the signs of all of the slope parameters (as) are reversed; this is equivalent to reversing the direction of the latent variable (θ). This lack of uniqueness is common to all IRT models that are parameterized with slopes, and it is the same as the indeterminacy of reflection in the single common factor model. While this obvious indeterminacy precludes the development of any formal proof of the uniqueness of the parameter estimates, it does not appear to affect the usefulness of the model in applied contexts, where the orientation of θ is usually determined by the selection of starting values for the iterative estimation procedure.

Similarly, there is no general proof of the existence of the maximum likelihood estimates of the parameters, nor is one possible, because there are obvious patterns of data for which finite estimates of the parameters (taken as a set) do not exist. For example, if x independent, then it follows that the MLEs of all of the as are zero, and the cs for the observed categories parametrize the marginal totals; there is no information left in the data for estimation of the latent DK class of the ds. As is generally the case with complex latent-variable models, the behavior of the parameters is highly data-dependent.

Fitting the multiple choice model, using procedures described by Thissen and Steinberg (1984) and Thissen et al. (1989), is both computationally intensive and fairly demanding of the data analyst. The focus of the problem is the large number of parameters involved: There are 11 free parameters per item for the four-alternative multiple-choice format, and 14 parameters per item for five-choice items. For the 80-item test that included the item shown in Fig. 1, fitting the model involved optimization of the likelihood in an 880-dimensional (parameter) space! The dimensions of the problem alone account for a good deal of the computer time required; using Multilog (Thissen, 1991), the 80-item calibrations for the examples used here, with about 1000 examinees, each required 1–2 hours on a 33MHz 80486-based MS-DOS computer.

The computational problem is exacerbated by the fact that the model is somewhat overparameterized for most test items and their associated data. Many multiple choice items, especially in the unselected sets usually used for item tryout, include distractors that are chosen by very few examinees. It is not unusual, even with a calibration sample size of 1000, for an alternative to be selected by fewer than 100 test takers. Nevertheless, the multiple choice model involves fitting a nonlinear function giving the expected proportion choosing that alternative; that would be unstable with a sample size of 100, even if the independent variable (θ) was fixed and known, but in this case it is a latent variable.

Further, for a four-alternative item, the model devotes three free parameters to distinguishing among the guessing levels for the four choices, and two more parameters to distinguish the DK curve from the rest of the response functions. However, if the item is relatively easy, most test takers know the answer and respond correctly; only a subset of the sample don't know, and guess. It is not possible to say precisely how large the guessing subset is; but it is not simply the proportion of the sample who respond incorrectly, because some of those select the correct response. Nevertheless, the effective sample size for the guessing parameters (the d_hs) and the DK parameters (the contrasts that yield a_0 and c_0) can be very small.

The result is that there may be very little information in the data about some of the parameters for many of the items, and the speed of the convergence of the EM algorithm is proportional to the information about the parameters (Dempster et al., 1977). The solution to the problem is obviously to reduce the number of parameters; but it is not clear, *a priori*, which parameters are needed to fit which items. A very difficult four-alternative item may well have sufficient information for all 11 parameters, while many of the easier items in a test may require different subsets of the parameters to be fitted properly. A partial solution to the problem is the use of subjective prior densities to constrain the estimates, computing MAPs in place of MLEs. In the item calibrations for the examples in this chapter, Gaussian prior densities were used for all three classes of parameters: the αs and γs were assumed $N(0,3)$, and the δs were assumed $N(0,1)$. These densities multiply the likelihood in Eq. (3), and their logs are added to the loglikelihood in Eq. (5); otherwise, the estimation algorithm is unchanged.

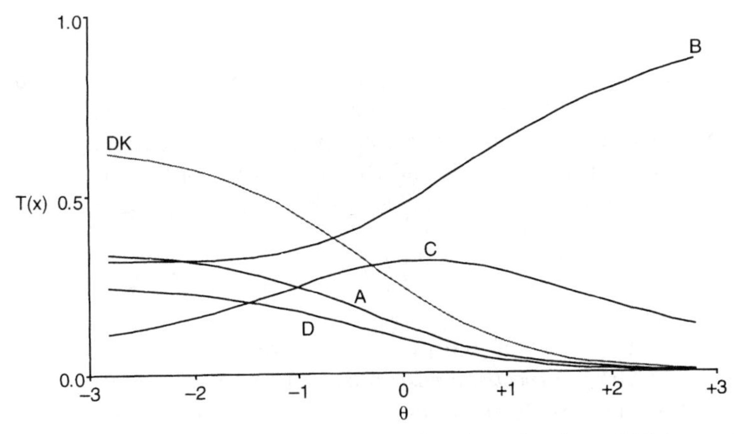

FIGURE 3. Multiple choice model response functions for item 62 (shown in Fig. 1), for third grade students, with the constraints on the parameters described in the text.

Often, upon inspection, the number of parameters for an item can be reduced without reducing the goodness of fit of the model. For instance, for the item in Fig. 1 with the curves in Fig. 2, after we observed that the response functions for alternatives A and D are very similar and roughly proportional to the DK curve, we re-fitted the model with the constraints $a_0 = a_1 = a_4$ and $d_1 = d_4$ (by fixing the values of α_1, α_4, and δ_3 equal to zero). These constraints reduced the number of free parameters from eleven to eight, and did not change the overall goodness of fit of the model for the 80-item test as measured by -2loglikelihood. The curves for the constrained estimation are shown in Fig. 3. There is little change in the forms of the curves between those shown in Figs. 2 and 3, except that the DK curve is monotonically decreasing in Fig. 3, as it should be (showing that the nonmonotonicity of the DK curve observed in Fig. 2 is not a reliable feature of the data).

At the present time, imposing such constraints to reduce the number of parameters estimated can only be done by the data analyst, on an item-by-item basis. It should be possible, in principle, to create an automated system that examines the item response data and imposes appropriate constraints on the multiple-choice model parameters before likelihood-based estimation is attempted. Because such an automated system requires response functions, it might well be based on Ramsay's (Abrahamowicz and Ramsay, 1992; Ramsay, 1991, 1992, this volume) much faster nonparametric system to provide those curves. With appropriate constraints, removing parameters for which there is little information, computational time for estimation may be reduced by factors of between two and ten.

Estimating θ

The response functions of the multiple-choice model may be used to compute scaled scores, in the same way that the response functions for any IRT model are used for that purpose. Given the response functions, which is to say, given the item parameters, and the assumption of local independence, the posterior density over θ for persons with response pattern $\mathbf{u}$ is

$$f(\mathbf{u} \mid \theta) = \left[\prod_{i=1}^{n} T_i(u_i \mid \theta)\right] \phi(\theta).$$

The mode or the mean of $f(\mathbf{u} \mid \theta)$ may be computed as the *maximum a posteriori* (MAP) or *expected a posteriori* (EAP) estimate of θ, respectively. The MAP is the most likely value of θ for persons with response pattern $\mathbf{u}$, and the EAP is the average value of θ for persons with response pattern $\mathbf{u}$; thus, either is a reasonable summary description, or scaled score. The mode of $f(\mathbf{u} \mid \theta)$ may be computed using any of a number of approaches to function maximization, maximizing $f(\mathbf{u} \mid \theta)$ as a function of θ. The mean of the posterior represented by $f(\mathbf{u} \mid \theta)$ requires numerical integration, as described by Bock and Mislevy (1982).

Bock (1972), Thissen (1976), Sympson (1983), Levine and Drasgow (1983), Thissen and Steinberg (1984), and Abrahamowicz and Ramsay (1992) have shown that some increased precision of measurement may be obtained when information in the incorrect alternatives on multiple-choice tests is included in the item response model. For the most part, the additional information obtained with models that take incorrect responses into account is limited to relatively low-ability examinees; with an appropriately-targeted test, most of the higher-ability examinees choose few incorrect alternatives, so there is little information available from that source for them.

There are, however, some potential difficulties with the use of the multiple choice model, or any model that incorporates a model for guessing, to compute scaled scores. As we noted at the time the model was originally presented (Steinberg and Thissen, 1984), the multiple-choice model may produce nonmonotonic response functions for correct responses. The use of nonmonotonic response functions in constructing the posterior density gives rise to potential problems: If the correct response function for an item is nonmonotonic on the right (e.g., it turns down), then examinees with some response patterns on the other items will be penalized by responding correctly to the item; they would have been assigned a higher scaled score if they had selected particular incorrect alternatives. Correct response functions that are nonmonotonic on the left similarly penalize examinees of low ability who respond correctly; conditional on the other item responses, a correct response to an item may not imply higher ability; rather, it may be more likely to be guessing or cheating. As measurement, this is all entirely satisfactory; but it may be a problem if the scoring system must be explained to the examinees, and the examinees are not adequately trained in psychometrics.

The software Multilog (Thissen, 1991) provides MML estimates of the item parameters for the multiple-choice model (as well as for those of several other logistic IRT models), or MAP estimates using Gaussian prior distributions. Multilog also computes MAP scaled scores for individual response patterns, or EAP scaled scores associated with response patterns in tabulated frequency data. The currently available version of Multilog operates under the MS-DOS operating system, and is limited to 50 items (with conventional memory), or 200 items (with extended memory), with up to nine response alternatives per item.

Goodness of Fit

Little formal work has been done on goodness-of-fit testing for any multiple-category models outside of the so-called Rasch family; so far, the problem appears fairly intractable. For fewer than three items, the multiple-choice model is simply not identified, so goodness of fit is an irrelevant concept. For a sufficiently large examinee sample and three, four, or five items, the m^n cross-classification of the responses produces a contingency table that may have expected values sufficiently large that the conventional Pearson's or likelihood ratio test statistics may be used to test the goodness of fit against the general multinomial alternative; that procedure was illustrated previously (Thissen and Steinberg, 1984; Thissen et al., 1989).

For six or more items, with any conceivable sample size, the m^n table becomes too sparse for the conventional test statistics to be expected to follow their conventionally expected χ^2 distributions, so that this approach does not generalize to long tests. The problem is that no specification of the distribution of responses in such a sparse table under some reasonably general alternative hypothesis has been done in any context. This leaves us with no general goodness-of-fit test for the model.

It is possible to use likelihood ratios to test the significance of the differences between hierarchically constructed parametrizations; indeed, that was done earlier in this chapter, when the equality constraints were imposed on the parametrization for the item shown in Fig. 1, to obtain the constrainted fit shown in Fig. 3. The conventional likelihood ratio test for the difference between the unconstrained model shown in Fig. 2 and the constrained model shown in Fig. 3 was 0.0 (computed to one decimal place) on three degrees of freedom (because the values of three contrast-coefficients, α_1, α_4, and δ_3, were constrained to be zero in the restricted model). Such likelihood ratio tests can be used generally to compare the fit of more versus less constrained models. Their use for examining differential item functioning (DIF) using the multiple choice model was illustrated in a paper by Thissen et al. (1993).

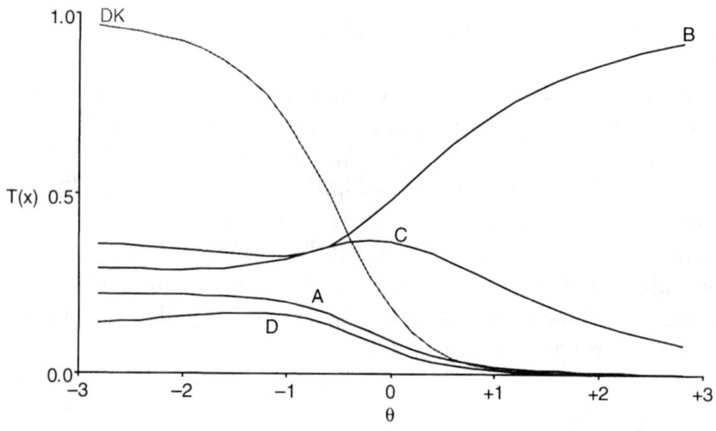

FIGURE 4. Multiple choice model response functions for item 62 (shown in Fig. 1), for fourth grade students.

Thus, as of this writing, the status of goodness-of-fit testing for the multiple-choice model is identical to that for the general linear model: There has been developed no overall goodness of fit against any general alternative; however, assuming that the fully parametrized model fits adequately, there are likelihood ratio tests of the significance of the null hypothesis that any of the component parameters in the model equal zero (or any other appropriate null value). Glas (1988) has developed some refined diagnostic statistics for Rasch family models; but no generalization of those statistics to models with differential slope and/or guessing parameters has yet appeared.

Example

As part of the scale-linking design used in the development of the North Carolina End of Grade Tests, the item tryout form including Item 62 (shown in Fig. 1) was also administered to a sample of about 1000 fourth grade students. The response function obtained in the calibration of that form with the fourth grade sample are shown in Fig. 4. Comparing Fig. 4 with Figs. 2 and 3, it is clear that the main features of the response functions are essentially the same, indicating that the results obtained are not specific to either sample. As expected, the response functions in Fig. 4 are shifted about 0.5 standard unit to the right, relative to Figs. 2 and 3; this is because when they are placed on a common scale, average mathematics ability in the fourth grade is about 0.5 standard unit higher than in the third grade.

Discussion

The principal use of the multiple-choice model is item analysis: Curves such as those shown in Figs. 2–4 provide more information to item analysts than do numerical summaries of item performance. In addition, the model and its associated graphics may provide information that may help item writers modify items that do not perform well, by indicating which of the distractors might be revised. The model also invites the more detailed analysis of DIF, by permitting the analyst to examine differences between alternative selection for different groups of examinees; see Green et al. (1989) for further motivation of this idea.

Given currently available software, the multiple-choice model is fairly difficult to apply routinely in large testing programs. The task of eliminating redundancies in the parametrization is a taxing one; before the model is likely to be widely applied, further research would be useful, to develop a system to reduce the parametrization for each item to a smaller set that is well identified. Nevertheless, interpretable results may be obtained without exhaustive model fitting and constraints. The multiple-choice model provides a complete IRT item analysis for multiple choice tests, with response functions for all of the response alternatives. Graphical presentation of the response functions provides information for thorough item analysis, which has much to recommend it. The item analysis is sufficiently flexible that even poorly designed items can be fitted and specific flaws can be exposed. These can then be observed and such items modified or eliminated in the course of test development.

References

Abrahamowicz, M. and Ramsay, J.O. (1992). Multicategorical spline model for item response theory. *Psychometrika* **57**, 5–27.

Bock, R.D. (1972). Estimating item parameters and latent ability when responses are scored in two or more latent categories. *Psychometrika* **37**, 29–51.

Bock, R.D. (1975). *Multivariate Statistical Methods in Behavioral Research.* New York: McGraw-Hill.

Bock, R.D. and Aitkin, M. (1981). Marginal maximum likelihood estimation of item parameters: An application of the EM algorithm. *Psychometrika* **46**, 443–449.

Bock, R.D. and Lieberman, M. (1970). Fitting a response model for n dichotomously scored items. *Psychometrika* **35**, 179–197.

Bock, R.D. and Mislevy, R.J. (1982). Adaptive EAP estimation of ability in a microcomputer environment. *Applied Psychological Measurement* **6**, 431–444.

Dempster, A.P., Laird, N.M., and Rubin, D.B. (1977). Maximum likelihood from incomplete data via the EM algorithm (with discussion). *Journal of the Royal Statistical Society*, Series B, **39**, 1–38.

Glas, C.A.W. (1988). The derivation of some tests for the Rasch model from the multinomial distribution. *Psychometrika* **53**, 525–546.

Green, B.F., Crone, C.R., and Folk, V.G. (1989). A method for studying differential distractor functioning. *Journal of Educational Measurement* **26**, 147–160.

Lazarsfeld, P.F. (1950). The logical and mathematical foundation of latent structure analysis. In S.A. Stouffer, L. Guttman, E.A. Suchman, P.F. Lazarsfeld, S.A. Star, and J.A. Clausen, *Measurement and Prediction* (pp. 362–412). New York: Wiley.

Levine, M.V. and Drasgow, F. (1983). The relation between incorrect option choice and estimated proficiency. *Educational and Psychological Measurement* **43**, 675–685.

Ramsay, J.O. (1991). Kernel smoothing approaches to nonparametric item characteristic curve estimation. *Psychometrika* **56**, 611–630.

Ramsay, J.O. (1992). *TESTGRAF: A Program for the Graphical Analysis of Multiple Choice Test and Questionnaire Data* (Technical Report). Montreal, Quebec: McGill University.

Samejima, F. (1968). *Application of the Graded Response Model to the Nominal Response and Multiple Choice Situations* (Research Report #63). Chapel Hill, N.C.: University of North Carolina, L.L. Thurstone Psychometric Laboratory.

Samejima, F. (1969). Estimation of latent ability using a response pattern of graded scores. *Psychometric Monograph*, No. 17.

Samejima, F. (1979). *A New Family of Models for the Multiple Choice Item* (Research Report #79-4). Knoxville, TN: University of Tennessee, Department of Psychology.

Steinberg, L. and Thissen, D. (1984, June). *Some Consequences of Non-Monotonic Trace Lines in Item Response Theory.* Paper presented at the meeting of the Psychometric Society, Santa Barbara, CA.

Sympson, J.B. (1983, June). *A New IRT Model for Calibrating Multiple Choice Items.* Paper presented at the meeting of the Psychometric Society, Los Angeles, CA.

Thissen, D. (1976). Information in wrong responses to the Raven Progressive Matrices. *Journal of Educational Measurement* **13**, 201–214.

Thissen, D. (1991). *MULTILOG User's Guide–Version 6.* Chicago, IL: Scientific Software.

Thissen, D. and Steinberg, L. (1984). A response model for multiple choice items. *Psychometrika* **49**, 501–519.

Thissen, D., Steinberg, L., and Fitzpatrick, A.R. (1989). Multiple choice models: The distractors are also part of the item. *Journal of Educational Measurement* **26**, 161–176.

Thissen, D., Steinberg, L., and Wainer, H. (1993). Detection of differential item functioning using the parameters of item response models. In P.W. Holland and H. Wainer (Eds.), *Differential Item Functioning* (pp. 67–113). Hillsdale, NJ: Lawrence Erlbaum Associates.

Wainer, H. (1989). The future of item analysis. *Journal of Educational Measurement* **26**, 191–208.

Wainer, H. and Thissen, D. (1987). Estimating ability with the wrong model. *Journal of Educational Statistics* **12**, 339–368.

4
The Rating Scale Model

Erling B. Andersen

Introduction

The rating scale model is a latent structure model for polytomous responses to a set of test items. The basic structure of the model is an extension of the Rasch model for dichotomous responses, suggested by Georg Rasch, 1961.

It is called a rating scale model because the response categories are scored such that the total score for all items constitute a rating of the respondents on a latent scale. It is assumed that the category scores are equally spaced, giving the highest score to the first or the last category. Thus, the phrasing of the response categories must reflect a scaling of the responses, e.g., "very good," "good," "not so good," "bad."

Presentation of the Model

The rating scale model is a special case of the polytomous model, first presented in Rasch (1961). It was reconstructed as a rating scale model by Andrich (1978a, 1978b). A similar model was presented in Andersen (1977). The main assumption for the rating scale model, apart from being a polytomous Rasch model, is that scoring of the response categories must be equidistant, i.e., their values must increase by a constant. In both Andersen (1977) and Andrich (1978a), convincing arguments were presented for specifying this condition. Andersen (1983) discussed a somewhat more general model, which is still a polytomous Rasch model but with less restrictive scoring of the response categories.

Consider n polytomous test items, $i = 1, \dots, n$. The response U_i on test item i can take the values $h = 1, \dots, m$. The response function for item i, category h is

$$P_{ih} = \text{Prob}(U_i = h).$$

The response pattern for an individual is defined as

$$\mathbf{U} = (U_1, \dots, U_n).$$

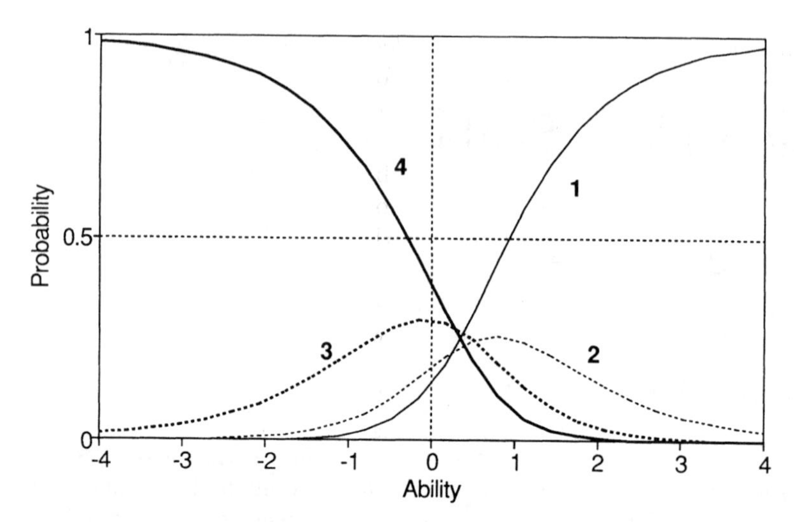

FIGURE 1. Response functions for four categories of an item (with parameter values 1.00, 0.75, 0.25, and 0.00).

It is sometimes convenient to introduce selection vectors

$$U_i^* = (U_{i1}, \ldots, U_{im}),$$

where $U_{ih} = 1$ if response h is chosen on item i, and 0 otherwise.

The response function is assumed to depend for each individual on the value of an ability parameter θ, describing the individual. Accordingly, we shall write

$$P_{ih} = P_{ih}(\theta).$$

Under the rating scale model, the response functions have the form

$$P_{ih}(\theta) = e^{w_i\theta - a_{ih}} \Big/ \sum_{h=1}^{m} e^{w_h\theta - a_{ih}}. \tag{1}$$

In this expression $w_1, \ldots, w_m$ are the category scores, which prescribe how the m response categories are scored, while a_{ih} are item parameters connected with the items and categories. Figure 1 shows the four response functions for a typical item with four possible responses. The category scores are chosen to be 3, 2, 1, and 0, and the item parameters were chosen to be $(a_{i1}, \ldots, a_{i4}) = (1.0, 0.75, 0.25, 0.0)$.

As can be seen in Fig. 1, and verified from the analytical form of the model in Eq. (1), the response function for the category with the highest category score tends to 1 as $\theta \to \infty$, and 0 as $\theta \to -\infty$, while the response function tends to 0 for $\theta \to \infty$ and to 1 for $\theta \to -\infty$, for the category with the lowest category score. It follows that individuals with high abilities will, with very high probability, choose category 1, while individuals with very low abilities most likely will choose category 4. For middle values of the ability, there are moderate probabilities for all four categories to be chosen. The role of the item parameters is to shift the response function to the left for small values of a_{ih} and to the right for larger values of a_{ih}. Thus, the higher the value of a_{ih}, the lower the probability of choosing category h for the category with the largest category score and the higher the probability of choosing category h for the item with the lowest category score. For categories with middle category scores, the probability of choosing category h will increase with a_{ih} for high θ-values and decrease for low θ-values with high probability for large θ-values and with low probability for small θ-values.

The rating scale model is based on the assumption that the category scores $w_1, \ldots, w_h$ are equidistant, i.e., the differences

$$d_h = w_h - w_{h-1}, \qquad h = 2, \ldots, m,$$

are all equal. This assumption was first suggested in Andersen (1977) based on certain properties connected with the sufficient statistic for θ, where θ is regarded as an unknown parameter to be estimated. When Andrich (1978a) introduced the rating scale model, he showed that $w_h = h$ could be interpreted as the number of the categories in which the response occurs, or as thresholds being exceeded [see also Andrich (1982)]. Any linear transformation

$$w'_h = c_0 + c_1 w_h$$

is, of course, equivalent to w_h, since this only entails a redefinition of the scale of the θ-axes.

In order to derive the probability of observing the response $\mathbf{u} = (u_1, \ldots, u_m)$, the assumption of local independence is needed, namely, that given the value of θ, the responses on the n items be independent. Thus, the required probability is

$$f(\mathbf{u} \mid \theta) = \text{Prob}(\mathbf{U} = \mathbf{u} \mid \theta) = \prod_{i=1}^{n} \text{Prob}(U_i = u_i \mid \theta)$$

$$= \prod_{i=1}^{n} \exp\left(\theta \sum_{h=1}^{m} u_{ih} - \sum_{h=1}^{m} a_{ih} u_{ih}\right) \Big/ C_i(\theta, \mathbf{a}), \qquad (2)$$

where

$$C_i(\theta, a) = \prod_{h=1}^{m} \exp(\theta w_h - a_{ih}).$$

The selection vector notation for u_{ih} is used in Eq. (2) to express which w_h and a_{ih} come into play, depends on the category h chosen by the individual. A rating scale model can thus be described as Eq. (1) combined with local independence.

Equation (2) can be rewritten as

$$f(\mathbf{u} \mid \theta) = \exp\left(\theta \sum_{i=1}^{n} \sum_{h=1}^{m} w_h u_{ih} - \sum_{i=1}^{n} \sum_{h=1}^{m} a_{ih} u_{ih}\right) biggl/C(\theta, \mathbf{a}), \quad (3)$$

where

$$C(\theta, \mathbf{a}) = \prod_{i=1}^{n} C_i(\theta, \mathbf{a}).$$

Since, obviously, $C(\theta, \mathbf{a})$ is just a normalization factor, Eq. (3) shows that the score

$$t = \sum_{i=1}^{n} \sum_{h=1}^{m} w_h u_{ih} = \sum_{i=1}^{n} w_{ih}$$

is sufficient for θ, where w_{ih} is the score of the category h, the individual chooses with item i. This result is clear from ordinary exponential family theory (Andersen, 1991, Chap. 3). It can also be seen directly from Eq. (3), which is the likelihood function pertaining to θ and factors into a factor containing only θ and t, a factor not containing θ, and a factor only containing parameters. Note that the total score for a given individual is simply the sum of the category scores of the chosen response categories. The category scores accordingly can also be regarded as a scoring of the n responses into the total score. In Andersen (1977), equidistant scoring was shown to be the only one allowing for a smooth variation over t values when a response was changed by changing just one category on one item.

The model is rather general as regards the item parameters. For inference purposes, there is no real advantage in assuming a more specified structure of the a's, but for many applications it is natural, as well as in accordance with the theory behind the items, to assume a structure. One may assume, for example, as in Andrich (1978a, 1982), that

$$a_{ih} = w_h a_i' - \sum_{\ell=1}^{h} d_\ell,$$

where $d_1, \ldots, d_{m-1}$ are threshold parameters, making the item parameters a_{ih} smaller (or larger for negative d's), depending on the threshold

$$d_h^* = \sum_{\ell=1}^{h} d_\ell.$$

Rasch (1961), in his first formulation of the model for polytomous items, argued that the item parameters a_{ih} should have the same multiplicative form

$$a_{ih} = w_h a_i^*$$

as the term θw_i, and even that the factor corresponding to category h should be the same as the category scores, although he assumed that w_h was a parameter to be estimated.

The description of the model is completed introducing the ability density $\varphi(\theta)$, which describes the variation of θ in the given population. The marginal distribution of any response pattern $\mathbf{u}$ is thus given by

$$f(\mathbf{u}) = \int f(\mathbf{u} \mid \theta)\phi(\theta)d\theta,$$

or, according to Eq. (3),

$$f(\mathbf{u}) = \exp\left(-\sum_i \sum_h a_{ih}u_{ih}\right) \cdot \int \exp\left(\theta \sum_{i=1}^{n} \sum_{h=1}^{m} w_h u_{ih}\right) C^{-1}(\theta, \mathbf{a})\phi(\theta)d\theta. \tag{4}$$

Extensions of the rating scale model can be found in Fischer and Parzer (1991) and in Glas (1989).

Parameter Estimation

The item parameters a_{ih} can be estimated by conditional maximum likelihood (CML) or by marginal maximum likelihood (MML). From Eq. (1) it follows that only $n(m-1)-1$ parameters are unconstrained, since $\sum_h P_{ih}(\theta) = 1$ and one a_{ih} can be changed by changing the θ-scale.

CML Estimation

From Eq. (3), it follows that the marginal distribution of t, i.e., the probability of observing score t, is equal to

$$f(t \mid \theta) = e^{t\theta} C^{-1}(\theta, \mathbf{a}) \sum_{(t)} e^{-a_{ih}u_{ih}}, \tag{5}$$

where the summation (t) is over all response vectors with

$$t = \sum_i \sum_h w_h u_{ih}.$$

The last factor in Eq. (5) is usually denoted $\gamma_t(\mathbf{a})$, so that using

$$\gamma_t(\mathbf{a}) = \sum_{(t)} e^{-a_{ih}u_{ih}},$$

the distribution of t can be given as

$$f(t \mid \theta) = e^{t\theta} C^{-1}(\theta, \mathbf{a}) \gamma_t(\mathbf{a}). \tag{6}$$

Hence the conditional probability of observing response pattern $\mathbf{u}$, given t, is

$$f(\mathbf{u} \mid t) = \exp\left(-\sum_i \sum_h a_{ih} u_{ih}\right) \Big/ \gamma_t(\mathbf{a}).$$

Now consider N individuals, who respond independently on the n items. If $u_{ijh} = 1$ when individual j responds in category h on item i, and 0 otherwise, the joint conditional distribution L_C is

$$L_C = \prod_{j=1}^{N} f(u_j \mid t_j) = \exp\left(-\sum_i \sum_h a_{ih} \sum_{j=1}^{N} u_{ihj}\right) \Big/ \prod_{j=1}^{N} \gamma_{t_j}(\mathbf{a})$$

$$= \exp\left(-\sum_i \sum_h a_{ih} y_{ih}\right) \Big/ \prod_t [\gamma_t(\mathbf{a})]^{N_t}, \tag{7}$$

where N_t is the number of individuals with score t and y_{ih} is the total number of responses h on item i.

Differentiation of the logarithm $\ln L_C$ of Eq. (7) with respect to a_{ih} gives the conditional likelihood equations

$$\partial \ln L_C / \partial a_{ih} = -y_{ih} - \sum_t N_t \partial \ln \gamma_t(\mathbf{a}) / \partial a_{ih}.$$

Hence, the CML estimates are obtained as solutions to

$$y_{ih} = -\sum_t N_t \partial \ln \gamma_t(\mathbf{a}) / \partial a_{ih}. \tag{8}$$

These likelihood equations have a unique set of solutions except for extreme sets of response patterns. Since Eq. (7) is an exponential family, it follows from a result by Barndorff–Nielsen (1978) that there is a unique solution unless the observed set of y's is a point on the convex hull of the set of y's with positive probability given the observed frequencies over score values [see also Andersen (1991), Chap. 3]. Unfortunately, it is not possible to describe the set of extreme response patterns in close form, as is the case for the dichotomous Rasch model [cf. Fischer (1981)].

The conditional likelihood equations are usually solved by a Newton–Raphson procedure, which also provides standard errors for the parameters. The CML method was suggested by Rasch (1961) and developed by Andersen (1972). Many more details are given in Glas (1989). The recursive procedure needed for the calculation of γ-functions is described in Andersen (1972).

MML Estimation

For MML estimation of the a's, the marginal likelihood L is needed. This likelihood is defined as the marginal probability of the responses $\mathbf{u}_j$ for $j = 1, \ldots, N$, i.e., for the N respondents.

From Eq. (4), assuming independence,

$$L = \prod_{j=1}^{N} f(u_j) = \exp\left(-\sum_i \sum_h a_{ih} y_{ih}\right) \cdot \prod_t \left[\int e^{\theta t} C(\theta, \mathbf{a}) \phi(\theta) d\theta\right]^{N_t}, \qquad (9)$$

where again y_{ih}, $i = 1, \ldots, n$, $h = 1, \ldots, m$ are the item totals and N_t is the size of score group t.

In order to maximize Eq. (9), assumptions concerning the form of $\phi(\theta)$ are needed. In the case of two parameters, it may be assumed that $\phi(\theta)$ belongs to a parametric family with parameters b_1, b_2. The log-likelihood function then becomes

$$\ln L = -\sum_i \sum_h a_{ih} y_{ih} + \sum_t N_t \ln \int e^{\theta t} C^{-1}(\theta, a) \phi(\theta \mid b_1, b_2) d\theta. \qquad (10)$$

From this likelihood simultaneous estimates of the a_{ih}'s, b_1 and b_2 can be obtained.

The maximization of Eq. (10) requires numerical integration of functions such as

$$e^{\theta t} - 1C^{-1}(\theta, \mathbf{a}) \partial \phi(\theta \mid b_1, b_2) / \partial b_j.$$

In case of a normal latent density, integration does not seem to be a serious numerical problem. More details can be found in Andersen (1991, Chap. 12) and Mislevy (1984).

If it as tried to maximize Eq. (10) for an unspecified latent density, only a set of discrete values for the ϕ-function can be identified. This important result is contained in Cressie and Holland (1983) and in de Leeuw and Verhelst (1986). In fact, nonparametric estimation of ϕ can be defined using the maximum likelihood estimate

$$\hat{\pi}_t = N_t / N, \qquad (11)$$

for the marginal probability of obtaining score t. The likelihood then becomes

$$\ln L = \ln L_C + \sum_t N_t \ln(N_t / N). \qquad (12)$$

For this nonparametric estimation of ϕ, it was first shown by Tjur (1982), that the results from MML and CML estimation coincides.

Goodness of Fit

Multinomial Tests

The most direct goodness of fit test is based on the multinomial distribution of response patterns, given the model holds true. Given n items with m

response categories for each item, there are n^m possible response patterns ranging from $(1, \ldots, 1)$ to $(m, \ldots, m)$. Let $\mathbf{u}$ be a typical response pattern, then the joint distribution of all response patterns has the same likelihood as the multinomial distribution

$$\{n_{\mathbf{u}}\} \sim \text{Mult}(N, \{\pi_{\mathbf{u}}\}), \tag{13}$$

where $n_{\mathbf{u}}$ is the observed number of individuals with response pattern $\mathbf{u}$, N is the total number of respondents and $\pi_{\mathbf{u}}$ is the probability of observing response pattern $\mathbf{u}$ given by Eq. (3). Many details on this approach can be found in Glas (1988a, 1988b, 1989).

For estimated call probabilities the fit of the multinomial model Eq. (13) is tested by the test quantity

$$Z = 2 \sum_{\mathbf{u}} n_{\mathbf{u}}[\ln n_{\mathbf{u}} - \ln(N\hat{\pi}_{\mathbf{u}})]. \tag{14}$$

Under suitable regularity conditions Z is approximately χ^2-distributed with

$$df = n^m - 1 - q \tag{15}$$

degrees of freedom, where q is the number of estimated parameters in the model. An equivalent test is the Pearson test quantity

$$Q = \sum_{\mathbf{u}} (n_{\mathbf{u}} - N\hat{\pi}_{\mathbf{u}})^2/(N\hat{\pi}_{\mathbf{u}}), \tag{16}$$

which is also approximately χ^2-distributed with a number of degrees of freedom given by Eq. (15). For the rating scale model in Eq. (4) there are $n(m-1) - 1 + s$ parameters to be estimated, where s is the number of parameters in $\phi(\theta)$. Hence, the number of degrees of freedom is

$$df = n^m - n(m-1) - 2 - s.$$

A critical condition for the approximation to the χ^2-distribution is that the expected number $N\pi_{\mathbf{u}}$ for the response patterns are not too close to zero. For many practical applications, it is rather safe to require that $N\pi_{\mathbf{u}} > 3$ for all $\mathbf{u}$. It is clear, on the other hand, that even for moderate values of n, especially if $m > 2$, a requirement like $N\pi_{\mathbf{u}} > 3$ is difficult to meet.

If the number of possible response patterns is very large, for example, $4^{20} = 1.0995 \cdot 10^{12}$, which is the number of possible patterns for $n = 20$ and $m = 4$, it is not likely that any expected number will satisfy the requirement, and we have to look for alternative tests. If the number of response patterns is moderately large, such as 243 (for $n = 5$ and $m = 3$), most response patterns will have low observed counts, but some response patterns may meet the requirement $N\pi_{\mathbf{u}} > 3$. In this case, one possibility is to group the response patterns with low counts into groups with similar response patterns and let grouped observed and expected numbers appear in Eq. (14) or (16) as a single item.

The degrees of freedom for Z and Q will then be equal to

$$df = N_G - 1 - q,$$

where N_G is the total number of terms corresponding to grouped or single response patterns appearing in the test quantities.

For a small set of items, where the number of response patterns is very limited, such as for $n = 5$, $m = 2$, grouping can be avoided, but in most cases a grouping is necessary.

A Likelihood-Ratio Test

If a goodness of fit test cannot be based on the multinomial distribution over response patterns, one may use the statistical test suggested by Andersen (1973).

Let $y_{ih}^{(t)}$ be the item totals for all respondents with score t, i.e., $y_{ih}^{(t)}$ is the number of respondents with score t, who respond h on item i. Then the conditional likelihood, Eq. (7), can be factored as

$$L_C(\mathbf{a}) = \prod_t L_C^{(t)}(\mathbf{a}) = \prod_t \exp\left(-\sum_i \sum_h a_{ih} y_{ih}^{(t)}\right) \Big/ [\gamma_t(\mathbf{a})]^{N_t}. \qquad (17)$$

In this expression, $L_C^{(t)}$ is the likelihood of all responses belonging to individuals with score t.

The CML estimates $\hat{a}_{ih}$ are the values of a_{ih} that maximize L_C given by Eq. (17). These estimates are the overall CML estimates. It is possible, on the other hand, to maximize the individual factors $L_C^{(t)}$ in L_C. This will result in a number of different sets of estimates called score-group CML estimates.

For practical reasons, one would often like to group the scores in interval groups such as $t_{g-1} < t < t_g$, but such a grouping does influence the argument below.

If the model holds true, the score-group estimates should only differ randomly from the overall estimates. If, on the other hand, the model does not hold, the factors L_C in Eq. (17) would depend on the distribution of the abilities in the score groups. In Andersen (1973), it was suggested to use the likelihood ratio test

$$Z_C = -2 \ln L_C(\hat{\mathbf{a}}) + 2 \sum_t \ln L_C^{(t)}(\hat{\mathbf{a}}^{(t)}). \qquad (18)$$

In this test statistic, the maximum of $\ln L_C$, with the overall estimates $\hat{a}_{ih}$ inserted, is compared with $\ln L_C$ with the score group estimates $\hat{a}_{ih}^{(t)}$

inserted. Clearly, Z_C is larger than zero, and the larger the value of Z_C, the less likely it is that the model fits the data. Under suitable regularity conditions

$$Z_c \sim \chi^2(df),$$

where

$$df = [n(m-1)-1](T-1),$$

where T is the number of score groups.

One has to be particularly careful with the approximation to the limiting χ^2-distribution in this case, since many score-group totals $y_{ih}^{(t)}$ are likely to be small. Hence, a grouping of scores into score intervals is necessary except for the case with a very small number of items.

A goodness-of-fit test based on Z_C given by Eq. (18) is less sensitive to model deviations than a test based on the multinomial tests Z or Q. But, as mentioned above, it is often the only practical possibility. It was discussed briefly in Andersen (1973), and further in Glas (1989), the types of model deviations that are likely to be detected by the test statistic Z_C. In Glas (1989), the use of Wald-type tests based on the score-group total $y_{ih}^{(t)}$ is suggested.

The likelihood-ratio test statistic Z_C checks only the part of the rating scale model contained in Eq. (2), since the conditional likelihood is independent of θ and, hence, of the form of the latent density $\phi(\theta)$. However, since the probability $f(\mathbf{u} \mid \theta)$ of response pattern $\mathbf{U}$, given by Eq. (4), can be factored as

$$f(\mathbf{u} \mid \theta) = f(\mathbf{u} \mid t) \cdot f(t \mid \theta),$$

where $f(\mathbf{u} \mid t)$ and $f(t \mid \theta)$ are given by Eq. (6) and the formula before Eq. (7), the total likelihood L factors into the conditional likelihood L_C and a term containing the marginal probabilities $f(t) = \pi_t$ of the scores, where π_t is given by

$$\pi_t = \gamma_t(\mathbf{a}) \int e^{\theta t} C^{-1}(\theta, \mathbf{a}) \phi(\theta) d\theta.$$

Hence, a two-stage procedure can be adopted, where in the first stage the item parameters are estimated based on $\ln L_C$ and the model fit is checked based on Z_C, while in the second stage the form of $\phi(\theta)$ is checked based on the multinomial distribution of the score t over its range. The relevant goodness-of-fit test statistic in stage two would be

$$Z_T = \sum_t N_t[\ln N_t - \ln(N\hat{\pi}_t)], \tag{19}$$

where $\hat{\pi}_t$ is π_t with its parameters estimated. It is safe, although not theoretically optimal in stage two, to use the CML estimates from stage one as estimates for the a_{ih}'s.

Analysis of Residuals

If a goodness of fit test has an observed level of significance so low that the model must be rejected, it is important to be able to identify data points contributing significantly to the lack of fit. Residuals are the appropriate tools for this purpose.

For the multinomial tests Z and Q, given by Eqs. (14) and (16), the residuals are defined as

$$r_u = \frac{(n_{\mathbf{u}} - N\hat{\pi}_{\mathbf{u}})}{\text{s.e.}\{n_{\mathbf{u}} - N\hat{\pi}_{\mathbf{u}}\}}. \tag{20}$$

The standard error, s.e.$\{n_{\mathbf{u}} - N\pi_{\mathbf{u}}\}$, is the square root of

$$\text{var}[n_{\mathbf{u}} - N\hat{\pi}_{\mathbf{u}}].$$

The precise form of this variance was derived by Rao (1973, Sec. 6b.3), and has the form

$$\text{var}[n_{\mathbf{u}} - N\hat{\pi}_{\mathbf{u}}] = N\pi_{\mathbf{u}}(1 - \pi_{\mathbf{u}})(1 - h_{\mathbf{u}}), \tag{21}$$

where $h_{\mathbf{u}}$ is a correction term that depends (on matrix form) on the response probabilities and their derivatives. Note that the variance is smaller than the multinomial variance $N\pi_{\mathbf{u}}(1 - \pi_{\mathbf{u}})$. The correction term $h_{\mathbf{u}}$ can be large, even close to 1, especially if a substantial percentage of the respondents choose response pattern $\mathbf{u}$.

For the test statistic Z_C, there are two possibilities for residuals. The first possibility is to standardize the differences

$$y_{ih}^{(t)} - E\left[Y_{ih}^{(t)}\right], \tag{22}$$

where the mean values are estimated using the overall estimates. Since Eq. (22) set equal to 0, for all i and h, are the likelihood equations for the score-group CML estimates, large values of these residuals would point to model deviations. The variance of the expression in Eq. (22) can, in principle, be derived from the response pattern variances and covariances, but actual computations are time consuming. As a second possibility, the overall CML estimates and the score-group CML estimates can be compared directly in the differences

$$\hat{a}_{ih}^{(t)} - \hat{a}_{ih}$$

for all i, h, and t.

It was proved in Andersen (1995) that approximately

$$\text{var}[\hat{a}_{ih}^{(t)} - \hat{a}_{ih}] = \text{var}[\hat{a}_{ih}^{(t)}] - \text{var}[\hat{a}_{ih}].$$

Thus, it is very easy to obtain the residuals

$$r_{ih}^{(t)} = \frac{(\hat{a}_{ih}^{(t)} - \hat{a}_{ih})}{\text{s.e.}\{\hat{a}_{ih}^{(t)} - \hat{a}_{ih}\}}. \tag{23}$$

Example

In order to illustrate the use of the rating scale model, 14 items from the *Symptoms Check List Discomfort* (SCL) scale were analyzed. These items were analyzed by Bech et al. (1992); see also Bech (1990) and Derogatis et al. (1974). Other applications of the rating scale model can be found, for example, in Fischer and Spada (1973), Andrich (1978b), Glas (1989), and Andersen (1983).

To obtain the scaling, psychiatric patients were presented with a number of items corresponding to problems or complaints people sometimes have. For each item, the patients were asked to describe how much that particular problem had bothered or distressed them during the last week. The response categories were: (1) Extremely; (2) Quite a bit; (3) Moderately; (4) A little bit; and (5) Not at all. For present purposes, Categories 1, 2, and 3 were merged.

The 14 items selected for illustrative purposes were the following:

1. Blaming yourself for things
2. Feeling critical of others
3. Your feelings being easily hurt
4. Feeling hopeless about the future
5. Feeling blue
6. Feeling lonely
7. Thoughts of ending your life
8. Having to do things very slowly
9. Difficulty making decisions
10. Trouble concentrating
11. Your mind going blank
12. Lack of sexual interest
13. Trouble falling asleep
14. Feeling low in energy

If a rating scale model fits the patients' responses to these 14 items, each patient's total score would represent a degree of discomfort, and thus implicitly provide a scaling of the patients.

TABLE 1. Item Totals, y_{ih}, and Score Group Counts N_t.

y_{ih}	$h=1$	2	3	t	N_t	t	N_t
$i=1$	117	155	526	0	151	15	12
2	154	235	409	1	70	16	10
3	142	149	507	2	54	17	10
4	161	226	411	3	48	18	12
5	187	237	374	4	54	19	7
6	72	126	600	5	40	20	12
7	67	101	630	6	32	21	8
8	76	135	587	7	40	22	7
9	147	206	445	8	37	23	4
10	91	177	530	9	40	24	5
11	120	164	514	10	36	25	6
12	173	213	412	11	24	26	5
13	27	53	718	12	19	27	6
14	76	116	606	13	22	28	4
				14	23		

Table 1 shows the item totals and score-group totals for the equidistant scores

$$w_h = m - h, \qquad h = 1, \ldots, m.$$

The minimum and maximum obtainable scores across the 14 items with this scoring of response categories were 0 and 28 (i.e., 14×2).

The minimum score corresponded to no symptoms, while a high score reflected a high degree of discomfort or a high indication of psychiatric problems. The CML estimates are given in Table 2.

The CML estimates show, as do the item totals, that Items 2, 4, 5, 9, and 12 contributed most to a high discomfort score, while Items 6, 7, 8, 13, and 14 were less often used as indicators of discomfort. Thus, in a rating scale model the item parameters reflected how strongly a given item tended to provoke a response contributing to a high score.

For $n = 14$ items with $m = 3$ response categories, there are close to 5 million possible response patterns. For this case, a goodness of fit test based on the multinomial distribution over response patterns was not possible. However, it was possible to use the test statistic Z_C given by Eq. (18) based on score groups. In order to ensure that the required approximations could be expected to hold, the following interval grouping of the score t was selected: 0–7, 8, 9–11, 12–13, 14, and 15–28. Figure 2 shows the score-group CML estimates plotted against the overall estimates. The main structure was satisfactory, but there were obvious deviations from the ideal identity line. The test statistic Z_C had observed value

$$z_c = 174.45, \quad df = 135$$

with a level of significance around 0.1%. There was no sound reason, there-

TABLE 2. CML Estimates With Standared Errors in Parentheses (With Normalizations $\hat{a}_{i3} = 0$).

$\hat{a}_{ih}$:	$h = 1$	2		$h = 1$	2
i=1	−0.032	0.138	$i = 8$	−1.003	−0.291
	(0.133)	(0.101)		(0.155)	(0.104)
2	1.048	1.120	9	0.761	0.806
	(0.125)	(0.097)		(0.125)	(0.097)
3	0.366	0.205	10	−0.432	0.222
	(0.125)	(0.103)		(0.144)	(0.097)
4	1.104	1.079	11	0.070	0.247
	(0.124)	(0.097)		(0.132)	(0.100)
5	1.578	1.351	12	1.211	1.028
	(0.122)	(0.100)		(0.122)	(0.099)
6	−1.153	−0.416	13	−3.371	−1.839
	(0.159)	(0.106)		(0.256)	(0.149)
7	−1.424	−0.756	14	−1.104	−0.514
	(0.165)	(0.114)		(0.156)	(0.109)

TABLE 3. Goodness of Fit Tests for Various Selections of Items.

Number of Items	Items Included	Items Excluded	Goodness of Fit Test	Degrees of Freedom	Level of Significance
14	1–14	None	174.45	135	0.013
11	1–4, 6–12	5, 13, 14	129.13	105	0.055
10	1–4, 6–7, 9–12	5, 8, 13, 14	124.50	114	0.236

fore, to accept the model, and, consequently, a rating scale based on all 14 items.

In order to inspect the lack of fit somewhat closer, the residuals in Eq. (23) were plotted against the item number. An inspection of this plot, Fig. 3, reveals that the significant residuals were concentrated in Items 5, 13, and 14. Hence, a set of items without these three items was expected to fit the model better. When the goodness of fit test was repeated for this set, and the residuals were plotted again, the level of significance for the Z_C test became 0.06, and the residual plot looked satisfactory. If Item 8 was also excluded from the set, the goodness of fit test Z_C had the observed value $z_c = 124.50$, with 114 degrees of freedom. This corresponded to a level of significance around 25%, and was judged to be a very satisfactory fit. It seemed that the rating scale model fitted the data well with 11 of the original 14 items included in the scoring of the responses, and very well with 10 items included. Table 3 provides a summary of the goodness of fit tests.

In order to illustrate the use of a normal latent density, consider the test statistic Z_T given by Eq. (19). In Table 4 the observed score-group counts N_t and their expected values $N_t\hat{\pi}_t$ for a normal latent density are given.

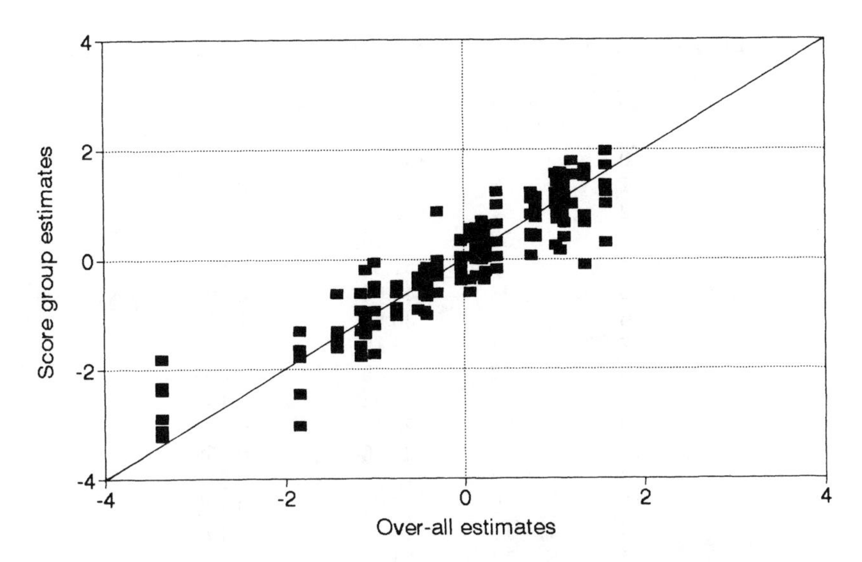

FIGURE 2. Score-group CML estimates plotted against overall CML estimates.

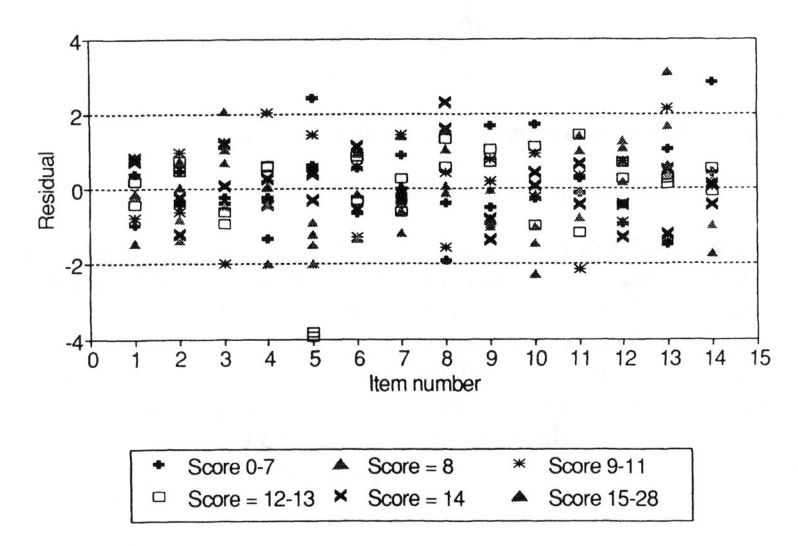

FIGURE 3. Residuals plotted against item number (14 items).

TABLE 4. Observed and Expected Score Group Counts for 10 Items.

Score	Observed Count	Expected Count	Standardized Residuals
$t = 0$	176	149.88	4.744
1	78	111.30	−3.586
2	61	82.22	−2.552
3	57	63.76	−0.912
4	57	51.55	0.808
5	48	43.03	0.800
6	45	36.82	1.414
7	48	32.12	2.920
8	47	28.45	3.605
9	20	25.53	−1.131
10	24	23.15	0.183
11	25	21.16	0.858
12	16	19.49	−0.813
13	19	18.04	0.233
14	16	16.77	−0.194
15	14	15.63	−0.428
16	11	14.58	−0.979
17	5	13.54	−2.455
18	9	12.39	−1.040
19	12	10.80	0.408
20	10	7.78	0.925

The estimated mean and variance were found to be

$$\hat{\mu} = -1.35 \quad \text{and} \quad \hat{\sigma}^2 = 2.96.$$

The observed value of Z_T was $z_t = 54.63$, with 18 degrees of freedom. This result was significant at 0.1%. Hence, a latent structure model seemed to fit the data but a normal latent density did not. The residuals given in Table 4, that is, the differences between observed and expected values divided by their standard errors, show that the lack of fit is primarily due to a clear overrepresentation of score 0 as compared to the model. The model, thus, to a large extent described the shape of the score distribution, but was not able, it seemed, to describe the frequency of the (not very interesting) respondents with score 0.

References

Andersen, E.B. (1972). The numerical solution of a set of conditional estimation equations. *Journal of the Royal Statistical Society, B* **34**, 42–54.

Andersen, E.B. (1973). A goodness of fit test for the Rasch model. *Psychometrika* **38**, 123–140.

Andersen, E.B. (1977). Sufficient statistics and latent trait models. *Psychometrika* **42**, 69–81.

Andersen, E.B. (1983). A general latent structure model for contingency table data. In H. Wainer and S. Messick (Eds.), *Principles of Modern Psychological Measurement* (pp. 117–139). New Jersey: Lawrence Erlbaum Associates.

Andersen, E.B. (1991). *The Statistical Analysis of Categorical Data* (2nd ed.). Heidelberg: Springer-Verlag.

Andersen, E.B. (1995). Residual analysis in the polytomous Rasch model. *Psychometrika* **60**, 375–393.

Andrich, D. (1978a). A rating formulation for ordered response categories. *Psychometrika* **43**, 561–573.

Andrich, D. (1978b). Application of a psychometric rating model to ordered categories which are scored with successive integers. *Applied Psychological Measurement* **2**, 581–594.

Andrich, D. (1982). An extension of the Rasch model to ratings providing both location and dispersion parameters. *Psychometrika* **47**, 105–113.

Barndorff-Nielsen, O. (1978). *Information and Exponential Families in Statistical Theory.* New York: Wiley and Sons.

Bech, P. (1990). Methodological problems in assessing quality of life as outcome in psychopharmacology: A multiaxial approach. In O. Benkert, W. Maier, and K. Rickels (Eds.), *Methodology of the Evaluation of Psychotropic Drugs* (pp. 79–110). Berlin-Heidelberg: Springer-Verlag.

Bech, P., Allerup, P., Maier, W., Albus, M., Lavori, P., and Ayuso, J.L. (1992). The Hamilton scale and the Hopkins Symptom Checklist (SCL-90): A cross-national validity study in patients with panic disorders. *British Journal of Psychiatry* **160**, 206–211.

Cressie, N. and Holland, P.W. (1983). Characterizing the manifest probabilities of latent trait models, *Psychometrika* **48**, 129–141.

de Leeuw, J. and Verhelst, N. (1986). Maximum likelihood estimation in generalized Rasch models. *Journal of Educational Statistics* **11**, 183–196.

Derogatis, L.R., Lipman, R.S., Rickels, K., Uhlenhuth, E.H., and Covi, L. (1974). The Hopkins Symptom Checklist (HSCL). In P. Pichot (Ed.), *Psychological Measurement in Psychopharmacology* (pp. 79–110). Basel: Karger.

Fischer, G.H. (1981). On the existence and uniqueness of maximum likelihood estimates in the Rasch model. *Psychometrika* **46**, 59–77.

Fischer, G.H. and Parzer, P. (1991). An extension of the rating scale model with an application to the measurement of change. *Psychometrika* **56**, 637–651.

Fischer, G.H. and Spada, H. (1973). *Die Psychometrischen Grundlagen des Rorschachtests under der Holtzman Inkblot Technique.* Bern: Huber.

Glas, C.A.W. (1988a). The derivation of some tests for the Rasch model from the multinomial distribution. *Psychometrika* **53**, 525–546.

Glas, C.A.W. (1988b). The Rasch model and multistage testing. *Journal of Educational Statistics* **13**, 45–52.

Glas, C.A.W. (1989). *Contributions to Estimating and Testing Rasch Models.* Doctoral dissertation, University of Twente, Enschede, The Netherlands.

Mislevy, R.J. (1984). Estimating latent distributions. *Psychometrika* **49**, 359–381.

Rao, C.R. (1973). *Linear Statistical Inference and Its Applications*, 2nd Ed. New York: Wiley and Sons.

Rasch, G. (1961). On general laws and the meaning of measurement in psychology, *Proceedings of the Fourth Berkeley Symposium on Mathematical Statistics and Probability* (Vol. 4, pp. 321–333). Berkeley: University of California Press.

Tjur, T. (1982). A connection between Rasch's item analysis model and a multiplicative Poisson model. *Scandinavian Journal of Statistics* **9**, 23–30.

5
Graded Response Model

Fumiko Samejima

Introduction

The graded response model represents a family of mathematical models that deals with ordered polytomous categories. These ordered categories include rating such as letter grading, A, B, C, D, and F, used in the evaluation of students' performance; strongly disagree, disagree, agree, and strongly agree, used in attitude surveys; or partial credit given in accordance with an examinee's degree of attainment in solving a problem.

Presentation of the Model

Let θ be the latent trait, or ability, which represents a hypothetical construct underlying certain human behavior, such as problem-solving ability, and this ability is assumed to take on any real number. Let i denote an item, which is the smallest unit for measuring θ. Let U_i be a random variable to denote the graded item response to item i, and u_i $(= 0, 1, \ldots, m_i)$ denote the actual responses. The category response function, $P_{u_i}(\theta)$, is the probability with which an examinee with ability θ receives a score u_i, that is,

$$P_{u_i}(\theta) \equiv \text{Prob}[U_i = u_i \mid \theta].$$

$P_{u_i}(\theta)$ will be assumed to be five times differentiable with respect to θ. For convenience, u_i will be used both for a specific discrete response and for the event $U_i = u_i$, and a similar usage is applied for other symbols.

For a set of n items, a response pattern, denoted by V, indicates a sequence of U_i for $i = 1, 2, \ldots, n$, and its realization v, can be written as

$$v = \{u_1, u_2, \ldots, u_i, \ldots, u_n\}'.$$

It is assumed that local independence (Lord and Novick, 1968) holds, so that within any group of examinees with the same value of ability θ the distributions of the item responses are independent of each other. Thus, the conditional probability, $P_v(\theta)$, given θ, for the response pattern v can be written as

$$P_v(\theta) \equiv \text{Prob}[V = v \mid \theta] = \prod_{u_i \in v} P_{u_i}(\theta), \tag{1}$$

which is also the likelihood function, $L(v \mid \theta)$, for $V = v$.

Samejima (1969) proposed the first graded response models: the normal-ogive model and the logistic model for graded response data (i.e., ordered polytomous categories). Later she proposed a broader framework for graded response models, distinguishing the *homogeneous* case, to which the normal-ogive and logistic models belong, and the *heterogeneous* case (Samejima, 1972).

General Graded Response Model

Suppose, for example, that a cognitive process, like problem solving, contains a finite number of steps. The graded item score u_i should be assigned to the examinees who successfully complete up to step u_i but fail to complete the step $(u_i + 1)$. Let $M_{u_i}(\theta)$ be the *processing function* (Samejima, 1995) of the graded item score u_i, which is the probability with which the examinee completes the step u_i successfully, under the joint conditions that (a) the examinee's ability level is θ and (b) the steps up to $(u_i - 1)$ have already been completed successfully. Let $(m_i + 1)$ be the next graded item score above m_i. Since everyone can at least obtain the item score 0, and no one is able to obtain the item score $(m_i + 1)$, it is reasonable to set

$$M_{u_i}(\theta) = \begin{cases} 1 & \text{for } u_i = 0 \\ 0 & \text{for } u_i = m_i + 1, \end{cases} \tag{2}$$

for all θ. For each of the other u_i's, it is assumed that $P_{u_i}(\theta)$ is nondecreasing in θ. This assumption is reasonable considering that each item has some direct and positive relation to the ability measured. Thus, the category response function, $P_{u_i}(\theta)$, of the graded item score u_i is given by

$$P_{u_i}(\theta) = \left[\prod_{s \le u_i} M_s(\theta)\right] [1 - M_{(u_i+1)}(\theta)]. \tag{3}$$

This provides the fundamental framework for the general graded response model.

Let $P^*_{u_i}(\theta)$ denote the conditional probability with which the examinee of ability θ completes the cognitive process successfully up to step u_i, or further. Then,

$$P^*_{u_i}(\theta) = \prod_{s \le u_i} M_s(\theta). \tag{4}$$

This function is called the *cumulative category response function* (Samejima, 1995), although cumulation is actually the usual convention. From

Eqs. (3) and (4), the category response function can also be expressed as

$$P_{u_i}(\theta) = P^*_{u_i}(\theta) - P^*_{(u_i+1)}(\theta). \tag{5}$$

Note that $P^*_{u_i}(\theta)$ becomes the response function, $P_i(\theta)$, of the positive response to item i, when the graded item score u_i is changed to the binary score, assigning 0 to all scores less than u_i and 1 to those score categories greater than or equal to u_i. It is obvious from Eqs. (2) and (4) that $P^*_{u_i}(\theta)$ is also nondecreasing in θ, and assumes unity for $u_i = 0$ and zero for $u_i = m_i + 1$ for the entire range of θ.

The general graded response model includes many specific mathematical models. In an effort to select a model interpretable within a particular psychological framework, it will be wise to examine whether the model has certain desirable features. Among others, a model should be examined as to whether (a) the principle behind the model and the set of assumptions agree with the psychological reality in question; (b) it satisfies the unique maximum condition (Samejima, 1969, 1972); (c) it provides the ordered modal points of the category response functions in accordance with the item scores; (d) additivity of the category response functions (Samejima, 1995) holds; and (e) the model can be naturally generalized to a continuous response model.

The unique maximum condition is satisfied if the *basic function*, $A_{u_i}(\theta)$, defined by

$$A_{u_i}(\theta) \equiv \frac{\partial}{\partial\theta} \log P_{u_i}(\theta) = \sum_{s \le u_i} \frac{\partial}{\partial\theta} \log M_s(\theta) + \frac{\partial}{\partial\theta} \log[1 - M_{(u_i+1)}(\theta)], \tag{6}$$

is strictly decreasing in θ and its upper asymptote is nonnegative and its lower asymptote is nonpositive (Samejima, 1969, 1972). Satisfaction of this condition ensures that the likelihood function of *any* response pattern consisting of such response categories has a unique local or terminal maximum. Using this basic function, a sufficient, though not necessary, condition for the strict orderliness of the modal points of the category response functions is that $A_{(u_i-1)}(\theta) < A_{u_i}(\theta)$ for all θ for $u_i = 1, 2, \ldots, m_i$.

Additivity of a model will hold if the category response functions still belong to the same mathematical model under finer recategorizations and combinations of two or more categories together, implying that the unique maximum condition will be satisfied by the resulting category response functions if it is satisfied by those of the original u_i's. Graded item scores, or partial credits, are more or less incidental. For example, sometimes letter grades, A, B, C, D, and F, are combined to pass–fail grades. Also, with the advancement of computer technologies, more abundant information can be obtained from an examinee's performance in computerized experiments, and thus finer recategorizations of the whole cognitive process are possible. Additivity of response categories and generalizability to a continuous model are, therefore, important criteria in evaluating models.

Homogeneous Case

The homogeneous case of the graded response model represents a family of models in which $P^*_{u_i}(\theta)$'s for $u_i = 1, 2, \ldots, m_i$ are identical in shape, and these m_i functions are positioned alongside the ability continuum in accordance with the item score u_i. Thus, it is obvious that additivity of the category response functions always holds for mathematical models that belong to the homogeneous case.

The *asymptotic basic function* $\tilde{A}_{u_i}(\theta)$ has been defined in the homogeneous case for $u_i = 1, 2, \ldots, m_i$ by

$$\tilde{A}_{u_i}(\theta) \equiv \lim_{\lambda_{(u_i+1)} \to \lambda_{u_i}} A_{u_i}(\theta) = \frac{\partial}{\partial\theta} \log\left[\frac{\partial}{\partial\theta} P^*_{u_i}(\theta)\right] - \frac{\frac{\partial^2}{\partial\theta^2} M_1(\theta - \lambda_{u_i})}{\frac{\partial}{\partial\theta} M_1(\theta - \lambda_{u_i})}, \quad (7)$$

with λ_{u_i} being zero for $u_i = 1$ and increases with u_i, which is identical in shape for all $u_i = 1, 2, \ldots, m_i$ except for the positions alongside the dimension θ (Samejima, 1969, 1972). Using this asymptotic basic function, Samejima (1972, 1995) demonstrated that, in the homogeneous case, the unique maximum condition is simplified: (a) the lower and upper asymptotes of $M_{u_i}(\theta)$ for $u_i = 1$ are zero and unity, respectively, (b) $\frac{\partial}{\partial\theta}\tilde{A}_{u_i}(\theta) < 0$ for the entire range of θ for an arbitrarily selected u_i, and (c) for this specific u_i, the upper and lower asymptotes of $\tilde{A}_{u_i}(\theta)$ have some positive and negative values, respectively.

When the unique maximum condition is satisfied, the mathematical model can be represented by

$$P^*_{u_i}(\theta) = \int_{-\infty}^{a_i(\theta - b_{u_i})} \psi(t)\, dt, \quad (8)$$

where the item discrimination parameter a_i is finite and positive, and the difficulty or location parameters, b_{u_i}'s, satisfy

$$-\infty = b_0 < b_1 < b_2 < \ldots < b_{m_i} < b_{m_i+1} = \infty,$$

and $\psi(\cdot)$ denotes a density function that is four times differentiable with respect to θ, and is unimodal with zero as its two asymptotes as θ tends to negative and positive infinities, and with a first derivative that does not assume zero except at the modal point.

In the homogeneous case, satisfaction of the unique maximum condition also implies:

1. A strict orderliness among the modal points of $P_{u_i}(\theta)$'s, for it can be shown that

$$A_{(u_i-1)}(\theta) < \tilde{A}_{u_i}(\theta) < A_{u_i}(\theta)$$

for $u_i = 1, 2, 3, \ldots, m_i$, throughout the whole range of θ (Samejima, 1972, 1995).

2. Additivity of the category response functions, for, even if two or more adjacent graded item scores are combined, or if a response category is more finely recategorized, the $\tilde{A}_{u_i}(\theta)$'s for the remaining u_i's will be unchanged, and those of the newly created response categories will have the same mathematical form as that of the $\tilde{A}_{u_i}(\theta)$'s for the original response categories.

3. A natural expansion of the model to a continuous response model by replacing u_i in Eq. (8) by z_i, which denotes a continuous item response to item i and assumes any real number between 0 and 1, and by defining the *operating density characteristic*

$$H_{z_i}(\theta) = \lim_{\Delta z_i \to 0} \frac{P^*_{z_i}(\theta) - P^*_{(z_i+\Delta z_i)}(\theta)}{\Delta z_i} = a_i \psi(a_i(\theta - b_{z_i})) \left[\frac{db_{z_i}}{dz_i}\right],$$

where b_{z_i} is the difficulty parameter for the continuous response z_i and is a strictly increasing function of z_i (Samejima, 1973). The basic function, $A_{z_i}(\theta)$, in the continuous response model is identical with the asymptotic base function $\tilde{A}_{u_i}(\theta)$ defined by Eq. (7) on the graded response level, with the replacement of u_i by z_i, and thus for these models the unique maximum condition is also satisfied on the continuous response level.

It is wise, therefore, to select a specific model from those which satisfy the unique maximum condition, if the fundamental assumptions in the model agree with the psychological reality reflected in the data.

Samejima (1969, 1972) demonstrated that both the normal-ogive model and the logistic model belong to this class of models. In these models, the category response function is given by

$$P_{u_i}(\theta) = \frac{1}{[2\pi]^{1/2}} \int_{a_i(\theta - b_{u_i+1})}^{a_i(\theta - b_{u_i})} \exp\left[\frac{-t^2}{2}\right] dt, \tag{9}$$

and

$$P_{u_i}(\theta) = \frac{\exp[-Da_i(\theta - b_{u_i+1})] - \exp[-Da_i(\theta - b_{u_i})]}{[1 + \exp[-Da_i(\theta - b_{u_i})]][1 + \exp[-Da_i(\theta - b_{u_i+1})]]}, \tag{10}$$

respectively. In both models, $M_{u_i}(\theta)$ is a strictly increasing function of θ with unity as its upper asymptote; the lower asymptote is zero in the former model, and $\exp[-Da_i(b_{u_i} - b_{u_i} - 1)]$ in the latter (see Fig. 5-2-1 in Samejima, 1972). The upper asymptote of the basic function $A_{u_i}(\theta)$ for $u_i = 1, 2, \ldots, m_i$ and the lower asymptote for $u_i = 0, 1, \ldots, m_i - 1$, are positive and negative infinities in the normal-ogive model, and Da_i and $-Da_i$ in the logistic model (Samejima, 1969, 1972).

Figure 1 illustrates the category response functions in the normal-ogive model for $m_i = 4$, $a_i = 1.0$ and b_{u_i}'s equal to: -2.0, -1.0, 0.7, 2.0 for $u_i = 1$

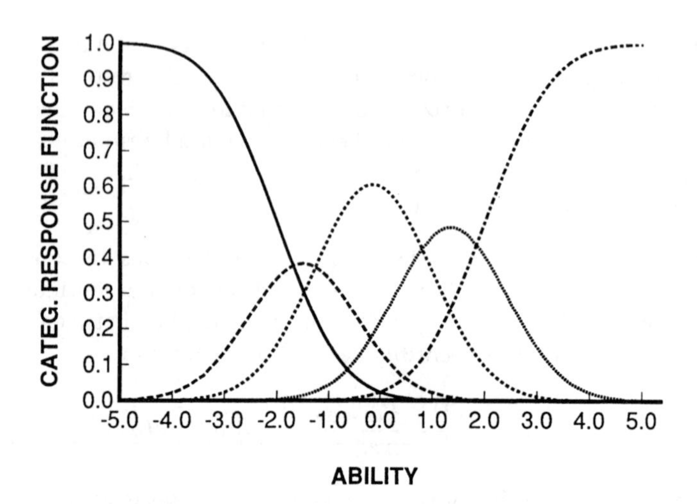

FIGURE 1. Example of a set of category response functions in the normal-ogive model for the item scores, 0, 1, 2, 3, and 4.

2, 3, 4, respectively. The corresponding category response functions in the logistic model with $D = 1.7$ are very similar to those in the normal-ogive model with the identical set of modal points; those curves are a little more peaked, however.

In the normal-ogive model for continuous response data, there exists a simple sufficient statistic, $t(v)$, for a specific response pattern v, and is provided by

$$t(v) = \sum_{z_i \in v} a_i^2 b_{z_i}, \tag{11}$$

so that the maximum likelihood estimate $\hat{\theta}$ is obtained directly from this simple sufficient statistic (Samejima, 1973). This fact suggests that, when m_i is substantially large, the normal-ogive model for continuous response data can be used as an approximation to the model for graded response data. In so doing, the value of m_i should be perhaps nine or greater.

Heterogeneous Case

The heterogeneous case of the graded response model represents all mathematical models that provide a set of cumulative category response functions $P^*_{u_i}(\theta)$'s *not all* of which are identical in shape, that is, those which do not belong to the homogeneous case. One example is Bock's nominal response model (Bock, 1972), represented by

$$P_{h_i}(\theta) = \frac{\exp[\alpha_{h_i}\theta + \beta_{h_i}]}{\sum_{s \in H_i} \exp[\alpha_s \theta + \beta_s]}, \tag{12}$$

where h_i denotes a nominal response to item i and H_i is the set of all h_i's, and α_{h_i} (> 0) and β_{h_i} are item category parameters. Samejima (1972) demonstrated that Bock's nominal response model can be considered as a graded response model in the heterogeneous case, if the nominal response h_i in Eq. (12) is replaced by the graded item response u_i and the parameter α_{u_i} satisfies

$$\alpha_0 \leq \alpha_1 \leq \alpha_2 \leq \ldots \leq \alpha_{m_i}, \tag{13}$$

where a strict inequality should hold for at least one pair of α values. Two examples are Masters' (1982; this volume) Partial Credit Model (PCM) and Muraki's (1992; this volume) Generalized Partial Credit Model (GPCM). This family of models satisfies the unique maximum condition, and the perfect orderliness of the modal points of the category response functions is realized with strict inequality held between every pair of α_{u_i}'s in Eq. (13). However, it does not have additivity or generalizability to a continuous response model, and thus applicabilities are limited because of the assumption used in Bock's model (Samejima, 1995).

Samejima (1995) proposed the *acceleration model* that belongs to the heterogeneous case of the graded response model. Consider a situation, such as problem solving, that requires a number of subprocesses be completed correctly before attaining the solution. It is assumed that there is more than one step in the process and the steps are observable. Graded item scores, or partial credits, 1 through m_i, are assigned for the successful completion of these separate observable steps. The processing function for each u_i ($= 1, 2, \ldots, m_i$) is given by

$$M_{u_i}(\theta) = [\Psi_{u_i}(\theta)]^{\xi_{u_i}}, \tag{14}$$

where ξ_{u_i} (> 0) is called the *step acceleration parameter*. The acceleration model is a family of models in which $\Psi_{u_i}(\theta)$ is specified by a strictly increasing, five times differentiable function of θ with zero and unity as its two asymptotes. Here a specific model in this family will be introduced, in which $\Psi_{u_i}(\theta)$ is given by

$$\Psi_{u_i}(\theta) = \frac{1}{1 + \exp[-D\alpha_{u_i}(\theta - \beta_{u_i})]}, \tag{15}$$

where $D = 1.7$ and α_{u_i} (> 0) and β_{u_i} are the discrimination and location parameters, respectively. It is assumed that the process leading to a problem solution consists of a finite number of *clusters*, each containing one or more steps, and within each cluster the parameters α and β in the logistic distribution function are common. Thus, if two or more adjacent u_i's belong to the same cluster, then the parameters α_{u_i}'s and β_{u_i}'s are the same for these u_i's, and, otherwise, at least one parameter is different.

It can be seen from Eqs. (14) and (15) that the roles of the step acceleration parameter, ξ_{u_i}, are to control (a) the general shape of the curve representing $M_{u_i}(\theta)$, (b) the steepness of the curve, and (c) the position

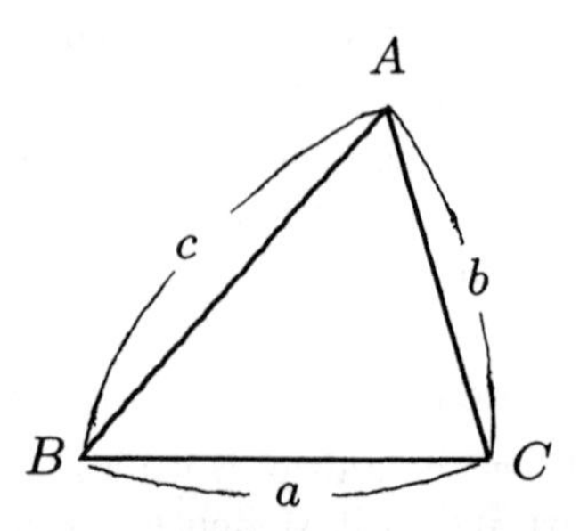

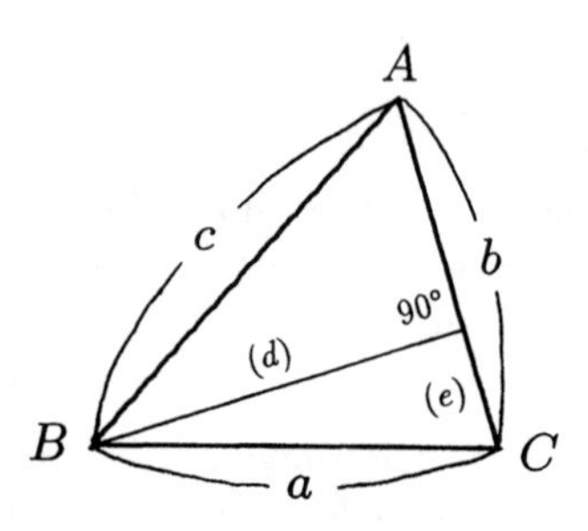

FIGURE 2. Triangle provided for the proof of the law of cosine (left), and the one after the perpendicular line has been drawn by the examinee (right).

of the curve alongside the ability continuum. When $\Psi_{u_i}(\theta)$ is given by Eq. (15), $M_{u_i}(\theta)$ is point-symmetric only when $\xi_{u_i} = 1$, and point-asymmetric otherwise. Let θ_{stp} denote the point of θ at which $M_{u_i}(\theta)$ is steepest. This is provided by

$$\theta_{\text{stp}} = \Psi_{u_i}^{-1}\left[\frac{\xi_{u_1}}{1+\xi_{u_i}}\right],$$

which increases with ξ_{u_i}. This maximum slope at $\theta = \theta_{\text{stp}}$ equals $Da_i[\xi_{u_i}/(1+\xi_{u_1})]^{\xi_{u_i}+1}$, which is also an increasing function of ξ_{u_i}. The value of $M_{u_i}(\theta)$ at $\theta = \theta_{\text{stp}}$ is $[\xi_{u_i}/(1+\xi_{u_i})]^{\xi_{u_i}}$, which decreases with ξ_{u_i}. The general position of the curve representing $M_{u_i}(\theta)$ is shifted to the positive side alongside the continuum as ξ_{u_i} increases, and in the limiting situation when ξ_{u_i} tends to positive infinity $M_{u_i}(\theta)$ approaches 0 for all θ, whereas in the other limiting situation where ξ_{u_i} tends to zero $M_{u_i}(\theta)$ approaches 1 for all θ.

Let w denote a subprocess, which is the smallest unit in the cognitive process. Thus, each step contains one or more w's. Let ξ_w (> 0) represent the *subprocess acceleration* parameter, and then the step acceleration parameter, ξ_{u_i}, for each of $u_i = 1, 2, \ldots, m_i$ is given as the sum of ξ_w's over all $w \in u_i$. The name, *acceleration parameter*, derives from the fact that, within each step, separate subprocesses contribute to accelerate the value of θ at which the discrimination power is maximal (Samejima, 1995).

Consider the following problem-solving example:

Using the triangle shown on the left-hand side of Fig. 2, prove that

$$a^2 = b^2 + c^2 - 2bc\cos A.$$

Five observable steps in solving this particular problem may be as shown below:

$a^2 = d^2 + e^2$ Step 1 [Pythagoras' theorem]

$a^2 = (c\sin A)^2 + (b - c\cos A)^2$ Step 2 [sine and cosine]

$$a^2 = c^2 \sin^2 A + b^2 - 2bc \cos A + c^2 \cos^2 A \quad \text{Step 3 } [(a-b)^2 = a^2 - 2ab_b^2]$$

$$a^2 = b^2 + c^2(\sin^2 A + \cos^2 A) - 2bc \cos A \quad \text{Step 4 } [ab + ac = a(b+c)]$$

$$a^2 = b^2 + c^2 - 2bc \cos A \quad \text{Step 5 } [\sin^2 A + \cos^2 A = 1],$$

where d and e are as shown in the right-hand side diagram of Fig. 2.

Each of the steps contain more than one substep or subprocess except for Step 5. For example, Step 1 includes three subprocesses, that is, (a) thinking of the use of the Pythagoras' theorem, (b) drawing the perpendicular line from B to b (or, alternatively, from C to c), and naming the perpendicular line d and the lower line sigment of be, and (c) applying the Pythagoras' theorem to the right triangle that includes C; Step 2 includes two subprocesses: the evaluation of d as $(c \sin A)$ and that of e as $(b - c \cos A)$.

It should be noted that in Eq. (15) the location parameter, β_{u_i}, does not necessarily increase with u_i. To illustrate an extreme case, assume that in the above problem-solving example Step 1 is the most critical step, and that for examinees who have completed the subprocesses of considering and using the Pythagoras' theorem, all other steps will be completed mechanically. In such a case, location parameter, β_{u_i}, for each of $u_i = 2$, 3, 4, 5 is likely to be substantially lower than β_i. As a result, with reasonably small values of ξ_{u_i} for $u_i = 2$, 3, 4, 5, the item will become practically a dichotomous item, with $P_{u_i}(\theta)$ for each of $u_i = 1$, 2, 3, 4, taking on very small values for all θ, and $P_5(\theta)$ will be close to $M_1(\theta)$. On the other hand, if the steps leading to a solution become progessively more difficult, then it is likely that β_{u_i} increases with u_i.

Note that in Step 2 the sequential order between the two subprocesses is arbitrary. Successful completion of the step does not depend on the order in which the subprocesses are completed. If there are two or more subprocesses within a step whose sequential order is arbitrary, then these subprocesses are said to be *parallel*, as distinct from *serial* subprocesses. It is assumed that for any number of parallel subprocesses the subprocesses acceleration parameters are invariant to shifts of the positions of the subprocesses in the sequence. Thus, the step acceleration parameter, ξ_{u_i} $(= \xi_{w_{u_1 1}} + \xi_{w_{u_i 2}} + \cdots)$, will be unchanged regardless of the sequential order of these parallel subprocesses.

Note that any grading system is arbitrary. If our experimental setting is improved and allows observation of the examinee's performance in more finely graded steps, then m_i will become larger. It is obvious from Eq. (14) and the definition of ξ_{u_i} that the resulting category response functions still belong to the acceleration model which partially satisfies the additivity criterion. It is also obvious that the model can be generalized to a continuous response model as the limiting situation in which the number of steps approaches infinity.

From Eqs. (4) and (14), the cumulative category response function,

$P^*_{u_i}(\theta)$, is given by

$$P^*_{u_i}(\theta) = \prod_{s=0}^{u_i} [\Psi_s(\theta)]^{\xi_s},$$

and from Eqs. (3) and (14), the category response function is obtained such that

$$P_{u_i}(\theta) = \prod_{s=0}^{u_i} [\Psi_s(\theta)]^{\xi_s} \left[1 - [\Psi_{(u_i+1)}(\theta)]^{\xi_{u_i+1}}\right]. \tag{16}$$

The basic function, $A_{u_i}(\theta)$, in this model is obtained from Eqs. (6), (14), and (15), so that

$$A_{u_i}(\theta) = D\left[\sum_{s \leq u_i} \xi_s \alpha_s [1 - \Psi_s(\theta)] - \xi_{u_i+1}\alpha_{u_i+1} \frac{[\Psi_{(u_i+1)}(\theta)]^{\xi_{u_i+1}}[1 - \Psi_{(u_i+1)}(\theta)]}{1 - [\Psi_{(u_i+1)}(\theta)]^{\xi_{u_i+1}}}\right], \tag{17}$$

for $u_i = 1, 2, \ldots, m_i - 1$, and for $u_i = 0$ and $u_i = m_i$ the first term and the second term on the right-hand side of Eq. (17) disappear, respectively. The upper and lower asymptotes of this basic function are $D\sum_{s \leq u_i} \xi_s \alpha_s$ (> 0) for $u_i = 1, 2, \ldots, m_i$, and $-D\alpha_{u_i+1}$ (< 0) for $u_i = 0, 1, \ldots, m_i - 1$, respectively, and the upper asymptote for $u_i = 0$ and the lower asymptote for $u_i = m_i$ are both zero. It has been demonstrated (Samejima, 1995) that $A_{u_i}(\theta)$ in Eq. (17) is strictly decreasing in θ. Thus, the unique maximum condition is satisfied for $u_i = 0, 1, \ldots, m_i$. It has also been shown (Samejima, 1995) that the orderliness of the modal points of the category response functions usually holds, except for cases in which the unidimensionality assumption is questionable, and additivity of the category response functions practically holds. Figure 3 illustrates the six category response functions by a solid line, with $m_i = 5$ and the parameters:

$$\begin{aligned}
\alpha_{u_i} &= 1.35119,\ 1.02114,\ 0.85494,\ 1.08080,\ 0.58824; \\
\beta_{u_i} &= -0.95996,\ -0.79397,\ -0.01243,\ 1.33119,\ 0.8000; \text{ and} \\
\xi_{u_i} &= 0.43203,\ 0.53337,\ 0.57260,\ 0.61858,\ 1.00000, \text{ for } u_i = 1, 2, 3, 4, 5.
\end{aligned}$$

The dashed lines in this figure represent those following Master's PCM or Muraki's GPCM with unity for the item parameters, using $\alpha_{u_i} = 1$, 2, 3, 4, 5, 6 and $\beta_{u_i} = 1.0$, 2.0, 3.0, 3.5, 1.8, 1.0 in Eq. (12) with h_i replaced by u_i for $u_i = 0$, 1, 2, 3, 4, 5, respectively.

Parameter Estimation

In estimating the item parameters of the normal-ogive model in the homogeneous case, if our data are collected for a random sample from an unscreened population of examinees, assuming a normal ability distribution,

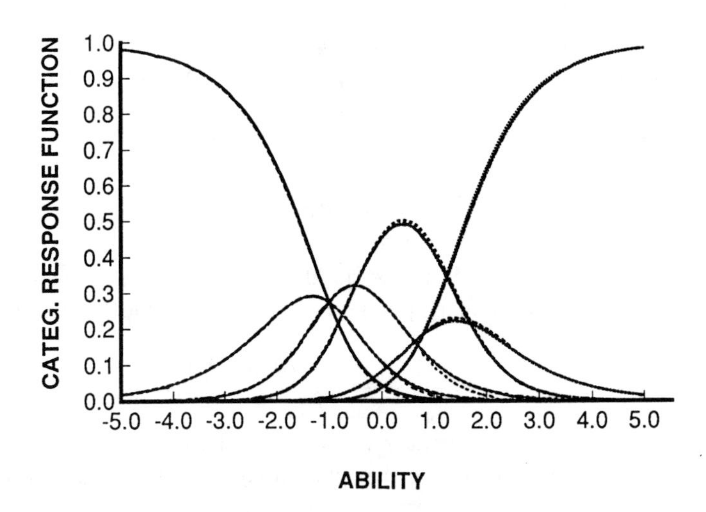

FIGURE 3. Example of a set of six category response functions following the acceleration model, which approximate those following the PCM (dotted line).

we can (a) compute the polychoric correlation coefficient for each pair of items, (b) factor analyze the resulting correlation matrix and confirm the unidimensionality, and (c) estimate a_i and b_{u_i} for $u_i = 1, 2, \ldots, m_i$, using the same method adopted by Lord (1952) and Samejima (1995). In the logistic model, item parameter estimation can be done by using the EM algorithm. Thissen wrote Multilog for this purpose, as well as for Bock's nominal response model, among others, with facilities for fixing parameter values at priors and imposing equality constraints (Thissen, 1991; Thissen and Steinberg, this volume).

Multilog is based on the EM solution of the marginal likelihood equations. Bock and Aitkin (1981) proposed a solution for dichotomous responses, and Multilog uses a direct expansion to handle graded responses in the homogeneous case. Unlike the joint likelihood solution, the marginal likelihood solution treats the parameter θ_j of the examinee j as incidental, and integrates it out from the likelihood function. Thus, the marginal likelihood function, $L(a_i, b_{u_i})$, can be written as

$$L(a_i, b_{u_i}) = \prod_{j=1}^{N} \int_{-\infty}^{\infty} g(\theta_j) P_{v_j}(\theta_j) d\theta_j = \prod_{j=1}^{N} P_{v_j} = \prod_{V} P_v^{r_v}, \tag{18}$$

where N is the number of examinees in the sample, $g(\theta_j)$ is the ability density function, v_j is the response pattern obtained by an examinee j, $P_{v_j}(\theta)$ given by Eq. (1) for an examinee i equals the joint likelihood function, $L(\theta_j, a_i, b_{u_i})$, P_{v_i} is the marginal probability for the response pattern v_j of an examinee j, r_v is the frequency of a specific response pattern v, and $\prod_v$ indicates the product over all possible response patterns. Actually, the continuous ability θ is replaced by q discrete latent classes, each characterized by θ_k ($k = 1, 2, \ldots, q$), and homogeneity is assumed within each class.

Let $\tilde{P}_v$ be an approximation for P_v, which is given by

$$\tilde{P}_v = \sum_{k=1}^{q} P_v(\theta_k)G(\theta_k), \tag{19}$$

where $G(\theta_k)$ is the Gauss–Hermite quadrature weight. The expected frequency, $\bar{r}_{u_i k}$, of the graded response u_i to item i in the latent class k is provided by

$$\bar{r}_{u_i k} = \frac{\sum_v r_v x_{v u_i} P_v(\theta_k)G(\theta_k)}{\tilde{P}_v}, \tag{20}$$

where x_{vu_i} ($=$ 0,1) is the indicator variable that assumes 1 if $u_i \in v$, and 0, otherwise. The expected sample size, $\bar{N}_k$, of the latent class k is given by

$$\bar{N}_k = \frac{\sum_v r_v P_v(\theta_k)G(\theta_k)}{\tilde{P}_v}. \tag{21}$$

Thus, in the E-step of the EM algorithm, $P_v(\theta_k)$ is computed for provisional a_i and b_{u_i}'s, and then $\tilde{P}_v$, $\bar{r}_{u_i k}$, and $\bar{N}_k$ are obtained, using Eqs. (19), (20), and (21), respectively. In the M-step, improved estimates of a_i and b_{u_i}'s are obtained by maximizing the approximated likelihood function, which is given by the last expression of Eq. (18), with P_v replaced by $\tilde{P}_v$. The cycles are continued until the estimates become stable to the required number of places. Muraki and Bock (1993) wrote Parscale, which includes the logistic model for graded response data, based on essentially the same EM algorithm.

Since the acceleration model was recently proposed, there is little software available. Parameter estimation can be done, however, using the following method when Eq. (15) is adopted for $\Psi_{u_i}(\theta)$. Suppose we have used a nonparametric estimation method like Levine's (1984) or Samejima's (1983, 1993, 1996), and estimated category response functions, $P_{u_i}(\theta)$'s, and they have tentatively been parametrized using a very general semiparametric method [see, for example, Ramsay and Wang, (1993)]. From these results, $\hat{M}_{u_i}(\theta)$ and its partial derivative with respect to θ can be obtained by means of Eqs. (4) and (5). Then select three arbitrary probabilities, p_1, p_2, and p_3, which are in an ascending order, and determine θ_1, θ_2, and θ_3 at which $\hat{M}_{u_i}(\theta)$ equals p_1, p_2, and p_3, respectively. From Eqs. (14) and (15), the estimated acceleration parameter $\hat{\xi}_{u_i}$ is obtained as the solution of

$$\frac{\theta_3 - \theta_2}{\theta_2 - \theta_1} = \frac{\log[(p_2)^{-1/\xi_{u_i}} - 1] - \log[(p_3)^{-1/\xi_{u_i}} - 1]}{\log[(p_1)^{-1/\xi_{u_i}} - 1] - \log[(p_2)^{-1/\xi_{u_i}} - 1]}. \tag{22}$$

The estimate, $\hat{\beta}_{u_i}$, is given as the solution of

$$\hat{M}_{u_i}(\beta_{u_i}) = \left[\frac{1}{2}\right]^{\xi_{u_i}}, \tag{23}$$

and from these results the estimate of α_{u_i} is obtained by

$$\hat{\alpha}_{u_i} = \frac{2^{\hat{\xi}_{u_i}+1}}{D\hat{\xi}_{u_i}} \frac{\partial}{\partial\theta}\hat{M}_{u_i}(\theta) \quad \text{at } \theta = \hat{\beta}_{u_i}. \tag{24}$$

Note that this method can be applied for any curve as long as $\frac{\partial}{\partial\theta}\hat{M}_{u_i}(\theta)$ (> 0) is available at $\theta = \hat{\beta}_{u_i}$. Actually, the parameters in the acceleration model used in Fig. 3 were obtained by this method from the $\hat{M}_{u_i}(\theta)$'s in Masters' or Muraki's model as the solutions of Eqs. (22)–(24), setting $p_1 = 0.25$, $p_2 = 0.50$, and $p_3 = 0.75$ in Eq. (22).

Goodness of Fit

For small numbers of items, the observed frequencies for each response pattern may be tabulated; Multilog (Thissen, 1991) computes the expected frequencies for each response pattern and then the likelihood-ratio statistic as a measure of the goodness of fit of the model. Parscale (Muraki and Bock, 1993) adopts the likelihood-ratio chi-square statistic as a measure of fit for each item, and the sum of these chi-square statistics provides the likelihood-ratio chi-square statistic for the whole test. When the polychoric correlation matrix is used for parameter estimation in the normal-ogive model, goodness of fit can be examined by the chi-square statistic using bivariate normal frequency for each of the $(m_i + 1)(m_h + 1)$ cells for a pair of items, i and h, as the theoretical frequency; when most of the $n(n-1)/2$ chi-square values are large, then we must conclude that one or more assumptions are violated; when large chi-square values are clustered around a relatively small number of items, exclusion of these items will usually improve the fit, although the psychological meaningfulness of the remaining items must be checked to be such that the construct has not been distorted or changed (Samejima, 1994). Note that goodness of fit of the curves should not be used as the *sole* criterion in accepting or rejecting a specified model; there are many models that are based on quite different principles and yet produce similar sets of curves.

Example

An interesting application of a graded response model was reported in the medical literature. Roche et al. (1975) applied the logistic model in the homogeneous case, represented by Eq. (10), for skeletal maturity. Children of the same chronological age and sex differ in maturity levels of body systems, and thus the skeletal age must be estimated using a skeletal maturity scale. The items were thirty-four carefully selected radiographically visible maturity indicators of the left knee joint, and the radiographs for

552 normal children were evaluated by experts in terms of their maturities with respect to each maturity indicator into two to five graded categories ($1 \leq m_i \leq 4$). An example of the items can be seen in item FEM-K, lateral capping, graded into three categories, that is, absent, incomplete, and complete. Capping refers to the way in which the epiphysis overlaps the metaphysis as maturation proceeds (Roche et al. 1975). This item is suitable for 7.5 to 16 year-old girls and 8 to 17 year-old boys.

The male and female data were analyzed separately, using Logog (Kolakowski and Bock, 1973), and 3,997 and 3,800 radiographs were involved for the two groups, respectively. For each group, the origin and unit of the skeletal maturity scale were set so that its mean and variance equal the mean and variance of the chronological age in the calibration sample, respectively. The resulting 34 discrimination parameters, a_i's, for the most part, ranged from 0.5381 to 3.8376 for males and from 0.4269 to 6.1887 for females, with two common outliers, item FEM-D (epiphyseal shape) and item TIB-C (metaphyseal shape), for both groups, of which a_i's are 8.1123 and 5.7874 for males and 8.8509 and 7.9769 for females. Overall configurations of a_i's were very similar between the two groups, and the same was also true with the configurations of the difficulty, or threshold, parameters. To give a couple of examples, out of the six items with $m_i = 4$, the item with the lowest b_1 was item FEM-A ([epiphyseal width]/[metaphyseal width]) for both groups, with 0.4927, 1.3556, 2.3016, and 3.2535 for b_{u_i} ($u_i = 1$, 2, 3, 4) for males and 0.4262, 0.9984, 1.7310, 2.2797 for females; and the item with the highest b_4 was item TIB-B ([epiphyseal width]/[epiphyseal height]) for both groups, with 5.0022, 6.3704, 8.2832, and 10.4988 for males and 3.8412, 4.8152, 6.3514, and 8.3020 for females.

The resulting skeletal maturity scale demonstrated assessibility to a high proportion of the participants in the Fels Longitudinal Study for each age group, that is, for most age groups the proportion is approximately 0.9 or greater, except for ages 0.1, 17.0, and 18.0. It was found that the regression of the skeletal age on the chronological age is almost linear, except for drops at the end showing the maximum drop of 16.88 against 18.0 for the female 18-year-old group. The distributions of skeletal age are skewed significantly within some chronological age groups in each sex with variable directions of skewness. The standard deviations of skeletal age increase until about 4.5 years in each sex, then more or less stabilize, and drop at 18 years for males and 17 and 18 years for females, the same tendencies observed in the regression of the skeletal age on the chronological age. There are many other interesting findings reported in Roche et al. (1975).

Discussion

It has been observed that in the homogeneous case, the models have features that satisfy the criteria for good models, while in the heterogeneous case, fulfillment of these criteria becomes more difficult. The heterogeneous case provides greater varieties in the configuration of the category response functions; and therefore model fit will be better. In certain situations, such as Likert scale attitude surveys, it will be reasonable to apply a model in the homogeneous case, which assumes invariance of the discrimination power of an item for every possible redichotomization of the graded categories. This is supported by the results by Koch (1983). In general, however, it will be wise to start with a nonparametric estimation of the category response functions, and let the data determine which of the cases is more appropriate.

Acknowledgments

The author would like to thank David Thissen for his assistance running Multilog and H. Paul Kelley and Mark Reckase for their assistance with a literature review on the topic of applications of graded response models. Part of the work in preparing this paper was supported by the Office of Naval Research, N00014-90-J-1456.

References

Bock, R.D. (1972). Estimating item parameters and latent ability when responses are scored in two or more nominal categories. *Psychometrika* **37**, 29–51.

Bock, R.D. and Aitkin, M. (1981). Marginal maximum likelihood estimation of item parameters: Application of an EM algorithm. *Psychometrika* **46**, 443–459.

Kolakowski, D. and Bock, R.D. (1973). *Maximum Likelihood Item Analysis and Test Scoring: Logistic Model for Multiple Item Responses.* Ann Arbor, MI: National Educational Resources.

Koch, W.R. (1983). Likert scaling using the graded response latent trait model. *Applied Psychological Measurement* **7**, 15–32.

Levine, M. (1984). *An Introduction to Multilinear Formula Scoring Theory* (Office of Naval Research Report, 84-4). Champaign, IL: Model-Based Measurement Laboratory, Education Building, University of Illinois.

Lord, F.M. (1952). A theory of mental test scores. *Psychometric Monograph*, No. 7.

Lord, F.M. and Novick, M.R. (1968). *Statistical Theories of Mental Test Scores.* Reading, MA: Addison Wesley.

Masters, G.N. (1982). A Rasch model for partial credit scoring. *Psychometrika* **47**, 149–174.

Muraki, E. (1992). A generalized partial credit model: Application of an

EM algorithm. *Applied Psychological Measurement* **16**, 159–176.

Muraki, E. and Bock, R.D. (1993). *Parscale.* Chicago, IL: Scientific Software.

Ramsay, J.O. and Wang, X. (1993). *Hybrid IRT Models.* Paper presented at the Meeting of the Psychometric Society, Berkeley, CA.

Roche, A.F., Wainer, H., and Thissen, D. (1975). *Skeletal Maturity: The Knee Joint As a Biological Indicator.* New York, NY: Plenum Medical Book.

Samejima, F. (1969). Estimation of ability using a response pattern of graded scores. *Psychometrika Monograph*, No. 17.

Samejima, F. (1972). A general model for free-response data. *Psychometrika Monograph*, No. 18.

Samejima, F. (1973). Homogeneous case of the continuous response model. *Psychometrika* **38**, 203–219.

Samejima, F. (1983). Some methods and approaches of estimating the operating characteristics of discrete item responses. In H. Wainer and S. Messick (Eds.), *Principles of Modern Psychological Measurement: A Festschrift for Frederic M. Lord* (pp. 159–182). Hillsdale, NJ: Lawrence Erlbaum.

Samejima, F. (1993). Roles of Fisher type information in latent trait models. In H. Bozdogan (Ed.), *Proceedings of the First US/Japan Conference on the Frontiers of Statistical Modeling: An Informational Approach* (pp. 347–378). Netherlands: Kluwer Academic Publishers.

Samejima, F. (1994). Nonparametric estimation of the plausibility functions of the distractors of vocabulary test items. *Applied Psychological Measurement* **18**, 35–51.

Samejima, F. (1995). Acceleration model in the heterogeneous case of the general graded response model. *Psychometrika* **60**, 549–572.

Samejima, F. (1996). Rationale and actual procedures of efficient nonparametric approaches for estimating the operating characteristics of discrete item responses. (In press.)

Thissen, D. (1991). *Multilog User's Guide — Version 6.* Chicago, IL: Scientific Software.

6
The Partial Credit Model

Geofferey N. Masters and Benjamin D. Wright

Introduction

The Partial Credit Model (PCM) is a unidimensional model for the analysis of responses recorded in two or more ordered categories. In this sense, the model is designed for the same purpose as several other models in this book, including Samejima's graded response model (Samejima, 1969). The PCM differs from the graded response model, however, in that it belongs to the Rasch family of models and so shares the distinguishing characteristics of that family: separable person and item parameters, sufficient statistics, and, hence, conjoint additivity. These features enable "specifically objective" comparisons of persons and items (Rasch, 1977) and allow each set of model parameters to be conditioned out of the estimation procedure for the other.

The PCM (Masters, 1982, 1987, 1988a, 1988b) is the simplest of all item response models for ordered categories. It contains only *two* sets of parameters: one for persons and one for items. All parameters in the model are *locations* on an underlying variable. This feature distinguishes the PCM from models that include item "discrimination" or "dispersion" parameters which qualify locations and so confound the interpretation of variables.

In this chapter, the PCM is introduced as a straightforward application of Rasch's model for dichotomies (Rasch, 1960) to pairs of adjacent categories in a sequence. The simplicity of the model's formulation makes it easy to implement in practice, and the model has been incorporated into a range of software packages.

The PCM can be applied in any situation in which performances on an item or an assessment criterion are recorded in two or more ordered categories and there is an intention to combine results across items/criteria to obtain measures on some underlying variable. Successful applications of the PCM to a wide variety of measurement problems have been reported in the literature. These include applications to the assessment of language functions in aphasia patients (Guthke et al., 1992; Willmes, 1992); ratings of infant performance (Wright and Masters, 1982); computerized patient simulation problems (Julian and Wright, 1988); ratings of writing samples (Pollitt and Hutchinson, 1987; Harris et al., 1988); measures of critical thinking (Masters and Evans, 1986); ratings of second language proficiency

(Adams et al., 1987); computer adaptive testing (Koch and Dodd, 1989); answer-until-correct scoring (Wright and Masters, 1982); measures of conceptual understanding in science (Adams et al., 1991); embedded figure tests (Pennings, 1987); self-ratings of fear (Masters and Wright, 1982); applications of the SOLO taxonomy (Wilson and Iventosch, 1988); self-ratings of life satisfaction (Masters, 1985); the diagnosis of mathematics errors (Adams, 1988); measures of conceptual understanding in social education (Doig et al., 1994); the construction of item banks (Masters, 1984); and statewide testing programs (Titmanis et al., 1993).

Presentation of the Model

The PCM is an application of Rasch's model for dichotomies. When an item provides only two scores 0 and 1, the probability of scoring 1 rather than 0 is expected to increase with the ability being measured. In Rasch's model for dichotomies, this expectation is modeled as

$$\frac{P_{ij1}}{P_{ij0} + P_{ij1}} = \frac{\exp(\theta_j - \delta_i)}{1 + \exp(\theta_j - \delta_i)}, \tag{1}$$

where P_{ij1} is the probability of person j scoring 1 on item i, P_{ij0} is the probability of person j scoring 0, θ_j is the ability of person j, and δ_i is the difficulty of item i defined as the location on the measurement variable at which a score of 1 on item i is as likely as a score of 0. The model is written here as a conditional probability to emphasize that it is a model for the probability of person j scoring 1 *rather than* 0 (i.e., given one of only two possible outcomes and conditioning out all other possibilities of the person–item encounter such as "not answered" and "answered but not scorable").

When an item provides more than two response categories (e.g., three ordinal categories scored 0, 1, and 2), a score of 1 is not expected to be increasingly likely with increasing ability because, beyond some point, a score of 1 should become *less* likely as a score of 2 becomes a more probable result. Nevertheless, it follows from the intended order $0 < 1 < 2, \ldots, < m_i$ of a set of categories that the *conditional* probability of scoring x rather than $x-1$ on an item should increase monotonically throughout the ability range. In the PCM, this expectation is modeled using Rasch's model for dichotomies:

$$\frac{P_{ijx}}{P_{ijx-1} + P_{ijx}} = \frac{\exp(\theta_j - \delta_{ix})}{1 + \exp(\theta_j - \delta_{ix})}, \quad x = 1, 2, \ldots, m_i \tag{2}$$

where P_{ijx} is the probability of person j scoring x on item i, P_{ijx-1} is the probability of person j scoring $x-1$, θ_j is the ability of person j, and δ_{ix} is an item parameter governing the probability of scoring x rather than $x-1$ on item i.

By conditioning on a pair of adjacent categories and so eliminating all other response possibilities from consideration, Eq. (2) focuses on the *local* comparison of categories $x-1$ and x. This local comparison is the heart of the PCM.

To apply the PCM it is conventional to rewrite the model as the unconditional probability of each possible outcome $0, 1, \ldots, m_i$ of person j's attempt at item i. This reexpression of the model requires only that person j's performance on item i is assigned one of the $m_i + 1$ available scores for that item, i.e.,

$$\sum_{h=0}^{m_i} P_{ijh} = 1. \tag{3}$$

The probability of person j scoring x on item i can then be written

$$P_{ijx} = \frac{\exp \sum_{k=0}^{x} (\theta_j - \delta_{ik})}{\sum_{h=0}^{m_j} \exp \sum_{k=0}^{h} (\theta_j - \delta_{ik})}, \quad x = 0, 1, \ldots, m_i, \tag{4}$$

where, for notational convenience,

$$\sum_{k=0}^{0} (\theta_j - \delta_{ik}) \equiv 0 \quad \text{and} \quad \sum_{k=0}^{h} (\theta_j - \delta_{ik}) \equiv \sum_{k=1}^{h} (\theta_j - \delta_{ik}).$$

For an item with only two categories, Eq. (4) simplifies to Rasch's model for dichotomies.

Response Functions

When the PCM is applied, it provides estimates of the item parameters $(\delta_{i1}, \delta_{i2}, \ldots, \delta_{im_i})$ for each item i. When these estimates are substituted into Eq. (4), the estimated probabilities of scoring $0, 1, \ldots, m_i$ on item i are obtained for any specified ability θ.

Figure 1(a) shows the model probabilities of scoring 0, 1, 2, and 3 on a four-category item calibrated with the PCM. Note that the maxima of the response curves are in the order $0 < 1 < 2 < 3$ from left to right. This is a basic feature of the model: the response curve maxima are always ordered $0 < 1 < 2 < \ldots < m_i$ on the measurement variable.

The item parameters $(\delta_{i1}, \delta_{i2}, \ldots, \delta_{im_i})$ have a simple interpretation in this picture. Each parameter δ_{ix} corresponds to the position on the measurement variable at which a person has the same probability of responding in category x as in category $x-1$ (i.e., $P_{ijx} = P_{ijx-1}$). The parameter estimates for the item in Fig. 1(a) are thus at the intersections of the response curves for categories 0 and 1, 1 and 2, and 2 and 3.

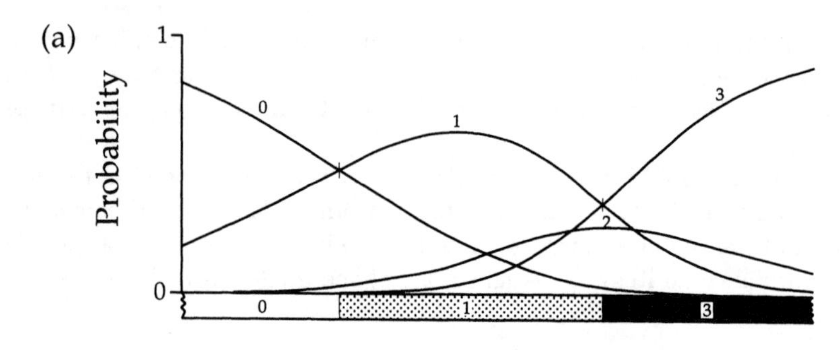

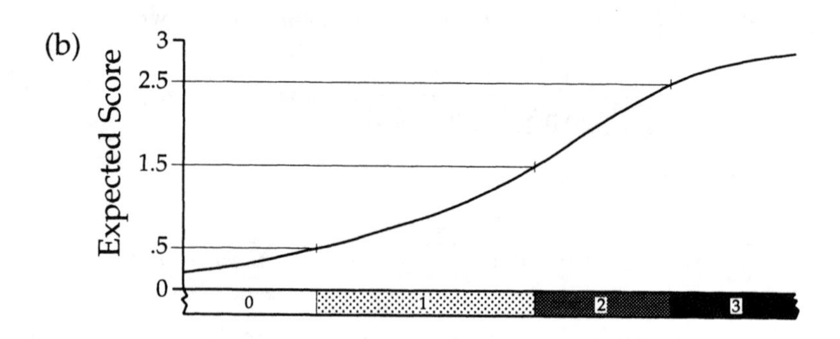

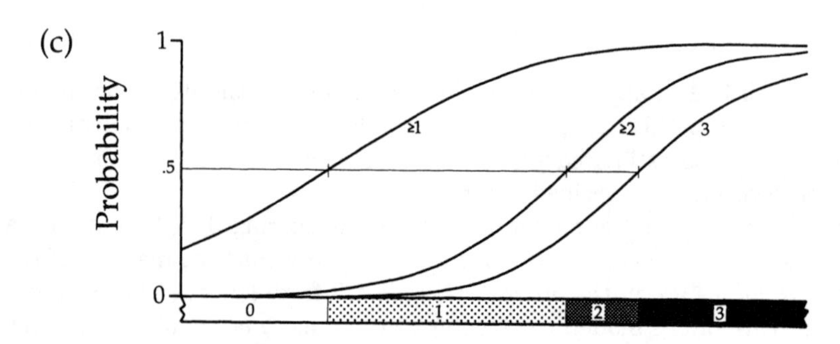

FIGURE 1. Three approaches to defining regions of a measurement continuum using the PCM.

Interpreting Parameters

The person ability parameter θ_j in the PCM is the modeled location of person j on the variable being measured. For each item i scored $0, 1, \ldots, m_i$, the PCM defines a set of m_i item parameters. These parameters, all of which are locations on the measurement variable, can be used to map the qualitative meaning of the variable and to interpret person parameters.

In the case of items scored right or wrong, only one parameter is estimated for each item and these item "difficulties" mark out and give qualitative meaning to a variable. Levels of ability are differentiated in terms of the kinds of items likely to be answered correctly. By convention, "likely" means with a probability ≥ 0.5, although in some testing programs higher probabilities of success (e.g., ≥ 0.7 or ≥ 0.8) are specified.

Open-ended and performance tasks of the kind the PCM is designed to analyze are usually intended to be accessible to a wide range of abilities and to differentiate among test takers on the basis of their levels of response. Response categories for each item capture this response diversity and thus provide the basis for the qualitative mapping of measurement variables and the consequent interpretation of ability estimates. For items with more than two response categories, however, the mapping of response categories on to measurement variables is a little less straightforward than for right/wrong scoring.

Because each item parameter in the PCM is defined locally with respect to just two adjacent categories (rather than globally taking into account all categories simultaneously), the item parameters in the model can take *any* order. For the item in Fig. 1(a) they are ordered $\delta_{i1} < \delta_{i3} < \delta_{i2}$. Because they have this property, these parameters may not, in themselves, be helpful in marking out regions of an underlying variable. Three useful alternatives are illustrated in Figs. 1(a), 1(b), and 1(c).

The first method, illustrated in Fig. 1(a), identifies regions of "single most probable response" to an item. The three shaded regions at the bottom of Fig. 1(a) indicate the single most probable response (0, 1, or 3) for the range of abilities shown.

A disadvantage of this method is that, in this case, it defines no region for a score of 2. In fact, it gives the impression that category 2 has "disappeared" entirely. This is not the case: a score of 2 on this item is a quite likely result ($p = 0.28$) for an ability at the junction of curves 1 and 3. When PCM item parameters are in the order $\delta_{i1} < \delta_{i2} < \delta_{i3}$, the parameters mark out regions of "single most probable response" for *all* categories. However, as can be seen from Fig. 1(a), other orders of PCM item parameters are possible.

Some caution is required in the interpretation of "most probably" statements. Toward the far right of the shaded region labeled "1" in Fig. 1(a), it is *not* the case that persons will "most probably" score 1. Because the sum of the probabilities for categories 2 and 3 exceeds the probability of a response in category 1, persons with abilities in this part of the continuum are more likely to score at least 2 than to score only 1. This observation makes it clear that the most useful method of mapping response categories onto underlying measurement variables is not obvious when items are scored in more than two categories.

The second method, illustrated in Fig. 1(b), is based on the calculation of the expected score

$$E_x = \sum_{h=0}^{m_i} h P_{ijh}. \tag{5}$$

In Fig. 1(b), the abilities at which $E_x = 0.5$, 1.5, and 2.5 are identified. These are used to mark out an alternative set of response regions along the horizontal variable.

An attraction of Method b is that it is consistent with procedures for testing model-data fit which contrast a person's observed score on an item with their expected score. For expected scores between, say, 1.5 and 2.5, the observed score that minimizes the observed-expected residual is a score of 2. In this sense it might be argued that the "2" region of the measurement variable is best defined as that range of abilities for which the expected score is between 1.5 and 2.5. A disadvantage of this method is that it provides category regions which may seem implausibly wide.

The third method, illustrated in Fig. 1(c), sums the curves in Fig. 1(a). The curve labeled "≥ 1" is the result of summing curves 1, 2, and 3 in Fig. 1(a). The curve labeled "≥ 2" is the result of summing curves 2 and 3. These cumulative ogives give the probability of scoring "1 or better," "2 or better," and "3" on this item. The abilities at which the cumulative probabilities equal 0.5 have been used to mark out a third set of regions. Persons with abilities in the "2" region in Fig. 1(c) will most probably (i.e., $p > 0.5$) score *at least* 2 on this item, but will most probably ($p > 0.5$) *not* score 3.

An attractive feature of Method c is that it parallels the interpretation of variables constructed from dichotomously scored items. On a variable defined by dichotomous items, a person's estimated location places them above items they will most probably ($p > 0.5$) pass and below items they will most probably ($p > 0.5$) fail. Method c similarly interprets an individual's location by reference to thresholds they will most probably ($p > 0.5$) pass and thresholds they will most probably ($p > 0.5$) fail. Method c also has the advantage of being consistent with Thurstone's approach to mapping response categories onto underlying measurement variables. Thurstone used cumulative probabilities to define "category boundaries" or "thresholds" on a latent continuum. The distance between cumulative ogives Thurstone described as the "width" of the corresponding response category [e.g., Edwards and Thurstone (1952)].

Relations to Other Models

The difference between the PCM and Samejima's (this volume) graded response model can be understood in terms of the cumulative ogives in Fig. 1(c). In the PCM, these cumulative probabilities are not modeled directly, but are the result of summing the category response functions in Fig. 1(a), which in turn are the result of applying Rasch's model for dichotomies separately to each pair of adjacent categories. In the graded response model, cumulative probabilities *are* modeled directly. Thus, while the PCM gives the probability of person j scoring x on item i, the GRM models the probability of person j scoring x *or better* on item i. As a result, the PCM is *not* a case of Samejima's graded response model (e.g., with equal item discriminations). This difference between the two models is sometimes misunderstood.

As a member of the Rasch family of item response models, the PCM is closely related to other members of that family. Masters and Wright (1984) describe several members of this family and show how each has as its essential element Rasch's model for dichotomies. Andrich's (1978) model for rating scales, for example, can be thought of as a version of the PCM with the added expectation that the response categories are defined and function in the same way for each item in an instrument. With this added expectation, rather than modeling a set of m_i parameters for each item, a single parameter δ_i is modeled for item i, and a set of m parameters $(\tau_1, \tau_2, \ldots, \tau_m)$ are proposed for the common response categories. To obtain the rating scale version of the PCM, each item parameter in the model is redefined as $\delta_{ix} = \delta_i + \tau_x$. Wilson (1992) and Muraki (1992) have proposed generalized versions of the PCM for other kinds of multicategory data.

Parameter Estimation

Conditional and joint maximum likelihood procedures for estimating PCM parameters are described by Masters (1982) and Wright and Masters (1982), who also describe a procedure based on the pairwise comparison of responses to items (PAIR) and a simplified procedure (PROX) based on the assumption that the effects of the person sample on item calibration and of the test on person measurement can be summarized by means and standard deviations on the variable. The essentials of the conditional and joint maximum likelihood procedures are summarized here.

Conditional Maximum Likelihood

The Conditional Maximum Likelihood (CML) procedure begins with the conditional probability of the response vector (x_i) given test score r

$$P\{(x_i);((\delta_{ik}))\mid r\} = \frac{\exp\left(-\sum_i^n \sum_{k=0}^{x_i} \delta_{ik}\right)}{\sum_{(x_q)}^r \exp\left(-\sum_i^n \sum_{k=0}^{x_q} \delta_{ik}\right)}, \tag{6}$$

where $\delta_{i0} \equiv 0$ and $\sum_{(x_q)}^r$ is the sum over all response vectors (x_q) that produce the score r.

The conditional probability of responding in category h of item i given score r is

$$P^*_{irh} = \frac{\exp\left(-\sum_{k=0}^h \delta_{ik}\right) \sum_{(x_{q\neq i})}^{r-h} \exp\left(-\sum_{q\neq i}^n \sum_{k=0}^{x_q} \delta_{qk}\right)}{\sum_{g=0}^{m_i} \left\{\exp\left(-\sum_{k=0}^g \delta_{ik}\right) \sum_{(x_{q\neq i})}^{r-g} \exp\left(-\sum_{q\neq i}^n \sum_{k=0}^{x_q} \delta_{qk}\right)\right\}}$$

$$= \frac{\exp\left(-\sum_{k=0}^h \delta_{ik}\right) \gamma_{r-h,i}}{\gamma_r}, \tag{7}$$

where $\sum_{(x_{q\neq i})}^{r-h}$ is the sum over all response vectors $(x_{q\neq i})$ that exclude item i and produce the score $r-h$.

The conditional likelihood over N persons with various scores is

$$\Lambda = \prod_j^N \left[\exp\left(-\sum_i^n \sum_{k=0}^{x_{ij}} \delta_{ik}\right) \Big/ \gamma_r\right]$$

$$= \exp\left[-\sum_j^N \sum_i^n \sum_{k=0}^{x_{ij}} \delta_{ik}\right] \Big/ \prod_r^{M-1} (\gamma_r)^{N_r}, \tag{8}$$

where $M = \sum_i^n m_i$ is the maximum possible score on the instrument, $\prod_j^N \gamma_r = \prod_r^{M-1} (\gamma_r)^{N_r}$, and N_r is the number of persons with a particular score r.

The log likelihood can then be written

$$\lambda \equiv \log \Lambda = -\sum_i^n \sum_{k=1}^{m_i} S_{ik}\delta_{ik} - \sum_r^{M-1} N_r \log \gamma_r, \tag{9}$$

where S_{ik} is the number of persons scoring k *or better* on item i.

The estimation equations for the CML procedure require the first and second derivatives of the log likelihood with respect to δ_{ih}. These are

$$\frac{\partial \lambda}{\partial \delta_{ih}} = -S_{ih} - \sum_r^{M-1} \frac{N_r}{\gamma_r} \left(\frac{\partial \gamma_r}{\partial \delta_{ih}}\right) = -S_{ih} + \sum_r^{M-1} N_r \sum_{k=h}^{m_i} P_{irk} \tag{10}$$

and

$$\frac{\partial^2 \lambda}{\partial \delta_{ih}^2} = -\sum_r^{M-1} N_r \left(\sum_{k=h}^{m_i} P_{irk} \right) \left(1 - \sum_{k=h}^{m_i} P_{irk} \right), \tag{11}$$

where $\sum_{k=h}^{m_i} P_{irk}$ is the probability of a person with score r scoring h or better on item i.

Joint Maximum Likelihood

The Joint Maximum Likelihood (JML) procedure begins by modeling the likelihood of an entire data matrix $[(x_{ij})]$ as the continued product of the probabilities P_{ijx} over all persons $j = 1, N$ and all items $i = 1, n$:

$$\Lambda = \prod_j^N \prod_i^n P_{ijx} = \frac{\exp \sum_j^N \sum_i^n \sum_{h=0}^{x_{ij}} (\theta_j - \delta_{ih})}{\prod_j^N \prod_i^n \left[\sum_{h=0}^{m_i} \exp \sum_{k=0}^{h} (\theta_j - \delta_{ik}) \right]}. \tag{12}$$

The log likelihood is

$$\lambda = \log \Lambda = \sum_j^N \sum_i^n x_{ij}\theta_j - \sum_j^N \sum_i^n \sum_{h=1}^{x_{ij}} \delta_{ih}$$

$$- \sum_j^N \sum_i^n \log \left[\sum_{h=0}^{m_i} \exp \sum_{k=0}^{h} (\theta_j - \delta_{ik}) \right],$$

which can be rewritten

$$\lambda = \sum_j^N r_j \theta_j - \sum_i^n \sum_{h=1}^{m_i} S_{ih}\delta_{ih} - \sum_j^N \sum_i^n \log \left[\sum_{h=0}^{m_i} \exp \sum_{k=0}^{h} (\theta_j - \delta_{ik}) \right], \tag{13}$$

where r_j is the score of person j on the instrument and S_{ih} is the number of persons scoring h or better on item i.

The first derivatives of λ with respect to θ_j and δ_{ih} are

$$\frac{\partial \lambda}{\partial \theta_j} = r_j - \sum_i^n \sum_{k=1}^{m_i} k P_{ijk}, \quad j = 1, N,$$

and

$$\frac{\partial \lambda}{\partial \delta_{ih}} = -S_{ih} + \sum_j^N \sum_{k=h}^{m_i} P_{ijk}, \quad i = 1, n, \quad h = 1, m_i.$$

The second derivatives of λ with respect to θ_j and δ_{ih} are

$$\frac{\partial^2 \lambda}{\partial \theta_j^2} = -\sum_i^n \left[\sum_{k=1}^{m_i} k^2 P_{ijk} - \left(\sum_{k=1}^{m_i} k P_{ijk} \right)^2 \right]$$

and

$$\frac{\partial^2 \lambda}{\partial \delta_{ih}^2} = -\sum_j^N \left[\sum_{k=h}^{m_i} P_{ijk} - \left(\sum_{k=h}^{m_i} P_{ijk} \right)^2 \right].$$

With these results, the JML estimation equations for the PCM are

$$\hat{\theta}_r^{(t+1)} = \hat{\theta}_r^{(t)} - \frac{r - \sum_i^n \sum_{k=1}^{m_i} kP_{irk}^{(t)}}{-\sum_i^n \left[\sum_{k=1}^{m_i} k^2 P_{irk}^{(t)} - \left(\sum_{k=1}^{m_i} kP_{irk}^{(t)} \right)^2 \right]}, \tag{14}$$

and

$$\hat{\delta}_{ih}^{(t+1)} = \hat{\delta}_{ih}^{(t)} - \frac{-S_{ih} + \sum_r^{M-1} N_r \sum_{k=h}^{m_i} P_{irk}^{(t)}}{-\sum_r^{M-1} N_r \left[\sum_{k=h}^{m_i} P_{irk}^{(t)} - \left(\sum_{k=h}^{m_i} P_{irk}^{(t)} \right)^2 \right]}, \tag{15}$$

where $\hat{\theta}_r^{(t)}$ is the estimated ability of a person with score r on the n-item instrument after t iterations, $\hat{\delta}_{ih}^{(t)}$ is the estimate of δ_{ih} after t iterations; N_r is the number of persons with score r, and M is the maximum possible score on the instrument (i.e., $M = \sum_i^n m_i$).

Of these two procedures, the conditional is preferable on theoretical grounds. The joint procedure has the advantage of being relatively easy to program, and for this reason is widely used in practice. The estimates it produces, however, contain a bias. Through simulation studies it has been shown that this bias—which is greatest for instruments with small numbers of items—can be significantly reduced by multiplying the final item estimates by $(n-1)/n$. For typical data sets, these "corrected" estimates are equivalent to those obtained from the conditional procedure.

In the implementation of partial credit analysis, it is possible to estimate all parameters for an item only if observations occur in each of the available response categories. Wilson and Masters (1993) have developed a procedure for automatically reparameterizing the model to provide JML estimates of a smaller number of item parameters when one or more response categories for an item are unused (i.e., "null").

Marginal Maximum Likelihood

Marginal maximum likelihood (MML) estimation was developed as an alternative to the joint estimation of person and item parameters. In models that do not have simple sufficient statistics for θ, and so do not permit CML estimates, the number of person parameters to be estimated increases with the number of persons, meaning that joint maximum likelihood may not provide consistent estimates of item parameters. MML treats person parameters as "incidental" or "nuisance" parameters and removes them from the likelihood function by assuming that persons are sampled randomly from a population in which ability is distributed according to some density function $g(\theta)$.

In the PCM, the person score $r_j = \sum_i^n x_{ij}$ is a sufficient statistic for θ and so the number of person parameters to be estimated is $\sum_i^n m_i - 1$, regardless of sample size. CML removes θ from the likelihood by conditioning on score, and so provides consistent estimates of the item parameters. Because CML does not require an assumption about the population distribution, it is more robust and is in general the procedure of choice.

An MML procedure for the PCM is developed in detail by Glas and Verhelst (1989) and Wilson and Adams (1993). The procedure follows Bock and Aitkin (1981).

If the probability of person j scoring x on item i is P_{ijx}, then the probability of person j's observed response vector $\underline{x}_j$ given θ_j and the set of PCM item parameters $\underline{\delta}$ is

$$P(\underline{x}_j \mid \theta_j, \underline{\delta}) = \prod_{i=1}^{n} P_{ijx_i}. \tag{16}$$

For a person sampled randomly from a population with a continuous distribution $g(\theta)$, the unconditional probability of response vector $\underline{x}_j$ is

$$P(\underline{x}_j \mid \underline{\delta}, \underline{\alpha}) = \int_\theta P(\underline{x}_j \mid \theta_j, \underline{\delta}) g(\theta \mid \underline{\alpha}) d\theta, \tag{17}$$

where $\underline{\alpha}$ is a set of population parameters, e.g., $\underline{\alpha} = (\mu, \sigma^2)$. When N persons are drawn at random from this population, the likelihood of their observed set of response patterns is

$$\Lambda = \prod_{j=1}^{N} P(\underline{x}_j \mid \underline{\delta}, \underline{\alpha}), \tag{18}$$

in which the incidental parameters θ have been eliminated.

MML finds the values of the structural (item and population) parameters that maximize the log likelihood $\lambda = \log \Lambda$, by solving the likelihood equations

$$\frac{\partial \lambda}{\partial \underline{\delta}} = 0 \tag{19}$$

and

$$\frac{\partial \lambda}{\partial \underline{\alpha}} = 0. \tag{20}$$

Rather than solving Eqs. (19) and (20) directly, it is possible, following Bock and Aitkin (1981), to apply an EM algorithm. When applied to the PCM, this approach is particularly straightforward because of the existence of sufficient statistics for the model parameters.

If it is assumed that, in addition to the response data, the person parameters $\underline{\theta}$ are known, then an expression can be written for the joint likelihood $\Lambda(\underline{\delta}, \underline{\alpha} \mid \underline{x}, \underline{\theta})$ and log-likelihood $\lambda = \log \Lambda(\underline{\delta}, \underline{\alpha} \mid \underline{x}, \underline{\theta})$. The joint log-likelihood cannot be maximized directly because it depends on a knowledge of $\underline{\theta}$. An alternative is to maximize its expectation $E[\lambda]$ given current estimates of $\underline{\theta}$. First, the marginal posterior density of θ_j given $\underline{x}_j$ is estimated using provisional estimates of the item and population parameters (the E-step). Then the expected value of the joint log-likelihood is maximized to obtain improved estimates of the item and population parameters (the M-step):

$$\frac{\partial E[\lambda]}{\partial \underline{\delta}} = 0, \qquad \frac{\partial E[\lambda]}{\partial \underline{\alpha}} = 0.$$

These two steps are repeated until convergence.

Partial credit analysis is now available in a range of software packages. Early programs to implement the PCM were *CREDIT* (University of Chicago), *PC-CREDIT* (University of Melbourne), and *PARTIAL* (University of Texas at Austin). Today, a number of programs are capable of implementing partial credit analysis, including *QUEST* (Adams and Khoo, 1992) and *BIGSTEPS* (Wright and Linacre, 1992).

Goodness of Fit

Tests of fit to the PCM are conducted at several different levels. Tests of *item fit* identify problematic items. These may be items that do not work to define quite the same variable as the other items in an instrument, or items that are ambiguous or flawed. Tests of *person fit* identify persons with responses that do not follow the general pattern of responses. Tests of *global fit* indicate the overall fit of a set of data to the PCM.

Most PCM computer programs address the goodness of fit question at all three levels. In addition to statistical tests of fit, some also provide graphical displays of model–data fit.

The two most widely used PCM programs provide tests of item and person fit as weighted and unweighted mean squares. Although the exact distributional properties of these statistics are unknown, weighted and unweighted mean squares are useful in practice for diagnosing sources of model–data misfit. These two statistics are exlained briefly here [see also Wright and Masters (1982, Chapter 5)].

When person j with ability θ_j responds to item i, that person's response x_{ij} takes a value between 0 and the maximum possible score on item i, m_i. Under the PCM, the probability of person j scoring h on item i is denoted

P_{ijh}. The expected value and variance of x_{ij} are

$$E_{ij} \equiv E[x_{ij}] = \sum_{k=0}^{m_i} kP_{ijk}$$

and

$$W_{ij} \equiv V[x_{ij}] = \sum_{k=0}^{m_i} (k - E_{ij})^2 P_{ijk}.$$

The standardized difference between person j's observed and expected response to item i is

$$z_{ij} = (x_{ij} - E_{ij})/\sqrt{W_{ij}}.$$

Unweighted ("Outfit") Mean Square

For each item i, an unweighted mean square is calculated as

$$u_i = \sum_{j}^{N} z_{ij}^2/N. \tag{21}$$

Analogously, an unweighted mean square can be calculated for each person j:

$$u_j = \sum_{i}^{n} z_{ij}^2/n. \tag{22}$$

In practice, these unweighted item and person mean squares can be overly sensitive to "outliers" (i.e., unexpected high scores on difficult items or unexpected low scores on easy items). To reduce the influence of outliers, a weighted mean square can be calculated by weighting z_{ij}^2 by the information available about person j from item i. This is the basis of the "infit" mean square.

Weighted ("Infit") Mean Square

For each item i, a weighted mean square is calculated as

$$v_i = \sum_{j}^{N} W_{ij} z_{ij}^2 \Big/ \sum_{j}^{N} W_{ij}. \tag{23}$$

For each person j, a weighted mean square is calculated as

$$v_j = \sum_{i}^{n} W_{ij} z_{ij}^2 \Big/ \sum_{i}^{n} W_{ij}. \tag{24}$$

A considerable volume of research has investigated methods for testing the fit of data to members of the Rasch family of models. Much of this research has sought diagnostic goodness-of-fit tests with known null distributions. The fact that Rasch models are members of the family of exponential models has facilitated the development of methods for testing model–data fit. Readers are referred to work by Molenaar (1983), van den Wollenberg (1982), Kelderman (1984), and Glas (1988).

Empirical Example

To illustrate the use of partial credit analysis, an application to the assessment of student essay writing is now described. These data were collected to investigate the consistency with which 70 markers were able to make holistic judgments of the quality of student essays using a 5-point scale. The 70 markers had applied for positions as essay markers in a major testing program. After initial training in the use of the 5-point grade scale (E, D, C, B, A), all markers were given the same set of 90 essays to mark. Analysis was undertaken of the grades allocated by the aspiring markers, and the results were used in appointing markers to the program.

In this analysis the quality θ_j of each student essay j is measured by treating the 70 markers as "items," each providing information about θ_j. In this way, all 70 markers are calibrated. This approach allows each marker to have his or her own interpretation of the 5-point grade scale and provides a basis for studying differences in marker behavior.

Measuring Essay Quality

The first result of the partial credit analysis is a set of estimates ($\hat{\theta}_1$, $\hat{\theta}_2, \ldots, \hat{\theta}_{90}$) for the 90 student essays. These are plotted along the line of the variable in Fig. 2. The essay with the highest $\hat{\theta}$ (about +2.0 logits) is Essay 61. The essay with the lowest $\hat{\theta}$ (about −2.6 logits) is Essay 53.

The grades awarded to five of the 90 essays are shown on the right of Fig. 2. Column heights indicate the number of markers giving each grade. For Essay 61, the most commonly assigned grade was an "A." Many markers assigned this essay a "B," some gave it a "C." A few assigned it a grade of "D." At the bottom of Fig. 2, Essay 21 was most often assigned a grade of "E." None of the 70 markers rated Essay 21 higher than "C."

Figure 2 provides insight into the basis of the $\hat{\theta}$ estimates. When the grade awarded by each marker is replaced by a score so that $0 = \text{E}$, $1 = \text{D}$, $2 = \text{C}$, $3 = \text{B}$, and $4 = \text{A}$, and this score is averaged over the 70 markers, then the ordering of essays by their average score is identical to their order by estimated θ shown in Fig. 2. (This is the case in this example because all 70 markers rated all 90 essays.)

The dotted lines on the right of Fig. 2 show the expected numbers of markers giving each grade to these essays under the PCM. This is obtained

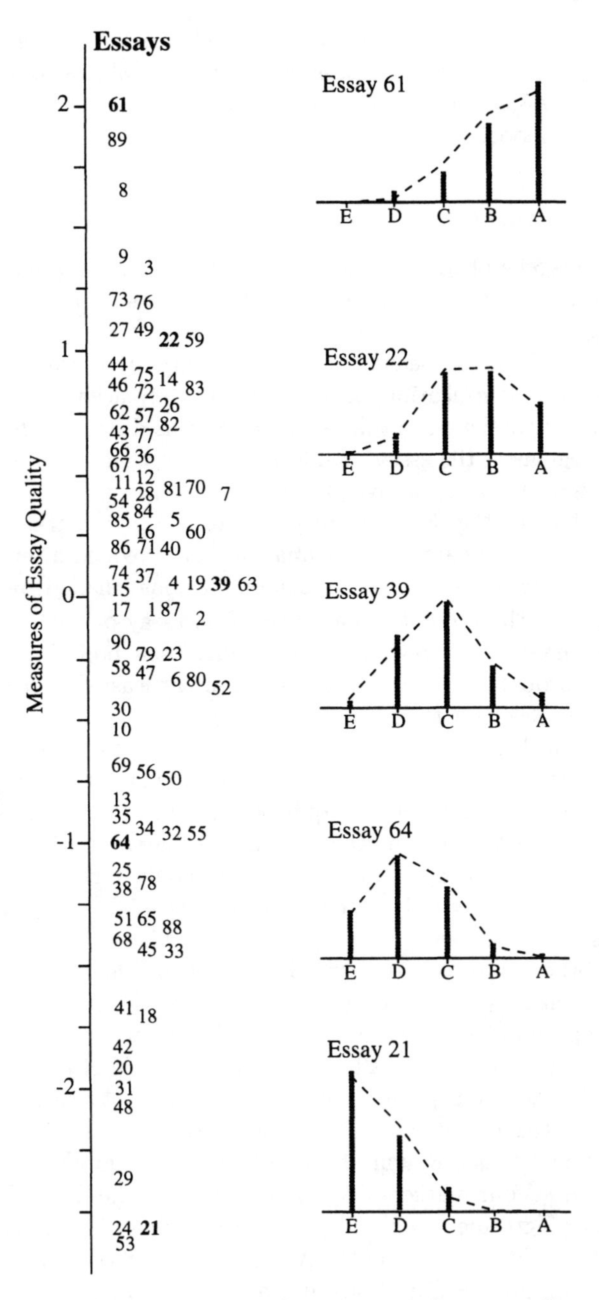

FIGURE 2. Partial credit measures of essay quality.

by calculating the model probability of each marker giving a particular grade to an essay and then summing these probabilities over the seventy markers. The essays on the right of Fig. 2 all show good fit to the expectations of the model.

Calibrating Markers

A second outcome of the partial credit analysis is a set of marker calibrations. Figure 3 illustrates the results of this process for four markers, #57, #25, #43, and #24.

On the left of Fig. 3, measures of essay quality are reproduced from Fig. 2. Each essay's identification number has been replaced here by the grade most commonly assigned to that essay. From this distribution it is possible to see the regions of the essay quality continuum that these 70 markers, as a group, associate with the five grades.

On the right of Fig. 3 the calibrations of the four markers are shown. For each marker the partial credit analysis has provided a set of threshold estimates that have been used to mark out regions (shaded) reflecting that marker's use of the 5-point grade scale. If an essay of quality $\hat{\theta}$ is located within a marker's "C" region, for example, then under the PCM, that marker will probably ($p > 0.5$) rate that essay at least C, but probably not ($p > 0.5$) rate it better than C.

The four markers in Fig. 3 have been selected because of their different uses of the grade scale. Marker 57 is a "typical" marker. His interpretation of the five grade points matches quite closely the distribution on the left of Fig. 3. Marker 25, on the other hand, is a 'harsh' marker. This marker typically gives Bs to essays that most commonly receive As, and Cs to essays that most commonly receive Bs. Marker 25 has higher than usual thresholds for all grades.

At the other extreme, Marker 43 is atypically lenient. But as Fig. 3 shows, this leniency applies only at lower grades: Marker 43 is not lenient in allocating As but is reluctant to award Es and allocates Ds only to very poor essays that would typically be assigned a grade of E.

Finally, Marker 24 displays an unusual tendency not to assign the highest grade, A, or the lowest grade, E. This marker shows a tendency to be noncommittal by making unusual use of the middle grades.

Each of these four markers displayed good fit to the PCM. Their ratings were in good agreement with the general ordering of these essays on the variable. Their different uses of the A to E grades, reflected in their different threshold estimates in Fig. 3, are not an indication of misfit, but suggest that they have different interpretations of these grades.

Partial credit analysis can be used in this way to identify differences among markers in their use of the provided grade points. Once markers are calibrated, differences in marker behavior can be taken into account automatically in future marking exercises.

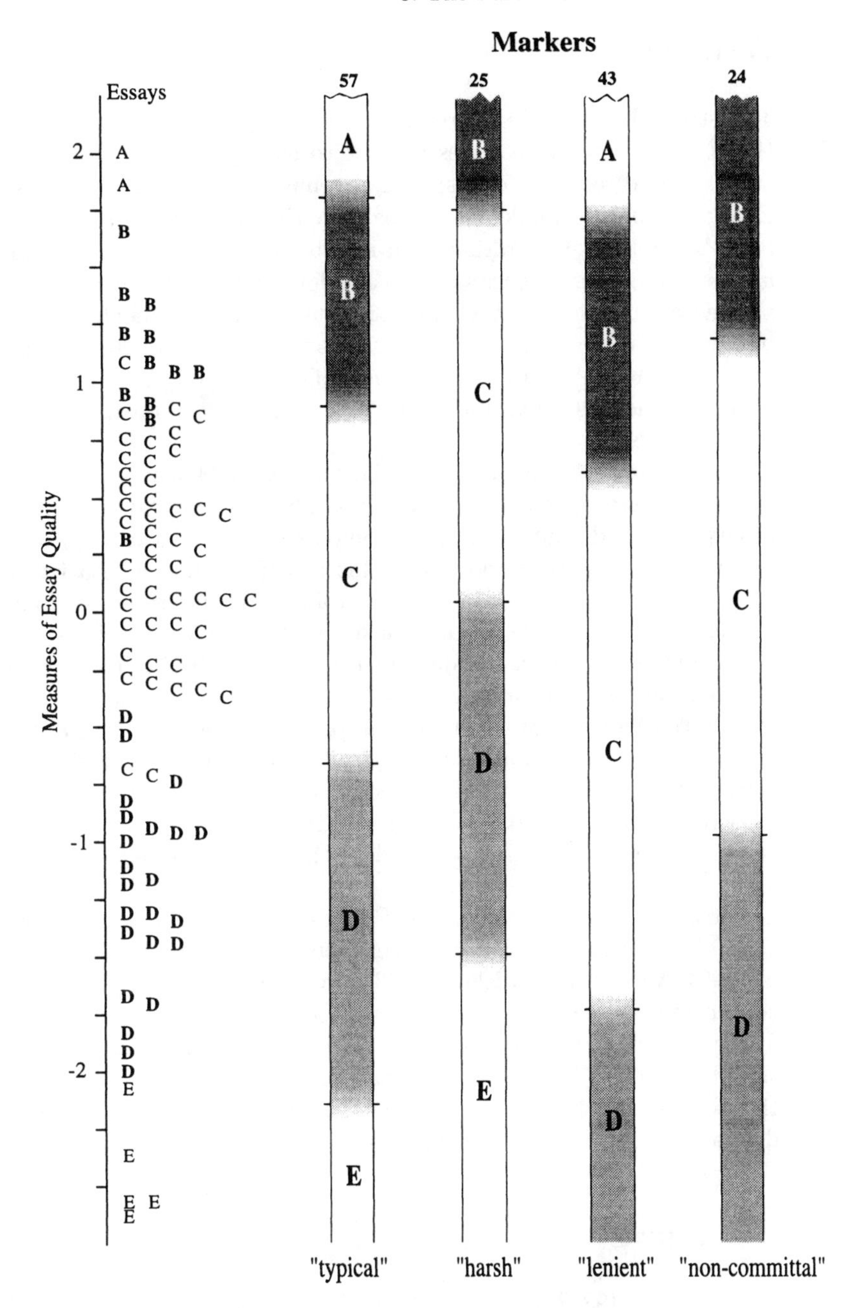

FIGURE 3. Partial credit calibrations of markers.

Discussion

The strength of the PCM resides in its simplicity. It is simply Rasch's (1960) model for dichotomies applied to each pair of adjacent categories in an ordered sequence of response alternatives. The use of Rasch's model for dichotomies to model the probability that person j's response to item i will be in category x rather than in category $x - 1$ means that the PCM has only *two* sets of parameters—one for persons and one for items; all parameters in the model are *locations* on the measurement variable; and, because it can be "repeated without modification in different parts of the measurement continuum" (Thurstone, 1931, p. 257), Rasch's simple logistic expression defines a *unit* for the PCM, which is maintained over the range of the variable.

As a result of its algebraic formulation, the PCM shares the distinguishing statistical properties of the Rasch family of item response models: separable person and item parameters, the possibility of "specifically objective" comparisons of persons and items (Rasch, 1977), sufficient statistics for all model parameters, and so, the conjoint additivity necessary for fundamental measurement. These features make the PCM easy to implement. Partial credit analysis is now a standard feature of many IRT software packages.

A number of recent applications of the PCM have been to the analysis of "alternative" assessments such as performances, projects, and portfolios. In these contexts, assessors typically rate student work either holistically or against a set of pre-specified criteria. Measures of achievement are constructed by aggregating ratings on different tasks or across assessment criteria. The PCM is ideally suited to the analysis of assessments of this kind.

Another promising application of the PCM is to the measurement of conceptual understanding. Several recent studies (Adams et al., 1991; Doig et al., 1994; Masters and Mislevy, 1993) have used the findings of "alternative conceptions" research to develop response categories for open-ended tasks. These categories represent different levels of conceptual understanding of the phenomenon the task is designed to address. The use of the PCM in this context provides a basis for constructing measures of conceptual understanding from diverse responses to open-ended tasks.

References

Adams, R.J. (1988). Applying the PCM to educational diagnosis. *Applied Measurement in Education* **4**, 347–362.

Adams, R.J., Doig, B.A., and Rosier, M.R. (1991). *Science Learning in Victorian Schools: 1990* (Monograph 41). Melbourne, Victoria: Australian Council for Educational Research.

Adams, R.J., Griffin, P.E., and Martin, L. (1987). A latent trait method for measuring a dimension in second language proficiency. *Language Testing* **4**, 9–27.

Adams, R.J. and Khoo, S.T. (1992). *QUEST: The Interactive Test Analysis System.* Melbourne, Victoria: Australian Council for Educational Research.

Andrich, D. (1978). A rating formulation for ordered response categories. *Psychometrika* **43**, 561–573.

Bock, R.D. and Aitkin, M. (1981). Marginal maximum likelihood estimation of item parameters: Application of an EM algorithm. *Psychometrika* **46**, 443–459.

Doig, B.A., Mellor, S., Piper, K., and Masters, G.N. (1994). *Conceptual Understanding in Social Education.* Melbourne, Victoria: Australian Council for Educational Research.

Edwards, A.L. and Thurstone, L.L. (1952). An internal consistency check for scale values determined by the method of successive intervals. *Psychometrika* **17**, 169–180.

Glas, C.A.W. (1988). The derivation of some tests for the Rasch model from the multinomial distribution. *Psychometrika* **53**, 525–546.

Glas, C.A.W. and Verhelst, N.D. (1989). Extensions of the PCM. *Psychometrika* **53**, 525–546.

Guthke, J., Wolschke, P., Willmes, K., and Huber, W. (1992). Leipziger Lerntest — Diagnostisches Programm zum begriffsanalogen Klassifizieren (DP-BAK). Aufbau und Konstruktionseigenschaften. *Heilpaedagogische Forschung* **18**, 153–161.

Harris, J., Laan, S., and Mossenson, L.T. (1988). Applying partial credit analysis to the construction of narrative writing tests. *Applied Measurement in Education* **4**, 335–346.

Julian, E.R. and Wright, B.D. (1988). Using computerized patient simulations to measure the clinical competence of physicians. *Applied Measurement in Education* **4**, 299–318.

Kelderman, H. (1984). Loglinear Rasch model tests. *Psychometrika* **49**, 223–245.

Koch, W.R. and Dodd, B.G. (1989). An investigation of procedures for computerized adaptive testing using partial credit scoring. *Applied Measurement in Education* **2**, 335–357.

Masters, G.N. (1982). A Rasch model for partial credit scoring. *Psychometrika* **47**, 149–174.

Masters, G.N. (1984). Constructing an item bank using partial credit scoring. *Journal of Educational Measurement* **21**, 19–32.

Masters, G.N. (1985). A comparison of latent trait and latent class analyses of Likert-type data. *Psychometrika* **50**, 69–82.

Masters, G.N. (1987). Measurement models for ordered response categories. In R. Langeheine and J. Rost (Eds.). *Latent Trait and Latent Class Models* (pp. 11–29). New York: Plenum Publishing Corporation.

Masters, G.N. (1988a), Partial credit models. In J.P. Keeves (Ed.). *Educational Research Methodology, Measurement and Evaluation* (pp. 292–296). Oxford: Pergamon Press.

Masters, G.N. (1988b). The analysis of partial credit scoring. *Applied Measurement in Education* **1**, 279–298.

Masters, G.N. and Evans, J. (1986). Banking non-dichotomously scored items. *Applied Psychological Measurement* **10**, 355–367.

Masters, G.N. and Mislevy, R. (1993). New views of student learning: Implications for educational measurement. In N. Frederiksen, R.J. Mislevy, and I.I. Begar (Eds.). *Test Theory for a New Generation of Tests* (pp. 219–242). Hillsdale, NJ: Erlbaum.

Masters, G.N. and Wright, B.D. (1982). Defining a fear-of-crime variable: A comparison of two Rasch models. *Education Research and Perspectives* **9**, 18–32.

Masters, G.N. and Wright, B.D. (1984). The essential process in a family of measurement models. *Psychometrika* **49**, 529–544.

Molenaar, I.W. (1983). Some improved diagnostics for failure of the Rasch model. *Psychometrika* **48**, 49–73.

Muraki, E. (1992). A generalized partial credit model: Application of an EM algorithm. *Applied Psychological Measurement* **16**, 159–176.

Pennings, A. (1987). *The Diagnostic Embedded Figures Test.* Paper presented at the Second Conference on Learning and Instruction of the European Association of Learning and Instruction, University of Tübingen.

Pollitt, A. and Hutchinson, C. (1987). Calibrating graded assessments: Rasch partial credit analysis of performance in writing. *Language Testing* **4**, 72–92.

Rasch, G. (1960). *Probabilistic Models for Some Intelligence and Attainment Tests.* Copenhagen: Denmarks Paedagogiske Institut.

Rasch, G. (1977). On specific objectivity: An attempt at formalizing the request for generality and validity of scientific statements. *Danish Yearbook of Philosophy* **14**, 58–94.

Samejima, F. (1969). Estimation of latent ability using a response pattern of graded scores. *Psychometrika*, Monograph Supplement No. 17.

Thurstone, L.L. (1931). Measurement of social attitudes. *Journal of Abnormal and Social Psychology* **26**, 249–269.

Titmanis, P., Murphy, F., Cook, J., Brady, K., and Brown, M. (1993). *Profiles of Student Achievement: English and Mathematics in Western Australian Government Schools, 1992.* Perth: Ministry of Education.

Van den Wollenberg, A.L. (1982). Two new test statistics for the Rasch model. *Psychometrika* **47**, 123–140.

Willmes, K. (1992). Psychometric evaluation of neuropsychological test performances. In N. von Steinbuechel, D.Y. von Cramon, and E. Poeppel (Eds.) *Neuropsychological Rehabilitation* (pp. 103–113). Heidelberg: Springer-Verlag.

Wilson, M.R. (1992). The ordered partition model: An extension of the PCM. *Applied Psychological Measurement* **16**, 309–325.

Wilson, M.R. and Adams, R.J. (1993). Marginal maximum likelihood estimation for the partial order model. *Journal of Educational Statistics* **18**, 69–90.

Wilson, M. and Iventosch, L. (1988). Using the PCM to investigate responses to structured subtests. *Applied Measurement in Education* **1**, 319–334.

Wilson, M. and Masters, G.N. (1993). The PCM and null categories. *Psychometrika* **58**, 87–99.

Wright, B.D. and Linacre, J.M. (1992). *BIGSTEPS Rasch Analysis Computer Program.* Chicago: MESA Press.

Wright, B.D. and Masters, G.N. (1982). *Rating Scale Analysis.* Chicago: MESA Press.

7
A Steps Model to Analyze Partial Credit

N.D. Verhelst, C.A.W. Glas, and H.H. de Vries

Introduction

The partial credit model (PCM) by Masters (1982, this volume) is a unidimensional item response model for analyzing responses scored in two or more ordered categories. The model has some very desirable properties: it is an exponential family, so minimal sufficient statistics for both the item and person parameters exist, and it allows conditional–maximum likelihood (CML) estimation. However, it will be shown that the relation between the response categories and the item parameters is rather complicated. As a consequence, the PCM may not always be the most appropriate model for analyzing data.

In this chapter, an alternative to the PCM, called the steps model, is presented, which is conceptually quite different. The presentation starts with a description of a multistage testing design with dichotomous items, where the choice of a follow-up test is a function of the responses on the previous items. It is shown that it is possible to view polytomous response data as a special case of data emanating from a multistage testing design with dichotomous items, where every test consists of one dichotomous item only. Next, it is shown that adopting the assumptions of marginal-maximum-likelihood (MML) estimation results in a comprehensive framework for parameter estimation. Finally, the results of several simulation studies designed to evaluate the extent to which the steps model can be distinguished from the PCM will be presented.

Presentation of the Model

Consider a situation where a person can complete an item at different performance levels and gets a credit equal to the level at which the item was completed. Within the class of exponential family models, this situation is captured by the PCM (Masters, 1982, this volume). To motivate the development of an alternative model, it is necessary to study the PCM in some detail. Consider the response of a person, indexed j, to an item, indexed i, which has $m_i + 1$ response categories indexed by $h = 0, \ldots, m_i$. Person j produces an m_i-dimensional response vector x_{ij} with elements

$$x_{ijh} = \begin{cases} 1 & \text{if person } j \text{ scores in category } h \text{ on item } i, \\ 0 & \text{if this is not the case,} \end{cases} \tag{1}$$

for $h = 1, \ldots, m_i$. So if the person scores in the zero category, $x_{ij} = (0, 0, \ldots, 0)$.

In the PCM, it is assumed that the probability of a person with parameter θ_j scoring in category h, $h = 1, \ldots, m_i$, on an item with parameter δ_i, $\delta_i = (\delta_{i1}, \ldots, \delta_{ih}, \ldots, \delta_{im_i})$, is given by

$$\psi_{ih}(\theta_j) = P(X_{ijh} = 1 \mid \theta_j, \delta_i) = \frac{\exp\left(h\theta_j - \sum_{g=1}^{h} \delta_{ig}\right)}{1 + \sum_{k=1}^{m_i} \exp\left(k\theta_j - \sum_{g=1}^{k} \delta_{ig}\right)}. \tag{2}$$

Although the properties of the model are most desirable, Molenaar (1983) has pointed out that interpretation of the parameters must be made carefully. From Eq. (1) it follows that the model is linear in the log odds of scoring in category h, $h > 0$, and category $h - 1$, that is,

$$\ln(P(x_{ijh} = 1 \mid \theta_j, \delta_i)/P(x_{ij(h-1)} = 1 \mid \theta_j, \delta_i)) = \theta_j - \delta_{ih}. \tag{3}$$

So δ_{ih} cannot be interpreted as the difficulty parameter of category h alone; the probability of completing the item in category $h-1$ must be taken into account also. In many instances, this requirement is of little significance. Especially if the interest of the test administrator is in the characteristics of the complete item, such as in test equating or item banking, the mathematical properties of the model prevail over the complicated interpretation of the item parameters. In theory-oriented research, however, interest may be especially in the difficulty of individual categories. However, one should be aware of the following restrictions. In the original development of the PCM, a polytomous item was taken to consist of a number of distinct sequential steps that can be either taken or not taken (Masters, 1982, this volume). So if an item has five categories, there are four distinct tasks that have to be performed in a certain succession. If the person fails at the first task, the response falls in the zero category, if the person completes the first task and fails the second, the response falls in the first category, etc. If all tasks are performed successfully, the response falls in the highest category. Now, as was pointed out above, the item parameters cannot be interpreted as the difficulties of distinct categories. So in the PCM, evaluating the hypothesis that a cognitive manipulation required to take a certain step is equally difficult as the manipulation required to take another step, will be quite difficult.

To develop a model where the response categories are independently parameterized, we proceed as follows. Again, it is assumed that a polytomous item consists of a sequence of item steps. Every item step is considered to be the conceptual equivalent of a dichotomous Rasch item. Furthermore, the person is only administered the next conceptual item if a correct response was given to the previous one. So it is assumed that the person keeps taking item steps until he or she stumbles. This process can be formalized in the following manner. Let item i consist of the conceptual items $h = 1, \ldots, m_i$, and let d_{ij} be a design vector with elements

$$d_{ijh} = \begin{cases} 1 & \text{if the conceptual item } h \text{ was administered to person } j, \\ 0 & \text{if this was not the case,} \end{cases} \tag{4}$$

for $h = 1, \ldots, m_i$. Furthermore, let y_{ij} be a response vector defined by

$$y_{ijh} = \begin{cases} 1 & \text{if } d_{ijh} = 1 \text{ and a correct response} \\ & \text{was given to conceptual item } h, \\ 0 & \text{if } d_{ijh} = 1 \text{ and an incorrect response} \\ & \text{was given to conceptual item } h, \\ c & \text{if } d_{ijh} = 0, \end{cases} \tag{5}$$

for $h = 1, \ldots, m_i$, where c is an arbitrary constant. This constant is a dummy to facilitate a simple mathematical formulation of the model; its value has no consequences for the solution of the likelihood equations and evaluation of model fit. It was assumed that if a conceptual item is administered, the Rasch model holds, so

$$P(y_{ijh} = 1 \mid d_{ijh} = 1; \theta_j, \beta_{ih}) = \frac{\exp(\theta_j - \beta_{ih})}{1 + \exp(\theta_j - \beta_{ih})}, \tag{6}$$

with β_{ih} the difficulty parameter of conceptual item h within i. Let r_{ij} be the number of item steps taken within i, that is, $r_{ij} = \sum_{h=1}^{m_i} d_{ijh} y_{ijh}$.

In Table 1, for some item with $m_i = 3$, all possible responses y_{ij}, $y_{ij} = (y_{ij1}, \ldots, y_{ijh}, \ldots, y_{ijm_i})$, are enumerated, together with the associated probabilities $P(y_{ij} \mid \theta_j, \beta_i)$, where $\beta_i = (\beta_{i1}, \ldots, \beta_{ih}, \ldots, \beta_{im_i})$ is a vector of item parameters.

It can be easily verified that in general

$$P(y_{ij} \mid \theta_j, \beta_i) = \frac{\exp\left(r_{ij}\theta_j - \sum_{h=1}^{r_{ij}} \beta_{ih}\right)}{\prod_{h=1}^{\min(m_i, r_{ij}+1)} (1 + \exp(\theta_j - \beta_{ih}))}, \tag{7}$$

where $\min(m_i, r_{ij} + 1)$ stands for the minimum of m_i and $r_{ij} + 1$ and $\sum_{h=1}^{0} \beta_{ih}$ is defined to be zero. Although Eq. (7) resembles the probability of a response pattern to dichotomous items in an incomplete design [see, for instance, Fischer (1981)], it is important to note that some differences exist because the design vector d_{ij} is not a prior fixed. In fact, the design vector depends on the responses given, which means that the design is controlled by the person. This fact gives rise to restrictions on the sample space. Considering again the example in Table 1, it can be verified that the response

TABLE 1. Representation of Responses to an Item With $m_i = 3$.

y_{ij}	r_{ij}	$P(y_{ij} \mid \theta_j, \beta_i)$
0,c,c	0	$\dfrac{1}{1+\exp(\theta_j - \beta_{i1})}$
1,0,c	1	$\dfrac{\exp(\theta_j - \beta_{i1})}{(1+\exp(\theta_j - \beta_{i1})(1+\exp(\theta_j - \beta_{i2})}$
1,1,0	2	$\dfrac{\exp(\theta_j - \beta_{i1})\exp(\theta_j - \beta_{i2})}{(1+\exp(\theta_j - \beta_{i1}))(1+\exp(\theta_j - \beta_{i2}))(1+\exp(\theta_j - \beta_{i3}))}$
1,1,1	3	$\dfrac{\exp(\theta_j - \beta_{i1})\exp(\theta_j - \beta_{i2})\exp(\theta_j - \beta_{i3})}{(1+\exp(\theta_j - \beta_{i1})(1+\exp(\theta_j - \beta_{i2}))(1+\exp(\theta_j - \beta_{i3}))}$

pattern $y_{ij} = (1, c, 0)$ is not possible under the test adminstration design considered here. For a general multistage test administration design, the implications of these restrictions have already been studied by Glas (1988), leading to the conclusion that conditional maximum likelihood (CML) estimation (Rasch, 1960; Fischer, 1974) is not possible in this situation. It was also shown that marginal maximum likelihood (MML) estimation (Bock and Aitkin, 1981; de Leeuw and Verhelst, 1986; Verhelst and Glas, 1993) will work for a multistage testing design, so it is within this framework that an estimation and testing procedure for the model will be developed.

Relation Between the PCM and the Steps Model at Fixed Ability Levels

Results from an investigation into the numerical relation between the item parameters of the PCM and the item parameters of the steps model at fixed ability levels will be reported next. In this study, the ability parameter θ and the step parameters β_i were fixed at various levels. Under the steps model, the probabilities of the item scores $h = 1, \ldots, m_i$, denoted by $f_h(\theta, \beta_i)$, were computed using Eq. (7). Under the PCM, the score probabilities, denoted by $g_h(\theta, \delta_i)$, were computed as $g_h(\theta, \delta_i) = \psi_{ih}(\theta)$, where $\psi_{ih}(\theta)$ is defined by Eq. (2). For a number of combinations of the ability parameter θ and the parameters in the Steps Model β_i, PCM parameters δ_i were computed such that

$$f_h(\theta, \beta_i) = g_h(\theta, \delta_i) \tag{8}$$

for $h = 1, \ldots, m_i$. An analytical solution to Eq. (8) is given in de Vries (1988). An interesting aspect of the solution is that it always held that $\delta_{im_i} = \beta_{im_i}$. Some results for an item with $m_i = 3$ are shown in Fig. 1. For

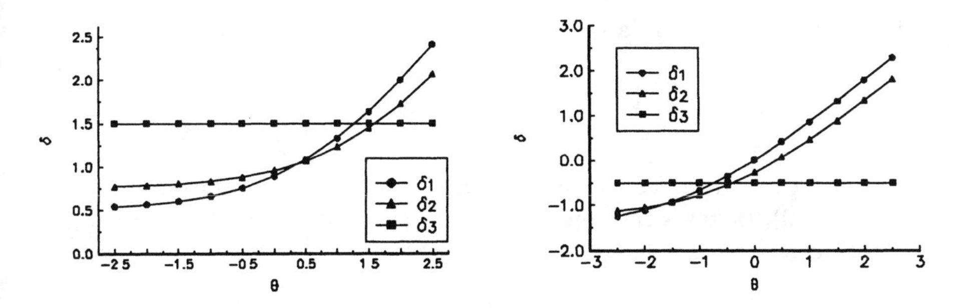

FIGURE 1. Relation between PCM and steps parameters at fixed ability levels.

the left-hand display the item parameters $\beta_i = (0.5, 0.75, 1.50)$ were used; for the right-hand display the item parameters were $\beta_i = (-1.5, -1.25, -0.50)$. The x-axis represents the values of θ, the y-axis the values of δ_{ih}, $h = 1, \ldots, 3$.

It can be seen that the relation between the PCM parameters varied with θ. Furthermore, it can be seen that there were no simple, invariant relations between the PCM parameters. Other simulations produced similar results.

Relation Between the PCM and the Steps Model under a Normal Ability Distribution

To distinguish between the PCM ability parameter and the steps model ability parameter, let the former be denoted ξ and the latter θ. It is assumed that the values of the ability parameter have a standard normal distribution. If it is assumed that the scales of the ability parameters of both models have interval properties, it holds that $\xi = a\theta + b$. As with the previous study, the step parameters β_i were fixed at various levels, and score probabilities $f_h(\theta, \beta_i)$ were computed. Next, values for a and δ_i were computed in such a way that they matched the score probabilities under the steps model. This was accomplished by minimizing the loss function

$$F(\delta_i, a) = \sum_{h=0}^{m_i} \int_{-\infty}^{\infty} [f_h(\theta, \beta_i) - g_h(a\theta, \delta_i)]^2 h(\theta)\, d\theta, \tag{9}$$

where $h(\theta)$ stands for the standard normal density function. A procedure and computer program for minimization of the loss function defined by Eq. (9) was developed by de Vries (1988).

Before discussing the results, the following consideration is needed. Although the differences between $f_h(\theta, \beta_i)$ and $g_h(\theta, \delta_i)$ should be as small as possible, it is plausible to weight the magnitude of the difference by the density of the latent variable, and minimize

$$H(\delta_i, a) = \sum_{h=0}^{m_i} \int_{-\infty}^{\infty} |f_h(\theta, \beta_i) - g_h(a\theta, \delta_i) \mid h(\theta)\, d\theta, \tag{10}$$

subject to a and δ_i. For an interpretation of the relation between Eqs. (9) and (10), Hölder's theorem [see, for instance, Abramowitz and Stegun (1974)] can be used. Let

$$O(\delta_i, a) = \sum_{h=0}^{m_i} \int_{-\infty}^{\infty} f_h(\theta, \beta_i) h(\theta)\, d\theta. \tag{11}$$

Since Eq. (11) is the sum of the manifest probabilities of the categories, it is always equal to one. Therefore, Hölder's theorem gives

$$H(\delta_i, a) \leq \sqrt{\frac{F(\delta_i, a)}{O(\delta_i, a)}} = \sqrt{F(\delta_i, a)}\,. \tag{12}$$

The left-hand side of Eq. (12) is an expression for the area of the difference between $f_h(\theta, \beta_i)$ and $g_h(\theta, \delta_i)$, and the right-hand side, which is the square root of the actual loss function that was minimized, is an upper bound for this area.

In Table 2, for a number of values of β_i, the values of δ_i, a, and the square root of $F(\delta_i, a)$ are given for items with $m_i = 3$. A more extensive report is given in de Vries (1988). In all replications, the values for the square root of $F(\delta_i, a)$ ranged between 0.0002 and 0.0049. So it was concluded that, under the assumption of a normal ability distribution, for every investigated item response function under the PCM, a closely matching item response function under the steps model could be found.

This conclusion can also be illustrated by Fig. 2, which shows a plot of the three item response functions generated using $\beta_i = (-0.5\ 0.5)$. Minimization of the loss function defined by Eq. (9) produced $\delta_i = (-0.0034, 0.4161)$, $a = 0.8043$, and a square root of $F(\delta_i, a)$ equal to 0.0011. The solid lines represent results for the PCM, the dotted lines are for the steps model. Figure 2 reveals that the item response functions under the two models closely match. Many replications showed similar results. Therefore, data fitting one model will usually also fit the other model. In the example section this conjecture will be supported further.

Parameter Estimation

As was mentioned above, the applicability of the MML estimation procedure follows from recognizing the analogy between the multistage testing design considered in Glas (1988) and the present design. Incidentally,

TABLE 2. Estimation of Item Parameters in the PCM Given the Parameters in the Steps Model.

β_1	β_2	β_3	δ_1	δ_2	δ_3	a	$\sqrt{F}$
−2.00	−2.00	−1.00	−0.35	−0.67	−0.95	0.64	0.0033
−1.50	−1.50	−0.50	−0.08	−0.41	−0.56	0.62	0.0033
−1.00	−1.00	0.00	0.19	0.16	−0.17	0.62	0.0028
−0.50	−0.50	0.50	0.46	0.11	0.22	0.62	0.0021
0.00	0.00	1.00	0.75	0.40	0.61	0.63	0.0013
0.50	0.50	1.50	1.05	0.72	1.03	0.65	0.0008
1.00	1.00	2.00	1.37	1.08	1.48	0.68	0.0005
−2.00	−1.00	−2.00	−0.81	1.09	−1.94	0.56	0.0008
−1.50	−0.50	−1.50	−0.55	1.25	−1.54	0.58	0.0008
−1.00	0.00	−1.00	−0.27	1.44	−1.13	0.60	0.0008
−0.50	0.50	−0.50	0.03	1.66	−0.69	0.64	0.0009
0.00	1.00	0.00	0.36	1.92	−0.22	0.68	0.0008
0.50	1.50	0.50	0.73	2.23	0.29	0.73	0.0007
1.00	2.00	1.00	1.13	2.60	0.84	0.79	0.0005
−1.00	−2.00	−2.00	0.97	0.25	−1.99	0.47	0.0014
−0.50	−1.50	−1.50	1.14	0.38	−1.61	0.47	0.0014
0.00	−1.00	−1.00	1.32	0.53	−1.24	0.48	0.0013
0.50	−0.50	−0.50	1.54	0.70	−0.86	0.50	0.0010
1.00	0.00	0.00	1.77	0.90	−0.47	0.52	0.0007
1.50	0.50	0.50	2.04	1.12	−0.06	0.55	0.0005
2.00	1.00	1.00	2.34	1.39	0.58	0.58	0.0003

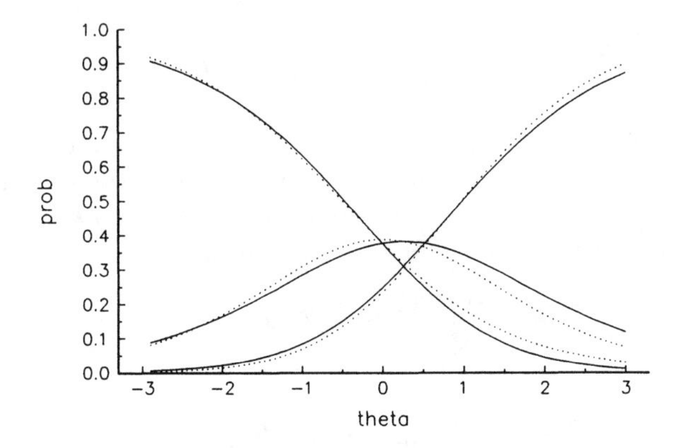

FIGURE 2. Item response functions under the PCM and the steps model.

the present model is not the only model where the analogy with a multistage testing design is utilized. Verhelst and Glas (1993) have used the same approach for the derivation of their dynamic test model. In the MML framework, it is assumed that the ability parameter θ is a stochastic variable with a density function $h(\cdot;\phi)$ indexed by a parameter vector ϕ. Glas (1988) shows that the dependency between the design and the responses does not result in a likelihood function that is different from the usual likelihood function for the Rasch model with data in an incomplete design. It is well known [see, for instance, Cressie and Holland (1983)] that IRT models can be viewed as parametric multinomial models. This fact will also be used here. Let $\{y\}$ be the set of all possible response patterns, and let n_y be the count of all persons producing y. The counts n_y have a parametric multinomial distribution with parameters N, which is the sample size, and $P(y;\beta,\phi)$, which is the probability of response pattern y given the parameters. Translated to the present problem, the log-likelihood to be maximized is thus given by

$$\ln L(\beta,\phi) = \sum_{\{y\}} n_y \ln P(y;\beta,\phi) = \sum_{\{y\}} n_y \int P(y \mid \theta,\beta) h(\theta;\phi)\, d\theta. \quad (13)$$

The equivalence of the log-likelihood function defined by Eq. (13) and the usual item response log-likelihood function with incomplete data makes it possible to directly use MML estimation with a normal distribution of ability (Bock and Aitkin, 1981; Mislevy, 1984; Glas and Verhelst, 1989), and nonparametric MML estimation (de Leeuw and Verhelst, 1986; Follmann, 1988; Verhelst and Glas, 1993).

For instance, if it is assumed that the ability distribution is normal with parameters μ and σ, and the test consist of K polytomous items, following Glas (1989), the likelihood equation for the item parameters can be derived as

$$\sum_{j=1}^{N} d_{ijh} y_{ijh} = \sum_{\{y\}} n_y E(\psi_{ih}(\theta) \mid y,\beta,\mu,\sigma), \quad (14)$$

for $i = 1,\ldots,K$ and $h = 1,\ldots,m_i$. So for every item i and category h, the parameters are estimated by equating the number of responses in category h of item i, $\sum_{j=1}^{N} d_{ijh} y_{ijh}$, to its expected value given the observed response patterns. For μ and σ, the likelihood equations are given by

$$\mu = N^{-1} \sum_{\{y\}} n_y E(\theta \mid y,\beta,\mu,\sigma) \quad (15)$$

and

$$\sigma^2 = N^{-1} \sum_{\{y\}} n_y E(\theta^2 \mid y,\beta,\mu,\sigma) - \mu^2. \quad (16)$$

So μ and σ are equated with the mean and standard deviation of the distribution of θ given the observed response patterns. To obtain a unique solution of Eqs. (14), (15), and (16), the latent scale must be fixed. This can be accomplished by setting μ equal to zero. For estimation errors and computational considerations, the reader is referred to Glas (1989).

Goodness of Fit

Like parameter estimation, testing the validity of the model presented above can be accomplished within the framework of parametric multinomial models. For example, Pearson's chi-square statistic and the likelihood-ratio statistics have direct applicability. The degrees of freedom associated with these statistics are given by the number of possible response patterns, minus the number of parameters to be estimated, minus one. However, the use of Pearson's chi-square statistic is rather limited because the number of response patterns grows exponentially with the number of items, so that even with a moderate number of items, many patterns will tend to have a very small expected frequency.

A more practical alternative can be based on the Lagrange multiplier (LM) statistic (Aitchison and Silvey, 1958). The idea underlying the LM statistic, as well as the equivalent efficient score statistic (Rao, 1948), will be summarized, before its application to the steps model is discussed. Let λ be the vector of parameters of some general model, and let λ_0 be the parameters of a special case of the general model. In the present case, it will be assumed that the restricted model is derived from the general model by fixing one or more parameters of the general model. So λ_0 is partitioned $\lambda_0' = (\lambda_{01}', \lambda_{02}') = (\lambda_{01}', c')$, where c is a vector of constants. Next, let $b_\lambda(\lambda^*)$ be the partial derivative of a log-likelihood function with respect to λ, evaluated at λ^*, that is, $(\partial/\partial\lambda)\ln L(\lambda)$ evaluated at λ^*. This partial derivative vector gives the rate of change in the log-likelihood at λ^*. Furthermore, $I_{\lambda,\lambda}(\lambda^*, \lambda^*)$ is defined as $-(\partial^2/\partial\lambda\partial\lambda')\ln L(\lambda, \lambda)$ evaluated at λ^*. The test statistic is defined as

$$LM = b(\hat{\lambda}_0)' I_{\lambda,\lambda}(\hat{\lambda}_0, \hat{\lambda}_0)^{-1} b(\hat{\lambda}_0). \tag{17}$$

This statistic is evaluated using the ML estimates of the parameters of the restricted model $\hat{\lambda}_0$, which is very convenient because in many instances the restricted model is much easier to estimate than the less restricted model.

The test statistic can be motivated as follows. The unrestricted elements of $\hat{\lambda}_0$, $\hat{\lambda}_{01}$ have a partial derivative zero, because their values originate from solving the likelihood equations. So the magnitude of the elements corresponding with fixed parameters determine the value of the statistic. The statistic itself has an asymptotic chi-square distribution with degrees of freedom equal to the number of parameters fixed. Since $b_\lambda(\hat{\lambda}_{01}) = \mathbf{0}$, the LM statistic can also be computed as

$$LM(c) = b_\lambda(c)' W^{-1} b_\lambda(c) \tag{18}$$

with

$$W = I_{\lambda_2,\lambda_2}(c,c) - I_{\lambda_2,\lambda_1}(c,\hat{\lambda}_{01}) I_{\lambda_1,\lambda_1}(\hat{\lambda}_{01},\hat{\lambda}_{01})^{-1} I_{\lambda_1,\lambda_2}(\hat{\lambda}_{01},c). \tag{19}$$

Note that if the restrictions are tested one at a time, W is a number easy to be inverted, and $I_{\lambda_1,\lambda_1}(\hat{\lambda}_{01},\hat{\lambda}_{01})$ needs to be inverted only once.

For application of the LM test to the steps model, a generalization of the model must be introduced. Let the probability of a correct response to a conceptual item be given by the two-parameter logistic model (Birnbaum, 1968), that is,

$$P(y_{ijh} = 1 \mid d_{ijh} = 1; \theta_j, \beta_{ih}, \alpha_{ih}) = \frac{\exp(\alpha_{ih}\theta_j - \beta_{ih})}{1 + \exp(\alpha_{ih}\theta_j - \beta_{ih})}, \tag{20}$$

where α_{ih} is a discrimination parameter. If the values of the discrimination parameter are considered to be known or imputed by hypothesis, the resulting model is known as the one-parameter logistic model (OPLM) (Verhelst and Eggen, 1989; Verhelst et al. 1993). From Eq. (20), it follows that Eq. (7) generalizes to

$$P(y_{ij} \mid \theta_j, \beta_i, \alpha_i) = \frac{\exp\left(s_{ij}\theta_j - \sum_{h=1}^{r_{ij}} \beta_{ih}\right)}{\prod_{h=1}^{\min(m_i, r_{jij}+1)} 1 + \exp(\alpha_{ih}\theta_j - \beta_{ih})}, \tag{21}$$

where $\alpha_i = (\alpha_{i1}, \ldots, \alpha_{ih}, \ldots, \alpha_{im_i})$, $s_{ij} = \sum_{h=1}^{m_i} d_{ijh}\alpha_{ih}y_{ijh}$, and $r_{ij} = \sum_{h=1}^{m_i} d_{ijh}y_{ijh}$. So s_{ij} is the sufficient statistic for the ability parameter, and r_{ij} stands for the number of steps taken. The likelihood function of the general model is now given by

$$\ln L(\beta, \phi, \alpha) = \sum_{\{y\}} n_y \ln \int P(y \mid \theta, \beta, \alpha) h(\theta; \phi)\, d\theta, \tag{22}$$

where α is a vector of values of the discrimination parameters for the items. The steps model can be considered as a restricted model where all discrimination indices are fixed to one and only the item difficulties β and the distribution parameters ϕ are free to vary. One of the possibilities is testing the constants α_{ih} one at a time. Using the above notation, $\lambda = (\beta, \phi, \alpha_{ih})$, and since only one restriction is imposed,

$$LM(\alpha_{ih}) = \frac{b(\alpha_{ih})^2}{W}, \tag{23}$$

where

$$W = I(\alpha_{ih}, \alpha_{ih}) - I(\alpha_{ih}, \hat{\lambda}_1) I(\hat{\lambda}_1, \hat{\lambda}_1)^{-1} I(\hat{\lambda}_1, \alpha_{ih}), \tag{24}$$

with $\lambda_1 = (\beta, \phi)$. Since the matrix $I(\hat{\lambda}_1, \hat{\lambda}_1)^{-1}$ is available as a result of the estimation procedure, computation of the statistic defined in Eq. (23) is easy.

The algebraic sign of $b(\alpha_{ih})$ gives an indication on how to change α_{ih} to obtain a better fit. A positive sign suggests a decrease, a negative value to an increase of α_{ih}. So, the test statistic

$$G_{ih} = \frac{|b(\alpha_{ih})|}{\sqrt{W}} \mathrm{sgn}(b(\alpha_{ih})) \tag{25}$$

is asymptotically standard normally distributed, and can be used to change the value of α_{ih} in case it is significant. In order to get a quick impression of the amount of change in α_{ih} needed, one might apply the univariate Newton–Raphson algorithm for α_{ih} at $\hat{\lambda}$, yielding the simple result that this change is equal to

$$\frac{b(\alpha_{ih})}{I(\alpha_{ih}, \alpha_{ih})}. \tag{26}$$

This procedure can, of course, also be extended to include more than one discrimination parameter. In that case, Eqs. (18) and (19) must be used, and the computation will become somewhat more elaborate. Furthermore, the procedure also gives rise to an extension of the model. One could, for instance, propose a model where items have fixed values for the discrimination parameter different from one, and then test the hypotheses implied by these alternative restrictions using the LM test. Just as the steps model is an alternative to the PCM, this steps model with imputed discrimination indices can be viewed as an alternative to the PCM with imputed values for the discrimination parameter or to the OPLM discussed earlier.

Example

An example will be given of the sensitivity, or rather the insensitivity, by which test statistics distinguish between the PCM and the steps model. The example concerns real data from examinations in Geography for HAVO (Higher General Education) in the Netherlands. The complete study also involved data from several examinations, but giving a full account of the findings is beyond the scope of the present chapter. Furthermore, for practical reasons, the presentation will be restricted to three items only. All three items have three response categories, that is, $m_i = 2$ for all three items. The sample of persons consisted of 1996 students. The results of the estimation procedure are shown in Table 3. In the column labeled "Score," the numbers of responses in the various item categories are given. In the following columns, the estimates of the item parameters and their asymptotic standard errors are given both for the PCM and the steps model, respectively. The estimates were computed using an MML procedure under the assumption of a normal ability distribution. The estimates of the standard deviation of these distributions are given at the bottom of the table. The means of the estimates were fixed to zero for identification of

TABLE 3. Overview of Parameter Estimates for the PCM and the Steps Model.

PCM Estimates			Steps Estimates					
Item	Cat	Score	δ_{ih}	Se(δ_{ih})	β_{ih}		Se(β_{ih})	G_{ih}
1	1	839	−1.897		0.079	−2.442	0.084	0.305
	2	920	0.021		0.088	0.020	0.058	−1.101
2	1	960	−1.564		0.073	−1.973	0.075	−0.772
	2	701	0.548		0.084	0.570	0.063	0.683
3	1	880	−0.210		0.057	−0.407	0.057	0.052
	2	278	1.737		0.097	1.825	0.091	−0.200
		N=1996	μ	:	0.000	μ	:	0.000
			σ	:	1.012	σ	:	1.138
			Se(σ)	:	0.037	Se(σ)	:	0.41

the two models. Again, there is no clear-cut relation between the item parameter estimates. In the last column of Table 3, the outcomes of the signed square-root Lagrange multiplier statistics G_{ih}, defined by Eq. (25), are given. It can be seen that none of these standard normally distributed statistics was significant, so the steps model needed not be rejected.

In Table 4, the fit of the steps model is evaluated using Pearson's chi-square statistic. In the column labeled "Response Pattern," the 27 possible response patterns are listed; in the column labeled "Score," the sum scores associated with the response patterns are given; the columns labeled "Observed" and "Expected" contain the observed and expected frequencies; whereas in the last column, the contributions of the differences between the observed and expected frequencies of response patterns to the Pearson's chi-square, given at the bottom of the table, are shown. Again, the steps model was not rejected. However, the same conclusion held for the PCM. The fit of the latter model was tested using two so-called generalized Pearson statistics proposed by Glas and Verhelst (1989), the R_0- and the R_{1m}-statistic. The R_0-statistic is based on the difference between the observed and expected distribution of the persons sum scores and has power against incorrect assumptions on the ability distribution. The data for the present example are given in Table 5. In the column labeled "Scaled Diff," the squared difference between observed and expected frequency divided by the expected frequency is given. R_0 is, however, not based on a simple addition of these scaled differences because the dependence between the terms and the effects of estimation of the parameters would produce a test statistic with an asymptotic distribution difficult to derive. To provide a solution, Glas and Verhelst (1989) introduced the class of generalized Pearson statistics. Roughly speaking, for these statistics the differences are combined into a quadratic form using the inverse of their covariance matrix. So, if $\hat{d}$ is a vector of the differences in Table 5, the R_0-statistic is

TABLE 4. Observed and Expected Frequencies of Response Patterns Under the Steps Model.

	Response Pattern	Score	Observed	Expected	Contribution
1	0c0c0c	0	57	54.05	0.16
2	0c0c10	1	21	17.95	0.51
3	0c0c11	2	1	1.37	0.10
4	0c100c	1	75	74.50	0.00
5	0c1010	2	41	42.49	0.05
6	0c1011	3	2	5.32	2.07
7	0c110c	2	18	17.99	0.00
8	0c1110	3	16	18.68	0.38
9	0c1111	4	6	4.54	0.46
10	100c0c	1	96	106.22	0.98
11	100c10	2	60	57.27	0.12
12	100c11	3	7	6.67	0.01
13	10100c	2	228	224.18	0.06
14	101010	3	169	185.35	1.44
15	101011	4	32	32.02	0.00
16	10110c	3	86	81.78	0.21
17	101110	4	128	112.28	2.19
18	101111	5	33	34.86	0.09
19	110c0c	2	52	41.70	2.54
20	110c10	3	31	40.57	2.25
21	110c11	4	10	9.11	0.08
22	11100c	3	143	141.77	0.01
23	111010	4	201	194.65	0.20
24	111011	5	69	60.43	1.21
25	11110c	4	83	95.96	1.75
26	111110	5	213	211.85	0.00
27	111111	6	118	122.31	0.15

TABLE 5. Information on the R_0-Statistic.

Score	Observed	Expected	Difference	Scaled Diff.
0	57	60.19	−3.19	−0.41
1	192	197.77	−5.77	−0.43
2	400	370.56	29.43	1.69
3	454	477.18	−23.18	−1.21
4	460	459.30	0.69	0.03
5	315	315.65	−0.65	−0.04
6	118	115.32	2.67	0.25

given by $\hat{d}'\hat{W}^{-1}\hat{d}$, where W is the covariance matrix of d and both d and W are evaluated using MML estimates. For the derivation of the asymptotic distribution, see Glas and Verhelst (1989). The R_{1m}-statistic is based on the difference between the observed and expected frequencies of scores in item categories evaluated at different score levels. Computation of R_0 resulted in a value of 4.01 (five degrees of freedom, pr. = 0.40), computation of R_{1m} produced 11.55 (14 degrees of freedom, pr. = 0.64). The PCM could not be rejected. The results presented here are typical of the results of the complete analysis: If model fit was obtained for one model, the other model would also fit. So for real data sets, it is also difficult to distinguish between the two models.

Discussion

Comparing the steps model with the PCM, the former has an advantage with respect to the interpretation of the item parameters, while the latter has more favorable mathematical properties. In the steps model, the item parameters are unambiguously related to the response categories of the items, and can legitimately be interpreted as their difficulty parameters. This fact opens up the possibility of further modeling of response behavior by imposing linear restrictions on the item parameters. On the other hand, the steps model lacks the possibility of CML estimation of the item parameters. But even if the model is extended with assumptions concerning the ability distribution, computation of the MML estimates is more laborious than for the PCM, because all possible response patterns are involved, while the PCM estimation equations are based only on the counts of the responses in the item categories and the frequency distribution of the person total scores (Glas and Verhelst, 1989).

In spite of the foregoing conclusions, simulation studies and studies with real data show that the item response functions of the models closely resemble each other. Therefore, if the interpretation of the item parameters prevails, that is, if each of the item parameter parameters should be related unequivocally to one, and only one, response category, the PCM parameters can be transformed to steps parameters using the procedure based on the minimization of the loss function defined in Eq. (9), whereas the rather heavy burden of computing MML estimates for the Steps Model can be shortened using the estimates for the PCM as starting values.

References

Abramowitz, M. and Stegun, I.A. (1974). *Handbook of Mathematical Functions.* New York: Dover Publications.

Aitchison, J. and Silvey, S.D. (1958). Maximum likelihood estimation of parameters subject to restraints. *Annals of Mathematical Statistics* **29**, 813–828.

Birnbaum, A. (1968). Some latent trait models and their use in inferring an examinee's ability. In F.M. Lord and M.R. Novick, *Statistical Theories of Mental Test Scores.* Reading, MA: Addison-Wesley.

Bock, R.D. and Aitkin, M. (1981). Marginal maximum likelihood estimation of item parameters: An application of an EM-algorithm. *Psychometrika* **46**, 443–459.

Cressie, N. and Holland, P.W. (1983). Characterizing the manifest probabilities of latent trait models. *Psychometrika* **48**, 129–141.

de Leeuw, J. and Verhelst, N.D. (1986). Maximum likelihood estimation in generalized Rasch models. *Journal of Educational Statistics* **11**, 183–196.

De Vries, H.H. (1988). *Het Partial Credit Model en het Sequentiële Rasch Model met Stochastisch Design* [The partial credit model and the sequential Rasch model with stochastic design]. Amsterdam, the Netherlands: Universiteit van Amsterdam.

Fischer, G.H. (1974). *Einführung in die Theorie psychologischer Tests* [Introduction to the Theory of Psychological Tests]. Bern: Huber.

Fischer, G.H. (1981). On the existence and uniqueness of maximum likelihood estimates in the Rasch model. *Psychometrika* **46**, 59–77.

Follmann, D. (1988). Consistent estimation in the Rasch model based on nonparametric margins. *Psychometrika* **53**, 553–562.

Glas, C.A.W. (1988). The Rasch model and multi-stage testing. *Journal of Educational Statistics* **13**, 45–52.

Glas, C.A.W. (1989). *Contributions to Estimating and Testing Rasch Models.* Doctoral dissertation, University of Twente, Enschede, The Netherlands.

Glas, C.A.W. and Verhelst, N.D. (1989). Extensions of the partial credit model. *Psychometrika* **54**, 635–659.

Masters, G.N. (1982). A Rasch model for partial credit scoring. *Psychometrika* **47**, 149–174.

Mislevy, R.J. (1984). Estimating latent distributions. *Psychometrika* **49**, 359–381.

Molenaar, I.W. (1983). *Item Steps* (Heymans Bulletins HB-83-630-EX). Groningen, The Netherlands: Psychologisch Instituut RU Groningen.

Rao, C.R. (1948). Large sample tests of statistical hypothesis concerning several parameters with applications to problems of estimation. *Proceedings of the Cambridge Philosophical Society* **44**, 50–57.

Rasch, G. (1960). *Probabilistic Models for Some Intelligence and Attainment Tests.* Copenhagen: Danish Institute for Educational Research.

Verhelst, N.D. and Eggen, T.J.H.M. (1989). *Psychometrische en Statistische Aspecten ven Peilingsonderzoek* [Psychometric and Statistical Aspects of Assessment Research] (PPON-Rapport, 4). Arnhem: Cito.

Verhelst, N.D. and Glas, C.A.W. (1993). A dynamic generalization of the Rasch model. *Psychometrika* **58**, 395–415.

Verhelst, N.D., Glas, C.A.W., and Verstralen, H.H.F.M. (1995). *OPLM: One Parameter Logistic Model: Computer Program and Manual.* Arnhem: Cito.

8
Sequential Models for Ordered Responses

Gerhard Tutz

Introduction

The model considered in this chapter is suited for a special type of response. First, the response should be from ordered categories, i.e., a graded response. Second, the categories or levels should be recorded successively in a stepwise manner. An example illustrates this type of item, which is often found in practice:

> Wright and Masters (1982) consider the item $\sqrt{9.0/0.3 - 5} =$? Three levels of performance may be distinguished: No subproblem solved (Level 0), $9.0/0.3 = 30$ solved (Level 1), $30 - 5 = 25$ solved (Level 2), $\sqrt{25} = 5$ (Level 3). The important feature is that each level in a solution to the problem can be reached only if the previous level is reached.

The main feature of a *sequential* or *step model* is that the stepwise manner of solving an item is exploited. The transition from one level to the next is modeled and item parameters are interpreted directly in terms of the difficulty of this transition. It should be emphasized that for sequential models, steps are *consecutive* steps in problem solving: The next step in the solution to a problem can be performed successfully only if the previous steps were completed successfully. Item difficulties refer to the difficulty of solving the next step.

A quite different concept of "steps" is used as the building block of the partial credit model (PCM) (Masters, 1982, this volume). This is seen from the PCM in the form

$$P(U_{ij} = h \mid U_{ij} \in \{h-1, h\}) = \exp(\theta_j - b_{ih})/(1 + \exp(\theta_j - b_{ih})),$$

where U_{ij} denotes the response, θ_j the ability of person j and b_{ih} the difficulty of "step h." It is seen that the response $U_{ij} = h$ probability is formalized as a dichotomous Rasch model. However, the difficulty b_{ih} is not the difficulty of a Rasch model for the step from $h-1$ to h *given* at least level $h-1$ is reached (which is the difficulty in sequential models). The step modeled by the PCM is a *local* step; it is conditioned on the response being in category $h-1$ or h.

Suppose a person solves $9.0/0.3 = 30$ (Level 1) in the example. The next step is the solving of the second subproblem $(30-5=25)$. Assuming a model like the Rasch model for this subproblem is the sequential approach, whereas the PCM assumes a Rasch model *given* the first and second subproblem but *not* the third one are solved. The difference between the two models is evident from the typical quote that in the PCM the Rasch model determines "how likely it is that a person will make a 2 *rather than* a 1" (Masters, 1982). This process should be clearly distinguished from modeling the process of sequential solving of subproblems.

In the regression context, models of this type are called models based on "adjacent categories logits" (Agresti, 1984, p. 133). For the PCM the adjacent categories logits have the form

$$\log(P(U_{ij}=h) \mid P(U_{ij}=h-1)) = \theta - b_{ih},$$

which clearly shows that the log-rate of adjacent categories is modeled instead of the next step. The PCM is well suited for the analysis of rating scales but less appropriate for modeling the process of subsequent solving of subproblems. For items as in the example above, the sequential model captures more adequately the underlying process. Sequential models have been considered previously in categorical regression (McCullagh, 1980, Agresti, 1984) and in discrete survival analysis (Kalbfleish and Prentice, 1980). In the context of item response theory (IRT) where regressors are not observed, sequential or item step approaches are found in Molenaar (1983) and Tutz (1990).

Presentation of the Model

Let the graded response for item i and person j be given by the response variable $U_{ij} \in \{0,\ldots,m_i\}$. Item i has levels $0,\ldots,m_i$, where 0 stands for the lowest and m_i stands for the highest level.

Item Steps and Response: The Sequential Mechanism

The basic assumption is that each item is solved step by step. Let U_{ijh}, $h = 1,\ldots,m_i$, denote the step from level $h-1$ to level h, where $U_{ijh}=1$ stands for successful transition and $U_{ijh}=0$ denotes an unsuccessful transition. Consider the response process step by step.

Step 1. The process always starts at level 0. If the transition to level 1 (response category 1) fails, the process stops and the examinee's score is $U_{ij}=0$. If the transition is successful, the examinee's score is at least level

1. Thus,

$$U_{ij} = 0 \quad \text{if} \quad U_{ij1} = 0.$$

Step 2. If $U_{ij1} = 1$ the person works on the second step from level 1 to level 2. Successful transition yields response $U_{ij} \geq 2$; when the person fails at the second step, the process stops. Thus,

$$U_{ij} = 1 \quad \text{given} \quad U_{ij} \geq 1 \quad \text{if} \quad U_{ij2} = 0.$$

The conditioning on $U_{ij} \geq 1$ is essential since the second step is only considered if the first step was successful ($U_{ij1} = 1$).

Step $h+1$. Step $h+1$ is under consideration only if $U_{ij1} = \ldots = U_{ijh} = 1$ or equivalently $U_{ij} \geq h$. In the same way as for previous steps, response h is obtained if the transition to $h + 1$ fails:

$$U_{ij} = h \quad \text{given} \quad U_{ij} \geq h \quad \text{if} \quad U_{ij,h+1} = 0. \tag{1}$$

Equation (1) gives the *sequential response mechanism*, which is based solely on the assumption of a step-by-step process.

Modeling of Steps

In order to obtain a model that links observed scores and abilities, the steps have to be modeled. One way of modeling the success of transitions is by assuming

$$U_{ijh}^* \equiv \theta_j + \varepsilon_{ijh}, \tag{2}$$

where θ_j is the ability of person j and ε_{ijh} a noise variable with distribution function F. The successful performance in the $(h+1)$th step is modeled by

$$U_{ij,h+1} = 1 \quad \text{if} \quad U_{ij,h+1}^* \geq b_{i,h+1}, \tag{3}$$

where $b_{i,h+1}$ is the difficulty of the $(h + 1)$th step of item i. Thus, the $(h + 1)$th step is given by the dichotomous response model

$$P(U_{ij,h+1} = 1) = F(\theta_j - b_{i,h+1}). \tag{4}$$

If F is the logistic function, $F(x) = \exp(x)/(1 + \exp(x))$, each step is modeled by the dichotomous Rasch model. Thus, instead of the derivation from latent random variables, a dichotomous Rasch model for steps could be assumed. However, the sequential mechanism in Eq. (1) together with the latent abilities assumption given in Eq. (2) and the threshold mechanism in Eq. (3) yield a larger class of models.

Using the equivalence of $U_{ij,h+1} = 1$ and $U_{ij} > h$ *given* $U_{ij} \geq h$, the sequential model (with distribution function F) has the form

$$P(U_{ij} > h \mid U_{ij} \geq h) = F(\theta_j - b_{i,h+1}), \quad h = 0, \ldots, m_i - 1, \tag{5}$$

or equivalently,

$$P(U_{ij}=h)=\begin{cases}\left(\prod_{s=0}^{h-1} F(\theta_j-b_{i,s+1})\right)(1-F(\theta_j-b_{i,h+1})), & \\ \qquad \text{for } h=0,\ldots,m_i-1 & \\ \prod_{s=0}^{m_i-1} F(\theta_j-b_{i,s+1}) & \\ \qquad \text{for } h=m_i. & \end{cases} \tag{6}$$

Equation (6) has a simple interpretation: The examinee's response is in category h ($h<m_i$) if the h steps $U_{ij1},\ldots,U_{ijh}$ are successful but the $(h+1)$th step is unsuccessful; for category m_i all the steps $U_{ij1},\ldots,U_{ijm_i}$ have to be successful. The model arising from the logistic distribution function F is called *sequential* or *stepwise Rasch model.* Figure 1 shows response functions for four categories or stages in an item. The first picture shows the probabilities for scores of 0, 1, 2, and 3 if item (step) difficulties are equal with $b_{i1}=b_{i2}=b_{i3}=0.0$. This means a person with ability $\theta_j=0.0$ has a probability of 0.5 at each step. As is seen, for this person $P(U_{ij}=0)=0.5$ and probabilities for the higher score levels of 1, 2, and 3 are very low. In the second picture, the second step is easy with $b_{i2}=-1.0$ and the third step is more difficult to perform with $b_{i3}=2.0$. The second threshold is unchanged ($b_{i2}=0.0$). Consequently, the probability for score category 2 is much higher now. For category 3 the probability is rather similar to that in the first picture. The reason is that, although the threshold b_{i3} is higher, the increased probability of categories 1 and 2 now has to be taken into account.

Interpretation of model parameters is simple and straightforward. Since the model is derived from a stepwise mechanism, interpretation may be done in terms of dichotomous response models, which are used to model the transitions. For example, in the stepwise Rasch model, θ_j is the usual ability that determines each step. For low b_{ih} the corresponding subproblem is easily solved; for high b_{ih} the specific step is hard to perform. It should be noted that the model is unidimensional. There is one latent scale for abilities and item difficulties, a unidimensional ability is measured. The ordered response is used to measure that ability more precisely than is possible with dichotomously scored items.

Relation to Special Cases of the Graded Response Model

In a simple version of the graded response model (Samejima, 1969), specialized to equal discrimination (Andrich, 1978), this cumulative model has the form

$$P(U_{ij}\geq h)=F(\theta_j-\tilde{b}_{ih}),\quad h=1,\ldots,m_i \tag{7}$$

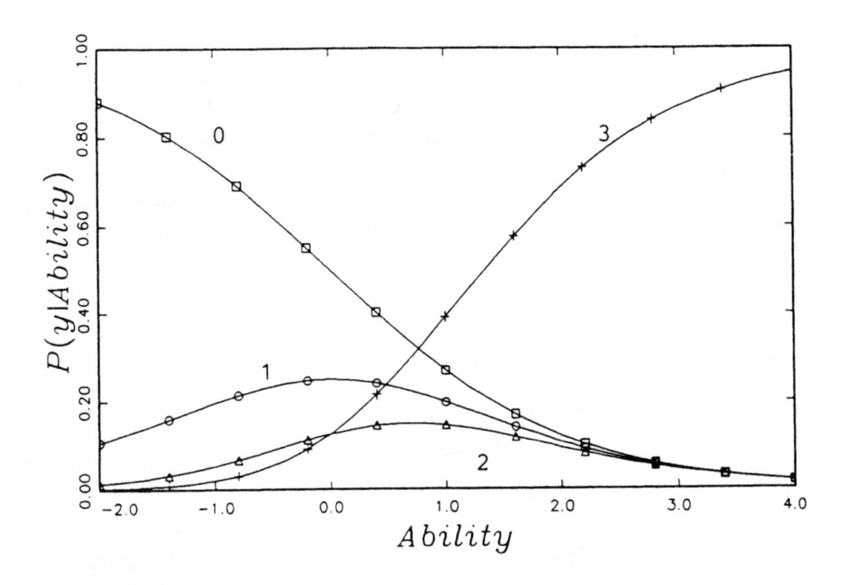

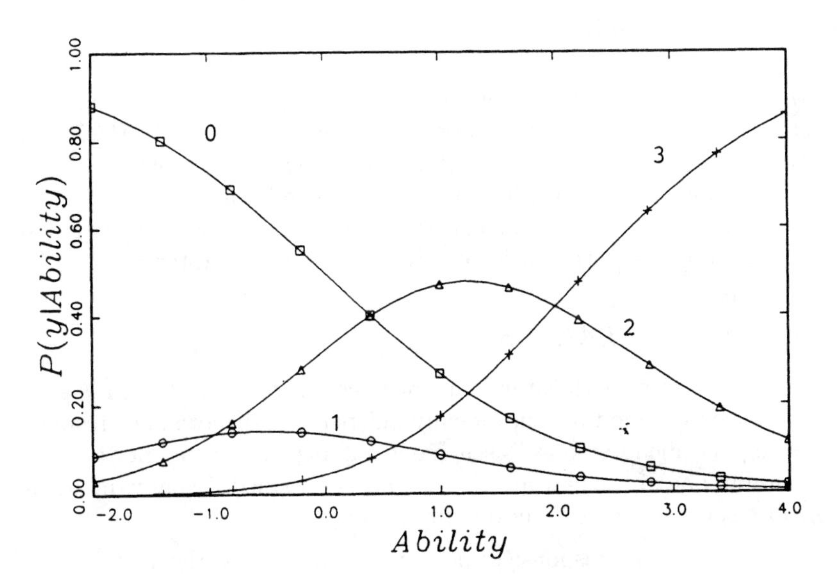

FIGURE 1. Category probabilities for two items, the first with $b_{i1} = b_{i2} = b_{i3} = 0$, the second with $b_{i1} = 0.0$, $b_{12} = -1.0$, $b_{i3} = 2.0$. (Numbers denote the category.)

where item parameters are ordered by $-\infty = \tilde{b}_{j0} < \ldots < \tilde{b}_{jm_i}$ and F is a distribution function (in Samejima's work, F is usually assumed to be of a logistic form). Item parameters may be interpreted as thresholds on the ability scale, where $U_{ij} = h$ is observed if the ability, which is randomized by the addition of a noise variable, lies between thresholds b_{ih} and $b_{i,h+1}$.

Consider the sequential model in Eq. (5) with the extreme-value distribution function $F(x) = \exp(-\exp(-x))$. A simple derivation shows that the sequential model

$$P(U_{ij} > h \mid U_{ij} \geq h) = F(\theta_j - b_{i,h+1})$$

is equivalent to the cumulative model

$$P(U_{ij} \geq h) = F(\theta_j - \tilde{b}_{ih}),$$

where $\tilde{b}_{ih} = \log(e^{b_{i1}} + \ldots + e^{b_{ih}})$. This means that for the special case of the extreme-value distribution function (and only for this case) the stepwise approach is equivalent to the cumulative approach [see also Tutz (1991)]. Then, the transformed item parameters $\tilde{b}_{ih}$ may again be interpreted as thresholds on a latent continuum and $-\infty = \tilde{b}_{i0} < \ldots < \tilde{b}_{im}$ holds.

Parameter Estimation

Two estimation methods are considered next, namely, joint maximum likelihood (JML) estimation and marginal maximum likelihood (MML) estimation based on a prior distribution. The alternative concept, which is often used for dichotomous Rasch models, is conditional maximum likelihood (CML) estimation. Although this principle may be used with some modification (Tutz, 1990), it is not presented in this chapter.

Joint Maximum Likelihood

It will be shown next that the joint (or unconditional) likelihood is equivalent to the likelihood of conditionally independent dichotomous responses following the dichotomous Rasch model. If person j attempts item i, a response in one of the categories $0, \ldots, m_i$ is obtained. Usually, multicategorical responses are given in dummy coding with

$$x_{ijh} = \begin{cases} 1 & \text{response of person } j \text{ to item } i \text{ in category } h \\ 0 & \text{otherwise.} \end{cases}$$

Thus, the vector $x_{ij} = (x_{ij0}, \ldots, x_{ijm_i})$ with just one "1" in the components is obtained. The kernel of the log-likelihood contribution from item i and person j has the common form

$$l_{ij} = \sum_{h=0}^{m_i} x_{ijh} \log \pi_{ijh}, \tag{8}$$

where $\pi_{ijh} = P(U_{ij} = h)$ is the probability of a response in category h. Here l_{ij} is an abbreviation for $\log L_{ij}$, where L_{ij} is the likelihood contributed by person j attempting item i.

For the sequential model, it is useful to do some recoding in terms of the transition process given by $U_{ij1}, \ldots$. The essential term in Eq. (5) is

$$\gamma_{ij,h+1} = P(U_{ij} > h \mid U_{ij} \geq h) = P(U_{ij,h+1} = 1 \mid U_{ij1} = \ldots = U_{ijh} = 1),$$

which represents the probability of the transition to category $h+1$ given all previous transitions were successful.

Equation (8) can be written with

$$\pi_{ijh} = P(U_{ij} = h \mid U_{ij} \geq h) \prod_{s=0}^{h-1} P(U_{ij} > s \mid U_{ij} \geq s) = (1-\gamma_{ij,h+1}) \prod_{s=1}^{h} \gamma_{ijs}.$$

Moreover, instead of $(x_{ij0}, \ldots, x_{ijm_i})$ the coding of transitions can be given by

$$u_{ijh} = 1 - (x_{ij0} + \ldots + x_{ij,h-1}), \quad h = 1, \ldots, m_i.$$

It is seen that $u_{ijh} = 1$ if transition to category h takes place and $u_{ijh} = 0$ if the response is in category $h-1$. For example, a response in category 3 is recorded as $x_{ij} = (0,0,0,1,0,\ldots,0)$ in "observation coding," but $u_{ij} = (1,1,1,0,\ldots,0)$ in "transition coding." If $m_i = 3$ and the response is in category 3, $x_{ij} = (0,0,0,1)$ in coding observations, and $u_{ij} = (1,1,1)$ in coding transition data. Using this recoding, after some derivation it can be shown that the log-likelihood expression in Eq. (8) has the form

$$\begin{aligned} l_{ij} &= \sum_{s=0}^{m_i-1} x_{ijs} \log(1-\gamma_{ij,s+1}) + (1 - x_{ij0} - \ldots - x_{ijs}) \log \gamma_{ij,s+1} \\ &= \sum_{s=1}^{\min(h_{ij}+1, m_i)} u_{ijs} \log \gamma_{ijs} + (1-u_{ijs}) \log(1-\gamma_{ijs}), \end{aligned} \tag{9}$$

where r_{ij} is the observed response category for individual j to item i. Since

$$\gamma_{ijs} = P(U_{ij} > s-1 \mid U_{ij} \geq s-1) = F(\theta_j - b_{is}), \tag{10}$$

represents the probability that the sth step is successful (transition from $s-1$ to s), l_{ij} is equivalent to the contribution to the likelihood of the dichotomous response model in Eq. (10) when person j meets the pseudo-items "transition from $s-1$ to s in item i" for $s = 1, \ldots, s_{ij} = \min(h_{ij} + 1, m_i)$. The number of pseudo-items is $s_{ij} = \min(h_{ij}+1, m_i)$; if $h_{ij} < m_i$, then the h_{ij} successful transitions and the last failing transition have to be included; if $h_{ij} = m$, all the m transitions were successful and have to be included. Thus, the total log-likelihood for persons $j = 1, \ldots, N$ and items $i = 1, \ldots, n$ given by

$$\log L = \sum_{ij} l_{ij}$$

is equivalent to the dichotomous transition model in Eq. (10), where person j has observations $u_{ij1}, \ldots, u_{ijs_{ij}}$, $i = 1, \ldots, n$. It should be noted that the items that are encountered by person j depend on the person. Thus, one has an incomplete design. The existence and uniqueness of estimates from this design were investigated by Fischer (1981). This embedding into the framework of dichotomous response models makes things easier. By considering transitions and the corresponding pseudo-items, standard software and inference procedures developed for dichotomous models may be used.

In order to use programs for regression models, the "regression term" $\theta_j - b_{is}$ should have the usual linear form $w_{ijs}^T\beta$, where β is an unknown parameter. The design vector corresponding to observation u_{ijs} is given by $w_{ijs}^T = (1(j)^T, z_{is})$, where the unit vector $1(j) = (0, \ldots, 1, \ldots, 0)^T$ with 1 in column j contains the coding of person j and the item is coded by $z_{ij}^T = -(z_{11}^{is}, \ldots, z_{im}^{is}, z_{21}^{is}, \ldots, z_{nm_n}^{is})$, where $z_{lm}^{is} = 1$ if $(i,s) = (l,m)$ and $z_{lm}^{is} = 0$ otherwise.

Marginal Estimates

The basic idea of marginal estimates is to consider the person ability θ_j as a random effect drawn from a distribution with density $g(\theta)$. Then integration over $g(\theta)$ yields the marginal likelihood.

By use of Eq. (9) the marginal likelihood for person j is given by

$$L_j^m = \int \prod_{i=1}^{n} \prod_{s=1}^{s_{ij}} F(\theta - b_{is})^{u_{ijs}} (1 - F(\theta - b_{is}))^{1-u_{ijs}} g(\theta) d\theta. \tag{11}$$

The marginal likelihood is again given in the form of dichotomous response models where instead of items $1, \ldots, n$ the pseudo-items corresponding to transition $u_{iy1}, \ldots, u_{ijs_{ij}}$, $i = 1, \ldots, n$ are considered.

In the same way as for the joint estimates in the sequential Rasch model, the methods for the dichotomous model may be applied (Bock and Aitkin 1981; Thissen 1982). A helpful device is the embedding of the estimation into the framework of generalized random effects regression models. Then the new methods and programs that have been developed in this area may be used.

The parameters to be estimated may be summarized into $b^T = (b_1^T, \ldots, b_n^T)$, where $b_i^T = (b_{i1}, \ldots, b_{im_i})$ are the difficulty parameters associated with the transition from one level to another for item i. The corresponding design vector when transition from level $s-1$ to level s for item i is considered may be chosen by $z_{is}^T = -(z_{11}^{is}, \ldots, z_{1m}^{is}, z_{21}^{is}, \ldots, z_{nm_n}^{is})$, where $z_{im}^{is} = 1$ if $(i,s) = (l,m)$ and $z_{lm}^{is} = 0$ otherwise.

Then the term in Eq. (11) that corresponds to the linear influence term in regression models may be written by $\theta - b_{is} = \theta + z_{is}^T b$. This assumption means for person j with random effect θ_j we have for $s = 1, \ldots, s_{ij}$, $i =$

$1, \ldots, n$

dichotomous response	u_{ijs}
linear regression term	$\theta + z_{is}^T b$
generalized random effects model	$P(U_{ijs} = 1) = F(\theta + z_{is}^T b)$,
	$\theta \sim N(0, \sigma^2)$.

For this model various estimation procedures are available. Numerical integration methods are based on maximizing the log-likelihood

$$l = \sum_j \log L_j^m \tag{12}$$

with respect to the unknown parameters b (item difficulties) and σ (heterogeneity of individuals). The integral in L is solved by Gauss–Hermite integration, or alternatively Monte Carlo methods may be used. Procedures for the estimation of nonrandom generalized linear models may be effectively used for the construction of the maximization algorithm. Alternatively, estimation of b and σ may be based on posterior modes yielding an EM type algorithm (Stiratelli et al. 1984). Details for both methods may be found in Fahrmeir and Tutz (1994, Chap. 7). Further methods are given by Anderson and Aitkin (1985), Anderson and Hinde (1988), Zeger et al. (1988), and Waclawiw and Liang (1993).

Goodness of Fit

Goodness of fit checks may be based on the dichotomous nature of transitions to higher levels. The basic idea is to consider only persons who have reached at least level $h_1, \ldots, h_n$ for items $1, \ldots, n$. Then, consider only the transition from h_1 to $h_1 + 1, \ldots, h_n$ to $h_n + 1$, which are determined by a dichotomous Rasch model. For the dichotomous model the local goodness of fit may be checked by all methods given in Hambleton and Swaminathan (1985), Andersen (1973), and Kelderman (1984). As an example consider the log-likelihood-ratio statistic, which is the basic statistic investigated in Kelderman (1984). It has the form

$$G^2(m, m^*) = 2 \sum m^* \log(m^*/m),$$

where m and m^* stand for the expected counts of model M and M^*, M being a submodel of M^*. Here, M stands for the Rasch model and M^* may be chosen as the saturated model that does not restrict the data.

The log-likelihood-ratio statistic gives a measure for the goodness of fit of the transitions from h_i to $h_i + 1$, $i = 1, \ldots, n$. Comparison with the asymptotic chi square distribution shows if the model is appropriate for these steps. Of course, testing all the possible combinations of binary transitions yields $m_1 \cdot \ldots \cdot m_n$ tests. The resulting multiple test procedure makes it necessary to adjust the significance level, e.g., by using closed test procedures (Bauer et al. 1988). By considering all the possible combinations of transitions each step is tested several times. Therefore, one may consider only specific groups of transitions. For example, one may build a group for the transitions from categories 0 to 1 for all items, for 1 to 2 for all items, etc. Then the number of transition groups is the maximal number of item steps. If $m_i = m$, the number of groups is m. Consequently, one has only m goodness of fit statistics G^2 corresponding to the steps in the items. This procedure is also used in the example below.

Example

The example refers to the solution of problems in statistics. Six items with three levels, 0, 1, 2, were presented to 99 students. For most of the items the first step was to find the proper statistical tool (e.g., Wilcoxon test) and the second step was to carry out the computations and interpret the results. For some of the items, finding a statistical procedure and using it was considered as one step, the second step required answering an additional question such as a question about the invariance properties of the procedure. The fitted model was the sequential Rasch model with F being the logistic distribution function. The parameters involved were the ability scores $\theta_j, j = 1, \ldots, 99$ and the item difficulties $b_{i1}, b_{i2}, i = 1, \ldots, 6$. In joint maximum likelihood estimation 111 parameters would be estimated. Since the primary interest in this example was in the item parameters, the focus here was on marginal estimation where only the 12 item parameters needed to be estimated. The estimation procedures considered were posterior mode estimation as well as Gauss–Hermite integration with 6 and 8 quadrature points [GH(6) and GH(8), respectively]. The underlying assumption was that abilities were drawn from $N(0, \sigma^2)$. Table 1 shows the estimated item difficulties with standard errors given in parentheses. Estimation was done by an easy to handle menu driven version of GLAMOUR (Fahrmeir et al., 1990).

The results of the marginal estimation procedures were quite similar, indicating that 6 to 8 quadrature points were sufficient. As is seen from the estimated standard deviation $\hat{\sigma}$, heterogeneity across individuals was quite high. Consider the first item with $b_{11} = -0.527$ and $b_{12} = -0.279$. Since $b_{11} < b_{12}$ the first step was easier than the second step. For a person with $\theta = 0$ the probability of performing the first step successfully was $F(0.527) = 0.845$; the probability of performing the second step successfully was $F(0.279) = 0.570$. The resulting probability of response categories 0, 1, 2 for this person is 0.155, 0.363, 0.489, respectively. The principle that the first step is easier than the second step holds for items 1, 3, 4, 5, and 6 but not for item 2. In item 2 for the second step the difficulty was very low and the probability of successful performance was $F(1.488) = 0.810$. From the

TABLE 1. Marginal estimates based on Gauss–Hermite quadrature [GH(6) and GH(8)] and posterior modes.

	GH(6)		GH(8)		Posterior Mode
b_{11}	−0.527	(0.276)	−0.530	(0.294)	−0.504
b_{12}	−0.279	(0.367)	−0.285	(0.394)	−0.297
b_{21}	−0.365	(0.295)	−0.369	(0.315)	−0.357
b_{22}	−1.448	(0.471)	−1.452	(0.503)	−1.385
b_{31}	−0.365	(0.288)	−0.369	(0.307)	−0.357
b_{32}	−0.421	(0.414)	−0.424	(0.439)	−0.426
b_{41}	−0.692	(0.292)	−0.695	(0.313)	−0.655
b_{42}	0.080	(0.344)	0.077	(0.367)	0.036
b_{51}	−0.748	(0.290)	−0.751	(0.314)	−0.706
b_{52}	0.958	(0.351)	0.955	(0.369)	0.838
b_{61}	−0.979	(0.322)	−0.983	(0.347)	−0.917
b_{62}	0.233	(0.330)	0.233	(0.352)	0.181
$\hat{\sigma}$	1.212	(0.140)	1.209	(0.151)	1.135

estimated standard error of parameters it is seen that $\sigma(b_{i1}) < \sigma(b_{i2})$ for each item. This is a natural consequence of the stepwise solution of items. All of the individuals attempted the first step whereas the second step was attempted only by individuals who had successfully completed step 1. Consequently, the precision of item parameter estimates for the second step was lower.

Goodness of fit was checked for the two steps separately. First, all individuals were included, and only the first step of items was considered. For this dichotomous Rasch model the likelihood ratio test versus the saturated model yielded a value of 36,199, with 56 degrees of freedom (Kelderman, 1984). Secondly, for the 22 individuals who succeeded in the first step of each item the second step was checked yielding a value for the likelihood-ratio statistic of 17.720. However, with only 99 individuals the use of the asymptotic distribution of the likelihood ratio test was not trustworthy. Therefore, the mixed Rasch model approach (Rost, 1991, this volume) was used as an additional check. For the assumption of two groups the values of the likelihood-ratio statistics were 4,420 (first steps) and 4.553 (second steps). The difference between the one group model and the two group model was 31.779 (first steps) and 12.767 (second steps) on 8 degrees of freedom. Hence, deviances with respect to the two class model suggested that it was doubtful that the Rasch model held for the first step of all items. All the computations of the goodness of fit checks as well as conditional estimates were done with MIRA (Rost and van Daviér, 1992).

Discussion

The sequential model is suited for the special type of item that is solved successively. This stepwise character of items is taken seriously and directly modelled by considering conditional transitions to higher levels. The reduction to dichotomous transitions makes accessible much of the theory and computational tools already developed for this case. This compensates for the lack of sufficient statistics which makes it difficult to obtain CML estimates.

References

Agresti, A. (1984). *Analysis of Ordinal Categorical Data.* New York: Wiley.

Andersen, E.B. (1973). A goodness of fit test for the Rasch model. *Psychometrika* **38**, 123–139.

Anderson, D.A. and Aitkin, M. (1985). Variance component models with binary responses: Interviewer variability. *Journal of the Royal Statistical Society B* **47**, 203–210.

Anderson, D.A. and Hinde, J. (1988). Random effects in generalized linear models and the EM algorithm. *Communications in Statistical Theory and Methodology* **17**, 3847–3856.

Andrich, D.A. (1978). A rating formulation for ordered response categories. *Psychometrika* **43**, 561–573.

Bauer, P., Hommel, G., and Sonnemann, E. (1988). *Multiple Hypotheses Testing.* Heidelberg: Springer-Verlag.

Bock, R.D. and Aitkin, M. (1981). Marginal maximum likelihood estimation of item parameters: Application of an EM algorithm. *Psychometrika* **46**, 443–459.

Fahrmeir, L., Frost, H., Hennevogl, W., Kaufmann, H., Kranert, T., and Tutz, G. (1990). *GLAMOUR: User and Example Guide.* Regensburg, Germany: University of Regensburg.

Fahrmeir, L. and Tutz, G. (1994). *Multivariate Statistical Modelling Based on Generalized Linear Models.* New York: Springer-Verlag.

Fischer, G.H. (1981). On the existence and uniqueness of maximum-likelihood estimates in the Rasch-model. *Psychometrika* **46**, 59–77.

Hambleton, R.K. and Swaminathan, H. (1985). *Item Response Theory: Principles and Applications.* Boston: Kluwer Academic Publishers.

Kalbfleisch, J. and Prentice, R. (1980). *The Statistical Analysis of Failure Time Data.* New York: Wiley.

Kelderman, H. (1984). Loglinear Rasch model tests. *Psychometrika* **49**, 223–245.

Masters, G.N. (1982). A Rasch model for partial credit scoring. *Psychometrika* **47**, 149–174.

McCullagh, P. (1980). Regression models for ordinal data. *Journal of the Royal Statistical Society A* **135**, 370–384.

Molenaar, I.W. (1983). *Item Steps* (Heymans Bulletin 83-630-EX). Groningen, The Netherlands: Psychologische Instituten, Rijksuniversiteit Groningen.

Rost, J. (1991). A logistic mixture distribution model for polychotomous item responses. *British Journal of Mathematical and Statistical Psychology* **44**, 75–92.

Rost, J. and Daviér, M.v. (1992). *MIRA: A PC Program for the Mixed Rasch Model* (User Manual). Kiel, Germany: Institute of Science Eduation (IPN).

Samejima, F. (1969). Estimation of latent ability using a response pattern of graded scores. *Psychometrika*, Monograph No. 17.

Stiratelli, R., Laird, N., and Ware, J.H. (1984). Random-effects models for serial observation with binary response. *Biometrics* **40**, 961–971.

Thissen, D.M. (1982). Marginal maximum likelihood estimation for the one-parameter logistic model. *Psychometrika* **47**, 175–186.

Tutz, G. (1990). Sequential item response models with an ordered response. *British Journal of Mathematical and Statistical Psychology* **43**, 39–55.

Tutz, G. (1991). Sequential models in categorical regression. *Computational Statistics Data Analysis* **11**, 275–295.

Waclawiw, M. and Liang, K.Y. (1993). Prediction of random effects in the generalized linear model. *Journal of the American Statistical Association* **88**, 171–178.

Wright, B.D. and Masters, G.N. (1982). *Rating Scale Analysis.* Chicago: MESA Press.

Zeger, S.L., Liang, K.Y., and Albert, P.S. (1988). Models for longitudinal data: A generalized estimating equation approach. *Biometrics* **44**, 1049–1060.

9
A Generalized Partial Credit Model

Eiji Muraki

Introduction

A generalized partial credit model (GPCM) was formulated by Muraki (1992) based on Masters' (1982, this volume) partial credit model (PCM) by relaxing the assumption of uniform discriminating power of test items. However, the difference between these models is not only the parameterization of item characteristics but also the basic assumption about the latent variable. An item response model is viewed here as a member of a family of latent variable models which also includes the linear or nonlinear factor analysis model, the latent class model, and the latent profile model (Bartholomew, 1987).

In Masters' PCM, the discrimination power is assumed to be common for all items. This model is a member of the Rasch family of item response models. The GPCM not only can attain some of the objectives that the Rasch model achieves but also can provide more information about the characteristics of test items than does the Rasch model.

Presentation of the Model

The PCM (Masters, this volume; Muraki, 1992) is formulated on the assumption that the probability of choosing the hth category over the $h-1$st category of item i is governed by the logistic dichotomous response model:

$$C_{ih} = P_{ih|h-1,h}(\theta) = \frac{P_{ih}(\theta)}{P_{i,h-1}(\theta) + P_{ih}(\theta)} = \frac{\exp[Z_{ih}(\theta)]}{1 + \exp[Z_{ih}(\theta)]}. \tag{1}$$

Eq. (1) can be written as

$$P_{ih}(\theta) = \frac{C_{ih}}{1 - C_{ih}} P_{i,h-1}(\theta) = \exp[Z_{ih}(\theta)] P_{i,h-1}(\theta). \tag{2}$$

Note that $C_{ih}/(1 - C_{ih})$ in Eq. (2) is the odds of choosing the hth category instead of the $h-1$st category, given two available choices, $h-1$ and h. Its log transformation, $Z_{ih}(\theta)$, is called the logit. After normalizing each

$P_{ih}(\theta)$ within an item such that $\sum P_{ih}(\theta) = 1$, the GPCM is written as

$$P_{ih}(\theta) = \frac{\exp\left[\sum_{v=1}^{h} Z_{iv}(\theta)\right]}{\sum_{c=1}^{m_i} \exp\left[\sum_{v=1}^{c} Z_{iv}(\theta)\right]} \tag{3}$$

and

$$Z_{ih}(\theta) = Da_i(\theta - b_{ih}) = Da_i(\theta - b_i + d_h), \tag{4}$$

where D is a scaling constant that puts the θ ability scale in the same metric as the normal ogive model ($D = 1.7$), a_i is a slope parameter, b_{ih} is an item-category parameter, b_i is an item-location parameter, and d_h is a category parameter. The slope parameter indicates the degree to which categorical responses vary among items as θ level changes. This concept of item discriminating power is closely related to the item reliability index in classical test theory (Muraki and Wang, 1992). This parameter captures information about differential discriminating power of the different items. $P_{ih}(\theta)$ in Eq. (3) is also called the item category response function (ICRF) of the GPCM.

If the number of response categories is m_i, only $m_i - 1$ item-category parameters can be identified. Any one of the m_i category threshold parameters can be arbitrarily defined as any value. The reason is that the term including the parameter is canceled out from both the numerator and denominator of the model (Muraki, 1992). We arbitrarily define $b_{i1} \equiv 0$.

As shown in Eqs. (2) and (4), the item-category parameters, b_{ih}, are the points on the θ scale at which the plots of $P_{i,h-1}(\theta)$ and $P_{ih}(\theta)$ intersect. These two ICRFs intersect only once, and the intersection can occur anywhere along the θ scale. Thus, under the assumption $a_i > 0$,

$$\begin{array}{lll} \text{if} & \theta = b_{ih}, & P_{ih}(\theta) = P_{i,h-1}(\theta) \\ & \theta > b_{ih}, & P_{ih}(\theta) > P_{i,h-1}(\theta) \\ \text{and} & \theta < b_{ih}, & P_{ih}(\theta) < P_{i,h-1}(\theta). \end{array} \tag{5}$$

Figure 1 shows the ICRFs for two GPCM items, each having three categorical responses. For item 1 with $a_1 = 1.0$, $b_{11} = 0.0$, $b_{12} = -1.5$, and $b_{13} = 2.0$, the ICRFs of $P_{11}(\theta)$ and $P_{12}(\theta)$ intersect at $\theta = -1.5$, and the ICRFs of $P_{12}(\theta)$ and $P_{13}(\theta)$ intersect at $\theta = 2.0$. If the second item-category parameter changes from -1.5 to -0.5 (item 2), the intersection of the first and second ICRFs moves from -1.5 to -0.5, as shown in Fig. 1. Since the first category probability becomes dominant over a wider range of θ values, the expected frequency of the first categorical response increases. Consequently, the ICRF of the second category is depressed. If the slope parameter is decreased, the intersections of ICRFs stay the same but the curves of the ICRFs become flat. Thus, the second category probability, $P_{22}(\theta)$, is further depressed. The categorical responses of examinees become more likely to fall into the first or third category. The cumulative response frequencies of these two items for 10,000 simulees were generated

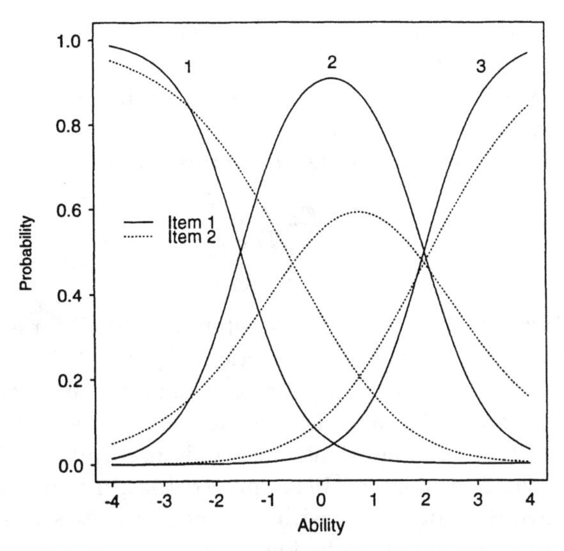

FIGURE 1. Item-category response functions of items 1 and 2.

based on the standard normal distribution of ability. In these generated data, the response frequencies of the first, second, and third categories were 1449, 7709, and 842 for item 1 and 3685, 4973, and 1342 for item 2, respectively.

In the GPCM the parameters b_{ih} may be additively decomposed as $b_{ih} = b_i - d_h$ in the same manner as in Andrich's (1978) rating scale model. The values of d_h are not necessarily ordered sequentially within an item. The parameter d_h is interpreted as the relative difficulty of category h in comparing other categories within an item or the deviate of each categorical threshold from the item location, b_i. The following location constraint is imposed to eliminate an indeterminacy:

$$\sum_{h=2}^{m_i} d_h = 0. \tag{6}$$

The sum of the $Z_{iv}(\theta)$ for item i in the GPCM can be written as

$$Z_{ih}^{+}(\theta) = \sum_{v=1}^{h} Z_{iv}(\theta) = a_i[T_h(\theta - b_i) + K_h], \tag{7}$$

where

$$K_h = \sum_{v=1}^{h} d_v, \tag{8}$$

and a scaling constant is set at $D = 1$. Andrich (1978) calls T_h and K_h the scoring function and the category coefficient, respectively (see Andersen, this volume). For the PCM, the scoring function T_h is a linear integer scoring function ($T_h = h$). The PCM becomes the model for ordered categorical responses only when the scoring function is increasing, that is, $T_h > T_{h-1}$ for any h within item i and $a_i > 0$.

The expected value of the scoring function is computed by

$$\bar{T}_i(\theta) = \sum_{h=1}^{m_i} T_h P_{ih}(\theta). \tag{9}$$

$\bar{T}_i(\theta)$ in Eq. (9) is called the item response function (IRF) for a polytomously-scored item with a given scoring function (T_h, $h = 1, 2, \ldots, m_i$) and it can be viewed as a regression of the item score onto the ability scale (Lord, 1980). For dichotomous IRT models, the IRF coincides with the ICRF. In the GPCM, the IRF is the conditional mean of item scores at a given θ (Muraki, 1993). Chang and Mazzeo (1944) proved that, if two polytomously-scored items have the same IRFs with the linear integer scoring function, then the model parameters must be identical.

Parameter Estimation

Estimating both person and item parameters simultaneously—the joint (Lord, 1980) or conditional maximum likelihood estimation method (Andersen, 1973; Fisher and Parzer, 1991; Wright and Masters, 1982)—by treating the person component as a fixed effect fails to produce numerically and statistically stable estimates (Neyman and Scott, 1948), especially when either the number of examinees or the number of items is very large. For this reason Bock and Lieberman (1970) proposed the marginal maximum likelihood (MML) method for the case of dichotomously-scored items. In their method, the latent trait is treated as a random component (Bartholomew, 1987) and integrated out of the likelihood by using the prior distribution. The MML parameter estimates are invariant in the same manner as coefficients of a regression function.

The Bock and Lieberman method, however, is computationally feasible only when the number of items is very small because of the necessity of inversion of the $2n \times 2n$ information matrix (n is the number of items). In 1981, Bock and Aitkin (1981) reformulated the MML method with the EM algorithm (Dempster, Laird, and Rubin, 1977). The MML-EM estimation method consists of two steps. The first is the expectation step (the E-step) where the provisional expected frequency, $\bar{r}_{ihf}$, and the provisional expected sample size, $\bar{N}_f$ ($\bar{N}_{if}$ if the sample size differs for each item), are computed. Then, in the maximization step (the M-step), the MML estimates are obtained by Fisher's scoring method (Kendall and Stuart, 1973, p. 51). The EM algorithm for the GPCM will now be presented.

The E-Step

We denote the number of examinees with response pattern l $(l = 1, 2, \ldots, S)$ by r_l where $S \le \min(N, J)$, $N = \sum r_l$, and $J = \prod m_i$. For the lth response pattern, let us denote $U_{ihl} = 1$ if the response to item i is in the hth category, otherwise $U_{ihl} = 0$. The provisional expected frequency of the hth categorical response of item i, $\bar{r}_{ihf}$, and the provisional expected sample size, $\bar{N}_f$, are computed at each quadrature point, f, by the following equations, respectively:

$$\bar{r}_{ihf} = \sum_{l=1}^{S} \frac{r_l L_l(X_f) A(X_f) U_{ihl}}{\tilde{P}_l}; \tag{10}$$

$$\bar{N}_f = \sum_{l=1}^{S} \frac{r_l L_l(X_f) A(X_f)}{\tilde{P}_l}, \tag{11}$$

where

$$\tilde{P}_l = \sum_{f=1}^{F} L_l(X_f) A(X_f) \tag{12}$$

and

$$L_l(X_f) = \prod_{i=1}^{n} \prod_{h=1}^{m_i} [P_{ih}(X_f)]^{U_{ihl}}. \tag{13}$$

Notice that Eq. (12) is the numerical approximation of the unconditional probability of the observed response pattern l where the prior distribution is assumed to be standard normal. $A(X_f)$ is the weight of the Gauss-Hermite quadrature, and X_f is the quadrature point (Stroud & Secrest, 1966). The quadrature weight $A(X_f)$ is approximately the standard normal probability density at the point X_f, such that where F is the total number of quadrature points:

$$\sum_{f=1}^{F} A(X_f) = 1 \tag{14}$$

Empirical weights can also be used in place of $A(X_f)$ is the condition in Eq. (14) is met.

The M-Step

The qth cycle of the iterative process can be expressed as

$$\boldsymbol{v}_q = \boldsymbol{v}_{q-1} + \mathbf{V}^{-1}\mathbf{t}, \tag{15}$$

where $\boldsymbol{v}_q$ and $\boldsymbol{v}_{q-1}$ are the parameter estimates of the qth and $q-1$st cycles respectively, $\mathbf{V}^{-1}$ is the inverse of the information matrix, and $\mathbf{t}$ is the gradient vector.

The elements of the gradient vector and the information matrix (2×2) for the slope and item-location parameters for the item i are given by

$$t_{a_i} = a_i^{-1} \sum_{f=1}^{F} \sum_{h=1}^{m_i} \bar{r}_{ihf} [Z_{ih}^{+}(X_f) - \bar{Z}_i^{+}(X_f)]; \tag{16}$$

$$t_{b_i} = a_i \sum_{f=1}^{F} \sum_{h=1}^{m_i} \bar{r}_{ihf} [-T_h + \bar{T}_i(X_f)]; \tag{17}$$

$$V_{a_i a_i} = a_i^{-2} \sum_{f=1}^{F} \bar{N}_f \sum_{h=1}^{m_i} P_{ih}(X_f) [Z_{ih}^{+}(X_f) - \bar{Z}_i^{+}(X_f)]^2; \tag{18}$$

$$V_{b_i b_i} = a_i^2 \sum_{f=1}^{F} \bar{N}_f \sum_{h=1}^{m_i} P_{ih}(X_f) [-T_h + \bar{T}_i(X_f)]^2; \tag{19}$$

$$V_{a_i b_i} = \sum_{f=1}^{F} \bar{N}_f \sum_{h=1}^{m_i} P_{ih}(X_f) [Z_{ih}^{+}(X_f) - \bar{Z}_i^{+}(X_f)][-T_h + \bar{T}_i(X_f)], \tag{20}$$

where $\bar{T}_i(X_f)$ is defined in Eq. (9) and

$$\bar{Z}_i^{+}(X_f) = \sum_{h=1}^{m_i} Z_{ih}^{+}(X_f) P_{ih}(X_f). \tag{21}$$

The entry of the gradient vector for the hth category parameter estimation is given by

$$t_{d_h} = \sum_{f=1}^{F} \sum_{i=1}^{n'} a_i \sum_{k=h}^{m_i} \left[\bar{r}_{ikf} - P_{ik}(X_f) \sum_{c=1}^{m_i} \bar{r}_{icf} \right]. \tag{22}$$

The entry of the information matrix for $h' \leq h$ is given by

$$V_{d_h d_{h'}} = \sum_{f=1}^{F} \bar{N}_f \sum_{i=1}^{n'} \sum_{k=1}^{m_i} \frac{1}{P_{ik}(X_f)} \frac{\partial P_{ik}(X_f)}{\partial d_h} \frac{\partial P_{ik}(X_f)}{\partial d_{h'}}$$

$$= \sum_{f=1}^{F} \bar{N}_f \sum_{i=1}^{n'} a_i^2 \left[\sum_{k=h}^{m_i} P_{ik}(X_f) \right] \left[1 - \sum_{k=h'}^{m_i} P_{ik}(X_f) \right], \tag{23}$$

where n' is the number of items included in a given block. A block of items is defined here as a set of items which share the same set of category parameters. When a set of category parameters is unique for each item, n' is 1 and the summation drops from Eqs. (22) and (23). Since d_1 is defined to be 0, the orders of the gradient vector $\mathbf{t}$ and the information matrix $\mathbf{V}$ are $m - 1$ and $(m - 1) \times (m - 1)$, respectively.

In the M-step, the provisional expected values computed in the E-step are used for Eqs. (16)–(20), and (22)–(23), and the parameters for each item are estimated individually and then the iterative process is repeated over the n items until the estimates of all items become stable to the required number of decimal places.

The optimal number of quadrature points for the calibration must be chosen by considering the number of items and categories under the restriction of available computing resources. For the polytomous item response model, more quadrature points are generally necessary as compared to the calibration of dichotomous items. However, the number of EM cycles to reach convergence and the memory requirements for the computation increase exponentially with the number of quadrature points. Although 30 to 40 quadrature points seem to be adequate, further empirical research is necessary.

The MML-EM estimation method described above is implemented in the PARSCALE program (Muraki & Bock, 1991). The PARSCALE program is also capable of estimating parameters of Samejima's normal and logistic models for graded responses (Muraki, 1990; Samejima, 1969). This program is particularly suitable for large-scale studies of rating data or performance assessments, and it operates both at the individual level and also at the group level to obtain scores for schools or other groups of examinees.

Goodness of Fit

The goodness of fit of the GPCM can be tested item by item. If the test is sufficiently long, the method of PC-BILOG 3 (Mislevy and Bock, 1990) can be used with minor modifications. In the method, the examinees in a sample of size N are assigned to intervals of the θ-continuum. The expected a posteriori (EAP) is used as the estimator of each examinee's ability score. The EAP estimate is the mean of the posterior distribution of θ, given the observed response pattern l (Bock and Mislevy, 1982). The EAP score of the response pattern l is approximated by

$$\hat{\theta}_l \cong \frac{\sum_{f=1}^{F} X_f L_l(X_f) A(X_f)}{\sum_{f=1}^{F} L_l(X_f) A(X_f)}. \tag{24}$$

After all examinees' EAP scores are assigned to any one of the predetermined W intervals on the θ-continuum, the observed frequency of the hth categorical responses to item i in interval w, r_{wih}, and the number of examinees assigned to item i in the wth interval, N_{wi}, are computed. Thus, the W by m_i contingency table for each item is obtained. Then, the estimated θ's are rescaled so that the variance of the sample distribution equals that of the latent distribution on which the MML estimation of the item parameters is based. For each interval, the interval mean, $\bar{\theta}_w$, based on the rescaled θ's, and the value of the fitted ICRF function, $P_{ih}(\bar{\theta}_w)$, are computed. Finally, a likelihood-ratio chi-square statistic for each item is computed by

$$G_i^2 = 2 \sum_{w=1}^{W_i} \sum_{h=1}^{m_i} r_{wih} \ln \frac{r_{wih}}{N_{wi} P_{ih}(\bar{\theta}_w)}, \tag{25}$$

where W_i is the number of intervals remaining after neighboring intervals are merged, if necessary, to avoid expected values, $N_{wi}P_{ih}(\bar{\theta}_w)$, less than 5. The number of degrees of freedom is equal to the number of intervals, W_i, multiplied by $m_i - 1$. The likelihood-ratio chi-square statistic for the test as a whole is simply the summation of the statistic in Eq. (25) over items. The number of degrees of freedom is also the summation of the degrees of freedom for each item.

Further research of the goodness-of-fit index for IRT models in general is needed. The method discussed above is quite sensitive to the number of classification intervals. If the number is too large, the expected values of the contingency table become fragmented and the fit statistics are inflated.

Example

The National Assessment of Educational Progress (NAEP) (Beaton & Zwick, 1992) is an ongoing survey designed to measure students' academic knowledge in various subject-areas. The GPCM was applied to the item calibration and scaling procedures of the 1992 cross-sectional writing assessment data of grades 8 and 12 (Grima & Johnson, 1992).

Among nine writing items for the grade 8 assessment, six items are common with grade 12 (linking items). Students' writings were scored by trained readers on a five-point scoring scale. Omitted responses were treated as the lowest categorical response (scored as 1). For some items, the highest category responses were combined with the next highest so that the observed frequency of any category response was at least 10. The resulting number of response categories and corresponding observed frequencies for grade 8 are presented in Table 1.

Two analyses were conducted using the PARSCALE computer program. For both analyses, 33 quadrature points were used for normal prior distributions and the precision level for the estimation convergence was set at 0.001. First, a set of item parameters were estimated based on the pooled response data of the grade 8 and 12 assessments (the pooled calibration). For the second analysis, calibrations were done separately for each grade group (the separate calibrations).

The total number of response vectors used for the item calibration of the grade 8 and grade 12 samples were 10167 and 9344, respectively. Seventy-six EM cycles were required for the pooled calibration, and 102 was needed for the separate calibrations of the grade 8 assessment. For the grade 8

TABLE 1. Frequencies of Categorical Responses (NAEP Cross-Sectional Writing, Grade 8, Year 1992).

Item	Response Categories						Total
	1	2	3	4	5	6	
1. Favorite Object	79	72	923	827	284	34	2219
2. Another Planet	54	376	827	787	151	18	2213
3. Lengthen School Year	67	566	1133	408	45		2219
4. Performance Review	249	87	1050	553	183		2122
5. Invention	147	421	1055	469	90		2182
6. Embarrassing Incident	97	640	757	579	99		2172
7. Grandchildren	68	703	721	607	85	14	2198
8. Rating Labels	101	658	1250	162			2171
9. Drug Search	156	732	1130	162			2180

TABLE 2. Slope, Item-Location, and Category Parameters (NAEP Cross-Sectional Writing, Grade 8, Year 1992).

Item	Slope	Location	Category				
	a	b	d_2	d_3	d_4	d_5	d_6
1	0.447	0.197	1.195	4.136	0.090	−1.732	−3.690
2	0.589	0.350	3.444	1.643	0.167	−2.071	−3.183
3	0.622	0.165	3.185	1.108	−1.227	−3.066	
4	0.311	0.086	−1.216	5.073	−1.273	−2.584	
5	0.315	0.257	2.857	2.167	−1.504	−3.520	
6	0.666	0.001	2.647	0.466	−0.564	−2.550	
7	0.408	0.735	4.874	1.008	0.203	−2.902	−3.183
8	0.519	−0.254	2.623	0.555	−3.178		
9	0.671	−0.051	2.098	0.379	−2.477		

assessment, the goodness-of-fit stàtistics were computed based on 10 intervals and were 4293.741 (degree of freedom = 123) for the pooled calibration and 3863.961 (degree of freedom = 124) for the separate calibration. The significant reduction in the chi-square, 429.780, when separate calibrations were performed suggests that the separate calibration estimates should be used. The parameters estimated in the separate calibrations are presented in Table 2.

Figures 2 and 3 present the ICRFs and IRFs of items 5 and 6, respectively. The IRF was computed by Eq. (9) based on the scoring function, $\underline{T} = (0, 1, 2, \ldots)$ and divided by the number of categories minus 1 so that both ICRFs and IRFs can be plotted on the same figures. For the computation of the ICRF, there is no difference if the successive increment of the scoring function is 1, that is, using either $\underline{T} = (0, 1, 2, \ldots)$, $\underline{T} = (1, 2, 3, \ldots)$, or $\underline{T} = (101, 102, 103, \ldots)$ produces the same probability of the GPCM.

Both items have five response categories, and their means of the item responses for the grade 8 sample are about 2.70. Based upon classical item statistics, these items seems to be equally difficult. However, their ICRFs show differences. Compared to item 6, the observed response frequency of

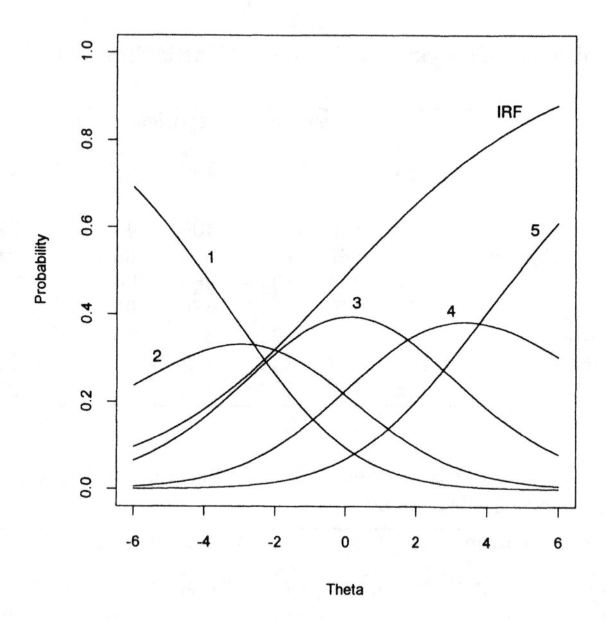

FIGURE 2. Item response function (IRF) and item-category response functions of item 5.

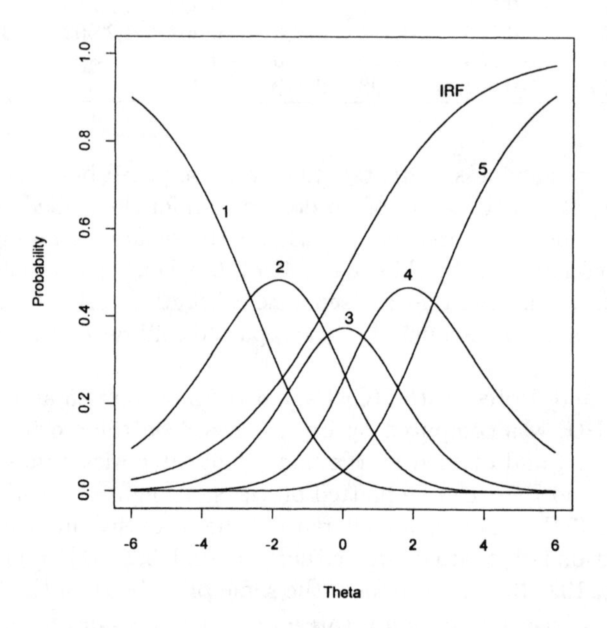

FIGURE 3. Item response function (IRF) and item-category response functions of item 6.

the third category of item 5 is very large, 757 versus 1055 (Table 1). Figure 2 also shows that the third ICRF of item 2 is quite dominant compared to that of item 6. Another distinct difference is that the ICRFs are relatively flat compared to the ICRFs of item 6. The polyserial correlations of items 5 and 6 with the total scores are 0.768 and 0.853, respectively. The difference of the overall discrimination between these items reflects on the slope of IRFs as well as the shapes of ICRFs. The IRF of item 6 is considerably steeper than that of item 5. Both items cover a wide range of the θ scale.

A major advantage of polytomously-scored items is that the assessment generally covers a wider range of the ability scale with a sufficient amount of information compared to an assessment with the same number of dichotomous items. For polytomous item response models, the parameter values should be interpreted with the aid of graphical presentations (Masters, 1982; Muraki, 1992; Muraki, 1993). Inspecting the plots of ICRFs, IRF, and item information functions for each item is an essential item analysis procedure (Muraki, 1993).

Acknowledgment

The work in this chapter was supported in part by a contract from the National Center for Educational Statistics, Office of Educational Research Improvement, U.S. Department of Education.

References

Andersen, E.B. (1973). Conditional inference for multiple-choice questionnaires. *British Journal of Mathematical and Statistical Psychology* **26**, 31–44.

Andrich, D. (1978). A rating formulation for ordered response categories. *Psychometrika* **43**, 561–573.

Bartholomew, D.J. (1987). *Latent Variable Models and Factor Analysis*. London: Charles Griffin & Company.

Beaton, A.E. and Zwick, R. (1992). Overview of the national assessment of educational progress. *Journal of Educational Statistics* **17**, 95–109.

Bock, R.D. and Aitkin, M. (1981). Marginal maximum likelihood estimation of item parameters: Application of an EM algorithm. *Psychometrika* **41**, 443–459.

Bock, R.D. and Lieberman, M. (1970). Fitting a response model for n dichotomously scored items. *Psychometrika* **35**, 179–197.

Bock, R.D. and Mislevy, R.J. (1982). Adaptive EAP estimation of ability in a microcomputer environment. *Applied Psychological Measurement* **6**, 431–444.

Chang, H. and Mazzeo, J. (1944). The unique correspondence of item response function and item category response functions in polytomously scored item response models. *Psychometrika* **59**, 391–404.

Dempster, A.P., Laird, N.M., and Rubin, D.B. (1977). Maximum likelihood from incomplete data via the EM algorithm. *Journal of the Royal Statistical Society, Series B* **39**, 1–38.

Fisher, G.H. and Parzer, P. (1991). An extension of the rating scale model with an application to the measurement of change. *Psychometrika* **56**, 637–651.

Grima, A.M. and Johnson, E.G. (1992). Data analysis for the writing assessment. In E.G. Johnson and N.L. Allen (Eds.), *The NAEP 1990 Technical Report.* Princeton, NJ: Educational Testing Service.

Kendall, M.G. and Stuart, A. (1973). *The Advanced Theory of Statistics*, vol. 2. New York, NY: Hafner Publishing Company.

Lord, F.M. (1980). *Application of Item Response Theory to Practical Testing Problems.* Hillsdale, NJ: Erlbaum.

Masters, G.N. (1982). A Rasch model for partial credit scoring. *Psychometrika* **47**, 149–174.

Mislevy, R.J. and Bock, R.D. (1990). *BILOG 3: Item Analysis and Test Scoring with Binary Logistic Models* [Computer program]. Chicago, IL: Scientific Software, Inc.

Muraki, E. (1990). Fitting a polytomous item response model to Likert-type data. *Applied Psychological Measurement* **14**, 59–71.

Muraki, E. (1992). A generalized partial credit model: Application of an EM algorithm. *Applied Psychological Measurement* **16**, 159–176.

Muraki, E. (1993). Information functions of the generalized partial credit model. *Applied Psychological Measurement* **17**, 351–363.

Muraki, E. and Bock, R.D. (1991). *PARSCALE: Parameter Scaling of Rating Data* [Computer program]. Chicago, IL: Scientific Software, Inc.

Muraki, E. and Wang, M. (1992). *Issues Relating to the marginal maximum likelihood estimation of the partial credit model.* Paper presented at the Annual Meeting of the American Educational Research Association, San Francisco, CA.

Neyman, J. and Scott, E.L. (1948). Consistent estimates based on partially consistent observations. *Econometrika* **16**, 1–32.

Samejima, F. (1969). Estimating of latent ability using a response pattern of graded scores. *Psychometrika Monograph Supplement*, No. 17.

Stroud, A.H. and Secrest, D. (1966). *Gaussian Quadrature Formulas.* Englewood Cliffs, NJ: Prentice Hall.

Wright, B.D. and Masters, G. (1982). *Rating Scale Analysis.* Chicago, IL: MESA Press.

Part II. Models for Response Time or Multiple Attempts on Items

An important distinction is the one between response processes invoked by *power* and *speed* tests. Two constraints are needed to describe the differences between such tests: (1) a constraint on the response time available; and (2) a constraint on the distribution of the difficulties of the items in the test.

In a power test, no constraints are imposed on the amount of time available or on the difficulties of the items in the test. In practice, the distribution of difficulties is often such that the items are presented in increasing order of difficulty. The reason for this is efficiency. If an examinee reaches items which are too difficult to solve, he or she may conclude that trying any of the remaining items is a waste of time and decide to stop. If the remaining items are scored as incorrect, the decision creates test scores with negligible bias.

In a speed test, however, both the time available and the distribution of the item difficulties are constrained. The examinee either knows in advance when he or she has to stop or that he or she will be informed to stop when the time has elapsed. With speed tests, the examinee's task is to solve as many items as possible. The difficulties of the individual items are constrained to be equal or approximately equal and of a low difficulty level. Given enough time, most examinees could answer all of the test items correctly. As a consequence, all items are expected to have the same response time for each examinee. Response processes on speed tests can therefore be conceived of as stationary processes with constant probability of success, to be modeled as series of observations of the values of identically distributed response variables which stops when the total response time is over. For such processes, the number of items solved in a certain time interval and the average response time per item are variables that differ only in their metric but basically convey the same information about the ability of the examinees. For this reason, Lord and Novick (1968, Chap. 5) were able to present the classical equations for the effects of test length on reliability and validity as a function of a generic length parameter which can be interpreted equally well as response time or the number of items in the test. Only practical reasons govern the choice between the experiment of counting the number of successes in a fixed period and the *inverse* or *negative* experiment in which the response time is recorded.

The concepts of power and speed tests exist only as idealizations. In practice, all power tests involve some kind of speededness. Even if examinees are not instructed to work at their own speed, they may choose to set tight targets for the time they want to spend on the test. Also, speed tests never have items which all have exactly the same difficulty level. It seems, therefore, safe to conclude that to analyze examinee behavior on most existing tests realistically, models of a *hybrid* nature are needed. The fact that these models should address both the power and speed aspects of tests has important consequences.

The first consequence is that, unlike pure speed tests, item responses and their latencies are no longer equivalent measures of examinee ability. Consequently, both have to be collected. In principle, the technology of computerized testing could help the test administrator to collect the desired information, but it is obvious that the time elapsed between key strokes is not necessarily identical to the time an examinee spends on solving the items. Second, the presence of omitted answers becomes a puzzle. In pure power tests, omitted answers point to items which the examinee does not know and can be scored as incorrect. In pure speed tests omitted responses may represent random carelessness not related to the ability measured by the test and can be neglected. For most current tests, which are somewhere between pure power and pure speed tests, the correct interpretation of blanks on the answer sheet is unknown, however. Third, with achievement, aptitude, and ability tests, examinees can normally be assumed to operate on the principle of score maximization. As soon as more than one score is recorded, e.g., response time and number of items correct, different strategies of maximization become possible. The choice of strategy, however, is likely to depend not only on the ability measured by the test but also on unknown personality factors. If these factors are ignored in the test model, the ability estimates will show different bias for examinees with different strategies. Finally, the choice of strategy seems to be the one between working at high speed or at a high level of accuracy. Intuitively, the relation between these two factors has the form of a tradeoff imposed by the ability level of the examinee. A realistic model has to deal with these factors. However, if separate parameters for speed and accuracy are adopted for each examinee, their unknown values may be impossible to identify from response data. The only solution seems to be to describe one factor in the model as a known mathematical function of the other factor. However, such a function has to be realistic to allow fit of the model to empirical data.

From the problem above, it is clear that realistic models for tests which are neither pure power nor pure speed test are difficult to develop. Practical difficulties hamper recording of exact response times. In addition, unlike the case of pure speed tests, simplifying assumptions with respect to the distribution of item difficulties are no longer possible, introducing the necessity to deal with incidental parameters in the model. As for the statistical treatment of the models, the problems listed above entail the complicated problems known to exist for models with unknown mixtures of distributions, multidimensionality, and problems of identifiability. Nevertheless, models for tests with items varying in difficulty and a time limit are badly needed, and it is a challenge to develop them.

Three chapters on promising models related to the speed-power problem are offered in this section. The chapter by Verhelst, Verstralen, and Jansen formulates a model for tests which have both speed and power aspects. The model has a logistic form which is derived as the result of the more basic assumptions of a gamma distribution for response time and a generalized extreme-value distribution for a latent response given response time. For a different choice of distributions, Roskam also presents a model for this class of tests. However, his model is formulated directly for manifest response variables. Experience has shown that common tests of psychomotor skills fit the constraint on item difficulties of pure speed tests. The final chapter by Spray considers several models to analyze data from psychomotor tests. Some of these models assume that the test produces numbers of successes in a fixed number of trials whereas others assume the inverse experiment of recording the number of trials needed to reach a prespecified level of success.

Additional reading on the problems addressed in this section is found in Rasch (1980) who proposed a Poisson model for errors in an oral reading test. A Bayesian treatment and marginal versions of this model are given in Jansen (1986, 1994) and Jansen and van Duijn (1992). Scheiblechner (1979, 1985) formulated an exponential model for response times with an additive decomposition of its single parameter into item and person parameters. Different parameter structures for gamma models for response time distributions are given in Maris (1993). Finally, Thissen (1983) presents several applications of a model which consists of the common two-parameter logistic model extended with the assumption of a log-normal distribution of response time.

References

Jansen, M.G.H. (1986). A Bayesian version of Rasch's multiplicative Poisson model for the number of errors on an achievement test. *Journal of Educational Statistics* **11**, 51–65.

Jansen, M.G.H. (1994). Parameters of the latent distribution in Rasch's Poisson counts model. In G.H. Fisher and D. Laming (Eds.). *Contributions to Mathematical Psychology, Psychometrics, and Methodology* (pp. 319–326). New York, NY: Springer-Verlag.

Jansen, M.G.H. and van Duijn, M.A.J. (1992). Extensions of Rasch's multiplicative Poisson model. *Psychometrika* **57**, 405–414.

Lord, F.M. and Novick, M.R. (1968). *Statistical Theories of Mental Test Scores.* Reading, MA: Addison-Wesley.

Maris, E. (1993). Additive and multiplicative models for gamma distributed random variables, and their application as psychometric models for response times. *Psychometrika* **58**, 445–469.

Rasch, G. (1980). *Some Probabilistic Models for Some Intelligence and Attainment Tests.* Chicago, IL: The University of Chicago Press. (Original work published in 1960.)

Scheiblechner, H. (1979). Specific objective stochastic latency mechanisms. *Journal of Mathematical Psychology* **19**, 18–38.

Scheiblechner, H. (1985). Psychometric models for speed-test construction: The linear exponential model. In S.E. Embretson (Ed.), *Test Design: Developments in Psychology and Education* (pp. 219–244). New York, NY: Academic Press.

Thissen, D. (1983). Timed testing: An approach using item response theory. In D.J. Weiss (Ed.), *New Horizons in Testing: Latent Trait Test Theory and Computerized Adaptive Testing.* New York, NY: Academic Press.

10
A Logistic Model for Time-Limit Tests

N.D. Verhelst, H.H.F.M. Verstralen, and
M.G.H. Jansen

Introduction

The purpose of the present chapter is to introduce a psychometric model for time-limit tests. Our point of departure is a practical one. The main problem involved in the use of time-limit tests may be illustrated by the following example. Assume that a test consists of a large number of equally difficult items, and that examinees are allowed to answer the items during a fixed amount of time τ. Suppose person A and person B both have the same proportion of correct answers, but have completed a different number of items. Should the ability estimates of A and B be equal? It may be argued that for several reasons the answer should be no. The most practical reason may be that if only the proportion correct is important, the optimal strategy in answering the test is to spend all the allotted time on the first item. But also in realistic settings, where examinees are urged to work fast but accurately, a response style which favors accuracy at the expense of speed is advantageous. It might seem that using the number of correct responses reflects both speed and accuracy, and is therefore a more sensible way of scoring the test performance. But with this approach, another problem crops up. If the test consists of n items, the number of correct responses can be expressed as a proportion relative to n, implying that items not reached and wrong responses are treated in the same way, an approach which may prejudice to persons working slowly but accurately.

So, both scoring rules—proportion correct and number correct—seem to favor a different response style. Although it may be argued that response style may be induced and manipulated by test instructions, two important questions remain. The first has to do with the effectiveness of the instruction to the test. To what extent can general test instructions overrule the personal response style of examinees, and thus justify a scoring rule which may be prejudicial to 'careful' people? The second problem, which is only a more general reformulation of the first, has to do with the construct validity of the test. To what extent is the trait measured by the test invariant under different speed conditions?

In the model to be presented below, this invariance has a central position. Speed as well as accuracy are seen as two complementary aspects of a more fundamental concept labelled mental power. The trade off between speed and accuracy follows automatically from the model. The scoring rule is not chosen a priori but implied by the model. Of course, the model is only a hypothesis which may be false or only true in some circumstances. Although fit of a model is an empirical question, it may be appropriate to describe the kind of test we had in mind when developing the model. The prototype is a test commonly labelled 'speed test,' where speed of performance is essential, while, at the same time, the questions are sufficiently easy that if time were available, an examinee would answer the questions correctly with high probability.

Presentation of the Model

In IRT models, the most elementary notion in the case of binary responses is the item response function, $f_i(\theta)$ which gives the probability of a correct response on item i as a function of the latent variable θ, as depicted in Fig. 1a. The item difficulty parameter ε_i corresponds to the value of the latent variable for which the probability of a correct response is some fixed value, for which often the value 0.50 is chosen. An equivalent formulation is based on the graph displayed in Fig. 1b. Here it is assumed that the mental activities of the examinee result in some value z, which may be considered as the realization of a random variable Z. The item is correctly answered if the realized value z is larger than the threshold ε_i. If the probability density function (pdf) of Z belongs to a shift family, such that for a particular person θ_j can be considered a location parameter, we have

$$f_i(\theta_j) = P_{\theta_j}(Z > \varepsilon_i) = \int_{\varepsilon_i}^{\infty} g_{\theta_j}(z)\, dz. \tag{1}$$

For example, if $g_\theta(\cdot)$ is chosen to be the logistic pdf, this choice results in a logistic IRT model. Introduction of the random variable Z explains to some extent the probabilistic character of the resulting IRT model. Once the value of Z is fixed, the model is deterministic. The relative position of z with respect to the threshold ε_i determines the observed response. The probabilistic character results from Z being a random variable, which might be called 'momentary ability.' Understanding the behavior of an examinee amounts to explaining the variation of Z. In general, then, it is assumed that the variation in time used to answer the item will explain part of the variance of Z.

The distribution of Z therefore is considered as the marginal distribution

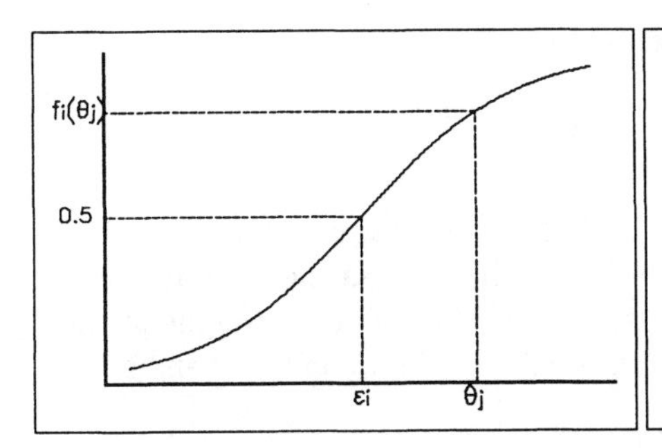

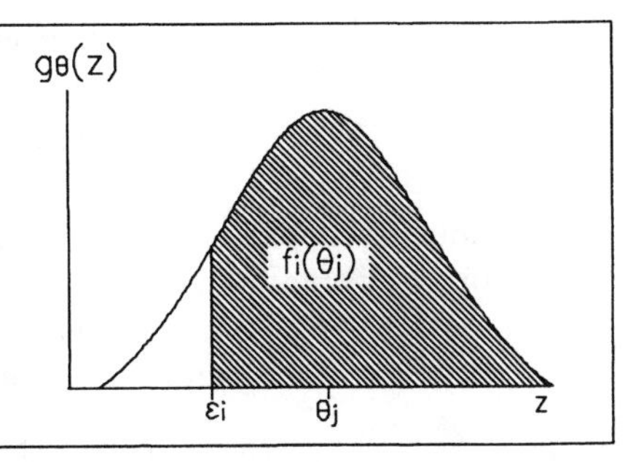

FIGURE 1. (a) Item response function. (b) pdf of momentary ability.

with time integrated out:

$$g_\theta(z) = \int_0^\infty h_\theta(z \mid t) q_\lambda(t)\, dt \tag{2}$$

where λ denotes the vector of parameters indexing the pdf of the time distribution. Given the popularity and the success of logistic IRT models in analyzing power tests, it is required that $g_\theta(\cdot)$ be the pdf of the logistic distribution. The main question then is the choice of suitable functions for the distribution of the time t and for the conditional distribution of Z given t. The distribution of response times is known to be positively skewed in general, with two inflection points, and the Weibull, the log-normal and the gamma p.d. functions seem to be reasonable choices. In view of a very elegant result by Dubey (1969), to be explained in the sequel, we choose the gamma distribution:

$$q_\lambda(t) = \frac{\beta^p}{\Gamma(p)} t^{p-1} e^{-\beta t}, \quad (\lambda = (\beta, p)). \tag{3}$$

It is asssumed, also in view of Dubey's result, that the conditional distribution of Z is a generalized form of the extreme-value distribution. Its distribution function is given by

$$1 - H_\theta(\varepsilon_i \mid t) = \int_{\varepsilon_i}^\infty h_\theta(z \mid t) dt = 1 - \exp\{-t\alpha \exp[(\theta - \varepsilon_i)/\alpha]\}, \ (\alpha > 0) \tag{4}$$

where t is formally introduced as an extra parameter. Bringing t within the argument of the inner exponential function gives

$$1 - H_\theta(\varepsilon_i \mid t) = 1 - \exp\left\{ - \exp\left[\frac{\theta}{\alpha} + \ln(t\alpha) - \frac{\varepsilon_i}{\alpha}\right]\right\}. \tag{5}$$

To arrive at an elegant interpretation of the model parameters, define

$$v = \exp(\theta/\alpha), \tag{6}$$

$$\rho_i = \exp(\varepsilon_i/\alpha), \tag{7}$$

and let

$$y(t) = \alpha t \frac{v}{\rho_i}. \tag{8}$$

Introducing metaphorical physical units for the measured cognitive concepts suggests an attractive interpretation. Think of v as the mental power of the person, expressed in Joules/second, ρ as the cognitive weight of the item, expressed in Newton, and t as physical time in seconds. Then

$$\alpha \frac{tv}{\rho} = \alpha \frac{t \text{ sec } v \text{ Joule/sec}}{\rho \text{ Newton}} = \alpha \frac{tv}{\rho} \text{ meter},$$

because Joule = Newton × meter. If we conceive of $y(t)$ as a dimensionless number it follows that α is expressed in meter^{-1}. The mentioned metaphorical units other than time are not yet standardized. We may do so by setting α equal to 1, and omit it as a parameter. In that case only for v or ρ a unit has to be fixed. However, if both v and ρ are standardized, for instance by setting their standard deviations equal to 1, then α must be explicitly kept as a parameter to be estimated.

The quantity α may also be conceived of as a dimensionless constant that depends on the 'size' of the units involved. As a consequence of this choice, $y(t)$ has dimension meter, and may be interpreted as 'cognitive height,' the distance the item has been lifted by the person into 'clarity' at time t, where the amount of clarity, measured in meters, determines the probability of a correct response according to Eq. (5). For ease of exposition the exponential parameters θ and ε will be called power and weight respectively.

The effect of spending more time on answering an item is shown in Fig. 2, where the conditional pdf's for $t = \alpha$ and $t = 2\alpha$ are displayed. The conditional distribution shifts with an amount $\alpha \ln(t\alpha)$. So a characteristic of the model is that the probability of a correct answer tends to unity if the time spent in answering it grows without bound. Although this assumption may be unrealistic in some situations, in most speeded tests the items are relatively easy, and errors are mainly caused by the time pressure.

Dubey (1969) shows that the compound distribution of the generalized extreme value distribution and the gamma distribution is a generalized logistic distribution. Applying this result to our model gives

$$1 - f_i(\theta, \beta, p) = \int_{\varepsilon_i}^{\infty} g_\theta(z)\, dz = \left[1 + \exp\left(\frac{\theta}{\alpha} - \ln\frac{\beta}{\alpha} - \frac{\varepsilon_i}{\alpha}\right)\right]^{-p}. \tag{9}$$

The right-hand side of this equation is a generalized logistic distribution function because of the parameter p. As to the interpretation of the model, several options are possible. Until now, it was assumed that θ is a characteristic of the person and that ε is a parameter characterizing the item. As to the parameters β and p of the time distribution, a choice has not been made yet. It may be argued that the time invested in responding to an item

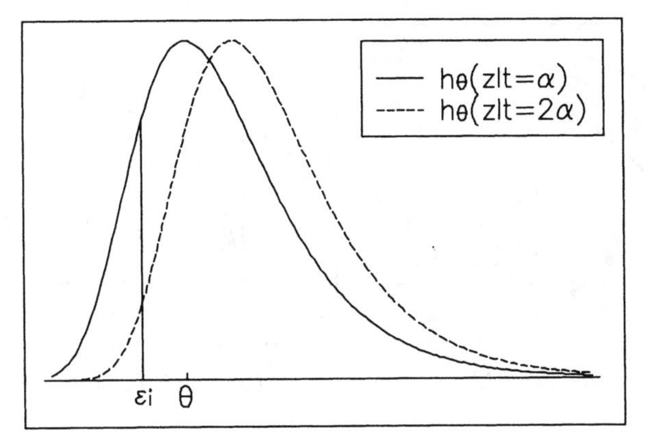

FIGURE 2. Conditional distributions $h_\theta(z \mid t = \alpha)$ and $h_\theta(z \mid t = 2\alpha)$.

is influenced by the difficulty of the item (Roskam, this volume). This is admittedly true, but our concern here is to also produce a model which is statistically elegant, that is, of which the parameters can be estimated with known accuracy. If the parameters β and p both depend on the person as well as on the item, and are to be interpreted as interaction parameters, it cannot be hoped that estimation procedures will ever be derived, given the inevitable constraint that every person answers the same item only once. As a first exploration of the features of the model, the parameter β will be considered person dependent and the parameter p item dependent. Using this convention, Eq. (9) can be rewritten as

$$1 - f_i(\theta_j, \beta_j, p_i) = \left[1 + \exp\left(\frac{\theta_j}{\alpha} - \ln\frac{\beta_j}{\alpha} - \frac{\varepsilon_i}{\alpha}\right)\right]^{-p_i} = [1 + \exp(\xi_j - \sigma_j)]^{-p_i}, \tag{10}$$

where

$$\sigma_i = \frac{\varepsilon_i}{\alpha} \tag{11}$$

and

$$\xi_j = \frac{\theta_j}{\alpha} - \ln\frac{\beta_j}{\alpha}. \tag{12}$$

If p_i is set equal to one, the common Rasch model with person parameter ξ_j results. Also, the time distribution specified in Eq. (3) is reduced to the exponential. Since the estimate of the person parameter in the Rasch model is a monotone function of the number of right items, and thus of the proportion correct if the number of attempted items is given, it seems reasonable to denote ξ as a measure of precision. Because the expected time to answer an item is given by $p_i/\beta_j = 1/\beta_j$, the parameter β_j, or any monotone increasing transformation of it, can be interpreted as a measure of speed. Rewriting Eq. (12) gives

$$\frac{\theta_j}{\alpha} = \xi_j + \ln\beta_j + c \tag{13}$$

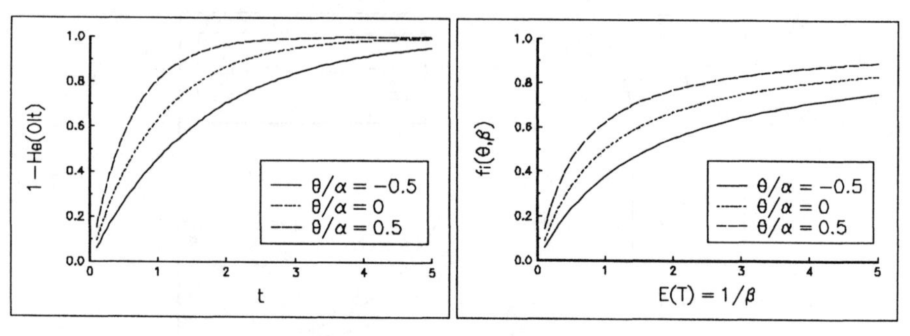

FIGURE 3. (a) CAF ($\varepsilon_i = 0$, $p_i = 1$). (b) SATF ($\varepsilon_i = 0$, $p_i = 1$).

or, in short, mental power is precision plus speed. This gives an answer to the problem stated in the introduction. If all items are equally difficult, and the proportion correct scores of two persons are equal, then Eq. (13) shows how the higher speed is to be combined with the same measure of precision, and leads to a higher measurement of mental power. The constant c is a function of α and of the arbitrary normalization of the item parameters σ_i.

It may be instructive to relate some of the functions studied here to two important functions discussed in the literature on time-limit tests: the speed-accuracy trade-off function (SATF) and the conditional accuracy function (CAF) (see, for example, Roskam, this volume). The latter expresses the probability of a correct response as a function of the time used to answer the item, and is given by $1 - H_\theta(\varepsilon_i \mid t)$ (Eq. (5)). The SATF expresses the (marginal) probability of a correct response as a function of the expected response time p_i/β_j. For fixed θ, ε_i and p_i, this relation is nothing else but the item response function $f_i(\theta_j, \beta_j, p_i)$ considered as a function of β_j. In Fig. 3a, three CAFs are displayed, and in Fig. 3b three SATFs. In case $p_i = 1$, the functional form of the latter is given by

$$f_i(\beta_j) = \frac{\beta_j^{-1} a_{ji}}{1 + \beta_j^{-1} a_{ji}}. \tag{14}$$

where a_{ji} depends on θ_j and ε_i. So the logit of the probability of a correct response is linear in the log of the expected response time, the same result as obtained for the Rasch-Weibull model (see Roskam, this volume).

Parameter Estimation

If the parameter p_i is set to 1 for all items, the distribution of the response time is exponential, which may appear unrealistic in many cases. However, it may be instructive to study the problems associated with parameter estimation in this simple case. The more general case will be commented upon later.

Case of $p_i = 1$

Estimation of β. Assume that the test is administered to J students, and let N_j, with realization n_j, denote the number of finished items in time τ by student j. Let the response variable be denoted by $\mathbf{U}_j = (U_{j1}, \ldots, U_{jn_j})$, with $U_{ji} = 1$ for a correct answer and $U_{ji} = 0$ for a wrong answer. The basic observation under the model consists of the pair (n_j, u_j), and the likelihood for one observation is proportional to the joint probability of this pair. Denote the set of observed response patterns by $\{\mathbf{u}\}$, and the set of numbers of items finished by the respondents by $\{\mathbf{n}\}$. Let $\theta = (\theta_1, \ldots, \theta_J)$. $\beta = (\beta_1, \ldots, \beta_J)$ and $\varepsilon = (\varepsilon_1, \ldots, \varepsilon_m)$, with $m = \max_j(n_j)$. Finally, denote the complete set of observations by $\{\mathbf{n}, \mathbf{u}\}$.

The exponential distribution has the following useful property for the estimation of the β-parameters. Let T_1, $T_2, \ldots$ be a sequence of independent random variables identically distributed as the exponential distribution with parameter β. Let τ be a fixed time interval, then the random variable N defined by

$$\sum_{i=1}^{N} T_i \leq \tau < \sum_{i=1}^{N+1} T_i$$

is Poisson distributed with parameter $\tau\beta$. The interpretation for our test situation is straightforward. If the limited test time equals τ and a student j has speed parameter β_j, then his number N_j of finished items has the indicated Poisson distribution. Moreover, the following derivation shows that the joint conditional density of the response times given the number n of finished responses is independent of β

$$\begin{aligned} f(t_1, \ldots, t_n; \beta \mid n) &= f(t; \beta \mid n) \\ &= \frac{\beta^n \exp\left(-\beta \sum_i^n t_i\right) \exp\left[-\beta\left(\tau - \sum_i^n t_i\right)\right]}{\frac{(\tau\beta)^n \exp(-\tau\beta)}{n!}} = \frac{n!}{\tau^n}. \end{aligned} \tag{15}$$

The numerator in the third member of Eq. (15) is the product of the joint density of the n exponentially distributed response times and the probability that the $(n+1)$th item is not finished in the remaining time $\tau - \sum_i t_i$. The denominator is the Poisson probability of having n items finished in time τ. Therefore n is sufficient for β, and its maximum likelihood estimator is n/τ. This estimator is unbiased.

Estimation of ε. The likelihood for the complete data now factors into

$$L(\theta, \beta, \varepsilon; \{\mathbf{n}, \mathbf{u}\}) = L_P(\beta; \{\mathbf{n}\}) \times L_c(\theta, \varepsilon; \{\mathbf{u}\} \mid \{\mathbf{n}\}), \tag{16}$$

where L_P is proportional to the above-mentioned Poisson probability mass function, and the conditional likelihood L_c is given by

$$L_c(\theta, \varepsilon; \{\mathbf{u}\} \mid \{\mathbf{n}\}) = \prod_j^J \Bigg[f(t_j \mid n_j) \int_{\Delta_j} \prod_i [1 - \exp(-y_{ji}(t)]^{u_{ji}}$$

$$\left. \cdot \exp[-y_{ji}(t)]^{1-u_{ji}} (dt)^{n_j} \right] \tag{17}$$

where y_{ji} is defined by Eq. (8). The parameter α is no longer mentioned in the variable list; it is treated here as an arbitrary but fixed scale parameter, equal to one. The integral sign in Eq. (17) denotes the multiple integral over the domain $\Delta_{n_j,\tau} \equiv \Delta_j$, which is the set of n_j-dimensional vectors $\{(t_1, \ldots, t_{n_j}); \sum t_i \leq \tau, t_i \geq 0\}$.

Now consider the conditional likelihood in Eq. (17). Because $f(t_j \mid n_j)$ is a constant, it can be discarded. However, Eq. (17) resists further simplification. The main obstacle is the constant density of t over Δ, which introduces an interdependency among the individual components t_i of t, due to the inequality constraint $\sum_i t_i \leq \tau$. Maximizing the likelihood function in Eq. (17) with respect to θ and ε therefore seems prohibitive. Moreover, it is not desirable either: The number of elements in θ grows at the same rate as the sample size, and therefore it is to be expected that consistency of the ML-estimators does not hold. So, the maximization of the likelihood function in Eq. (17) is abandoned as an estimation procedure.

Arnold and Strauss (1988) showed that consistent estimates of model parameters can be obtained if a product of marginal and conditional likelihoods is maximized instead of the likelihood function. In order to estimate the parameters, the pseudo-likelihood function

$$PL(\xi, \beta, \varepsilon; \{\mathbf{n}, \mathbf{u}\}) = L_P(\beta; \{\mathbf{n}\}) \times L(\xi, \varepsilon; \{\mathbf{u}\}), \tag{18}$$

wil be maximized. The second factor in Eq. (18) is proportional to the product of the marginal probabilities of the J response patterns, with the response times integrated out. For a single response pattern u_j the marginal likelihood is given by

$$L(\xi_j, \varepsilon; u_j) = \prod_{i=1}^{n_j} [f_i(\xi_j)]^{u_{ji}} [1 - f_i(\xi_j)]^{1-u_{ji}} \tag{19}$$

where $f_i(\cdot)$ is defined by Eq. (9) with a single argument ξ_j, which is defined by Eq. (12). Let $s_j = \sum_i^{n_j} u_{ji}$, the score of respondent j, and let $\{s\}$ denote the set of observed scores, then Eq. (18) can be written as

$$PL(\xi, \beta, \varepsilon; \{\mathbf{n}, \mathbf{u}\}) = L_P(\beta; \{\mathbf{u}\} \mid \{s\}) \times L_c(\varepsilon; \{\mathbf{u}\} \mid \{s\}) \times L(\xi, \varepsilon; \{s\}). \tag{20}$$

The second factor in the right-hand side of this equation is the conditional likelihood of the response pattern conditional on the raw score. It should be understood that the number of items responded to also belongs to the condition, but the restriction that the items have been answered within a time interval τ no longer holds. It is well known (e.g., Fischer, 1974) that this conditional likelihood can be written as

$$L_c(\varepsilon; \{\mathbf{u}\} \mid \{s\}) = \frac{\prod_j^J \prod_{i=1}^{n_j} \exp(-\varepsilon_i u_{ji})}{\prod_j^J \gamma_{s_j}(e^{-\varepsilon})} \tag{21}$$

where $\gamma_s(\cdot)$ represents the well known basic symmetric functions, and the argument $e^{-\varepsilon}$ denotes $(\exp(-\varepsilon_1), \ldots, \exp(-\varepsilon_{n_j}))$. So the item parameters may be estimated by maximizing Eq. (21) which is nothing more than CML estimation in an incomplete design. Andersen (1970) has shown that this estimation procedure is asymptotically efficient. The fact that the third factor on the right-hand side of Eq. (20) is also a function of ε, does not mean that information is lost with respect to these parameters when CML is used.

Estimation of ξ. In order to estimate the subject parameters ξ, it is common use among practitioners of the Rasch model to maximize the likelihood function Eq. (19) with respect to ξ, while keeping the item parameters fixed at their CML estimates. This amounts to a procedure, known as Restricted Maximum Likelihood estimation (REML) (Amemiya, 1986), which in general does not affect the consistency of the estimates. Unfortunately, finite ML estimates for ξ do not exist if all or none of the items are correctly solved, and moreover ML estimates are biased in the sense that extreme scores get too extreme parameter estimation (Lord, 1983). Warm (1989) proposed an estimation procedure which removes the bias up to the order $1/n$. This procedure is called weighted maximum likelihood. In the case of the Rasch model, the estimate of ξ is obtained by maximizing the product W of the likelihood function and the square root of the test information function:

$$W(\xi) = \prod_{i}^{n_j} [f_i(\xi)]^{u_i} [1 - f_i(\xi)]^{1-u_i} \times \left[\sum_{i}^{n_j} f_i(\xi)[1 - f_i(\xi)] \right]^{1/2}. \qquad (22)$$

Another possibility is to work with a simpler model. If the items do not differ very much in difficulty, it might be reasonable to assume that all items are equally difficult. Without loss of generality, one can set $\varepsilon_i = 0$. In that case, maximization of Eq. (22) leads to the remarkable result

$$\xi = \ln \frac{s + \frac{1}{2}}{n - s + \frac{1}{2}}.$$

Combining this result with the bias correction from the simulation study in the Example section below (Eq. (35)), leads to the very simple estimation formula for θ:

$$\hat{\theta}_j = \ln\left(s_j + \frac{1}{2}\right) + \ln\left(n_j + \frac{1}{2}\right) - \ln\left(n_j - s_j + \frac{1}{2}\right). \qquad (23)$$

Summary of Estimation Procedure

The full estimation procedure comprises the following four steps:

(1) β_j is estimated from the number of answered items n_j. Its estimate is proportional to this number.

(2) The item parameters are estimated using the CML-procedure in an incomplete design. This can be accomplished by standard software, for example, the package OPLM (Verhelst, Glas, and Verstralen, 1995).

(3) The precision parameter ξ_j is estimated by maximizing Eq. (22). This also can be routinely done in OPLM.

(4) The estimate of the mental power θ_j is then given by applying Eq. (13) to the estimates of β_j and ξ_j:

$$\hat{\theta}_j = \hat{\xi}_j + \ln \hat{\beta}_j = \hat{\xi}_j + \ln n_j - \ln \tau. \tag{23}$$

Case of $p_i \neq 1$

If only the response patterns are observed, estimating one parameter p for each item is very hard. An approximation is therefore suggested. If p is taken to be a positive integer, using Eq. (12), the marginal probability of a wrong answer on item i in Eq. (9) can be written as

$$\begin{aligned} 1 - f_i(\xi, p) &= \left[1 + \sum_{h=1}^{p} \binom{p}{h} \exp(h\xi - h\varepsilon_i)\right]^{-1} \\ &= \left[1 + \sum_{h=1}^{p} \exp\left[h\xi - h\varepsilon_i + \ln \binom{p}{h}\right]\right]^{-1} \\ &= \left[1 + \sum_{h=1}^{p} \exp\left(h\xi - \sum_{g=1}^{h} \delta_{ig}\right)\right]^{-1}, \end{aligned}$$

where

$$\delta_{ig} = \varepsilon_i + \ln \frac{g}{p - g + 1}, \quad (g = 1, \ldots, p). \tag{28}$$

It is easily seen that Eq. (27) is formally identical to the probability of earning zero points on item i in the Partial Credit Model (PCM) (Masters, this volume). As shown in Eq. (28), the p category parameters are simple functions of the single item parameter ε_i. Since the responses are binary, the probability of an observed correct response equals the probability of a nonzero response in the partial credit interpretation. The model can be interpreted as a PCM with the nonzero categories collapsed.

The approximation now consists in replacing Eq. (27) by the complement of a logistic function that is characterized by a location parameter σ_i and a steepness parameter a_i. These steps result in

$$1 - f_i(\xi, p) \approx \left[1 + \exp[a_i(\xi - \sigma_i)]\right]^{-1}. \tag{29}$$

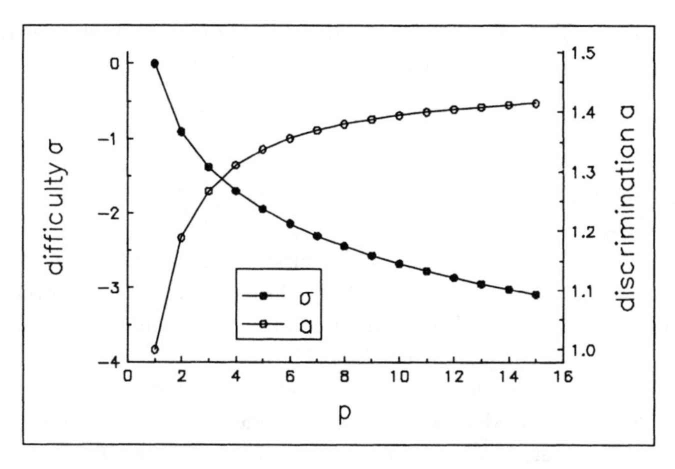

FIGURE 4. Best fitting values of σ_i and a_i as a function of p_i.

In a numerical study, several approximations were computed, all based on the weighted least squares principle, with different weight functions for the ξ-variate. These weight functions could be considered as proportional to a distribution density function of ξ. The results for different weight functions did not differ. The results of one approximation are displayed in Fig. 4. The values of σ_i are almost linear in $\ln(p)$. The steepness parameter increases monotonically with p, but seems to approach an asymptote which is less than 1.5 times its value at $p = 1$. This rather modest variation in steepness as a function of p makes it reasonable to work with a further approximation, namely, to fix the steepness parameter a_i at a common value. But this approach is equivalent to using the Rasch model.

With respect to the estimation of β_j, the following simple approximation may be used. The total response time is distributed as a sum of n_j gamma-distributed variates plus a nonnegative amount of time which is spent on the $(n_j + 1)$th item of which the response is not observed. Since all the n_j gamma distributions have the same shape parameter β_j, the likelihood equation for β_j is given by

$$\beta_j = \sum_i^{n_j} p_i \Big/ \sum_i^{n_j} t_{ji}. \tag{30}$$

If there is no correlation between the p_i-parameters and the rank number i of the items, a reasonable estimator of β is given by

$$\beta_j = \frac{\bar{p}(n_j + 0.5)}{\tau}. \tag{31}$$

where $\bar{p}$ is the average p-parameter, and where it is assumed that the time spent to the $(n_j + 1)$th item equals half of the average time spent to the completed items. The value of the average p-parameter is irrelevant because in the estimation of θ its logarithm is absorbed into an arbitrary additive constant.

Goodness of Fit

The fit of the Rasch component of the model may be tested both at test and item level. A fairly extensive battery of statistical tests is implemented in the program OPLM, and a detailed discussion is contained in Glas and Verhelst (1995) and Verhelst and Glas (1995).

When applying tests for item fit, it should be noted, however, that collecting data under speeded conditions has one aspect that may influence the power of the test. If the order of presentation of the items is the same for all examinees in the sample, the number of observations made on the items will decrease monotonically with their rank number, with the risk that some item parameters will not be estimable, for example, if they are responded to by very few examinees who all happen to give the same answer. Moreover, the standard error of the item parameter estimates will increase with their rank number, and as a consequence, the power of the test at the item level will decrease with the rank number of the item. To avoid this complication, one might consider presenting the items in different orders, such that the number of answers to the items is distributed more uniformly.

Testing the Constancy of β_j

To test the validity of the response time assumptions thoroughly, individual response times per item are needed. However, an elegant procedure can be constructed to test the constancy of the β-parameter in the gamma distribution during the response process. If the p-parameters are constant or their magnitude is uncorrelated with the item rank number, it follows from the model that expected number of items answered in the first half of the testing time is equal to number answered in the second half. This extra observation is quite easy to collect, for example, by asking the examinees to put a mark on their answer sheet at the place where they have arrived when a sign is given. Thus two numbers of items completed are collected for each examinee. n_{j1} and n_{j2} say, which together can be arranged in a $J \times 2$ contingency table. Because of experimental independence between examinees, the following simple log-linear model should fit:

$$\ln C(n_{jh}) = \mu + \alpha_j + \gamma_h, \quad (j = 1, \ldots, N;\ h = 1, 2), \tag{32}$$

with two additional restrictions, for example, $\alpha_1 = \gamma_1 = 0$. The hypothesis of equal expected numbers of items is then easily translated into the following linear restriction on the model parameters:

$$\gamma_1 = \gamma_2. \tag{33}$$

Estimating the model in Eq. (32) both with and without the restrictions yields two log-likelihoods, which by standard methods can be used to construct a likelihood-ratio test with one degree of freedom to test the hypothesis in Eq. (33).

Example

As an example of data analysis under the model, the results from a simulation study into the bias of the estimator of θ in Eq. (23) are given. Although the estimator of β is unbiased, and care was given to reduce the bias in the estimator of the precision parameter ξ, the conclusion that the estimator of the mental power is unbiased may be incorrect for at least two reasons. First, the whole estimation procedure on which Eq. (23) is based is an amalgam of different procedures which guarantees consistency but not automatically unbiasedness. For example, the estimator of β is unbiased, but in Eq. (23) the logarithm of β is used, and this transformed parameter is estimated by $\ln \hat{\beta}$, which is not an unbiased estimator of $\ln \beta$. Second, the remaining bias of the Warm estimator is not uniformly low (Verhelst and Kamphuis, 1989). In general, the bias increases with decreasing number of items in the test and with decreasing test information with respect to the precision parameter ξ.

In order to get an impression of the bias of the θ-estimate a small simulation study with a test consisting of 50 items was carried out. The item parameters ε of the first five items were equal to -2, -1, 0, 1, and 2, respectively. For the remaining items in the test, this sequence was repeated ten times, so that at whatever point test taking was finished, reasonable information is obtained over a broad range of the latent variable. The study comprised two other facets: (1) 21 different values of θ, equally spaced in the interval $[-2, 2]$ were used; (2) the number of items finished, n, took the values 5(5)50. So for every combination of θ and n an estimate of the bias, defined as

$$\text{bias}(\theta, n) = \theta - E(\hat{\theta} \mid \theta, n), \tag{34}$$

was wanted. The time limit of the test (τ) was 30 (unspecified) units. Since the bias, conditional on the number of finished items was investigated, the value of β was irrelevant; α was set to 1. For each of the $21 \times 10 = 210$ (θ, n) combinations, 3000 response patterns were generated according to the model, which in turn yielded 3000 estimates of θ. The averages of the 3000 estimates of θ were used as estimates of the expected value in Eq. (34). For further technical details of the simulation study, see Verhelst, Verstralen, and Jansen (1992). The results are displayed in Fig. 5. The first plot shows

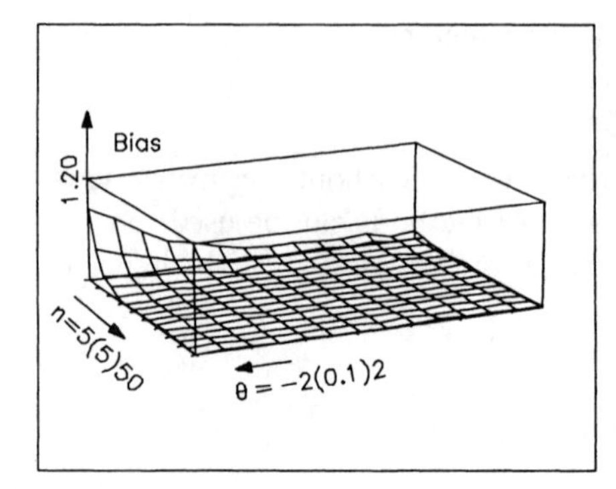

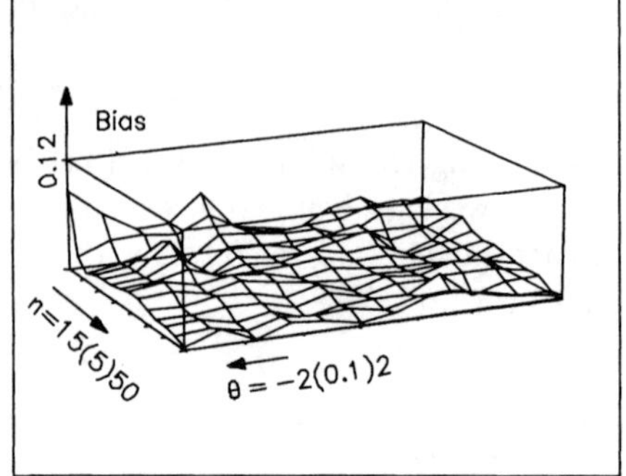

FIGURE 5. Estimated bias in the simulation study. Case 1: Well balanced information.

that there was considerable bias for combinations of large θ and small n. Small n means that the average response time was large, and, as explained earlier, a large response time acts as a positive shift of the distribution of the momentary mental power Z (see Fig. 2). So, in these cases the test becomes relatively easy, and a high proportion of correct responses will occur. As shown by Verhelst and Kamphuis (1989), a positive bias of the precision parameter results. The second plot displays the bias for values of n ranging from 15 to 50. The pattern of the surface is quite irregular, the irregularities being caused by sampling error.

It is remarkable that the estimated bias was positive for all (θ, n) combinations, meaning that mental power was systematically underestimated. This result can be explained by pointing at the fact that the expected response time per item conditional on the event that n items have been answered, actually represents examinees who were processing the $(n+1)$th item at the moment the total responding time τ has elapsed. It can be shown that this expected response time equals $\tau/(n+1)$. Using the reciprocal of this fraction as an estimator of β, however, resulted for a large n in a negative bias of about the same magnitude as the positive bias found in the simulation study. By a simple argument (see Verhelst, Verstralen, and Jansen, 1992), it was found that the estimator

$$\beta_j^* = \frac{n_j + \frac{1}{2}}{\tau} \tag{35}$$

removed the bias almost completely provided n was not too small.

Of course, the design of the simulation study was optimal to eliminate bias because of the special order in which the items were presented. In a second simulation study, the same items were presented in increasing order of difficulty, so that the expected difficulty of the finished items increased with n. As a consequence, as shown in Fig. 6, considerable bias for moderate and high θ-values results was found, even for moderate n. The second plot

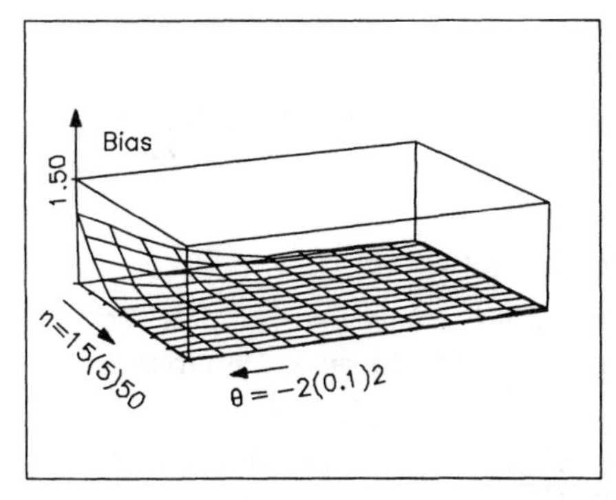

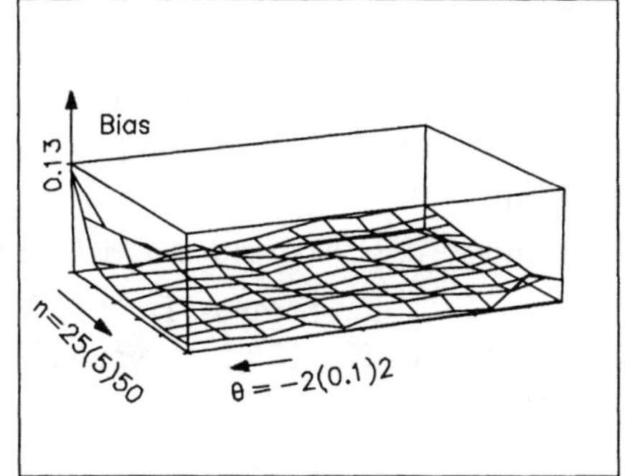

FIGURE 6. Estimated bias in the simulation study. Case 2: Items ordered with increasing difficulty.

in Fig. 6 shows that about the same bias resulted from $n = 25$ in this condition as for $n = 15$ in the first condition.

Discussion

Although the discussion of the model took the speed test as a paradigm, the results are with minor modifications, also valid for the so-called task-limit tests, where all examinees answer all items. The only extra observation needed is the total response time per respondent, τ_j. In this case, parameter estimation becomes even easier because one knows exactly the sum of the n_j item response times, so that the hard problem of the dependence of response times, due to the conditioning on n_j, does not exist.

In the Introduction it was stated that speed and accuracy can be considered as complementary aspects of the concept of mental power. This does not mean, however, that these concepts should be abandoned altogether. For example, it may be worthwhile to study the bivariate distribution of power and speed in some population of examinees, and to estimate their covariance, or the regression of one variable on the other. The model presented here offers the possibility to collect observations for the two variables with a single well designed speed test.

As in our approach mental power appears to be a more fundamental concept than speed and accuracy, one might raise the question whether a 'power test' with the number of correct responses as score measures mental power or only accuracy. Even in cases where there is (almost) no external time pressure, it seems reasonable to assume that examinees may have their own internal time restrictions and work at their own rate. Recording individual response time, and combining it with the usual number-right score as suggested in Eq. (23), might raise the predictive validity of the test. Empirical research into such options is a challenging area indeed.

References

Andersen, E.B. (1970). Asymptotic properties of conditional maximum likelihood estimation. *Journal of the Royal Statistical Society B* **32**, 283–301.

Amemiya, T. (1986). *Advanced Econometrics.* Oxford: Blackwell.

Arnold, B.C. and Strauss, D. (1988). *Pseudolikelihood Estimation* (Technical Report No. 164). Riverside: University of California, Department of Statistics.

Dubey, S.D. (1969). A new derivation of the logistic distribution. *Naval Research Logistics Quarterly* **16**, 37–40.

Fischer, G.H. (1974). *Einführung in die Theorie psychologischer Tests* [Introduction to the Theory of Psychological Tests]. Bern: Huber.

Glas, C.A.W. and Verhelst, N.D. (1995). Testing the Rasch model. In G.H. Fischer and I.W. Molenaar (Eds.), *Rasch Models: Foundations, Recent Developments and Applications* (pp. 69–95). New York: Springer-Verlag.

Lord, F.M. (1983). Unbiased estimation of ability parameters, of their variance, and of their parallel-forms reliability. *Psychometrika* **48**, 233–245.

Masters, G.N. (1982). A Rasch model for partial credit scoring. *Psychometrika* **47**, 149–174.

Rasch, G. (1980). *Probabilistic Models for Some Intelligence and Attainment Tests.* Chicago: The University of Chicago Press (original work published in 1960).

Roskam, E.E.Ch.I. (1987). Towards a psychometric theory of intelligence. In E.E.Ch.I. Roskam and R. Suck (Eds.), *Progress in Mathematical Psychology,* Vol. 1 (pp. 151–174). Amsterdam: North-Holland.

Van Breukelen, G.J.P. (1989). *Concentration, Speed and Precision in Mental Tests: A Psychometric Approach.* Doctoral dissertation, University of Nijmegen, The Netherlands.

Verhelst, N.D. and Kamphuis, F.H. (1989). *Statistiek met Theta-Dak* [Statistics with Theta-hat] (Bulletin series, 77). Arnhem: Cito.

Verhelst, N.D., Glas, C.A.W., and Verstralen, H.H.F.M. (1995). *OPLM: One Parameter Logistic Model. Computer Program and Manual.* Arnhem: Cito.

Verhelst, N.D. and Glas, C.A.W. (1995). The one-parameter logistic model. In G.H. Fischer and I.W. Molenaar (Eds.), *Rasch Models: Foundations, Recent Developments and Applications* (pp. 215–237). New York: Springer.

Verhelst, N.D., Verstralen, H.H.F.M., and Jansen, M.G.H. (1992). *A Logistic Model for Time Limit Tests.* (Measurement and Research Department Reports, 92-1). Arnhem: Cito.

Warm, Th.A. (1989). Weighted likelihood estimation of ability in item response theory. *Psychometrika* **54**, 427–450.

11
Models for Speed and Time-Limit Tests

Edward E. Roskam

Introduction

There is a long tradition in the ability testing literature, going back at least to Spearman (1927) and Thorndike et al. (1927), that response speed is as much an indicator of ability as is the correctness of responses to items of increasing difficulty (Berger, 1982; Eysenck, 1982; Brand and Dreary, 1982). Some tests are pure speed tests (consisting of items that are virtually always correctly solved, and where completion time is the recorded variable), others are pure power tests (consisting of items of increasing difficulty, administered without time limit, where the number of correct responses is the recorded variable), but most tests are a mixture: They consist of items of varying difficulty and are administered with a time limit.

Item response theory (IRT) essentially assumes that the test is a pure power test: The person attempts all items, and only the correctness of the response is modeled. Response time is ignored. Polytomous, partial credit, and related models are based on the same assumption, although the polytomous model may be adapted to take response time into account by scoring the item according to the time needed for a correct response. However, polytomous models such as the partial credit model are not invariant under a change of categorizing the response (time) continuum (Jansen and Roskam, 1986; Roskam and Jansen, 1989).

The principles of IRT can be adapted to response times, notably in pure speed tests. These models assume that all responses are correct, or simply ignore the (in)correctness of the response. Essentially, the pertinent models state that the probability (density) of the response time to an item is a function of the item difficulty and the person's (mental) speed, assuming an exponential response time distribution. The Weibull distribution (Scheiblechner, 1979, 1985) and a generalized gamma distribution (Maris, 1993) have also been considered. Each of these models assume that the rate of responding is an additive function of item difficulty ε_i and mental speed θ_j. Conditional maximum likelihood estimators are given by Scheiblechner (1979, 1985). For a more basic discussion, see Fischer and Kisser (1983).

Scheiblechner's model is related to Rasch' (1960; see also Fischer, 1991; Jansen and Van Duijn, 1992) Poisson model. The latter is concerned with tests of different difficulties rather than with single items. "Items" within tests are assumed to be equivalent. Rasch has proposed and applied the Poisson model notably for analyzing reading speed, e.g., the number of words read aloud from a given text within a time limit. It may apply more generally to any condition where the observed variable is the number of times that a particular response is given during a (fixed) time interval. In Rasch' Poisson model, the completion times for each item from test q are assumed to be exponentially distributed with parameter $\lambda_{jq} = \theta_j \varepsilon_q$, that is, the probability density function (pdf) of the response time, t, is given by $f_{jq}(t) = \theta_j \varepsilon_q e^{(-\theta_j \varepsilon_q t)}$. The parameter θ_j is the person's speed, ability, or propensity in performing the task, and ε_q is the easiness of the test or condition q. The total number K_{jq} of items completed within a time limit L_q is then Poisson distributed.

In this chapter, we address time-limit tests which are a mixture of "speed" and "power." To take both correctness and response time into account, some assumptions have to be made concerning the relation between response time and the correctness of the response. Early attempts to do so date back to Thurstone (1937), Furneaux (1960) and White (1982). Subsequent models developed by Roskam (1987), Van Breukelen (1989), and Verhelst et al. (1992, this volume) assume that the probability of a correct response increases with response time. This is a strong assumption, implying that given infinite time, any item will be answered correctly (though the probability of infinite response time is zero, and some provision might be modelled to put an upper limit on the probability of a correct response even if response time gets infinitely large). Both Van Breukelen (1989) and Verhelst et al. (1992) assume that the response time is governed by "persistence," or the tendency to spend (more) time on an item, and by one or more parameters representing the person's ability and/or the item's difficulty.

Speed-Accuracy Trade-Off (SAT) and Conditional Accuracy Function (CAF)

There is a trade-off between speed and accuracy: If a person tends to complete many items within the time limit, he will give more incorrect responses, and vice versa. The relation between the mean response time and the probability of a correct response across (experimental) conditions is called the Speed-Accuracy Trade-off Function (SATF). It is usually depicted as an increasing ogive-like function (see Fig. 1), but specific models may predict a different shape. Time pressure and other factors will affect the speed vs. accuracy preference of the person. The SATF should be distinguished from the Conditional Accuracy Function (CAF), which represents

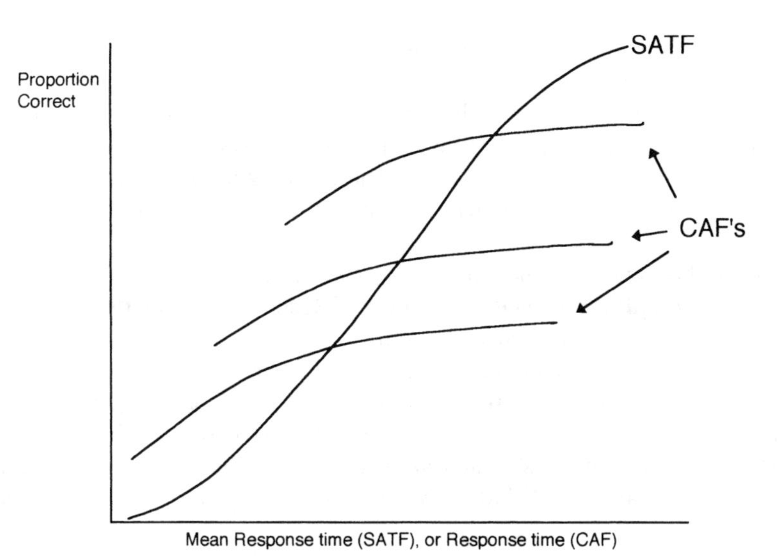

FIGURE 1. Examples of a Speed-Accuracy Trade-off Function (SATF) and Conditional Accuracy Functions (CAF).

the probability of a correct response conditional upon the response time (see Fig. 1) within a fixed SAT. Both SATF and CAF concern a given person ability and item difficulty.

A distinction should also be made between conditions where the response time is subject (person) and task controlled, and conditions where the response time is experimenter controlled. The latter is sometimes called 'inspection time' or "deadline". However, the CAF concerns the task- and subject-controlled response time. An accuracy function based on inspection time is a CAF only if the CAF is independent of the experimental condition. This is the case in the Rasch-Weibull model to be discussed below, which is even a stricter case since its CAF and SATF have the same functional form.

Constant, increasing, and decreasing CAFs have been described in the literature. For instance, if the subject's strategy is either to guess or to solve the problem, the CAF is likely to be increasing, but the subject's tendency to guess may depend on the time pressure, so the CAF is not independent of that strategy.

The psychometric models proposed by Van Breukelen and Roskam (1991), and by Verhelst et al. (1992) assume an increasing CAF: As the actual response time increases, the probability of correct response increases. Moreover, they assume that the CAF is independent of the SAT strategy of the subject. Such models are called Adjustable Timing Models (ATM; Ollman, 1977; Luce, 1986, pp. 249–252): Strategy parameters determine only the response time distribution, not the CAF. The probability of a correct response, then, depends on the strategy of the subject only via the response time distribution. Both the response time distribution and the CAF may depend on difficulty and ability parameters.[1]

The foregoing makes clear that two sets of parameters should be distinguished: (a) Strategy parameters concerning the speed-accuracy trade-off; and (b) task[2] parameters concerning the person's ability and the item difficulty. A crucial question is whether or not the CAF depends on strategy parameters.

As to the general structure of models which take response time into account, the following issues must be addressed: (a) What determines response time? (b) How is correctness of a response related to the response time? (c) How is the probability of correct responses $P[+ \mid \underline{\theta}]$ for given item and person parameters ($\underline{\theta}$) related to the conditional probability $P[+ \mid \underline{\theta}, t]$ (where t is the response time)? (d) What is the psychological interpretation of the person parameters? (mental speed, persistence, accuracy, "ability," or otherwise); and (e) What is it that is actually measured by speeded tests?

Analysis of Time-Limit Tests as Structurally Incomplete Design

The Rasch model property of sample independence can serve to analyze a time-limit test. Depending on their speed, persons complete different subsets of items, but according to the property of sample independence, the estimated item parameters should be independent of which persons have completed those items, and the person parameters should be independent of which items are completed by the person (except for calibration of the scale). Accordingly, the sample of persons can be partitioned into groups of persons completing the same subset of items, that is, the sample of persons is partitioned into "speed" groups. For instance, if the test contains $n = 20$ items, some persons have completed only the first 10 items within the time limit, others have completed only the first 11 items, and so forth. Let j denote a person, and let K_j denote the last completed item. The partitioning is based on K_j, assuming that all persons take the items in the same order, and that missing responses prior to the last completed item are considered as incorrect. Algorithms suitable for such a structurally incomplete design, e.g., RIDA (Glas, 1989) and RSP (Glas and Ellis, 1993) can be used to estimate simultaneously all n item parameters, and from the estimated item parameters the person parameters can be estimated.

---

[1] Ollman's original definition of ATM is more restrictive: It requires that the CAF depends only on task parameters and the response time distribution depends only on strategy parameters.

[2] The term 'task' in the psychonomic literature refers to everything concerning the solution process, as distinct from strategy and other parameters which are alien to the solution process.

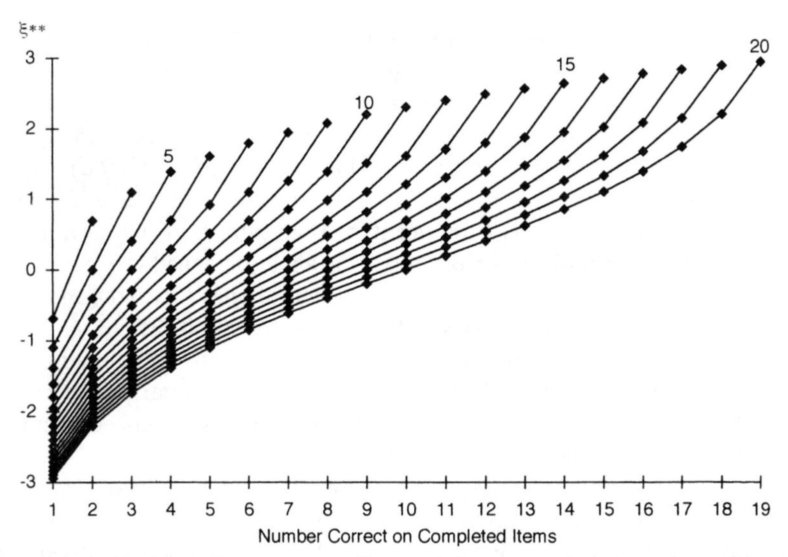

FIGURE 2. Estimated precision, ξ^{**}, as a function of the number of correct responses, for various numbers of items completed, and for a hypothetical test with equal item difficulties. (The symbol ξ^{**} is explained in the text at Eqs. (14) and (17). Curves for different numbers of items completed).

Van den Wollenberg (1979, 1983) estimated in each speed group separately the parameters of the items completed by those persons. After eliminating only a few items and persons, five of the six subtests of the ISI test analyzed by Van den Wollenberg turned out to be Rasch homogeneous both within and across speed groups. Once this was established, Van den Wollenberg then combined the speed groups into groups of persons who had completed *at least* k items and re-estimated all 1 through k item parameters in each of those groups, calibrating the scales by setting the sum of the first ten items parameters, $\Sigma\sigma_i$, for $i = 1, \ldots, 10$, equal to zero, and found virtually identical item parameters across these groups. This shows that (at least for the tests at hand) item and person parameters can be estimated independent of the person's speed. Note that algorithms for structurally incomplete designs can do all this simultaneously.

Estimation of the person parameters was based on the items actually completed by that person, using the estimated item parameters. As a consequence, the regression of the estimated person parameter on the number of correct responses was different in different speed groups. This is illustrated in Fig. 2.

Van den Wollenberg used the generic term "precision" for the person parameter, rather than "ability." Figure 2 shows the reason. The estimated person parameters, denoted as ξ^{**}, decreased with the speed of the person (see also Eq. (17), below). It was higher for persons producing r correct responses while completing k items than it was for persons producing the same number of correct responses but completing more than k items. With more items completed, i.e., increasing "raw" speed, the same number of correct responses indicated *less* precision. The estimated person parameter was a (nonlinear) function of the *proportion* correct responses. For the same number, r, of correct responses, increased speed ($K_{j_2}/L > K_{j_1}/L$) implies decreased precision ($r/K_{j_2} < r/K_{j_1}$). And since $K_{j_2}/L > K_{j_1}/L$ meant that person j_2 had used less time per item than person j_1, equal numbers of correct responses indicated that person j_2's mental speed is greater than person j_1's. An approximate estimation of mental speed, corresponding to Fig. 2, is based on the Rasch-Weibull model and given in Fig. 3.

Time-limit tests yield two scores: The number of items completed can be taken as a measure of "speed," and the estimated person parameter can be taken as a measure of "precision," and both depend on the speed-accuracy trade-off attitude of the person.

However, for various reasons, these terms may not be appropriate. The estimated precision is a function of the speed, and although that is in accordance with the speed-accuracy trade-off principle, it depends on the test-taking strategy of the person, and therefore it cannot be taken as a pure person ability parameter. The same holds for the number of items completed as a measure of speed. Only the item parameters appear to be justifiably interpretable as "item difficulty." With respect to the person parameters, task parameters (ability) and strategy parameters (SAT) are confounded.

Van den Wollenberg (1985) showed that speed (number of items completed within the time limit) and precision (the expected score on the first 10 items of a test as a function of the person parameter and the item parameters), were not uncorrelated over persons. This indicates that whatever the distribution of response times, and whatever the conditional accuracy function, speed and precision depend on a common person parameter. This would appear to be "something" which may appropriately be called "mental speed."

Presentation of the Model

The model[3] to be presented consists of two logically independent submodels. One submodel presents the Rasch response time model, which is a CAF with mental speed, θ, and item difficulty, ε, as its parameters. The basic idea is that a person's effective ability in solving an item increases with the time invested in solving it. The rate of that increase is 'mental speed.' The other submodel specifies the response time distribution as a Weibull distribution parameterized as a function of the person's mental speed, his

[3]Much of this section is a summary of Van Breukelen and Roskam (1991).

or her persistence in attempting to solve an item, and the item difficulty. More difficult items will take more time, mentally faster persons will use less time, and more persistent persons will take more time. Persistence is a strategy parameter. The more persistent person will invest more time in each item, and so will increase the probability of correct responses. Both submodels share Rasch' principle of "equivalent subjects" and "equivalent items" in comparing persons and items, respectively, either by the response times or by the correctness of the responses. The marginal probability of a correct response is obtained by integrating out the response time distribution, yielding (to a fair approximation) again a Rasch model where the (effective) person parameter is a function of both mental speed and persistence. Finally, it will be shown that the SATF is again a Rasch model with its shape dependent on mental speed and item difficulty, and the actual trade-off between precision and speed depending on the person's persistence.

The Rasch Response Time Model

Roskam (1987) proposed a model integrating response time and correctness:

$$P(U_{ij} = 1 \mid t_{ij}, j, i) = \frac{\theta_j t_{ij}}{\theta_j t_{ij} + \varepsilon_i} = \frac{\exp(\xi_j + \tau_{ij} - \sigma_i)}{1 + \exp(\xi_j + \tau_{ij} - \sigma_i)}, \tag{1}$$

where θ is person ability, ε is item difficulty, and t is the response time, and ξ, σ, and τ are the logarithms of θ, ε, and t, respectively. Equation (1) expresses that the effective ability parameter for item i is mental speed times processing time. Obviously, the sufficient statistic for the person parameter, ξ_j, is $\sum_i u_{ij}$, and the known t_{ij}'s enter into the conditional likelihood function (see Eq. (8) below). Equation (1) is illustrated in Fig. 5(a) below.

For a more general formulation of Eq. (1), we can replace $\theta_j t_{ij}$ by $\theta_j(t_{ij})$, where $\theta_j(t)$ is some monotonely increasing function of time, and t_{ij} is the actual response time such that $\theta_{j_1}(t^*) > \theta_{j_2}(t^*)$ for some $t^* \Leftrightarrow \forall t$: $\theta_{j_1}(t) > \theta_{j_2}(t)$. We can call $\theta(t)$ the 'effective ability.' This is useful if the model is tested experimentally and t is an experimenter controlled response deadline. Using an experimental controlled response deadline is compatible with the model if it is assumed that the response time distribution is a Weibull distribution as in Eq. (3), below, since that makes the CAF (Eq. (1)) and the SATF (Eq. (7), below) the same.

The Weibull Model

In standard administration of time-limit tests, the t_{ij} are not observed and only the total test time (or the time limit) is known. In that case, some assumption has to be made about the distribution of t_{ij}. Any distribution is fully characterized by its so-called hazard function. In terms of the duration of a response process, the hazard function, $h(t)$, is defined as the probability density that the response is given at time t, conditional upon not been given yet. Formally, $h(t)$ is the limit of $P(t < T < t + \Delta t) \mid t < T)/\Delta t$ as $\Delta t \to 0$. Van Breukelen (1989) proposed a hazard function which increases with time, proportional to the person's mental speed θ, and inversely proportional to the item difficulty (ε), and to the person's "persistence" (δ) in continuing working on the item (see Van Breukelen and Roskam, 1991, for details):

$$h_{ij}(t) = \frac{\theta_j}{\varepsilon_i \delta_j} t. \tag{2}$$

This hazard function expresses that more difficult items will take more time, mentally faster persons will use less time, and more persistent persons will take more time. The hazard function in Eq. (2) defines the probability density and probability distribution functions)[4]

$$f(t) = \lambda t \exp\left(-\frac{\lambda}{2}t^2\right), \tag{3a}$$

and

$$F(t) = 1 - \exp\left(-\frac{\lambda}{2}t^2\right), \tag{3b}$$

(where $\lambda = \frac{\theta}{\varepsilon\delta}$, omitting subscripts), which is a Weibull distribution.

'Specific Objectivity' and the Proportional Hazard Function

A pair of hazard functions $h_g(t)$ ($g = 1, 2$) is said to be proportional if they have the form $h_g(t) = \lambda_g b(t)$, where $b(t)$ is a function of t independent of g. For independent random variables with proportional hazard functions, it is easily shown[5] that $P(T_1 < T_2)$ is equal to $\frac{\lambda_1}{\lambda_1 + \lambda_2}$. When the parameters of hazard functions are multiplicative functions of person and item parameters, it follows that the odds of one person's response time to an item being shorter than another person's depends on the persons' parameters

[4]Because $f(t) = dF(t)/dt$, the hazard function $h(t)$ is equal to $f(t)/[1 - F(t)]$, where $f(t)$ is the probability density function, and $F(t)$ is the cumulative distribution function. Let $H(t) = \int_0^t h(x)dx$. Then $F(t) = 1 - e^{-H(t)}$, and $f(t) = h(t)e^{-H(t)}$. The Weibull distribution is defined by its hazard function $h(t) = \lambda t^{(\beta-1)}$, and so its pdf is $f(t) = \lambda t^{\beta-1} \exp\left(-\frac{\lambda}{\beta}t^{\beta}\right)$. For $\beta > 1$, the hazard rate increases. For $\beta = 2$, as in Eq. (2), it increases linearly. For $\beta = 3.6$, the distribution is approximately normal. For $\beta = 1$, the hazard function is constant, and the distribution is equal to the exponential distribution.

[5]The probability of $T_{g^*} = \min\{T_1, T_2, T_3, \ldots\}$ is equal to $f_{g^*}(t)$ times the product of the probabilities $P(T_g \geq t)$, $g \neq g^*$, integrated over t. Using the formulas in the previous footnote, and if hazard rates are proportional, that is, if $h_g(t) = \lambda_g b(t)$, the integral simplifies into $\lambda_{g^*}/\sum \lambda_g$.

only. Taking Eq. (2) as an example, comparing two persons j_1 and j_2:

$$\frac{P(T_{j_1 i} < T_{j_2 i})}{P(T_{j_2 i} > T_{j_1 i})} = \frac{\theta_{j_1}/\delta_{j_1}}{\theta_{j_2}/\delta_{j_2}} \quad \text{for all items } i. \tag{4a}$$

Similarly, comparing two items, i_1 and i_2:

$$\frac{P(T_{ji_1} < T_{ji_2})}{P(T_{ji_2} > T_{ji_1})} = \frac{\varepsilon_{i_2}}{\varepsilon_{i_1}} \quad \text{for all persons } j. \tag{4b}$$

So, response time distributions with proportional hazard functions which are multiplicative functions of person and item parameters share Rasch' principle of "equivalent subjects" and "equivalent items" in comparing persons and items, respectively, by their response times.

The Marginal Probability of a Correct Response

Multiplying Eq. (1) by the Weibull density and integrating yields the marginal probability of a correct response:

$$P(U_{ij} = 1 \mid j, i) = \int_0^\infty \frac{\theta_j t}{\theta_j t + \varepsilon_i} f(t)\, dt = \int_0^\infty \frac{\theta_j t}{\theta_j t + \varepsilon_i} h(t) e^{-H(t)}\, dt$$

$$= \int_0^\infty \frac{\theta_j t}{\theta_j t + \varepsilon_i} \frac{\theta_j}{\varepsilon_i \delta_j} t \exp\left\{ \frac{\theta_j}{2\varepsilon_i \delta_j} t^2 \right\} dt. \tag{5}$$

An approximation to this integral is obtained by assuming that t in Eq. (1) is equal to its mode. The mode of a Weibull distribution with hazard function λt is: $1/\sqrt{\lambda}$. Hence:

$$P(U_{ij} = 1 \mid j, i) \approx \frac{\theta_j \,\text{Mode}[T_{ij}]}{\theta_j \,\text{Mode}[T_{ij}] + \varepsilon_i} = \frac{\theta_j \sqrt{\varepsilon_i \delta_i / \theta_j}}{\theta_j \sqrt{\varepsilon_i \delta_j / \theta_j} + \varepsilon_i} = \frac{\sqrt{\theta_j \delta_j}}{\sqrt{\theta_j \delta_j} + \sqrt{\varepsilon_i}}. \tag{6}$$

Van Breukelen (1989) showed that Eq. (6) is quite close to the result obtained by numerical integration of Eq. (5). Obviously, Eq. (6) is a standard Rasch model but with a different meaning of the person parameter. Note that the square root in Eq. (6) is merely a matter of parameterization: Redefining the hazard function in terms of $\theta_j^* \equiv \sqrt{\theta_j \delta_j}$, and $\varepsilon_i^* \equiv \sqrt{\varepsilon_i}$, we obtain $h_{ij}(t) = \left(\frac{\theta_j^* \varepsilon_i^*}{\delta_j}\right)^2 t$, and $P(U_{ij} = 1 \mid j, i) = \frac{\theta_j^*}{\theta_j^* + \varepsilon_i^*}$.

The latter is a fascinating result. Equation (1) appears to be incompatible with Van den Wollenberg's (1979, 1983) finding that Rasch homogeneity can exist across persons who invest different amounts of time in each item. Equation (1) implies that the response times should have been taken into account in estimating the item parameters. These response times are certainly different between speed groups. Equation (6), however, shows that Rasch homogeneity can be found despite such differences. It also shows that the person parameter obtained in analyzing time-limit tests by means of a structurally incomplete design, is a function of mental speed and persistence. The parameter $\theta_j^* \equiv \sqrt{\theta_j \delta_j}$ might be called the person's *effective test ability*.

In comparing the right and middle members of Eq. (6), it may appear puzzling whether the item parameter should be defined as ε or as $\sqrt{\varepsilon}$. If the person's effective *test* ability is defined as $\theta_j^* \equiv \sqrt{\theta_j \delta_j}$, then $\sqrt{\varepsilon_i}$ is the corresponding *effective item* difficulty. If the model is interpreted in terms of mental speed, θ_j, then ε_i is the corresponding item difficulty. The reason for this apparent discrepancy is that the effective *item* ability is $\theta_j \operatorname{Mode}[T_{ij}] = \sqrt{\theta_j \varepsilon_i \delta_j}$, due to the definition of the hazard function, which makes the time spent on an item (and hence the effective *item* ability) a function of the item difficulty.

The Speed-Accuracy Trade-Off Function (SATF)

The marginal probability of a correct response in Eq. (6) was obtained by replacing t in Eq. (1) by its mode. The expected response time of the Weibull distribution with hazard function $h(t) = \lambda t$ is $\sqrt{\frac{\pi}{2\lambda}}$, where $\lambda = \frac{\theta}{\varepsilon\delta}$. So, Mode$[T]$ is $\sqrt{\frac{2}{\pi}}$ times the mean, and obviously the SATF of the Rasch–Weibull model has the same form as the CAF in Eq. (1):

$$P(U = 1 \mid \varepsilon, \theta) = \frac{\theta \operatorname{E}[T]\sqrt{2/\pi}}{\theta \operatorname{E}[T]\sqrt{2/\pi} + \varepsilon} = \frac{\operatorname{E}[T]}{\operatorname{E}[T] + \frac{\varepsilon}{\theta}\sqrt{\pi/2}}. \tag{7}$$

The log-odds of a correct response is a linear function of ln E$[T]$ or ln Mode$[T]$ with slope 1, and intercept $\ln(\frac{\varepsilon}{\theta}\sqrt{\pi/2})$, or $\ln(\frac{\varepsilon}{\theta})$, respectively.

Parameter Estimation

No methods are available for estimating the parameters taking both the Rasch response time model in Eq. (1) and the Weibull response time distribution in Eq. (3) simultaneously into account. We present a two-stage estimation procedure, details of which are given below. This procedure assumes that response times are recorded. Without any assumption about the response time distribution, the item difficulty parameters in Eq. (1) can be estimated by the method of conditional maximum likelihood (CML). This will also allow a test of the goodness of fit of the model in Eq. (1). Once the item parameters are estimated, and if the Rasch response time model fits, the mental speed parameters ($\theta \equiv \exp \xi$) can be estimated. Next, without any assumption about the conditional accuracy function in Eq. (1), but assuming the item difficulty parameters ($\varepsilon \equiv \exp \sigma$) and the mental speed parameters (θ) known, the persistence parameter (δ) can be estimated maximizing the likelihood of the observed response times.

We will also present another estimation procedure, for which individual item response times need not to be observed. It uses only the number of items completed within the time limit, and is based on either Eq. (6) or Eq. (7).

Estimation When Response Times Are Observed: (1) Item Parameters

The estimation procedure is essentially the same as in the dichotomous Rasch model: The parameters are estimated by conditional maximum likelihood, that is, by maximizing the likelihood of the data conditional upon the person's raw scores (cf. Fischer, 1974, p. 234).

Let $\underline{u}_j = \{u_{ij},\ i = 1, \ldots, K_j\}$ be the vector of binary scored responses of person j, $\underline{t}_j = \{t_{ij},\ i = 1, \ldots, K_j\}$ the associated vector of observed response times, and $\tau_{ij} = \ln(t_{ij})$. Let K_j be the number of items completed by person j, and r_j the number of positive responses (raw score). We assume that all persons attempt the items in the same order, but that assumption is not necessary (simply replace i in the following equations by $i(j)$, that is, the item completed at the ith position in the set of items completed by person j). The likelihood associated with $\underline{u}_j$ is:

$$P(\underline{u}_j \mid \underline{t}_j, K_j; \xi_j, \underline{\sigma}) = \prod_{i=1}^{K_j} \frac{\exp[u_{ij}(\xi_j + \tau_{ij} - \sigma_i)]}{1 + \exp[\xi_j + \tau_{ij} - \sigma_i]}$$

$$= \frac{\exp\left[r_j\xi_j + \sum_i^{K_j} u_{ij}(\tau_{ij} - \sigma_i)\right]}{\prod_{i=1}^{K_j}\{1 + \exp[\xi_j + \tau_{ij} - \sigma_i]\}}.$$

Let $\{\underline{s}_p(r_j, K_j)\}$ be the set of all distinct response patterns $\underline{s}_p$ ($p = 1, \ldots, \binom{K_j}{r_j}$) on items $i = 1, \ldots, K_j$, containing r_j positive responses, where $s_i = (0 \mid 1)$ and $\sum_i^{K_j} s_i = r_j$ (omitting the subscript p). The probability of the number of positive responses, r_j, is:

$$P(r_j \mid \underline{t}_j, K_j; \xi_j, \underline{\sigma}) = \frac{\exp(r_j\xi_j)}{\prod_i^{K_j}\{1 + \exp[\xi_j + \tau_{ij} - \sigma_i]\}}$$

$$\times \sum_{\{\underline{s}(r_j, K_j)\}} \exp\left[\sum_i^{K_j} s_i(\tau_{ij} - \sigma_i)\right].$$

Hence, the conditional likelihood associated with $\underline{u}_j$, given the raw score r_j is:

$$P(\underline{u}_j \mid r_j, \underline{t}_j, K_j; \xi_j, \underline{\sigma}) = \frac{\exp\left[\sum_i^{K_j} u_{ij}(\tau_{ij} - \sigma_i)\right]}{\sum_{\{\underline{s}(r_j, K_j)\}} \exp\left[\sum_i^{K_j} s_i(\tau_{ij} - \sigma_i)\right]}$$

$$= P(\underline{u}_j \mid r_j, \underline{t}_j, K_j; \underline{\sigma}). \tag{8}$$

The item parameter estimates are obtained by maximizing $\prod_{j=1}^{N} P(\underline{u}_j \mid r_j,$ $\underline{t}_j$, K_j; $\underline{\sigma}$) with respect to $\underline{\sigma}$. The estimation comes down to equating the persons' raw scores to their expected value conditionally on the frequency of the persons' raw scores. This estimator is essentially the same as the usual CML estimator in the dichotomous Rasch model (Fischer, 1974, pp. 241–245; Glas, 1989; Gustafsson, 1980), but with $\sigma_i - \tau_{ij}$ replacing the item parameter σ_i. This makes it hardly feasible for practical application, since the denominator in Eq. (8) must be evaluated for each person separately, and not merely for each different raw score. A practically feasible approximation to Eq. (8) is obtained by replacing τ_{ij} by the logarithm of the mean response time over items, as is given in Eq. (16), below.

Equation (8) becomes much more practicable in case of an experimenter controlled response deadline per item and person, limiting the variety of t_{ij} values. A deadline experiment is compatible with the model if the response time distribution is a Weibull distribution as in Eq. (3) since that makes the CAF and the SATF the same.

Estimation When Response Times Are Observed: (2) Person Parameters

Having estimated the item parameters, σ, the persons' mental speed parameters, ξ, can be obtained by solving:

$$\sum_{i}^{K_j} \frac{\exp(\xi_j + \tau_{ij} - \sigma_i)}{1 + \exp(\xi_j + \tau_{ij} - \sigma_i)} = r_j \tag{9}$$

for ξ_j (Fischer, 1974, p. 251). Unfortunately, this estimator can be seriously biased and unreliable. More robust methods have been developed by Warm (1990) and Mislevy (1984, 1986). These can be used if σ_i in their formulas is replaced by $\sigma_i - \tau_{ij}$.

Finally, the persistence parameter δ_j can be estimated by maximizing the log-likelihood, L, of the response time vector $\underline{t}_j$. This log-likelihood is obtained from Eq. (3) (remember that $\theta = e^{\xi}$, and $\varepsilon = e^{\sigma}$):

$$\mathrm{L} = \sum_{i=1}^{K_j} \ln(f_{ij}(t_{ij}))$$

$$= K_j(\ln \theta_j / \delta_j) + \sum_{i=1}^{K_j} \left(-\ln \varepsilon_i + \ln t_{ij} - \frac{1}{2} \frac{\theta_j}{\delta_j \varepsilon_i} t_{ij}^2 \right). \tag{10}$$

Taking the derivative of the log-likelihood in Eq. (10) with respect to $\phi_j \equiv$

θ_j/δ_j gives:

$$\partial \mathrm{L}/\partial\phi_j = \partial\left[K_j \ln \phi_j - \frac{1}{2}\sum_{i=1}^{K_j} \frac{\phi_i}{\varepsilon_i} t_{ij}^2\right] / \partial\phi_j = K_j/\phi_j - \frac{1}{2}\sum_{i=1}^{K_j} \frac{1}{\varepsilon_i} t_{ij}^2. \quad (11)$$

Setting the derivative in Eq. (11) to zero and solving for ϕ_j gives:

$$\phi_j = 1/G_j, \quad \text{where } G_j \equiv \frac{1}{K_j}\frac{1}{2}\sum_{i=1}^{K_j}\frac{1}{\varepsilon_i} t_{ij}^2. \quad (12)$$

Using the estimates of $\varepsilon = \ln\sigma$ and $\theta = \ln\xi$ obtained through Eqs. (8) and (9), δ_j is then estimated by $\delta_j = G_j e^{-\xi_j}$.

Estimation Not Using Item Response Times

The expectation of the Weibull distribution with hazard function $\lambda_{ij}t$ is $\sqrt{\frac{\pi}{2\lambda_{ij}}}$. If the time limit L occurs after the person has completed K_j items but before he has completed $K_j + 1$ items, the following relations will approximately hold (Van Breukelen, 1989; Donders, 1990):

$$L \approx \sum_{1}^{K_j} \sqrt{\frac{\pi}{2\lambda_{ij}}} \quad \text{and} \quad s_j \equiv \sqrt{\theta_j/\delta_j} \approx L^{-1}\sqrt{\pi/2}\sum_{1}^{K_j}\sqrt{\varepsilon_i}. \quad (13)$$

Taking Eq. (6) as the item response model and estimating $\theta^* \equiv \sqrt{\theta\delta}$ and $\varepsilon^* \equiv \sqrt{\varepsilon}$ in the way Van den Wollenberg (1979, 1983) did (or by means of a structurally incomplete design), the parameters θ and δ can be estimated from θ_j^* and s_j. Unfortunately, simulation studies (Donders, 1990) have shown that the estimates of θ_j and δ_j are seriously biased and unreliable. A person parameter estimator such as defined by Eq. (9) is known to be biased (Warm, 1989), and this fact probably also seriously affects the estimation of δ.

A coarser but possibly more robust approximation might be this: Assume the conditional probability in Eq. (1) is reasonably approximated by the marginal probability in Eq. (7). Next, assume that the item difficulties ε_i as far as the hazard functions are concerned, are close enough to set $\lambda_{ij} \approx \lambda_j$ allowing $E[T_{ij}]$ to be approximated by the mean response time over items, L/K_j. Substituting the latter in Eq. (7) yields:

$$P(U_{ij} = 1 \mid \varepsilon_i, \theta_j) \approx \frac{\theta_j(L/K_j)\sqrt{2/\pi}}{\theta_j(L/K_j)\sqrt{2/\pi} + \varepsilon_i}. \quad (14)$$

The item parameters can then be estimated by standard methods for a structurally incomplete design (Glas, 1989; Glas and Ellis, 1993). Estimating the person precision parameters $\theta_j^{**} = \theta_j(L/K_j)\sqrt{2/\pi}$, by any robust method, e.g., the Warm (1989) estimator, or the Mislevy (1984, 1986) expected a posteriori estimator, it suffices to divide this expression by $(L/K_j)\sqrt{2/\pi}$ to estimate θ_j. Note that Eq. (14) is equal to Eq. (6) if $(L/K_j)\sqrt{2/\pi}$ is equal to Mode$[T_{ij}] = \sqrt{\varepsilon_i \delta_j / \theta_j}$. Equation (14) demonstrates that the Rasch-Weibull model allows to apply Rasch analysis for incomplete designs to time-limit tests, and then to correct the estimated person precision parameter to obtain an estimate of the person's mental speed θ_j.

Equation (14) can be rewritten into logistic form by defining: $\kappa_j = \ln(K_j)$, and $\alpha_q = \ln(L_q\sqrt{2/\pi})$, a time limit dependent scaling constant, with L_q the time limit imposed on test q expressed in arbitrary time units:

$$P(U_{ij} = 1 \mid i, j, L_q) \approx \frac{\exp(\xi_j - \kappa_j + \alpha_q - \sigma_i)}{1 + \exp(\xi_j - \kappa_j + \alpha_q - \sigma_i)}. \tag{15}$$

Because the time unit is arbitrary, α_q can be set to zero unless the same test is administered with different time limits L_q to the same persons. Note that $-\kappa_j + \alpha_q$ is the logarithm of the mode of the response time, which is added to ξ_j. Conversely, if $\xi_j^{**} = \xi_j - \kappa_j + \alpha_q$ is defined as the person parameter, the mental speed ξ_j is obtained by subtracting $-\kappa_j + \alpha_q$ from ξ_j^{**}.

Making the simplifying assumption that the response time is concentrated at its mode, the CML estimator of the item parameters can also be obtained by simplifying the conditional likelihood in Eq. (8), replacing τ_{ij} by κ_j:

$$P(\underline{u}_j \mid r_j, \underline{t}_j, K_j; \underline{\sigma}) \approx \frac{\exp\left[\sum_i^{K_j} u_{ij}(-\kappa_j - \sigma_i)\right]}{\sum_{\{\underline{s}(r_j, K_j)\}} \exp\left[\sum_i^{K_j} s_i(-\kappa_j - \sigma_i)\right]}, \tag{16}$$

which makes only a minor modification of the algorithm for a structurally incomplete design.

Goodness of Fit

Tests of goodness of fit of the model in Eqs. (1), (6), or (14), are exactly the same as for the dichotomous Rasch model (cf. Van den Wollenberg, 1982; Glas, 1988; Glas and Ellis, 1993). In particular, these tests are based on partitioning the sample into groups, by, e.g., raw score, or by the number of items completed, and test the equality of item parameter estimates across groups, that is, whether there is no interaction between the estimates and the partitioning criterion. This is done by evaluating the likelihood of the data or the numbers of positive item responses, given the estimated item parameters and the sufficient statistics for the person parameters.

A complete test of goodness of fit of the Rasch-Weibull model requires taking into account the response times per person and item, and to consider the likelihood $f(\{t_{ij}\}, \{u_{ij}\})$ as a function of the parameters. No such test exists as yet.

Empirical Examples

No empirical examples which fully demonstrate all aspects of the Rasch-Weibull model are available yet. Van den Wollenberg's (1979) analyses corrobate the result in Eq. (16). Experiments by Van Breukelen (1989) using an experimenter controlled inspection time corrobate Eq. (1).

Van den Wollenberg's Analysis

The validity of Eq. (16) is corroborated by Van den Wollenberg's (1979) analyses, discussed in the Introduction to this chapter. He found approximately the same item parameters across 'speed groups' (by number of items completed), analyzing each 'speed group' separately, except, of course, for a nonidentificable shift κ_j of the σ scale. Subsequently, Van den Wollenberg estimated the item parameters in each group of persons who had *at least* completed k items ($k = \min\{K_j\}, \ldots, n\}$ setting $\Sigma\sigma_i = 0$ ($i = 1, \ldots, 10$), to calibrate the scales and found nearly the same item parameter estimates. This calibration incorporates κ_j into the person parameter as can be seen from the estimator, $\hat{\theta}_j$ or $\hat{\xi}_j$, of the person parameter (see Eqs. (9) and (15)):

$$r_j = \sum_{i=1}^{K_j} \frac{\hat{\theta}_j}{\hat{\theta}_j + (\varepsilon_i K_j)} = \sum_{i=1}^{K_j} \frac{\hat{\theta}_j^{**}}{\hat{\theta}_j^{**} + \varepsilon_i}, \tag{17}$$

with $\hat{\theta}_j^{**} = \exp(\hat{\xi}_j - \kappa_j)$; and $\varepsilon_i = \exp(\sigma_i)$. Figure 3 illustrates the estimation of ξ according to Eq. (17).

An Experimental Test of the Rasch Response Time Model

Van Breukelen (1989) tested the validity of the model in Eq. (1) experimentally, using Metzler and Shepard's (1974) mental rotation task. Each item consists of two pairs of geometric figures: One pair being the same figure except for a plane rotation, the other pair being different figures which can not be rotated to congruence (Fig. 4). The subject must indicate which one is a "same" pair. In this experiment, response time was an experimenter controlled inspection time, using a backward mask after stimulus presentation. Items of different difficulty (4 angles of rotation) were used, distinct (e.g., mirror imaged) but equally difficult replicas of each item being presented at each of four different inspection times. Details are given in Van

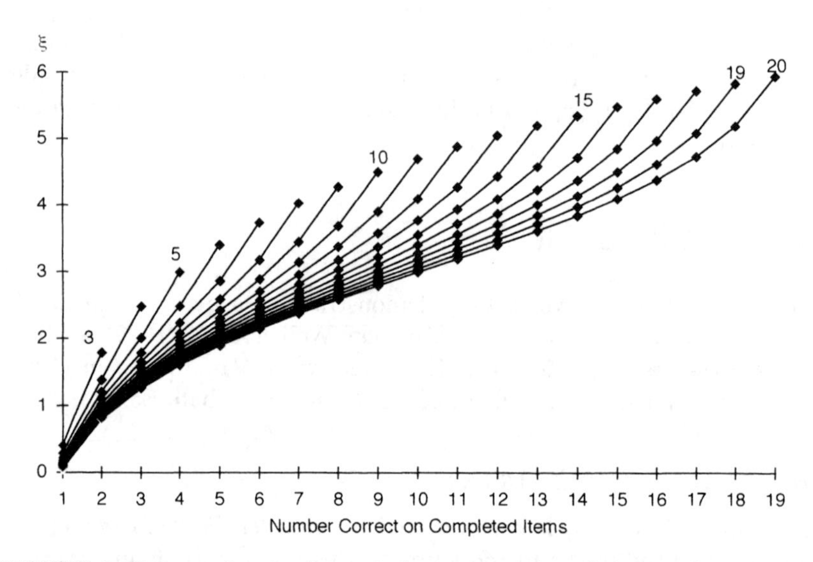

FIGURE 3. Estimated mental speed, ξ, as a function of the number of correct responses, for a hypothetical test with equal item difficulties, $\sigma_i = 0$. The scale of ξ is arbitrary. (Cf. Eq. (17); $\alpha = 0$. Curves for different numbers of items completed).

Breukelen (1989) and Van Breukelen and Roskam (1991). Each subject received 16 replications of each of four difficulty levels at each of four levels of inspection time, in randomized order. Each subject-by-presentation time replication was treated as a 'virtual' subject. In doing so, the virtual subject parameter was defined as $\theta_{jh}\tau(t)$, where t indicates the inspection time, h indicates the replication, and τ is some unspecified monotone function.

The item parameters were estimated using CML parameter estimation for the dichotomous Rasch model. The findings support the hypothesis that for experimentally controlled inspection time, the model in Eq. (1) with $\theta_{jh}\tau(t)$ as the virtual subject parameter is valid for this set of items. Applying Van den Wollenberg's (1982) Q_1 test and Andersen's (1973) likelihood-ratio test based on partitioning the data by raw score, by (real) subject, or by inspection time, yielded a good fit of the Rasch model. Furthermore, ANOVA analysis of the estimated "effective ability," $\theta_{jh}\tau(t)$, at four levels of inspection time (300, 400, 500, and 600 msecs) showed that the effective ability increased linearly with inspection time, that is, it could be written as $\theta_j t$. No significant nonlinear trend was found.

These results provide only partial evidence for the model in Eq. (1), because inspection time and response time are equivalent only if the assumption of an Adjustable Timing Model holds. In fact, Van Breukelen's experiment did not test the Weibull part of the model, or at best did so indirectly. Considering that Eq. (15) is also valid for tests consisting of a single item presented with time limit $L_i = t_i$, the Rasch-Weibull model

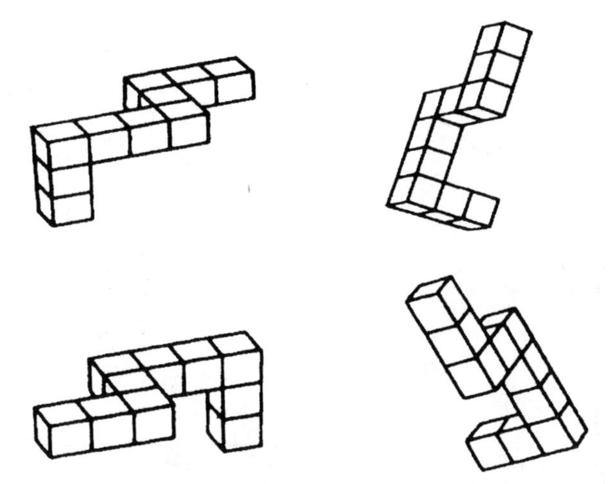

FIGURE 4. Example of Metzler-Shepard rotation items, 'different' and 'same' pairs, respectively. The angle of rotation of the 'same' pair is approximately 65 degrees.

predicts that Eq. (15) holds to the extent that T_{ij} is well approximated by its mode, that is, $\kappa_j = 0$, and α_q is the logarithm of the inspection time L_q of item i (except for an additive scale constant).

In another experiment, Van Breukelen (1989) found that the mean response time T_{ij}, obtained under free response time conditions by averaging over replicas of items of the same difficulty, divided by $\sqrt{\varepsilon_i}$ as estimated from fixed inspection time conditions, was not significantly different across difficulty levels—a result in accordance with the Rasch-Weibull model.

Discussion

A Comparison of the Roskam-Van Breukelen and Verhelst-Verstralen-Jansen Models

Verhelst, Verstralen and Jansen (1992, this volume) aimed at a Rasch model for the marginal probability of a correct response, with response time integrated out. By contrast, the Roskam-Van Breukelen model aimed at a Rasch model for the conditional probability of a correct response given the response time. Both models assume an increasing CAF. Verstralen-Verstralen-Jansen assumed exponentially distributed response times with individuals' 'speed' parameters λ_j, and their model is an ATM model in the strict sense (see Footnote 1). Their basic idea is straightforward and appears psychologically very sound: Let ζ_j be the person's effective ability given (response) time t, whose probability density function is a generalized

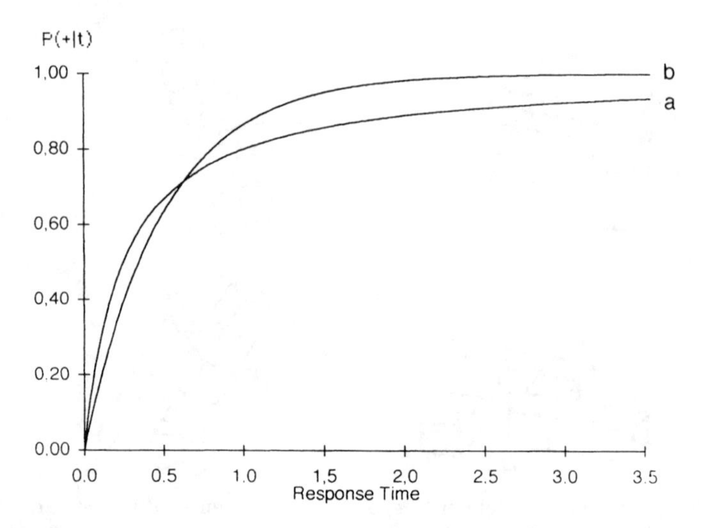

FIGURE 5. (a) The conditional accuracy function $\frac{\theta t}{\theta t+\varepsilon}$ of the Roskam-Van Breukelen model for $\theta/\varepsilon = 4$. (b) The conditional accuracy function in Verhelst et al.'s model, $1 - e^{-(\theta/\varepsilon)t}$, for $\theta/\varepsilon = 2$. Note that the parameters here are comparable to the square roots of the parameters of the Roskam-Van Breukelen model.

double-exponential pdf)[6] (omitting subscripts):

$$f(\zeta \mid t) = t\exp([-(\zeta - \xi)]\exp[-t\exp([-(\zeta - \xi)]]. \tag{18}$$

The probability of a positive response is then formalized as the probability that ζ exceeds the item difficulty σ. Reparameterizing, one obtains the CAF:

$$P[+ \mid \theta, \varepsilon, t] = P[\zeta > \sigma \mid t] = 1 - e^{-(\theta/\varepsilon)t} = 1 - e^{-te^{(\xi-\sigma)}}, \tag{19}$$

where $\theta = \exp(\xi)$ and $\varepsilon = \exp(\sigma)$ are person ability (mental speed) and item difficulty, as before. Equation (19) is illustrated in Fig. 5(b). Integrating out the exponentially distributed t:

$$P(+ \mid \theta, \varepsilon] = \int_0^\infty [1 - e^{-(\theta/\varepsilon)t}]\lambda e^{-\lambda t} dt = \frac{\theta/\lambda}{\theta/\lambda + \varepsilon}. \tag{20}$$

Obviously, λ_j is a speed (persistence) parameter and $1/\lambda_j$ is the expected time per item. The only reasonable interpretation is that λ is in fact 'persistence'-inverse. Due to the assumption of exponentially distributed

[6]We have adapted the derivation and notation of Verhelst et al. so as to be consistent and easily comparable to the Rasch-Weibull model. Also, we omitted the parameter α in their model, which does not appear to be identificable, and—to the opinion of the present author—does not appear to have a clear interpretation.

response times, the number, K_j, of items completed within a fixed time limit, L, is Poisson distributed with parameter $\lambda_j L$, and K_j is a sufficient statistic for λ_j.

The correspondence and the difference with the Roskam-Van Breukelen model are striking. Except for a change of scale ($\theta \to \sqrt{\theta}$, $\varepsilon \to \sqrt{\varepsilon}$) and $\lambda = 1/\sqrt{\delta}$, Eq. (20) is the same as Eq. (6). The difference, of course is, that Eq. (6) is a close approximation for Weibull distributed response times, depending on both mental speed, item difficulty, and persistence, whereas Eq. (20) is exact for exponentially distributed response times depending only on persistence.

Van den Wollenberg's (1979) results corroborate the Rasch-Weibull model virtually as much as they corroborate the Rasch-Exponential model of Verhelst et al.

The Psychological Validity of Models for Time-Limit Tests

The crucial question with respect to time limit tests appears to be: What do persons really do when confronted with performance items under time pressure? Owen White's assumption was that persons have a fixed level of accuracy, spend more time on more difficult items in order to maintain a constant level of correctness, but will give up if an item takes too much time. The other models all assume that the response time is a random variable depending on the person's persistence, but possibly also on their mental speed and on the item difficulty, and that the probability of a correct response increases with "invested time." These models permit of partialling out the person's speed-accuracy strategy, since ability parameters ("mental speed" and/or "mental accuracy") are modelled independent of strategy parameters ("persistence," "continuance"). These models also assume that the conditional accuracy function is increasing and independent of the strategy of the person. If that hypothesis would turn out to be invalid, none of these models discussed in this chapter can be appropriate.

Acknowledgments

The author expresses his gratitude to Eric Maris and to Rogier Donders for their advice in preparing this chapter. Many invaluable contributions were made by Gerard van Breukelen, Arnold van den Wollenberg, Jo Pieters, and Rogier Donders, in developing the approaches and concepts presented in this chapter. In order not to overload this chapter with references, their work has been referenced only with respect to essentials.

References

Andersen, E.B. (1973). A goodness of fit test for the Rasch model. *Psychometrika* **38**, 123–140.

Berger, M. (1982). The scientific approach to intelligence: An overview of its history with special reference to mental speed. In H.J. Eysenck (Ed.), *A Model for Intelligence* (pp. 13–43). Berlin, New York: Springer-Verlag.

Brand, C.R. and Dreary, I.J. (1982). Intelligence and 'inspection time.' In H.J. Eysenck (Ed.), *A Model for Intelligence* (pp. 133–148). Berlin, New York: Springer-Verlag.

Donders, A.R.T. (1990). Estimation problems in the Rasch-Weibull model. Unpublished masters dissertation, University of Nijmegen, Department of Mathematical Psychology.

Eysenck, H.J. (1982). Introduction. In H.J. Eysenck (Ed.), *A Model for Intelligence* (pp. 1–10). Berlin, New York: Springer-Verlag.

Fischer, G.H. (1974). *Einführung in die Theorie psychologischer Tests* [*Introduction to Test Theory*], Bern, Stuttgart, Wien: Huber.

Fischer, G.H. (1991). On power series models and the specifically objective assessment of change in event frequencies. In J.-P. Doignon and J.-C. Falmagne (Eds.), *Mathematical Psychology, Current Developments* (pp. 293–310). New York: Springer-Verlag.

Fischer, G.H. and Kisser, R. (1983). Notes on the exponential latency model and an empirical application. In H. Wainer and S. Messick (Eds.), *Principals of Modern Psychological Measurement* (pp. 139–157). Hillsdale: Lawrence Erlbaum.

Furneaux, W.D. (1960). Intellectual abilities and problem solving behavior. In H.J. Eysenck (Ed.), *Handbook of Abnormal Psychology* (pp. 167–192). New York: Basic Books.

Glas, C.A.W. (1988). The derivation of some tests for the Rasch model from the multinomial distribution, *Psychometrika* **53**, 525–547.

Glas, C.A.W. (1989). *Contributions to Estimating and Testing Rasch Models.* Unpublished doctoral dissertation, University of Twente, Enschede, The Netherlands.

Glas, C.A.W. and Ellis, J. (1993). *Rasch Scaling Program: User's Manual.* Groningen: Iec-ProGamma.

Gustafsson, J.E. (1980). A solution for the conditional estimation problem for long tests in the Rasch model for dichotomous items. *Educational and Psychological Measurement* **40**, 377–385.

Jansen, M.G.H. and Van Duijn, M.A.J. (1992). Extensions of Rasch' multiplicative Poisson model. *Psychometrika* **57**, 405–414.

Jansen, P.G.W. and Roskam, E.E. (1986). Latent trait models and dichotomization of graded responses. *Psychometrika* **51**, 69–92.

Luce, R.D. (1986). *Response Times: Their Roles in Inferring Elementary Mental Organization.* New York, Oxford: Oxford University Press.

Maris, E. (1993). Additive and multiplicative models for gamma distributed random variables, and their application as psychometric models for response times. *Psychometrika* **58**, 445–471.

Metzler, J. and Shepard, R.N. (1974). Transformational studies of the internal representation of three-dimensional objects. In R.L. Solso (Ed.), *Theories in Cognitive Psychology* (pp. 147–201). New York, Wiley.

Mislevy, R.J. (1984). Estimating latent distributions. *Psychometrika* **49**, 359–381.

Mislevy, R.J. (1986). Bayes modal estimation in item response models. *Psychometrika* **51**, 177–195.

Ollman, R.T. (1977). Choice reaction time and the problem of distinguishing task effects from strategy effects. In S. Dornic (Ed.), *Attention and Performance, VI* (pp. 99–113). Hillsdale, NJ: Erlbaum, 1977.

Rasch, G. (1960). *Probabilistic Models for Some Intelligence and Attainment Tests.* Copenhagen: Nielsen & Lydiche.

Roskam, E.E. (1987). Toward a psychometric theory of intelligence. In E.E. Roskam and R. Suck (Eds.), *Progress in Mathematical Psychology* (pp. 151–174). Amsterdam: North-Holland.

Roskam, E.E. and Jansen, P.G.W. (1989). Conditions for Rasch-dichotomizability of the unidimensional polytomous Rasch model. *Psychometrika* **54**, 317–333.

Scheiblechner, H. (1979). Specific objective stochastic latency mechanisms. *Journal of Mathematical Psychology* **19**, 18–38.

Scheiblechner, H. (1985). Psychometric models for speed-test construction: the linear exponential model. In S.E. Embretson (Ed.), *Test Design, Developments in Psychology and Psychometrics* (pp. 219–244). New York, NY: Academic Press.

Spearman, C. (1927). *The Abilities of Men.* London: MacMillan.

Thorndike, E.L., Bregman, E.O., Cobb, M.V., and Woodyard, E. (1927). *The Measurement of Intelligence.* New York: Teachers College of Columbia University.

Thurstone, L.L. (1937). Ability, motivation, and speed. *Psychometrika* **2**, 249–254.

Van Breukelen, G.J.P. (1989). *Concentration, Speed, and Precision in Mental Tests.* Unpublished doctoral dissertation, University of Nijmegen, The Netherlands.

Van Breukelen, G.P.J. and Roskam, E.E. (1991). A Rasch model for speed-accuracy trade-off in time limited tests. In J.-Cl. Falmagne and J.-P. Doignon (Eds.), *Mathematical Psychology, Current Developments* (pp. 251–272). New York: Springer-Verlag.

Van den Wollenberg, A.L. (1979). *The Rasch Model and Time-Limit Tests.* Unpublished doctoral dissertation, University of Nijmegen, The Netherlands.

Van den Wollenberg, A.L. (1982). Two new test statistics for the Rasch model. *Psychometrika* **47**, 123–141.

Van den Wollenberg, A.L. (1983). Measuring subjects on a joint scale by means of time-limit tests. *Tijdschrift voor Onderwijsresearch* **8**, 145–156.

Van den Wollenberg, A.L. (1985). Speed and precision: Facts or artefacts? *Tijdschrift voor Onderwijsresearch*, **10**, 69–81.

Verhelst, N.D., Verstralen, H.H.F.M., and Jansen, M.G.H. (1992). *A Logistic Model for Time-Limit Tests* (Measurement and Research Department Reports 92-1). Arnhem: CITO.

Warm, T.A. (1990). Weighted maximum likelihood estimation of ability in item response theory. *Psychometrika* **54**, 427–450.

White, P.O. (1982). Some major components in general intelligence. In H.J. Eysenck (Ed.), *A Model for Intelligence* (pp. 44–90). Berlin, Heidelberg, New York: Springer-Verlag.

12
Multiple-Attempt, Single-Item Response Models

Judith A. Spray

Introduction

The psychomotor literature has seen the appearance of several papers that have described the proposed or actual use of item resonse theory (IRT) models in the measurement of psychomotor skills (Costa et al., 1989; Safrit et al., 1989; Spray, 1987, 1989). These IRT models were originally developed for use with the assessment of either cognitive or affective behaviors but could be used on psychomotor responses in some situations. In order to use these models with psychomotor responses, the data have been frequently treated as though the responses had been obtained from mental tests. For example, a study by Safrit et al. (1992) examined the number of sit-ups that an examinee could perform within a 60-second time limit. The number of sit-ups completed were dichotomized as pass/fail or 1/0 responses according to a cutoff or criterion score, so that the data could be used in an IRT model commonly used for multiple-choice items. Several sit-up tests were administered to an examinee and each test varied by difficulty. This series of sit-up tests resulted in a response vector or string of dichotomous responses for each examinee, which were then treated as typical 1/0 or right/wrong responses to a cognitive test. The dichotomized responses were subsequently fitted to a two-parameter logistic model (2-PLM).

Any psychomotor response that could be dichotomized in this manner could be treated as a cognitive test item and modeled with one of the typical *item* response models. However, the frequently arbitrary nature of establishing such a criterion or cutoff score would introduce an additional source of variability into any dichotomous response modeling. Other tests of gross psychomotor skills result in dichotomous responses naturally and would not require the establishment of a pass/fail criterion. These tests, such as a basketball free-throw test, could be scored as either a miss (0) or a success (1). The resulting response *pattern* could be then modeled using a product of cognitive *item* response models.

Most tests of cognitive behaviors are mental tests that present multiple, written test items to an examinee who then is given a single attempt to answer each item correctly. Any test of this general type will be referred to in the present context as a single-attempt, multiple-item (SAMI) test. A popular IRT model for many written multiple-choice SAMI tests is the three-parameter logistic model (3-PLM). IRT models also have been developed to model nominal responses to more than two categories (Bock, 1972), ordered responses to more than two categories (Andrich, 1978a, 1978b; Samejima, 1969), and even continuous responses (Samejima, 1973). Some of these SAMI IRT models might be appropriate for responses to psychomotor tests. However, many tests of psychomotor skills require an examinee to repeat the same skill (i.e., *item*) over and over again, resulting in a *multiple-attempt, single-item* (MASI) test.

Within the context of IRT modeling, MASI tests would differ from the typical cognitive SAMI test in several important ways. In many psychomotor testing situations, a possible change in the skills of the examinees through learning or fatigue may be a negligible phenomenon. Basically, such tests can therefore be considered as to consist of only a single item with a single difficulty parameter. In addition, there would be no need for a discrimination parameter because such a parameter would only redefine the unit of scale. Finally, it would be nonsensical to consider guessing behavior in a test of psychomotor skills. In this special case, when all items or attempts are equally discriminating and have equal difficulty, the test consists of a series of Bernoulli trials. It is known for Bernoulli trials that they imply probabilistic models in which the number of successes is a sufficient statistic for the success parameter in the model. This feature makes sense for models of psychomotor tests because it is intuitively clear that for such tests the response *pattern* does not contain any additional information about the skill of the examinee once his or her number of successes is known.

There exists a family of one-parameter IRT models as kernel that have the number of successes as a sufficient statistic for the skill parameter in the model. The purpose of these MASI IRT models is to describe the examinee-by-test-interaction for a psychomotor test and to facilitate the estimation of ability and/or test difficulty from the observed test scores $x_1, x_2, \ldots, x_N$ of the N examinees.

These MASI models include the two models that have been presented elsewhere by Masters and Wright (1984), the *Binomial Model* and the *Poisson (Counts) Model*, and the *Inverse Binomial Model*, also called trials-to-criterion testing in classical or non-IRT form, by Feldt and Spray (1983) and Shifflett (1985). All three models assume that a test has been given to an examinee with some latent or unobserved unidimensional ability or skill θ_j. In the Binomial Model, the observed test score X_j is the total number of correct responses observed out of n possible attempts of a single task. In the Poisson Model, the observed test score X_j is the total number of correct responses observed in a finite length of time (rather than a fixed number of attempts). For the Inverse Binomial Model, the observed test score X_j is the number of attempts or trials it takes an examinee to achieve s successes.

It should be noted that, statistically, these three models are *parametric* models in that the success parameter in the (inverse) binomial and Poisson probability functions is further modeled as a function of a parameter representing the skills of the examinees and the difficulty of the psychomotor task. This feature makes it possible to estimate skills that are defined independently of the difficulty of the task. The practical consequences of this feature are explained below. Also, the three models belong to the *exponential family*, implying the availability of attractive procedures to estimate the parameters and test the goodness of fit of the models. For some theory on parametric models in this family, see Andersen (1980, Chap. 4).

Specifically, the three MASI models presented in this chapter could be used to estimate (1) a single test difficulty parameter b and (2) an examinee's psychomotor latent trait or skill θ_j. The b-parameter can be used to tailor testing to an individual examinee's ability, or to compare tests and/or groups of examinees. If, for example, many different versions of some test existed so that different b values identified a complete set or continuum of tests, then one might want to consider measuring each examinee with the test that best "matches" his or her ability to the difficulty of the test. Borrowing once again from the sport of basketball, consider that basketball sizes vary according to playing rules. The difficulty of the shooting task under different ball sizes (or other conditions) could be measured and b-parameter differences could be estimated. Similarly, changes or growth in examinee ability from pretest to posttest, as measured on the latent ability scale, θ, could be estimated using a response-modeling approach to psychomotor testing.

These MASI IRT models, like most known IRT models, make two strong assumptions regarding the latent trait being measured and the repeated attempts by an examinee. First, the models assume that θ is unidimensional, or that the test measures only a single trait or skill. In practice, this assumption is probably violated because most psychomotor skills, especially those observed in gross motor tasks, are likely to be multidimensional. In the basketball shooting example, a free-throw shooting test probably measures upper arm strength and coordination, as well as pure shooting ability. However, as long as the combination of traits remains the same for each attempt of the test, then one could always redefine or transform the multidimensional trait combination as a "new" unidimensional ability measure, α (e.g., $\alpha_j = \theta_{1j} + \theta_{2j} + \theta_{3j}$, where θ_{1j}, θ_{2j}, θ_{3j} are measures of traits 1, 2, and 3 for examinee j, respectively). The assumption of unidimensionality would still be satisfied because α would represent a new, transformed unidimensional trait.

A second assumption concerning IRT models is also likely to be violated in the repeated, multiple-attempt format frequently encountered in psychomotor skill testing. This is the assumption of local independence which requires that the individual trials or attempts be independent for a given examinee. This implies that the results of trial or attempt i, for example, cannot affect the next trial, $i+1$. In practice, there probably is some small effect between trial responses for a given examinee, especially those trials that occur close together in time. However, as already noted, these effects are often negligible. Research attempts to measure or estimate this dependency in real data sets have not succeeded except in instances where certain conditions of the task were experimentally manipulated (Spray and Newell, 1986). Studies that have reported the results of simulated response or trial dependency (Looney and Spray, 1992) have demonstrated that the degree or severity of the response dependency would have to be significantly large before estimation is seriously affected. Therefore, for the purpose or usefulness of the models for real psychomotor data, this assumption of local independence can probably be waived.

Presentation of the Model

Binomial Model

The success parameter in the model, that is, the probability that an examinee with latent ability θ_j successfully completes a single attempt of a task with difficulty b can be denoted by $P(\theta_j)$. Assume that this probability can be represented by a one-parameter logistic model (sometimes referred to as a Rasch model), or

$$P(\theta_j) = \frac{\exp[\theta_j - b]}{1 + \exp[\theta_j - b]}. \tag{1}$$

If it is assumed that the examinee can take n repeated attempts of this same task and that this probability stays constant from one attempt to another for all examinees with $\theta = \theta_j$, then the total number of successes X_j can be assumed to follow a binomial distribution. The probability of this examinee scoring x_j can then be written as

$$P(X_j = x_j \mid \theta_j, n) = \binom{n}{x_j} P(\theta_j)^{x_j}[1 - P(\theta_j)]^{n-x_j}, \ x_j = 0, 1, 2, \ldots, n. \tag{2}$$

Substituting Eq. (1) into Eq. (2) and simplifying gives

$$P(X_j = x_j \mid \theta_j, n, b) = \binom{n}{x_j} \frac{\exp[x_j(\theta_j - b)]}{\{1 + \exp(\theta_j - b)\}^n}, \ x_j = 0, 1, 2, \ldots, n, \tag{3}$$

which is the MASI IRT form of the Binomial Model. An example of trials that could be modeled by a Binomial Model would be the basketball free-throw shooting test where each repeated, independent trial could be scored dichotomously as a pass or fail.

Poisson Model

If there exists no upper limit, n, to the number of successes that a person can achieve in a testing situation, as when the test consists of a fixed time limit in which the repeated trials must be performed, then the number of observed successes, X_j, within this fixed period of time may be modeled by a Poisson process. An obvious example of such a psychomotor test is the bar pull-up test. The probability of a single observed success on any one trial can be denoted by the expression given in Eq. (1). This expression could still represent the probability of observing a success on a single or Bernoulli trial. However, in the Poisson model, it is usually assumed that the number of fixed trials, n, approaches infinity. If the probability in Eq. (1) is small enough so that $nP(\theta_j)$ is moderate, the number of successes observed is approximately a Poisson random variable X_j with parameter λ_j. This value (λ_j) is equal to the expected number of successes for the individual with ability θ_j on the test with difficulty, b.

The probability of this examinee scoring x_j can be written as

$$P(X_j = x_j \mid \lambda_j) = \frac{\lambda_j^{x_j}}{x_j! \exp[\lambda_j]}, \quad x_j = 0, 1, 2, \dots . \tag{4}$$

Masters and Wright (1984) suggested the following parameterization: $\lambda_j = \exp[\theta_j - b]$. Substituting this expression into Eq. (4) yields

$$P(X_j = x_j \mid \theta_j, b) = \frac{\exp[x_j(\theta_j - b)]}{x_j! \exp[\exp(\theta_j - b)]}, \quad x_j = 0, 1, 2, \dots , \tag{5}$$

which is the MASI IRT form of the Poisson Model.

Inverse Binomial Model

If, instead of fixing the number of trials to be performed in a repeated attempts tests, the number of successes to be observed s is fixed and the number of trials it takes each examinee to achieve this number of successes, or X_j, is observed, then this value can be assumed to be distributed as an inverse binomial random variable. The probability of an examinee with latent ability θ_j scoring x_j is given by

$$P(X_j = x_j \mid \theta_j, s) = \binom{x_j - 1}{s - 1} P(\theta_j)^s [1 - P(\theta_j)]^{x_j - s},$$
$$x_j = s, s+1, s+2, \dots, \tag{6}$$

where $P(\theta_j)$ is given by Eq. (1). The probability function in Eq. (6) is also known as the negative binomial function. Substituting Eq. (1) into Eq. (6) yields

$$P(X_j = x_j \mid \theta_j, s, b)$$

$$= \binom{x_j - 1}{s - 1} \frac{\exp[x_j(\theta_j - b)]}{[1 + \exp(\theta_j - b)]^{x_j}}, \quad x_j = s, s+1, s+2, \ldots, \tag{7}$$

which is the MASI IRT form of the Inverse Binomial Model. Any test that can be administered in a Binomial Model format can also be given in an Inverse Binomial setting. The Inverse Binomial format offers optimal properties for examinee populations with negatively skewed true scores (Feldt and Spray, 1983).

Parameter Estimation

If either the difficulty or the ability parameters are known, model parameter estimation can be performed by using maximum likelihood estimation (MLE). When all parameters are unknown, a suggested procedure for the estimation of the difficulty parameter is via marginal maximum likelihood estimation (MMLE) in conjunction with the estimation of ability via a Bayesian procedure.[1]

Maximum Likelihood Estimation

Generally, for a model in the exponential family a possible form of the likelihood equations is the one in which a sufficient statistic is equated to its expected value (Andersen, 1980, Sec. 3.2). In this section, this type of likelihood equation will be derived for the Binomial Model. Then the likelihood equations for the remaining models will be given.

If L is the likelihood function for the Binomial Model,

$$L = \prod_{j=1}^{N} P(X_j = x_j \mid \theta_j, n, b)$$

$$= \prod_{j=1}^{N} \binom{n}{x_j} \frac{\exp[x_j(\theta_j - b)]}{[1 + \exp(\theta_j - b)]^n}, \tag{8}$$

and the natural logarithm of L, or the log likelihood is

$$\log(L) = \sum_{j=1}^{N} \log[P(X_j = x_j \mid \theta_j, n, b)] = \sum_{j=1}^{N} \log \binom{n}{x_j} \frac{\exp[x_j(\theta_j - b)]}{[1 + \exp(\theta_j - b)]^n}, \tag{9}$$

[1] A computer program written by the author to perform the MASI IRT model parameter estimation discussed in this chapter is available at no charge from the author. The program is suitable for all IBM-compatible microcomputers. To obtain a copy of the program in executable form, please write the author, c/o ACT, P.O. Box 168, Iowa City, IA 52243, USA. A manual is included at no charge.

then the appropriate parameter (i.e., θ or b) may be estimated implicitly by taking the partial derivative of the log-likelihood equation with respect to that parameter, setting the resulting equation to zero, and solving for the parameter using some numerical analysis technique such as the Newton–Raphson procedure. The equations for the partial derivatives of the log-likelihood equations with respect to b and θ_j for the Binomial Model are given, respectively, by

$$\frac{\partial \log(L)}{\partial(b)} = -\sum_{j=1}^{N} x_j + n \sum_{j=1}^{N} [\exp(\theta_j - b)][1 + \exp(\theta_j - b)]^{-1} \tag{10}$$

and

$$\frac{\partial \log(L)}{\partial(\theta_j)} = x_j - n[\exp(\theta_j - b)][1 + \exp(\theta_j - b)]^{-1}. \tag{11}$$

Equating these two derivatives to zero, the following likelihood equations are obtained:

$$\sum_{j=1}^{N} x_j = n \sum_{j=1}^{N} [\exp(\theta_j - b)][1 + \exp(\theta_j - b)]^{-1} \tag{12}$$

and

$$x_j = n[\exp(\theta_j - b)][1 + \exp(\theta_j - b)]^{-1}. \tag{13}$$

The likelihood function for the Poisson Model is

$$L = \prod_{j=1}^{N} P(X_j = x_j \mid \theta_j, b) = \prod_{j=1}^{N} \frac{\exp[x_j(\theta_j - b)]}{x_j! \exp[\exp(\theta_j - b)]}. \tag{14}$$

Using the same derivation as in the previous case, the following two likelihood equations are obtained:

$$\sum_{j=1}^{N} x_j = \sum_{j=1}^{N} [\exp(\theta_j - b)] \tag{15}$$

and

$$x_j = \exp(\theta_j - b), \tag{16}$$

both of which can be solved explicitly.

And finally, the likelihood function for the Inverse Binomial Model is

$$L = \prod_{j=1}^{N} P(X_j = x_j \mid \theta_j, s, b) = \prod_{j=1}^{N} \binom{x_j - 1}{s - 1} \frac{\exp[s(\theta_j - b)]}{[1 + \exp(\theta_j - b)]^{x_j}}, \tag{17}$$

which gives the following two likelihood equations:

$$N \cdot s = \sum_{j=1}^{N} x_j [\exp(\theta_j - b)][1 + \exp(\theta_j - b)]^{-1} \tag{18}$$

and

$$s = x_j[\exp(\theta_j - b)][1 + \exp(\theta_j - b)]^{-1}, \tag{19}$$

which can be solved numerically.

Marginal Maximum Likelihood Estimation

When the difficulty and ability parameters are unknown, but the density that defines the ability distribution in the population of examinees is known, MMLE can be used to provide a point estimate of b. Given this estimate of b, a Bayesian procedure can then be used to estimate the ability of the individual examinees.

The steps necessary to complete the MMLE estimation of b for a MASI model *in general* are given below.

Step 1. Specify some hypothesized or known density, $g(\theta)$, for the distribution of the ability parameters (e.g., the standard normal density). Next, write the marginal likelihood function for the realization of the sufficient statistic, $X_j = x_j$, for a random examinee as

$$P(X_j = x_j \mid b) = \int P(X_j = x_j \mid b, \theta_j) g(\theta)\, d\theta. \tag{20}$$

Step 2. For all N examinees, the marginal likelihood is

$$L = \prod_{j=1}^{N} [P(X_j = x_j \mid b)]. \tag{21}$$

The natural logarithm can be written as

$$\log(L) = \sum_{j=1}^{N} [P(x_j = x_j \mid b)]. \tag{22}$$

Step 3. The partial derivative of $\log(L)$ with respect to b is taken and set equal to zero, or

$$\frac{\partial[\log(L)]}{\partial(b)} = 0. \tag{23}$$

The value of b that satisfies this equation is the one that maximizes the $\log(L)$, or it is the marginal maximum likelihood estimate (MMLE) of b, or $\hat{b}$. The general form of the derivative of the $\log(L)$, where L is a marginal likelihood function w.r.t. the b parameter [see Eq. (23)], omitting the subscript j, is

$$\frac{\partial \log(L)}{\partial(b)} = \frac{\partial\{\sum \log[P(X = x \mid b)]\}}{\partial(b)}. \tag{24}$$

$$= \sum \left(\frac{\partial \log[P(X = x \mid b)]}{\partial(b)} \right) \tag{25}$$

$$= \sum P^{-1} (X = x \mid b) \frac{\partial[P(X = x \mid b)]}{\partial(b)} \tag{26}$$

$$= \sum P^{-1}(X = x \mid b) \frac{\partial\{\int P(X = x \mid \theta, b) g(\theta) d\theta\}}{\partial(b)}. \tag{27}$$

Using the relationship

$$\frac{\partial[P(X = x \mid \theta, b)]}{\partial(b)} = \frac{\partial\{\log[P(X = x \mid \theta, b)]\}}{\partial(b)} P(X = x \mid \theta, b) \tag{28}$$

in Eq. (27), gives

$$\frac{\partial[\log(L)]}{\partial(b)}$$

$$= \sum P^{-1}(X = x \mid b) \int \frac{\partial\{\log[P(X = x \mid \theta, b)]\}}{\partial(b)} P(X = x \mid \theta, b) g(\theta) d\theta \tag{29}$$

$$= \sum \int \left(\frac{\partial \log[P(X = x \mid \theta, b)]}{\partial(b)} \right) \left(\frac{P(X = x \mid \theta, b) g(\theta)}{P(X = x \mid b)} \right) d\theta, \tag{30}$$

$$= \sum \int \left(\frac{\partial[\log P(X = x \mid \theta, b)]}{\partial(b)} \right) P(\theta \mid X = x, b)\, d\theta, \tag{31}$$

according to Bayes' theorem. Numerical algorithms, such as the Newton–Raphson procedure, can be used to evaluate Eq. (31) to yield the MMLE of b.

Bayesian Estimation of Ability

The ability of an individual examinee is estimated in a Bayesian fashion using the density of the population of examinees, $g(\theta)$, as the prior density. The procedure is as follows:

With the MMLE of b from Step 3, evaluate the posterior distribution of θ_j, given $X_j = x_j$ and $\hat{b}$. The expected value of this distribution is the *expected a posteriori* or EAP estimate of θ_j. The EAP estimate of θ_j can be obtained for each examinee using an appropriate algorithm for numerical integration. Estimates are needed only for each different value of X.

The general form of the posterior distribution of θ_j given X and $\hat{b}$ is

$$P(\theta \mid X = x, \hat{b}) = \frac{P(X = x \mid \theta, \hat{b}) g(\theta)}{\int P(X = x \mid \theta, \hat{b}) g(\theta) d\theta}. \tag{32}$$

An EAP estimate of ability can also be obtained when b is known (rather than use the MLE procedure described previously). There are some advantages to using EAP over MLE when b is known. For example, with the Binomial Model, test scores of $X_j = n$ or $X_j = 0$ are possible. The use of MLE in these situations produces undetermined (i.e., infinite) estimates of θ; however, finite estimates are obtained using EAP methods. Similarly, with the Inverse Binomial Model, perfect scores of $X_j = s$ would also yield an undetermined (i.e., infinite) estimate of ability, but an EAP ability estimate would be finite. For these reasons, the EAP approach is preferred over MLE when b is known and an estimate of θ_j is desired.[2]

Goodness of Fit

A natural approach to evaluate the goodness of fit of parametric models such as the ones described in this chapter is Pearson's Q or chi-squared test (Andersen, 1980, Sec. 4.4). The null hypothesis to be tested is that X follows the distribution specified in Eqs. (3), (5), or (7). Once the difficulty parameter b has been estimated (either by MLE or MMLE) or is known, Eq. (20) provides estimates of $P(X_j = x_j \mid b)$, $x_j = x_1, x_2, \ldots, x_K$, where K is either equal to the number of possible values of X_j, or a number of finite, disjoint intervals used to pool the data. Computation of $P(X_j = x_j \mid b)$ for $x_j = x_1, x_2, \ldots, x_K$ is again accomplished using an algorithm for numerical integration, assuming that $g(\theta)$ has been specified. These predicted values of $P(X_j = x_j \mid b)$, $x_j = x_1, x_2, \ldots, x_K$ can then be compared to the observed frequencies $F(X_j = x_j)$, $x_j = x_1, x_2, \ldots, x_K$, from a one-way table with the chi-squared statistic,

$$Q = N \sum_{j=1}^{K} \frac{[F(X_j = x_j) - P(X_j = x_j \mid b)]^2}{P(X_j = x_j \mid b)}. \tag{33}$$

This statistic has a limiting distribution $\chi^2_{(K-1)}$ under the null hypothesis if b is known, and $\chi^2_{(K-2)}$ if b is estimated, as $N \to \infty$.

The choice for K is relatively easy using the Binomial Model. In this case, $K = n + 1$ would be logical, provided N was large enough so that no empty intervals or cells [i.e., $F(X_j = x_j) = 0$] would result. If empty cells occur, cells can be collapsed so that $K < n + 1$. Likewise, for the Poisson Model and the Inverse Binomial Model, the data should be collapsed so that zero cell frequencies do not exist.

In the case of the MLE situation where θ_j is known and b is estimated, a similar procedure can be performed. However, the observed frequencies and predicted probabilities have to be tabulated in a two-way table (i.e., X_j, $j = 1, 2, \ldots, K$ by θ_m, $m = 1, 2, \ldots, M$, where M is the number of distinct θ values given). The resulting statistic Q has a limiting $\chi^2_{(K-1)(M-1)}$, as $N \to \infty$, where Q is now defined as

[2]The EAP approach is used in the computer program that is available from the author.

TABLE 1. Binomial Data for Goodness-of-Fit Example.

K	X	$F(X)$	$P(X \mid b)$
1	0	0.14000	0.11915
2	1	0.15000	0.17271
3	2	0.14000	0.17461
4	3	0.16000	0.15332
5	4	0.13000	0.12459
6	5	0.15000	0.09550
7	6	0.04000	0.06897
8	7	0.06000	0.04615
9	8–10	0.03000	.04500

$$Q = N \sum_{j=1}^{K} \sum_{m=1}^{M} \frac{[F(X_j = x_j \mid \theta_m) - P(X_j = x_j \mid \theta_m, b)]^2}{P(X_j = x_j \mid \theta_m, b)}. \tag{34}$$

Example

For a test of $n = 10$, $N = 100$ test scores were generated from a Binomial Model with a true test difficulty parameter $b = 1.0$ and a standard normal ability distribution. The 100 observed test scores yielded an MMLE of $b = 0.976$. Observed and predicted frequencies of total test score, X, are given in Table 1. Because scores of $x = 9$ and $x = 10$ were not observed, the last three score intervals were collapsed so that $K = 9$. Substituting these frequencies into Eq. (33) yields $Q = 6.6448$. This statistic Q is compared to some critical value c for which $\Pr[\chi^2_{(7)} > c] = \alpha = 0.05$, for example. Because $Q < c = 14.1$, the null hypothesis is not rejected (i.e., the model fit is acceptable).

References

Andersen, E.B. (1980). *Discrete Statistical Models with Social Science Applications.* Amsterdam, The Netherlands: North-Holland.

Andrich, D. (1978a). A rating formulation for ordered response categories. *Psychometrika* **43**, 561–573.

Andrich, D. (1978b). Application of a psychometric rating model to ordered categories which are scored with successive integers. *Applied Psychological Measurement* **2**, 581–594.

Bock, R.D. (1972). Estimating item parameters and latent ability when responses are scored in two or more nominal categories. *Psychometrika* **37**, 29–51.

Costa, M.G., Safrit, M.J., and Cohen, A.S. (1989). A comparison of two item response theory models used with a measure of motor behavior. *Research Quarterly for Exercise and Sport* **60**, 325–335.

Feldt, L.S. and Spray, J.A. (1983). A theory-based comparison of the reliabilities of fixed-length and trials-to-criterion scoring of physical education skills tests. *Research Quarterly for Exercise and Sport* **54**, 324–329.

Looney, M.A. and Spray, J.A. (1992). Effects of violating local independence on IRT parameter estimation for the binomials trials model. *Research Quarterly for Exercise and Sport* **63**, 356–359.

Masters, G.N. and Wright, B.D. (1984). The essential process in a family of measurement models. *Psychometrika* **49**, 529–544.

Safrit, M.J., Costa, M.G., and Cohen, A.S. (1989). Item response theory and the measurement of motor behavior. *Research Quarterly for Exercise and Sport* **60**, 325–335.

Safrit, M.J., Zhu, W., Costa, M.G., and Zhang, L. (1992). The difficulty of sit-ups tests: An empirical investigation. *Research Quarterly for Exercise and Sport* **63**, 277–283.

Samejima, F. (1969). Estimation of latent ability using a response pattern of graded scores. *Psychometric Monograph*, No. 17.

Samejima, F. (1973). Homogeneous case of the continuous response model. *Psychometrika* **38**, 203–219.

Shifflett, B. (1985). Reliability estimation for trials-to-criterion testing. *Research Quarterly for Exercise and Sport* **56**, 266–274.

Spray, J.A. (1987). Recent developments in measurement and possible applications to the measurement of psychomotor behavior. *Research Quarterly for Exercise and Sport* **58**, 203–209.

Spray, J.A. (1989). New approaches to solving measurement problems. In M.J. Safrit and T.M. Wood (Eds.), *Measurement Concepts in Physical Education and Exercise Science* (pp. 229–248). Champaign, IL: Human Kinetics.

Spray, J.A. and Newell, K.M. (1986). Time series analysis of motor learning: KR versus no-KR. *Human Movement Science* **5**, 59–74.

Part III. Models for Multiple Abilities or Cognitive Components

Historically, multidimensionality in test data has been handled in three ways. First, clustering techniques such as factor analysis are used to identify groups of items from the larger pool of items of interest that are relatively homogeneous among themselves and rather different from other clusters in the pool. Then, each group of items is treated as a separate unidimensional test or subtest. Any useful information about intercorrelations among the groups of items is sacrificed with this approach. A second solution is to fit a multifactor analysis model to obtain vectors of factor scores for examinees and a multidimensional representation of items in the factor space adopted to fit the data. This solution preserves information about the interrelatedness of factors or clusters but, as with the first approach, fails to provide descriptors of, for example, item difficulty that are needed in the practice of testing. The third solution, which only has merit when the assumption is adequately met by the data, is to assume unidimensionality and proceed forward with an IRT approach. The consequence in the extreme is a totally unacceptable representation of examinees and items. However, it may be a tolerable solution in some instances.

Measurement practices are changing today to accommodate the informational needs of curriculum specialists, policy-makers, special educators, psychologists, and researchers. In earlier sections of this volume, the impact of new item formats was emphasized and valid arguments were made for new IRT models to handle polytomous response data. But the presence of polytomous response data is not the only feature introduced by new formats. The fact is that many of these new formats often require examinees to use more than one skill such as problem solving, critical thinking, reasoning, organization, and writing. Not only will polytomous response models be needed, but it is quite possible that these models will have to permit the assessment of multiple abilities. Certainly, a surface review of many new forms of assessment and the associated scoring protocols, such as represented in portfolio assessments, performance tasks, standardized patients methodology, clinical skills assessments, writing assessments, oral presentations, projects, etc., leave the impression that multidimensional IRT models will be needed to adequately account for examinee test performance.

Lord and Novick (1968), McDonald (1967), and Samejima (1974) were among the first to put forward multidimensional IRT models. However, it has not been until quite recently that these and related models have been developed to any great extent and software was made available for model parameter estimation. In Chapter 15, McDonald extends the unidimensional normal-ogive model introduced in Chapter 1 [developed originally by Lord (1952)] to the multidimensional case, albeit for dichotomous response data. In Chapter 16, Reckase provides a parallel development for the multidimensional extension of unidimensional logistic models. This work is a direct extension of the work by Lord and Birnbaum with unidimensional logistic models [see, for example, Lord (1980)]. Finally, in Chapter 19 Fischer provides multidimensional extensions of the unidimensional dichotomous and polytomous Rasch models. Three differences between McDonald and Reckase's models and Fischer's models are: (1) Fischer restricts his work to a consideration of Rasch models; (2) Fischer's models are designed to measure change and need examinee data on two test occasions; and (3) Fischer's models provide a detailed accounting of the cognitive processes that are involved in responding to items in a test. The contrast in the models is really between statistical and psychological modeling of test and person data.

This section of the volume also introduces two additional multidimensional IRT models. Kelderman describes a loglinear multidimensional IRT model to handle polytomous data. The flexibility of loglinear models with well-developed estimation procedures and statistical tests appear to make this line of model building very attractive. The relative advantages and disadvantages of various formulations of multidimensional IRT models (e.g., Kelderman versus McDonald, Reckase, and Fischer) remains to be determined and represents a very important line of research for the near future.

In Chapter 14, Zwinderman does not offer a multidimensional IRT model per se but he does allow for the estimation of a unidimensional ability score from a set of independent variables or covariates, which may themselves tap rather different characteristics. Ability scores become a weighted composite of these independent variables. The result is an instance of logistic regression analysis that is finding considerably wider use in educational and psychological data analysis today [see, for example, Swaminathan and Rogers (1990)].

This section of the volume also introduces what are called cognitive component models. Test item writing has always been a fairly pragmatic enterprise. Drafts of test items are prepared to fit a set of content specifications. Some of the items prove to be useful and others must be discarded based upon an item analysis. At some point, a study may be done to determine what actually is being measured by the test items. This process gets repeated over and over again by test developers. But what makes an item difficult? Would it be possible to systematically construct items by incorporating varying amounts of cognitive skills or components? These are the sorts of questions which Fischer in Chapter 13 and Embretson in Chapter 18 are attempting to answer.

Fischer, for example, introduces a model in which the item difficulty parameter is decomposed in the course of analysis into parameters for the cognitive skills or components (he calls these the "basic parameters") needed to solve the item. Such models permit a more careful analysis of assessment material and provide the basis for a more systematic approach to test development where item validity is built into the test development process rather than something that is searched for after the test has been completed. Embretson, for example, attempts to advance multidimensional models to account for examinee performance on complex tasks by estimating examinee ability on each of the subtasks needed to complete the more complex task. The work by Fischer and Embretson and their colleagues has the potential of redesigning the way tests are constructed and analyzed in the future.

References

Lord, F.M. (1952). A theory of test scores. *Psychometric Monographs*, No. 7.

Lord, F.M. (1980). *Application of Item Response Theory to Practical Testing Problems.* Hillsdale, NJ: Lawrence Erlbaum Associates.

Lord, F.M. and Novick, M.R. (1968). *Statistical Theories of Mental Test Scores.* Reading, MA: Addison-Wesley.

McDonald, R.P. (1967). Non-linear factor analysis. *Psychometric Monograph*, No. 15.

Samejima, F. (1974). Normal ogive model on the continuous response level in the multidimensional latent space. *Psychometrika* **39**, 111–121.

Swaminathan, H. and Rogers, H.J. (1990). Detecting differential item functioning using logistic regression procedures. *Journal of Educational Measurement* **27**, 361–370.

13
Unidimensional Linear Logistic Rasch Models

Gerhard H. Fischer

Introduction

This chapter gives an overview of a family of unidimensional Rasch models where the item parameters are linearly decomposed into certain "basic" parameters. The latter are attached—depending on the particular kind of application—to cognitive operations required for solving the items, to testing situations, or to treatments given to the persons between testing occasions. Typical applications (see below) have sought to assess the difficulty of cognitive operations as elements of the solution process, but the models can just as well be used for measuring the effects of experimental conditions on item difficulty, or the impact of educational treatments on an ability, of therapies on a personality trait, or of communication on an attitude. Such models are available both for cases of dichotomous and for polytomous items.

Their development originated from the following considerations: The Rasch model (RM) explains person S_j's probability of solving item I_i in terms of the difference of an ability parameter θ_j and an item difficulty parameter β_i,

$$P(+ \mid \theta_j, \beta_i) = P_{ij} = \frac{\exp(\theta_j - \beta_i)}{1 + \exp(\theta_j - \beta_i)}. \tag{1}$$

Equivalently, the RM can also be written as a logit model where the so-called "reaction parameter" of S_j with respect to I_i is

$$\rho_{ij} = \ln\left(\frac{P_{ij}}{1 - P_{ij}}\right) = \theta_j - \beta_i. \tag{2}$$

The RM for a complete item response matrix of items $\times$ persons can therefore be called a complete "two-factorial logit model": One factor is the item factor with level parameters β_i, the other the person factor with level parameters θ_j. It was obvious to extend this two-factorial model into a multi-factorial one in the following manner: Rasch (1965), Micko (1969,

1970), Falmagne [cited in Micko (1970)], and in more detail and explicitly, Scheiblechner (1971) and Kempf (1972) appended additional factors, $L, M, \ldots$, with respective level parameters $\lambda_l, \mu_m, \ldots$, characterizing the effects of prevailing experimental conditions that influence the response probabilities,

$$\rho_{ijlm} = \theta_j - \beta_i + \lambda_l + \mu_m + \ldots . \quad (3)$$

Scheiblechner (1971) shows that the model in Eq. (3) can easily be determined via the usual conditional maximum likelihood (CML) method—which is well understood in the RM—by considering, in a purely formal sense, any of the factors the "item factor" (factor L with parameters λ_l, say), and each and every combination of all other levels of factors, $\theta_j \times \beta_i \times \mu_m \times \ldots$, as a separate level of only one "person factor." Practically, this amounts to rearranging the data in an item score matrix with rows corresponding one–one to parameters λ_l (formally now considered as "item parameters") and columns corresponding to combinations $\theta_j \times \beta_i \times \mu_m \times \ldots$ (now called "person parameters"). The λ_l are then estimable separately from all other factors in the same way as the item parameters β_i in an RM are separated from the person parameters θ_j via CML; that is, in estimating the λ_l the combinations $\theta_j \times \beta_i \times \mu_m \times \ldots$ are conditioned out. In order to estimate all factors in turn, however, this approach requires a design comprising all combinations of factors, that is, a complete multifactorial design. In the models to be described below, on the other hand, we shall always condition out only the θ_j and estimate all other parameters simultaneously. The motivation for this is that (a) there typically are many θ_j and comparatively few other parameters and (b) the main goal of freeing the estimation from influences of the θ-distribution is reached in this way.

Presentation of the Models

The Linear Logistic Test Model

The "Linear Logistic Test Model" (LLTM) is obtained by decomposing the item parameters β_i of Eq. (1) as

$$\beta_i = \sum_{l=1}^{p} w_{il}\alpha_l + c, \quad (4)$$

where the α_l, $l = 1, \ldots, p$, are so-called "basic parameters," the w_{il} are given weights of the α_l for each of the items, and c is the usual normalization constant. Clearly, the multifactorial model in Eq. (3) is a special case of that defined in Eq. (4). The α_l in Eq. (4) may represent the effects of the levels of experimental or other factors influencing item difficulty. These factors are assumed to be the source of difficulty *differences* between items. It follows immediately from Eq. (4) that, for any pair of items (I_i, I_k), the difference $\beta_i - \beta_k$ is fully explained by the α_l, given the w_{il}, as

$$\beta_i - \beta_k = \sum_{l=1}^{p} (w_{il} - w_{kl})\alpha_l. \tag{5}$$

Hence, for the model to hold it is necessary that all factors contributing to differences *between* items are taken into account; this does not apply to factors that are constant *across* all items, which only enter in the normalization constant c. The decomposition of the β_i in Eq. (4) was first suggested by Scheiblechner (1972), who applied ordinary regression analysis to the RM item parameter estimates $\hat{\beta}_i$ in a logical reasoning test. (The items were logical propositions presented in graphical form. Three logical operations sufficed for explaining item difficulty. The w_{il} were derived from the formal structure of the logical propositions: If an item required, e.g., the logical operation "disjunction," the respective weight w_{il} was set to 1, otherwise to 0.) Fischer (1973, 1983) studied the formal properties of the model jointly defined by Eqs. (1) and (4).

The LLTM usually is considered an RM with constraints imposed on the item parameters. It can be shown, though, that the LLTM is the more general formal structure: The RM is a special LLTM where the matrix of weights, $\mathbf{W}$, is diagonal. An alternative interpretation is that the LLTM is a Bradley–Terry–Luce model with constraints imposed on the object parameters [cf. Fischer and Tanzer (1994) or Fischer (1995a)].

The LLTM for Change

Another way of using the LLTM is as a model for change of a unidimensional ability: Suppose that a test is given to the same person S_j repeatedly at time points $T_1, T_2, \ldots, T_z$. Any single item I_i can then be viewed formally as a set of "virtual items" $I_{i1}^*, I_{i2}^*, \ldots, I_{iz}^*$, with different difficulty parameters $\beta_{i1}^*, \beta_{i2}^*, \ldots, \beta_{iz}^*$ mapping the change that occurs in S_j, e.g., due to the treatments given between testing occasions. The idea behind this formalization is to project change of S_j into the virtual item parameters; the latter can then be decomposed, e.g., as

$$\begin{aligned} \beta_{i1}^* &= \beta_i, \\ \beta_{i2}^* &= \beta_i + \eta_1, \\ &\vdots \\ \beta_{it}^* &= \beta_i + \eta_1 + \eta_2 + \cdots + \eta_{t-1}, \\ &\vdots \end{aligned} \tag{6}$$

where the β_{it}^*, $i = 1, \ldots, n$, $t = 1, 2, 3, \ldots, z$, are the nz virtual item parameters of an LLTM, and the β_i, $i = 2, \ldots, n$, and the $\eta_1, \ldots, \eta_{z-1}$ are the $n + z - 2$ basic parameters (β_1 being assumed to be zero for normalization). This LLTM as a model for change was first suggested in Fischer (1976, 1977a, 1977b), see also Fischer (1995b).

Polytomous Extensions of the LLTM

More recently, Fischer and Parzer (1991) and Fischer and Ponocny (1994) undertook to generalize the LLTM-approach to polytomous items, starting out from two well-known polytomous *unidimensional* Rasch-type models: the rating scale model [RSM; Andrich (1978a, 1978b)] and the partial credit model [PCM; Masters (1982)]. Here the term 'unidimensional' refers both to the understanding that the categories C_h are ordered levels of one underlying continuum and that all items are indicators of the same latent dimension. These models are more typically applied to rating scale data than to achievement tests, e.g., for measuring attitudes, or job complaints, or well-being vs. illness. The person parameters therefore are to be considered representations of attitudes or latent traits rather than of abilities.

The more general of the two models is the PCM. It states that

$$P(h \mid S_j, I_i) = \frac{\exp(h\theta_j + \beta_{ih})}{\sum_{l=0}^{d_i} \exp(l\theta_j + \beta_{il})}, \tag{7}$$

for $h = 0, \ldots, d_i$ response categories C_h of item I_i, and for $i = 1, \ldots, n$. The θ_j denote person parameters as before; β_{ih} describes the attractiveness of response category C_h of item I_i, or the availability of a reaction in category C_h of item I_i, or the prevalence of category C_h of symptom I_i, but can also be interpreted as a sum of thresholds between categories preceding C_h [cf. Masters (1982)]. Note that in this model the number of response categories, d_i, may differ between items I_i.

In order to adapt the PCM to many applied research questions, like the measurement of change, of treatment effects, or the like, the β_{ih} are again decomposed into weighted sums of basic parameters,

$$\beta_{ih} = \sum_{l=1}^{p} w_{ihl}\alpha_l + hc, \tag{8}$$

where

> α_l are the basic parameters,
>
> w_{ihl}, $l = 1, \ldots, p$, are weights of the α_l for item parameter β_{ih}, assumed to be given *a priori* as part of the model, and
>
> c is the usual normalization constant.

The model defined by Eqs. (7) and (8) is called the "linear partial credit model" [LPCM; Fischer and Ponocny (1994, 1995)].

The LPCM can be used as a framework for modeling change by employing again the virtual items concept: Item I_i, given at T_1, and the same item presented at later time points, $T_2, T_3, \ldots, T_z$, are formally treated as different items, $I^*_{i1}, I^*_{i2}, \ldots$, with parameters $\beta^*_{ih1}, \beta^*_{ih2}, \ldots$, etc. To simplify the notation, however, we arrange the virtual items in a vector rather than a matrix and hence distinguish "real" items I_i with item parameters β_{ih} from virtual items I^*_k, $k = 1, \ldots, v$, with associated virtual-item parameters β^*_{kh}. The β^*_{kh} are decomposed as

$$\beta^*_{kh} = \sum_{l=1}^{p} w_{khl}\alpha_l + hc, \tag{9}$$

for $k = 1, \ldots, v$ virtual items. As an example, suppose that an n-items test is given at two time points, T_1 and T_2, resulting in $v = 2n$ virtual items, with parameters

$$\beta^*_{kh} = \beta_{ih} + hc, \quad \text{for time point } T_1, \tag{10}$$

for $k = i = 1, \ldots, n$ and $h = 0, \ldots, d_i$, and

$$\beta^*_{kh} = \beta_{ih} + h\sum_{l} q_{gl}\eta_l + hc, \quad \text{for time point } T_2, \tag{11}$$

for $k = i + n$, $i = 1, \ldots, n$, and $h = 0, \ldots, d_i$, where q_{gl} is the dosage of treatment B_l in the respective treatment group G_g, and η_l the effect of B_l. (For $h = 0$, we get $\beta^*_{k0} = \beta_{i0} = 0$ according to the usual normalization conditions in the PCM.) The generalizability of Eqs. (10) and (11) to any number of time points is obvious.

As a special case of the LPCM we can define the "linear rating scale model' [LRSM; Fischer and Parzer (1991)] by setting $\beta_{ih} = h\beta_i + \omega_h$, and $d_i = d$. Staying within the framework of the previous example, for time point T_1 Eq. (10) becomes

$$\beta^*_{kh} = h(\beta_i + c) + \omega_h, \tag{12}$$

for $i = k = 1, \ldots, n$, and similarly, for time point T_2, Eq. (11) now is

$$\beta^*_{kh} = h(\beta_i + c) + h\sum_{l} q_{gl}\eta_l + \omega_h, \tag{13}$$

for $k = i + n$, $i = 1, \ldots, n$, and $h = 0, \ldots, d$.

The use of the LRSM for measuring change is essentially the same as that of the LPCM. The differences between these models are that (a) the LPCM allows for a different attractiveness of the response categories in different items, so that it is more flexible and thus easier to fit to data; (b) if the LRSM does hold, however, its parameters are more stable statistically, so that smaller samples suffice, and are easier to interpret. The generalizability of Eqs. (12) and (13) to any number of time points is obvious.

It is an easy matter to show that the dichotomous RM and the LLTM are special cases of the LPCM. This particularly implies that a procedure capable of computing CML estimates for the LPCM can estimate all these models. Similarly, the conditional likelihood ratio statistics are completely analogous in all four models.

Parameter Estimation

Linear Logistic Test Model

Fischer (1973) derived CML estimation equations for the parameters α_l of the LLTM by conditioning on the person raw scores:

$$\sum_{i=1}^{n} w_{il} \left(u_{i+} - \sum_{r=1}^{n-1} N_r \frac{\varepsilon_i \gamma_{r-1}^{(i)}}{\gamma_r} \right) = 0, \tag{14}$$

for $l = 1, \ldots, p$, where p is the number of basic parameters, n is the number of items, w_{il} the weight of basic parameter α_l for item I_i, N_r is the number of persons with raw score r, and

$r_j = \sum_i u_{ij}$ the sum of S_j's item responses u_{ij}, $i = 1, \ldots, n$, i.e., the raw score,

$u_{i+} = \sum_j u_{ij}$ the marginal sum of item I_i,

$\varepsilon_i = \exp(-\beta_i)$ an easiness parameter of item I_i,

γ_r the elementary symmetric function of order r of $\varepsilon_1, \ldots, \varepsilon_n$, and

$\gamma_{r-1}^{(i)}$ the elementary symmetric function of order $r-1$ of $\varepsilon_i, \ldots, \varepsilon_{i-1}$, $\varepsilon_{i+1}, \ldots, \varepsilon_n$, i.e., of all easiness parameters ε_i except for that of the ith item.

For many purposes it is important to generalize the CML equations such that incomplete data sets are admissible. Let a design matrix $\mathbf{B} = ((b_{ij}))$ be introduced with $b_{ij} = 1$ if person S_j has taken item I_i, and $b_{ij} = 0$ otherwise. It can then be shown (Fischer, 1983) that the CML Eqs. (14) generalize to

$$\sum_{i=1}^{n} w_{il} \left(s_i - \sum_{j} \frac{\varepsilon_i b_{ij} \gamma_{r_j-1}^{(i)}}{\gamma_{r_j}} \right) = 0, \tag{15}$$

for $l = 1, \ldots, p$, where u_{ij} is defined equal to a dummy u, $0 < u < 1$, whenever $b_{ij} = 0$; $s_i = \sum_j b_{ij} u_{ij}$ is the marginal sum of item I_i, $r_j =$

$\sum_i b_{ij}u_{ij}$ is person S_j's raw score, γ_{r_j} is the elementary symmetric function of order r_j of $\varepsilon_1 b_{1j}, \ldots, \varepsilon_n b_{nj}$, defined for each person S_j separately (or for groups of persons who have been presented the same item sets), and $\gamma_{r_j-1}^{(i)}$ the elementary symmetric function of order $r_j - 1$ of $\varepsilon_1 b_{1j}, \ldots, \varepsilon_{i-1} b_{i-1,j}$, $\varepsilon_{i+1} b_{i+1,j}, \ldots, \varepsilon_n b_{nj}$. (Note that γ_{r_j} and $\gamma_{r_j-1}^{(i)}$ actually depend on j, not only on r_j, but we refrain from introducing a more-complicated notation.)

Estimating the basic parameters α_l (and at the same time the item parameters β_i) via CML by means of Eqs. (14) or (15) is the most preferred method, making the estimators $\hat{\alpha}_l$ consistent independent of the distribution form of the θ_j; this holds under a mild regularity condition given by Hillgruber (1990), namely, that the sequence of the θ_j for $N \to \infty$ satisfies

$$\sum_{j=1}^{\infty} \exp(-|\theta_j|) = \infty, \tag{16}$$

cf. Pfanzagl (1994). Equation (16) prevents the pathological case that, as $N \to \infty$, only N_0 and/or N_n tend to ∞, while all other N_r, $r = 1, \ldots, n-1$, remain bounded.

Fischer (1983) gives a necessary and sufficient (n.s.) condition for Eq. (15) to have a unique solution $\hat{\alpha}$ for a given finite data set. This condition, however, is both complicated to formulate and to apply. Fortunately, for most practical purposes a special case of the condition suffices. The special case is that of "well conditioned" data. The data are well-conditioned if, for any partition of the items into two subsets J_1 and J_2, there is an item $I_i \in J_1$ and an item $I_k \in J_2$ such that some person S_j has given a correct response to I_i and an incorrect response to I_k. [This is the well known n.s. condition for obtaining a unique CML solution in the RM, cf. Fischer (1981). Well-conditionedness will occur almost surely in most standard applications of the RM or LLTM with at least moderate sample sizes.] Under this weak condition, it is n.s. for the existence of a unique CML solution of Eq. (15) that the $n \times (p+1)$ matrix $\mathbf{W}^+ = (\mathbf{W}, \mathbf{1})$, that is, the matrix $\mathbf{W}$ extended by a column of ones, has rank $p + 1$. This ensures that the decomposition of any given set of item parameters into the α_l and c in Eq. (4) will be unique. [Note, however, that the result is not trivial: Uniqueness of the decomposition in Eq. (4) does not *per se* imply uniqueness of the CML solution $\hat{\alpha}$.]

Polytomous Extensions of the LLTM

The technique of CML estimation for the LPCM is more complicated than that for the dichotomous LLTM and hence is beyond the scope of this chapter. The interested reader is referred to Fischer and Ponocny (1994, 1995) who present both numerically stable recurrence relations for the combinatorial functions involved and an efficient iteration method for solving the CML equations. A computer program under DOS is available from the author.

The LPCM algorithm enables one to estimate the parameters β_{ih} (= item $\times$ category parameters) and α_l (= effect parameters) in Eq. (8). Note that this model still is unidimensional in the sense that individual differences are measured on one latent dimension. Hypotheses on the α_l can be tested in exactly the same manner as in the LLTM using the conditional likelihood ratio statistic given below in Eq. (17).

Goodness of Fit

If the β_i of an RM are estimated by CML and the resulting $\hat{\beta}_i^{(RM)}$ are regressed on the (given) w_{il} of an LLTM, as was done by Scheiblechner (1972), the multiple correlation between the $\hat{\beta}_i^{(RM)}$ and the $\hat{\beta}_i^{(LLTM)}$ reproduced by means of Eq. (4) can be expected to be rather high. Such correlations seemingly suggest a good fit of the LLTM. That impression, however, may be quite misleading, because the regression analysis is based on only n "observed" $\hat{\beta}_i$ and np "predictor" values, corresponding to a sample size of n. It is well known that multiple regression in small samples considerably capitalizes on chance. Moreover, applying a significance test to the multiple correlation $R(\hat{\beta}_i^{(RM)}, \hat{\beta}_i^{(LLTM)})$ would be wholly misleading as it would refer to the H_0: $\rho = 0$, which is irrelevant in the present case: The hypothesis we are concerned with is H_0: $\beta_i^{(RM)} = \beta_i^{(LLTM)} + c$. Another equally damaging objection is that the sample size underlying the test statistic, n, would be independent of the actual sample size N.

The recommended method for testing of fit of the LLTM consists of two steps:

(a) Test the RM for fit. This is necessary because the LLTM is based on the RM defined by Eq. (1) and cannot fit empirically unless the RM does. (This seems to contradict the statement made above that the LLTM is more general than the RM. There is no contradiction, though, because the LLTM is more general as a *formal* model, but more restrictive *empirically*.)

(b) If the RM fits, test the linear decomposition in Eq. (4) by means of the following likelihood ratio procedure: Compare the conditional likelihood obtained under the RM (as H_1) with that under the LLTM (as H_0), using the statistic

$$-2\ln\lambda = -2\ln\left\{\frac{L(\mathbf{U} \mid H_0)}{L(\mathbf{U} \mid H_1)}\right\} \overset{as.}{\sim} \chi^2 \quad \text{with } df = n - 1 - p, \qquad (17)$$

where $n-1$ is the number of independent item parameters under H_1, and p the number of (independent) basic parameters.

The same procedure can be applied to testing one LLTM with p_0 basic parameters (H_0) against another one with p_1 parameters (H_1), if the latter is believed to be true, and $p_0 < p_1$. [In fact, the test of an LLTM (H_0) against the RM (H_1) formally is a test of an LLTM with p basic parameters against another LLTM with $n-1$ parameters, where $p < n-1$; this holds because the RM is an LLTM with basic parameters α_l coinciding with item parameters β_i, for $l = i = 2, \ldots, n$, and $\beta_1 = 0$ for normalization.]

Experience with applications of the LLTM has shown that, in most cases, the H_0 formulated in Eq. (4) had to be rejected. This is not too astonishing because fit of an LLTM depends upon the completeness and correctness of the researcher's hypotheses regarding *all* factors contributing to differences between items. It is therefore a natural question to ask whether the LLTM still is useful in spite of the significance of the statistic in Eq. (17). Often the answer will be "yes," because the LLTM (a) forces the researcher to make his/her hypotheses about the item material explicit, (b) allows the researcher to test his/her hypotheses, and (c), even if the explanation of item difficulty in terms of basic parameters (referring to facets of the item design) is not perfect, the LLTM still allows one to predict item difficulty of new items at least approximately. The LLTM can then be employed for generating a homogeneous item universe with predetermined item difficulties, e.g., for computerized adaptive testing [cf. Fischer and Pendl (1980)]. An interesting experiment about the predictability of item difficulty was made by Nährer (1980): Using the results of a previous LLTM application to matrices items, he constructed a set of new matrices items and presented these to a new sample of persons. Then he compared the predicted item parameters, based on Eq. (4) and the $\hat{\alpha}_l$ obtained from the old data (denoted $\hat{\beta}_i^{(LLTM)}$, with the Rasch item parameter estimates $\hat{\beta}_i^{(RM)}$ computed independently from the new data. The correspondence between both sets of estimates indicated that the prediction was successful, if by no means perfect. Note that this is a prediction in a strict sense where no capitalization on chance occurs.

Examples

Early applications aimed at testing cognitive hypotheses about the item material and constructing homogeneous item sets where a limited number of cognitive operations accounts for item difficulty. Scheiblechner (1972) showed that three cognitive operations, "negation," "disjunction," "asymmetry," sufficed for roughly explaining the difficulty of logical propositions. Similarly, Fischer (1973) analyzed the difficulty of tasks from calculus in terms of differentiation rules; Kubinger (1979) the difficulty of student's decisions in solving statistical problems; Spada (1976), Spada and Kluwe (1980), and Spada and May (1982) investigated tasks from elementary mechanics; several authors studied matrices tests (Formann, 1973; Formann and Piswanger, 1979; Embretson, 1985; Hornke and Habon, 1986; Hornke and Rettig, 1988) and spatial ability tests (Gittler and Wild, 1988; Gittler, 1990; Smith et al., 1992).

This "classical" LLTM approach is limited to item domains for which the researcher has valid hypotheses about the cognitive steps required for each item. Misspecifications of the **W**-matrix, however, should entail serious consequences. [Misspecification effects have not been investigated systematically so far; an exception is Baker (1993).]

Besides the explanation and prediction of item difficulty, the LLTM also enables one to identify and to model practicing effects within test-taking occasions: Already Scheiblechner (1972) reported that the actual item difficulty (measured by $\hat{\beta}_i^{(RM)}$) as compared to the item difficulty in the LLTM (measured by $\hat{\beta}_i^{(LLTM)}$) tended to decrease gradually in the course of the test. This pointed to learning/practice effects. He therefore incorporated a practice effect parameter λ into the model,

$$\beta_i = \sum_{l=1}^{p} w_{il}\alpha_l + (i-1)\lambda + c, \tag{18}$$

where item I_i is the ith item in the test and thus the term $(i-1)\lambda$ represents the total practice effect of having worked on $i-1$ items prior to I_i. Similar effects were reported by Spada (1976). Note, however, that these practice effects are independent of the person's success on the previous items, that is, the LLTM cannot model response contingent learning. [On response contingent or "dynamic" models of learning, see Kempf (1977) and Verhelst and Glas (1993, 1995).]

Another novel aspect in applications of the LLTM was the evidence of cultural influences on the availability of cognitive functions: By means of the LLTM, differential item functioning (DIF) can be *explained* by showing that certain cognitive operations are more readily available in one culture than in another. Piswanger (1975) [see also Fischer and Formann (1982)] gave the WMT ["Wiener Matrizentest"; Formann and Piswanger (1979)] to Austrian, Togolese, and Nigerian samples. All cognitive operations showed roughly the same difficulty in the Austrian (Mid-European) and the African samples, except for the operation "applying a rule in the horizontal direction." For the Austrian persons, apparently it was much more obvious to try a matrices item from left to right (i.e., in a horizontal direction) than from top to bottom (i.e., in a vertical direction). The Africans, on the other hand, found both directions equally easy (or obvious). The most plausible explanation of this finding is that, in the African culture, Arabian writing is still prominent: Arabs write from right to left; however, matrices items that require the horizontal direction cannot be solved from right to left, but only from left to right, owing to their design. Hence, the "horizontal direction" was not as easy for the Africans as for the Europeans. [A later study dealt more explicitly with this particular problem, Mohammadzadeh-Koucheri (1993)]. Further LLTM studies on cross-cultural differences are due to Whitely and Schneider (1981); Mislevy (1981); and van de Vijver (1988). These examples demonstrate that the LLTM is a very useful tool for gaining psychologically relevant insights into the process of test taking and factors influencing test performance.

An interesting application of the LLTM for change has recently been made by Gittler (1994): The objective was to assess the effect of taking classes in mechanical geometry on the development of spatial ability. A 17-items cubes test designed for measuring spatial ability [3DW; Gittler (1990)] was given to senior high school students of both sexes, some of whom attended classes in mechanical geometry ("treatment group"), while the rest took courses on other topics, such as biology ("control group"). The items considered in the analysis were items no. 2–18 of the 3DW, henceforth denoted $I_1, \ldots, I_{17}$ for convenience, while item no. 1 served only for warming up. All students were tested twice, aged 16 (T_1) and 18 (T_2), i.e., before and after the treatment period. The model comprising 85 virtual items with parameters β^*_{il} was

$\beta^*_{i1} = \beta_i$	for all persons at T_1; virtual items $1, \ldots, 17$;
$\beta^*_{i2} = \beta_i + \eta_1$	for males of the control group at T_2; virtual items $18, \ldots, 34$;
$\beta^*_{i3} = \beta_i + \eta_1 + \eta_2$	for males of the treatment group at T_2; virtual items $35, \ldots, 51$;
$\beta^*_{i4} = \beta_i + \eta_1 + \eta_3$	for females of the control group at T_2; virtual items $52, \ldots, 68$;
$\beta^*_{i5} = \beta_i + \eta_1 + \eta_2 + \eta_3 + \eta_4$	for females of the treatment group at T_2; virtual items 69–85.

The meaning of the basic parameters is as follows: The β_i are the item parameters of the items I_i; η_1 is the effect of natural cognitive development between T_1 and T_2 in students not receiving training in spatial abilities, including a possible practice effect of taking the test twice; η_2 is the effect of taking mechanical geometry ("treatment") rather than another subject; η_3 measures the effect of a possibly different speed of maturation of spatial ability in females as compared to males; and η_4 accounts for an interaction between gender and treatment. Although Gittler (1994) found a general difference in test performance between males and females in the 3DW, as expected, η_4 was positive (but insignificant), indicating that females improved at least as much under the training as males. Taking mechanical geometry can therefore be recommended for females at least as much as for males (in contradiction to an old tradition in Austrian high schools).

In the next section we reanalyze a subset of the data of Arrer (1992) who investigated whether the computerized version of a spatial ability test is comparable in difficulty to the older paper–pencil form: The 3DW test (mentioned above) was split in two blocks, items $I_1, \ldots, I_8$ and $I_9, \ldots, I_{17}$,

TABLE 1. Design of the Study of Arrer (1992).

Virtual Items and Virtual Item Parameters			
$I^*_{1,1},\ldots,I^*_{8,1}$	$I^*_{9,1},\ldots,I^*_{17,1}$	$I^*_{1,2},\ldots,I^*_{8,2}$	$I^*_{9,2},\ldots,I^*_{17,2}$
$\beta^*_{1,1},\ldots,\beta^*_{8,1}$	$\beta^*_{9,1},\ldots,\beta^*_{17,1}$	$\beta^*_{1,2},\ldots,\beta^*_{8,2}$	$\beta^*_{9,2},\ldots,\beta^*_{17,2}$
$I_1,\ldots,I_8$	$I_9,\ldots,I_{17}$	$I_1,\ldots,I_8$	$I_9,\ldots,I_{17}$
C	PP	PP	C
Group G_1		Group G_2	

Virtual Items and Virtual Item Parameters			
$I^*_{9,3},\ldots,I^*_{17,3}$	$I^*_{1,3},\ldots,I^*_{8,3}$	$I^*_{9,4},\ldots,I^*_{17,4}$	$I^*_{1,4},\ldots,I^*_{8,4}$
$\beta^*_{9,3},\ldots,\beta^*_{17,3}$	$\beta^*_{1,3},\ldots,\beta^*_{8,3}$	$\beta^*_{9,4},\ldots,\beta^*_{17,4}$	$\beta^*_{1,4},\ldots,\beta^*_{8,4}$
$I_9,\ldots,I_{17}$	$I_1,\ldots,I_8$	$I_9,\ldots,I_{17}$	$I_1,\ldots,I_8$
C	PP	PP	C
Group G_3		Group G_4	

and one block was presented in the usual paper–pencil form, the other in computerized form. Both the order of presentation of the two blocks of items and the order of the form of presentation (computerized vs. paper–pencil) were varied systematically, such that the design comprised four independent groups of testees, resulting in $4 \times 17 = 68$ virtual items (see Table 1).[1] For the present reanalysis, the data of 55 testees are taken from each group.

The 3DW is believed to be unidimensional and conforming to the RM (Gittler, 1990). The LLTM for change therefore appears to be the appropriate tool for measuring the effect of computerized vs. paper–pencil presentation and of a possible practice effect.

For formulating and testing several hypotheses, the following notation will be employed (see also Table 1):

β_i, $i = 1,\ldots,17$, are the difficulty parameters of the ("real") items,

β^*_{ig}, $i = 1,\ldots,17$ and $g = 1,\ldots,4$, are the difficulty parameters of the virtual items for the 4 groups G_g,

η_C is the effect of computerized presentation (as compared to paper–pencil presentation),

[1] *Note.* I_i, for $i = 1,\ldots,17$, denote the real test items; I^*_{ig}, for $i = 1,\ldots,17$ and $g = 1,\ldots,4$, the virtual items; C the computerized form; and PP the paper–pencil form of the 3DW.

η_T is the effect of the block of items presented first on the subsequent block.

The most general model (Model 1), against which more restrictive hypotheses will be tested, is defined by the set of equations

$$\begin{aligned}
\beta^*_{i1} &= \alpha_i, & i &= 1,\dots,17, \text{ for Group } G_1;\\
\beta^*_{i2} &= \alpha_{i+17}, & i &= 1,\dots,17, \text{ for Group } G_2;\\
\beta^*_{i3} &= \alpha_{i+34}, & i &= 1,\dots,17, \text{ for Group } G_3;\\
\beta^*_{i4} &= \alpha_{i+51}, & i &= 1,\dots,17, \text{ for Group } G_4.
\end{aligned}$$

This model assumes independent basic parameters for each of the four person groups, $\alpha_1,\dots,\alpha_{17}$; $\alpha_{18},\dots,\alpha_{34}$; $\alpha_{35},\dots,\alpha_{51}$; $\alpha_{52},\dots,\alpha_{68}$. It implies that the different forms and orders of presentation may interact with item difficulty in any way whatsoever. Note that, because the four groups are disjoint, four normalization conditions are required. We set $\alpha_1 = \alpha_{18} = \alpha_{35} = \alpha_{52} = 0$, eliminating the corresponding colums from the weight matrix $\mathbf{W}$ and thus equating the first virtual item parameter within each test to zero: $\beta^*_{1,1} = \beta^*_{1,2} = \beta^*_{1,3} = \beta^*_{1,4} = 0$.

The next hypothesis (Model 2) is more restrictive in that it assumes constant item parameters β_i, $i = 1,\dots,17$, over groups plus one effect of computerized presentation (as compared with paper–pencil presentation), η_C, plus one transfer effect parameter (transfer effect from the first block of items to the second block), η_T. Hence, Model 2 becomes

$$\begin{aligned}
\beta^*_{i1} &= \beta_i + \eta_C, & i &= 1,\dots,8, & &\text{for Group } G_1;\\
\beta^*_{i1} &= \beta_i + \eta_T, & i &= 9,\dots,17, & &\text{for Group } G_1;\\
\beta^*_{i2} &= \beta_i, & i &= 1,\dots,8, & &\text{for Group } G_2;\\
\beta^*_{i2} &= \beta_i + \eta_C + \eta_T, & i &= 9,\dots,17, & &\text{for Group } G_2;\\
\beta^*_{i3} &= \beta_i + \eta_C, & i &= 9,\dots,17, & &\text{for Group } G_3;\\
\beta^*_{i3} &= \beta_i + \eta_T, & i &= 1,\dots,8, & &\text{for Group } G_3;\\
\beta^*_{i4} &= \beta_i, & i &= 9,\dots,17, & &\text{for Group } G_4;\\
\beta^*_{i4} &= \beta_i + \eta_C + \eta_T, & i &= 1,\dots,8, & &\text{for Group } G_4.
\end{aligned}$$

For normalization, $\beta_1 = 0$ is assumed, hence Model 2 has $16 + 2 = 18$ independent basic parameters.

Now there are three ways of specializing Model 2 further:

$$\begin{aligned}
\eta_T &= 0, \text{ Model 3},\\
\eta_C &= 0, \text{ Model 4},\\
\eta_T = \eta_C &= 0, \text{ Model 5}.
\end{aligned}$$

The meaning of these models is obvious: Model 3 assumes an effect of computerized item presentation, but no transfer effect; Model 4 a transfer effect, but no effect of computerized presentation; Model 5 assumes neither effect, that is, the virtual item parameters β^*_{ig} are set equal to β_i, for $g = 1,\dots,4$. The normalizations in these three models are the same as

TABLE 2. Item Marginal Sums and Raw Score Frequencies in the Four Groups of Testees for the Data of the Example (Taken from Arrer, 1992).

Real	u_{i+}		Real	u_{i+}		N_r				Raw
Item	G_1	G_2	Item	G_3	G_4	G_1	G_2	G_3	G_4	Score
$i=1$	32	39	$i=9$	15	25	1	7	4	4	$r=1$
$i=2$	27	32	$i=10$	7	13	0	1	6	3	$i=2$
$i=3$	21	23	$i=11$	10	16	4	1	1	3	$r=3$
$i=4$	31	21	$i=12$	31	33	4	2	2	0	$r=4$
$i=5$	13	17	$i=13$	36	31	3	3	5	4	$r=5$
$i=6$	41	39	$i=14$	24	30	4	6	4	3	$r=6$
$i=7$	24	23	$i=15$	20	20	5	3	4	2	$r=7$
$i=8$	23	28	$i=16$	33	32	3	5	5	8	$r=8$
$i=9$	24	14	$i=17$	22	19	5	4	4	7	$r=9$
$i=10$	21	12	$i=1$	39	39	8	2	6	5	$r=10$
$i=11$	20	18	$i=2$	26	26	3	2	1	2	$r=11$
$i=12$	37	28	$i=3$	26	25	3	3	2	5	$r=12$
$i=13$	41	38	$i=4$	21	26	2	2	2	0	$r=13$
$i=14$	35	28	$i=5$	17	11	4	6	3	3	$r=14$
$i=15$	30	24	$i=6$	32	36	3	2	3	1	$r=15$
$i=16$	38	30	$i=7$	26	20	1	2	1	0	$r=16$
$i=17$	23	21	$i=8$	19	19	1	1	0	2	$r=17$

TABLE 3. Results of the Analysis of the Data Taken from Arrer (1992).

Model	p	$\hat{\eta}_C$	$\hat{\eta}_T$	$\log L$	Sign
1	64	–	–	−1434.13	–
2	18	0.283	−0.010	−1463.13	n.s.
3	17	0.287	–	−1463.91	n.s.
4	17	–	−0.109	−1469.36	s.
5	16	–	–	−1470.29	s.

in Model 2. Therefore, Models 3 and 4 each have 17, and Model 5 has 16 independent parameters.

The summary statistics of the data underlying the analysis are given in Table 2.[2] Since the item marginal sums and the raw score distributions of the four groups are sufficient statistics, the entries in Table 2 suffice for the analysis. The results of the analysis are to be found in Table 3.[3]

[2] *Note.* The u_{i+} are the item marginal sums, r the raw scores, N_r the frequencies of the raw scores, $G_1, \ldots, G_4$ the four groups.

[3] *Note.* Symbol p denotes the number of parameters per model, $\hat{\eta}_C$ and $\hat{\eta}_T$ the CML estimates of η_C and η_T, $\log L$ the logarithm of the conditional likelihood function at the CML solution, and sign the significance of the test of the respective model against Model 1 as H_1, for $\alpha = .05$.

First we test Model 2 against Model 1:

$$\chi^2 = -2(-1463.13 + 1434.13) = 58.00,$$

with $df = 64 - 18 = 46$, $\chi^2_{.95} = 62.83$, which is nonsignificant. Hence, we may assume that the item parameters β_i are constant across groups [which, by the way, is in accordance with the observation that the test is Rasch-homogeneous, see Gittler (1990)].

Next we test Model 3 against Model 1:

$$\chi^2 = -2(-1463.91 + 1434.13) = 59.56,$$

with $df = 64 - 17 = 47$, $\chi^2_{.95} = 64.00$, which again is nonsignificant. Hence we conclude that there is no transfer effect [again in accordance with general experiences with the 3DW, Gittler (1990)].

Model 4, however, has to be rejected:

$$\chi^2 = -2(-1469.36 + 1434.13) = 70.46,$$

with $df = 64-17 = 47$, $\chi^2_{.95} = 64.00$, which is significant. We conclude that there is an effect of computerized presentation of the 3DW, namely that the paper–pencil version is easier. The CML estimate $\hat{\eta}_C$ based on Model 3 is 0.287, and from the asymptotic standard error of $\hat{\eta}_C$ it can further be concluded that the 95% confidence interval for η_C is [0.129, 0.444].

Finally, for completeness we test Model 5 against Model 1:

$$\chi^2 = -2(-1470.29 + 1434.13) = 72.32,$$

with $df = 64-16 = 48$, $\chi^2_{.95} = 65.17$, which again is significant as expected; the hypothesis of constant β_i across groups and no effects of presentation nor of item order has to be rejected.

References

Andrich, D. (1978a). A rating formulation for ordered response categories. *Psychometrika* **43**, 561–573.

Andrich, D. (1978b). Application of a psychometric rating model to ordered categories which are scored with successive integers. *Applied Psychological Measurement* **2**, 581–594.

Arrer, S. (1992). *Unterschiede zwischen Computer- und Papier-Bleistift-Vorgabe des 3DW.* [Differences Between Computerized and Paper–Pencil Forms of the 3DW. In German.] Unpublished master's thesis, University of Vienna, Vienna.

Baker, F.B. (1993). Sensitivity of the linear logistic test model to misspecification of the weight matrix. *Applied Psychological Measurement* **17**, 201–210.

Embretson, S.E. (1985). Introduction to the problem of test design. In S.E. Embretson, *Test Design: Developments in Psychology and Psychometrics* (pp. 3–18). Orlando: Academic Press.

Fischer, G.H. (1973). The linear logistic test model as an instrument in educational research. *Acta Psychologica* **37**, 359–374.

Fischer, G.H. (1976). Some probabilistic models for measuring change. In D.N.M. de Gruijter and L.J.Th. van der Kamp (Eds), *Advances in Psychological and Educational Measurement* (pp. 97–110). New York: Wiley.

Fischer, G.H. (1977a). Some probabilistic models for the description of attitudinal and behavioral changes under the influence of mass communication. In W.F. Kempf and B. Repp (Eds), *Mathematical Models for Social Psychology* (pp. 102–151). Berne: Huber and New York: Wiley.

Fischer, G.H. (1977b). Linear logistic latent trait models: Theory and application. In H. Spada and W.F. Kempf (Eds), *Structural Models in Thinking and Learning* (pp. 203–225). Berne: Huber.

Fischer, G.H. (1981). On the existence and uniqueness of maximum-likelihood estimates in the Rasch model. *Psychometrika* **46**, 59–77.

Fischer, G.H. (1983). Logistic latent trait models with linear constraints. *Psychometrika* **48**, 3–26.

Fischer, G.H. (1995a). The linear logistic test model. In G.H. Fisher and I.W. Molenaar (Eds), *Rasch Models, Foundations, Recent Developments, and Applications* (pp. 131–155). New York: Springer-Verlag.

Fischer, G.H. (1995b). Linear logistic models for change. In G.H. Fischer and I.W. Molenaar (Eds), *Rasch Models, Recent Developments, and Applications* (pp. 158–180). New York: Springer-Verlag.

Fischer, G.H. and Formann, A.K. (1982). Some applications of logistic latent trait models with linear constraints on the parameters. *Applied Psychological Measurement* **4**, 397–416.

Fischer, G.H. and Parzer, P. (1991). An extension of the rating scale model with an application to the measurement of change. *Psychometrika* **56**, 637–651.

Fischer, G.H. and Pendl, P. (1980). Individualized testing on the basis of the dichotomous Rasch model. In L.J. Th. van der Kamp, W.F. Langerak, and D.N.M. de Gruijter (Eds), *Psychometrics for Educational Debates* (pp. 171–188). New York: Wiley.

Fischer, G.H. and Ponocny, I. (1994). An extension of the partial credit model with an application to the measurement of change. *Psychometrika* **59**, 177–192.

Fischer, G.H. and Ponocny, I. (1995). Extended rating scale and partial credit models for assessing change. In G.H. Fisher and I.W. Molenaar

(Eds), *Rasch Models, Foundations, Recent Developments, and Applications* (pp. 353–370). New York: Springer-Verlag.

Fischer, G.H. and Tanzer, N. (1994). Some LLTM and LBTL relationships. In G.H. Fischer and D. Laming (Eds), *Contributions to Mathematical Psychology, Psychometrics, and Methodology* (pp. 277–303). New York: Springer-Verlag.

Formann, A.K. (1973). *Die Konstruktion eines neuen Matrizentests und die Untersuchung des Lösungsverhaltens mit Hilfe des linear logistischen Testmodells.* [The Construction of a New Matrices Test and the Investigation of the Response Behavior by Means of the Linear Logistic Test Model. In German.] Unpublished doctoral dissertation, University of Vienna, Vienna.

Formann, A.K. and Piswanger, K. (1979). *Wiener Matrizen-Test. Ein Rasch-skalierter sprachreier Intelligenztest.* [Viennese Matrices Test. A Rasch-Scaled Culture-Fair Intelligence Test. In German.] Weinheim: Beltz-Test.

Gittler, G. (1990). *Dreidimensionaler Würfeltest (3DW). Ein Rasch-skalierter Test zur Messung des räumlichen Vorstellungsvermögens.* [The Three-Dimensional Cubes Test (3DW). A Rasch-Scaled Test for Spatial Ability. In German.] Weinheim: Beltz-Test.

Gittler, G. (1994). Intelligenzförderung durch Schulunterricht: Darstellende Geometrie und räumliches Vorstellungsvermögen. [The promotion of intelligence via teaching: Mechanical geometry and spatial abilities. In German.] In G. Gittler, M. Jirasko, U. Kastner-Koller, C. Korunka, and A. Al-Roubaie (Eds), *Die Seele ist ein weites Land* (pp. 103–122). Vienna: WUV-Universitätsverlag.

Gittler, G. and Wild, B. (1988). Der Einsatz des LLTM bei der Konstruktion eines Item-pools für das adaptive Testen. [Usage of the LLTM for the construction of an item pool for adaptive testing. In German.] In K.D. Kubinger (Ed), *Moderne Testtheorie* (pp. 115–139). Weinheim and Munich: Beltz Test Gesellschaft/Psychologie Verlags Union.

Hillgruber, G. (1990). *Schätzung von Parametern in psychologischen Testmodellen.* [Parameter estimation in psychological test models. In German.] Unpublished master's thesis, University of Cologne, Cologne.

Hornke, L.F. and Habon, M.W. (1986). Rule-based item bank construction and evaluation within the linear logistic framework. *Applied Psychological Measurement* **10**, 369–380.

Hornke, L.F. and Rettig, K. (1988). Regelgeleitete Itemkonstruktion unter Zuhilfenahme kognitionspsychologischer Überlegungen. [Rule-based item construction using concepts of cognitive psychology. In German.] In K.D. Kubinger (Ed), *Moderne Testtheorie* (pp. 140–162). Weinheim: Beltz.

Kempf, W. (1972). Probabilistische Modelle experimentalpsychologischer Versuchssituationen. *Psychologische Beiträge*, **14**, 16–37.

Kempf, W. (1977). Dynamic models for the measurement of "traits" in social behavior. In W. Kempf and B.H. Repp (Eds), *Mathematical Models for Social Psychology* (pp. 14–58). Berne: Huber.

Kubinger, K.D. (1979). Das Problemlöseverhalten bei der statistischen Auswertung psychologischer Experimente. Ein Beispiel hochschuldidaktischer Forschung. [The task-solving behavior in the statistical analysis of psychological experiments. An example of research in didactics. In German.] *Zeitschrift für Experimentelle und Angewandte Psychologie* **26**, 467–495.

Masters, G.N. (1982). A Rasch model for partial credit scoring. *Psychometrika* **47**, 149–174.

Micko, H.C. (1969). A psychological scale for reaction time measurement. *Acta Psychologica* **30**, 324–335.

Micko, H.C. (1970). Eine Verallgemeinerung des Messmodells von Rasch mit einer Anwendung auf die Psychophysik der Reaktionen. [A generalization of Rasch's measurement model with an application to the psychophysics of reactions. In German.] *Psychologische Beiträge* **12**, 4–22.

Mislevy, R.J. (1981). *A general linear model for the analysis of Rasch item threshold estimates.* Unpublished doctoral dissertation, University of Chicago, Chicago.

Mohammadzadeh-Koucheri, F. (1993). *Interkultureller Vergleich mit einer variierten Form des Matrizentests von Formann.* [Cross-cultural comparisons using a variation of the matrices test of Formann. In German.] Unpublished master's thesis, University of Vienna, Vienna.

Nährer, W. (1980). Zur Analyse von Matrizenaufgaben mit dem linearen logistischen Testmodell. [On the analysis of matrices items by means of the linear logistic test model. In German.] *Zeitschrift für Experimentelle und Angewandte Psychologie* **27**, 553–564.

Pfanzagl, J. (1994). On item parameter estimation in certain latent trait models. In G.H. Fischer and D. Laming (Eds), *Contributions to Mathematical Psychology, Psychometrics, and Methodology* (pp. 249–263). New York: Springer-Verlag.

Piswanger, K. (1975). *Interkulturelle Vergleiche mit dem Matrizentest von Formann.* [Cross-cultural comparisons by means of the matrices test of Formann. In German.] Unpublished doctoral dissertation, University of Vienna, Vienna.

Rasch, G. (1965). *Statistisk Seminar.* [Statistical Seminar.] Copenhague: University of Copenhague, Department of Mathematical Statistics. (Notes taken by J. Stene.)

Scheiblechner, H. (1971). *CML-parameter-estimation in a generalized multifactorial version of Rasch's probabilistic measurement model with two categories of answers*, Research Bulletin No. 4. Vienna: Department of Psychology, University of Vienna.

Scheiblechner, H. (1972). Das Lernen und Lösen komplexer Denkaufgaben. [The learning and solving of complex reasoning tasks. In German.] *Zeitschrift für Experimentelle und Angewandte Psychologie* **3**, 456–506.

Smith, R.M., Kramer, G.A., and Kubiak, A.T. (1992). Components of difficulty in spatial ability test items. In M. Wilson (Ed), *Objective Measurement: Theory into Practice*, Vol. 1 (pp. 157–174). Norwood, NJ: Ablex.

Spada, H. (1976). *Modelle des Denkens and Lernens.* [Models of Thinking and Learning. In German.] Berne: Huber.

Spada, H. and Kluwe, R. (1980). Two models of intellectual development and their reference to the theory of Piaget. In R. Kluwe and H. Spada (Eds), *Developmental Models of Thinking* (pp. 1–30). New York: Academic Press.

Spada, H. and May, R. (1982). The linear logistic test model and its application in educational research. In D. Spearritt (Ed), *The Improvement of measurement in Education and Psychology* (pp. 67–84). Hawthorne, Victoria: Australian Council for Educational Research.

van de Vijver, F.J.R. (1988). Systematizing item content in test design. In R. Langeheine and J. Rost (Eds), *Latent Trait and Latent Class Models* (pp. 291–307). New York: Plenum.

Verhelst, N.D. and Glas, C.A.W. (1993). A dynamic generalization of the Rasch model. *Psychometrika* **58**, 395–415.

Verhelst, N.D. and Glas, C.A.W. (1995). Dynamic generalizations of the Rasch model. In G.H. Fischer and I.W. Molenaar (Eds), *Rasch Models, Foundations, Recent Developments, and Applications* (pp. 181–201). New York: Springer-Verlag.

Whitely, S.E. and Schneider, L.M. (1981). Information structure for geometric analogies: A test theory approach. *Applied Psychological Measurement* **5**, 383–397.

14
Response Models with Manifest Predictors

Aeilko H. Zwinderman

Introduction

Every test or questionnaire, constructed with either classical test theory or modern IRT, is ultimately meant as a tool to do further research. Most often the test is used to evaluate treatments or therapies or to see whether the abilities underlying the test are associated to other constructs, and sometimes test scores are used to make individual predictions or decisions. Whatever the ultimate goal, the immediate interest is usually to estimate correlations between the abilities underlying the test and other important variables.

A straightforward way to compute the correlations of interest is to use the estimated person parameters according to some (IRT) model. However, these person parameter estimates may be subject to considerable error and consequently the correlations are often estimated too low. Of course, this problem is well known and so is its general solution. In classical test theory, the correlations between the test scores and other variables may be disattenuated for the unreliability of the test scores or, more complicated, one may develop a structural equations model. The general idea presented in this paper, however, is to combine the measurement model and the structural model such that the correlations between the ability (or abilities) measured by the test and the other constructs are estimated directly from the model.

Several investigators have formulated such models in association with item response theory, with different goals in mind, and only allowing for one ability underlying the item responses and only manifest extraneous variables. Mislevy (1987) formulated a structural model for the two-parameter logistic or Birnbaum model, but was primarily interested in minimizing the estimation error of the item and person parameters. Verhelst and Eggen (1989) and Zwinderman (1991) formulated a structural model for the Rasch or one parameter logistic model assuming that the item parameters are known (or estimated with conditional maximum likelihood). Finally, Hoijtink (1993) formulated a structural model for the three-parameter logistic model also assuming that the item parameters are known. The work of these authors will be elaborated upon and generalized in this chapter.

Presentation of the Model

The structural model offered in this chapter is based on the unidimensional polytomous Rasch model (UPRM) with equidistant scoring of the categories (Andersen, 1973, this volume). This model will be introduced first in order to clarify notation.

Assume there is a sample of persons responding to a set of items underlying which there is a single unidimensional ability (θ). Let U_{ij} be the stochastic response of person j to item i with realization u_{ij}, which can attain values $0, \ldots, h, \ldots, m_i$. The conditional probability that U_{ij} is equal to h given j's value of θ, is given by

$$p(U_{ij} = h \mid \theta_j) = \frac{\exp(\psi_h + h(\theta_j + \alpha_i))}{1 + \sum_{g=1}^{m_i} \exp(\psi_g + g(\theta_j + \alpha_i))}, \tag{1}$$

where α_i is the easiness parameter of item i and Ψ_h is the intercept parameter of category h. The properties of this model are well known. The structural parameters (α, Ψ, and parameters of the distribution of θ) can be estimated consistently under mild conditions with either the conditional or marginal maximum likelihood method, and the estimates are unique under mild conditions (Fischer, 1981, 1990, this volume) except for normalizing constants. Usually, both Ψ_0 and the mean of the item parameters are fixed at zero. Furthermore, it is neither necessary that all persons respond to all items nor that all items have the same number of categories; however, the design must be connected (Glas, 1989). Note that the Rasch model for dichotomous items is a special case of Eq. (1).

A structural model is constructed by including extraneous variables, called covariates in the remainder of this chapter, in the model. The first step is to model θ as a function of a vector of covariates observed at the level of the person ($\mathbf{X}_j$):

$$\theta_j = \beta_1 X_{1j} + \cdots + \beta_p X_{pj} + \varepsilon_j, \tag{2}$$

where β is the vector of regression parameters and ε_j is the usual error term. Substituting Eq. (2) into (1) and direct estimation of β facilitates estimation of the (multiple) correlation of θ with X without estimating the person parameters (θ_j).

Of course it is a straightforward generalization to combine Eq. (2) with a LLTM-type model for the item parameters (Fischer, 1983, this volume) allowing its weight matrix to vary among persons. So if $\mathbf{X}_{ij}$ is a vector of covariates observed with the response of j to item i, then

$$\theta_j + \alpha_i = \beta_1 X_{ij1} + \cdots + \beta_p X_{ijp} + \varepsilon_j = \beta' X_{ij} + \varepsilon_j. \tag{3}$$

Substituting Eq. (3) into (1) yields the conditional probability that U_{ij} is h given $\mathbf{X}_{ij}$ and ε_j:

$$p(U_{ij} = h \mid X_{ij}, \varepsilon_j) = \frac{\exp(\psi_h + h(\beta' X_{ij} + \varepsilon_j))}{1 + \sum_{g=1}^{m_i} \exp(\psi_g + g(\beta' X_{ij} + \varepsilon_j))}. \tag{4}$$

This model is most flexible and can be used to tackle several research questions, but it is important to distinguish among three types of covariates:

1. covariates varying between persons, but not within persons (e.g., sex, age, other test scores),
2. covariates varying within persons, but equal for all persons (e.g., items, LLTM weights), and
3. covariates varying both within and between persons (e.g., item response time, interactions between type 1 and 2 covariates, functions of preceding item responses).

This distinction is important because both conditional (CML) and marginal maximum likelihood (MML) methods may be employed to estimate the parameters in Eq. (4). However, the regression parameters associated with type 1 covariates cannot be estimated with CML; they are conditioned out of the inference problem.

As was already mentioned, Eq. (4) is most flexible and leads to several special cases. An obvious special case is the unidimensional polytomous Rasch model in Eq. (1), which is the case when there are no covariates, only different items. In that case, the random variable ε is equal to θ, and the regression parameters β can be interpreted as item parameters: when there are k different items, $k-1$ type 2 dummy covariates suffice (Molenaar and Verhelst, 1988). In this formulation, the contrasts between the items are free to be chosen; usually deviation contrasts are used (mean of the parameters equals zero), but other types may also be chosen (simple, Helmert, polynomial contrast). Also the traditional LLTM is a special case of Eq. (4): again ε equals θ, and the regression parameters β can be interpreted as Fischer's basic parameters.

Another special case of Eq. (4) may be used to test whether there is differential item functioning (DIF) in a test. This happens when a test item has different difficulty parameters for persons with different covariate vectors but otherwise the same ability. For instance, if item i^* is suspected of differential functioning between males and females (type 1 covariate), then an additional covariate may be included in the model which equals 1 if j is female and i is i^* and zero otherwise (type 3 covariate: interaction between gender and items). It suffices to test whether the associated regression parameter equals zero.

Another interesting special case of Eq. (4) is modeling "learning during test taking." This is a violation of the usual assumption of local stochastic independence, and this can be accounted for if functions of preceding item responses are used as covariates in Eq. (4). Some hints on how to do this will be discussed next, but for a general treatment of dynamic models the reader is referred to Verhelst and Glas (1993).

Given θ_j (or given the covariates and ε_j) the U_{ij}'s are assumed to be independent in Eq. (4), meaning that marginally there is a constant correlation between U_i and U_{i^*} for any i and i^* (compound symmetry). Therefore, the sum score $u_{.j} = \sum_i u_{ij}$ is a sufficient statistic for θ_j. Hence, a consequence of using $u_{.j}$ as a (type 1) covariate in Eq. (4) is that there should be no correlation left between, for instance, u_{ij} and u_{ij+1} if the model fits. When, however, u_{ij} (or other preceding item responses: type 3 covariates) is a significant covariate for U_{ij+1} in addition to $u_{.j}$, this means that local stochastic independence is violated. When this is the case, a compound symmetry correlation structure cannot be true. Alternatives may be autoregressive structures if learning during test taking occurred, or factor-analytic structures if unidimensionality is violated.

To finalize this section, the assumptions underlying Eq. (4) will be summarized. The most important assumptions are that $u_{.j}$ is a minimal sufficient statistic for θ_j, and that the item responses are locally independent given θ. As already mentioned, this means that the marginal correlation between the item responses is constant. This correlation is a function of the variance of θ (σ^2) and may be approximated as (van Houwelingen et al., 1991)

$$\rho \approx \frac{\sigma^2}{(1.7)^2 + \sigma^2}. \tag{5}$$

ρ is an intra-class correlation and may be interpreted in the same way as the classical reliability coefficient. It is easy to see that ρ has the same flaw as its classical counterpart: if θ has little variation ρ will be low, and if θ has considerable variation, ρ will be high. But note that ρ is only a reliability coefficient if θ equals ε; after all, if covariates enter the model, the variance of ε will decrease, and ultimately the variance of ε may even become zero. When that is the case, the item responses are not only locally but also globally independent (conditional on the covariates), in which case Eq. (4) is equal to the ordinary polytomous logistic regression model with equal odds ratio's for every pair of adjacent categories (Dixon et al., 1990).

Parameter Estimation

In this section some mathematical details of the procedures to estimate the parameters of Eq. (4) are given. As mentioned before, both CML and MML methods can be used. However, as CML has the disadvantage that the effects of type 1 covariates cannot be estimated, only MML will be discussed.

When using MML, it is necessary to assume a density function for the random terms in the model: either for θ or for ε. Although any density function will do [parametric or nonparametric: Hoijtink (1993)], usually the normal density function is used with unknown variance. The mean must be fixed to zero because it is not identified: it is intertwined with the category parameters (Ψ).

The estimation of (β, Ψ, and σ^2) takes place by maximizing the conditional marginal loglikelihood of the item responses given the covariates. Define $u_{ijh} = 1$ if $u_{ij} = h$ and zero otherwise, let p_{ijh} be the probability that j responds in category h to item i according to Eq. (4), and let $g(\varepsilon)$ be the normal density function with mean zero and variance σ^2. The conditional density of the item responses $\mathbf{U}$ given ε and the covariate values $\mathbf{X}$ is given by

$$f_c(\mathbf{U} \mid \varepsilon, \mathbf{X}) = \prod_{j=1}^{N} f_{c_j}(\mathbf{U}_j \mid \varepsilon_j, \mathbf{X}_j) = \prod_{i=1}^{n_j} \prod_{j=1}^{N} \prod_{h=1}^{m_i} p_{jih}^{u_{jih}} (1 - p_{jih})^{u_{jih}}, \quad (6)$$

and the joint density of $(\mathbf{U}, \varepsilon)$ given $\mathbf{X}$ by

$$f_j(\mathbf{U}, \varepsilon \mid \mathbf{X}) = \prod_{j=1}^{N} (f_{j_j}(\mathbf{U}_j, \varepsilon_j \mid \mathbf{X}_j) = \prod_{j=1}^{N} f_{c_j}(\mathbf{U}_j \mid \varepsilon_j, \mathbf{X}_j) g(\varepsilon), \quad (7)$$

and finally the conditional marginal likelihood of (β, Ψ, and σ^2) given $(\mathbf{U}, \mathbf{X})$

$$L_m(\beta, \psi, \sigma^2 \mid \mathbf{U}, \mathbf{X}) = \prod_{j=1}^{N} \int_{-\infty}^{\infty} f_{c_j}(\mathbf{U}_j \mid \varepsilon_j, \mathbf{X}_j) g(\varepsilon) d\varepsilon. \quad (8)$$

The conditional marginal likelihood in Eq. (8) is a function of (β, ψ, and σ^2) only, the random effect terms ε are integrated out. There are many possible iterative algorithms to maximize the log of Eq. (8); the most commonly used algorithm is Newton's, but the Fisher-scoring, and the Davidon–Fletcher–Powell algorithms are good alternatives (Isaacson and Keller, 1966). Also a generalized EM algorithm has been suggested (Zwinderman, 1991), which is based on maximizing the expectation of the logarithm of Eq. (7). All algorithms require first-order and some second-order partial derivatives of the log of Eq. (8) or the expectation of the log of Eq. (7). This requires some mathematical skill and good bookkeeping, but is in itself not very complex. Here, the first-order partial derivatives of the log of Eq. (8) are given:

$$\frac{\partial \log L_m(\beta, \psi, \sigma^2 \mid \mathbf{U}, \mathbf{X})}{\partial \beta_q} = \sum_{i=1}^{nn_j} \sum_{j=1}^{N} \sum_{h=1}^{m_i} \int_{-\infty}^{\infty} (u_{ijh} - p_{ijh}) X_{ijq} \frac{p_j(\varepsilon)}{\int_{-\infty}^{\infty} p_j(\varepsilon) d\varepsilon} d\varepsilon,$$

$$\frac{\partial \log L_m(\beta, \psi, \sigma^2 \mid \mathbf{U}, \mathbf{X})}{\partial \sigma^2} = \sum_{j=1}^{N} \int_{-\infty}^{\infty} \varepsilon_j^2 \frac{p_j(\varepsilon)}{\int_{-\infty}^{\infty} p_j(\varepsilon) d\varepsilon} d\varepsilon,$$

where

$$p_j(\varepsilon) = \frac{\exp(u_{j.}\varepsilon_j - \frac{1}{2}\varepsilon_j^2/\sigma^2)}{\prod_{i=1}^{n_j} 1 + \sum_{g=1}^{m_i} \exp(\psi_g + g(\beta' X_{ji} + \varepsilon_j))}, \tag{9}$$

and n_j is the number of items j responsded to.

The integral in the above expression is usually evaluated with Gauss–Hermite quadrature methods (Abramowitz and Stegun, 1965). When using Newton's algorithm, the asymptotic covariance matrix of the parameter estimates is immediately available as the inverse of the negative matrix of second-order partial derivatives.

The conditions under which the parameters of Eq. (4) can be identified have as yet not been established as firmly as for the Rasch model for dichotomous item responses. Some necessary conditions are that (1) every response category must be observed at least once; (2) the sum scores ($u_{.j}$) must have "sufficient" variance; (3) the covariates must have "sufficient" variance; and (4) the correlation between the covariates and the responses must be less than perfect (Albert and Anderson, 1984; Fischer 1981, 1990; Glas, 1989).

In general, the estimation process is rather laborious for two reasons. First, the estimation process is sensitive to the choice of starting values for the parameters of Eq. (4). However, good candidates are usually provided by the estimates of the fixed effects polytomous logistic regression model [Eq. (4) without the random effect term ε] which is available in BMDP's PR module. Second, estimation may take a long time, especially when continuous covariates are involved. When there are only items and no other covariates in the model, the contributions to the likelihood of persons with the same sum score are equal, and can therefore be grouped together. If, however, there are covariates in the model that vary among all item responses, the contribution of each item response to the likelihood must be evaluated separately. For example, when you have 1000 persons and 10 dichotomous items, only the evaluation of the likelihood contributions of 11 sum score groups is needed, but if you have in addition a covariate varying with all responses, 10,000 likelihood contributions must be evaluated. When the main interest of the investigation is to see whether the covariates are correlated with the item responses, a marginal model for the item responses may be more practical (Prentice, 1988; van Houwelingen et al., 1991; Zeger et al., 1988; Zeger and Liang, 1986).

Goodness of Fit

As yet no global goodness of fit tests for the most general model in Eq. (4) have been developed. But tests are available for special cases such as the unidimensional polytomous Rasch model in Eq. (1) (Glas, 1989; Glas and Verhelst, 1989). The best strategy for testing the goodness of fit of the model is, therefore, to start fitting and testing the fit of the UPRM. After obtaining a satisfactory fit, the UPRM may be extended to include covariates. The effects of covariates and the usual assumptions underlying regression models may then be tested by Score, Wald or likelihood ratio tests (Rao, 1973). Some caution is needed when testing the hypothesis $H_0: \sigma^2 = 0$, because σ^2 cannot be negative, therefore a one-sided test is called for.

Examples

Two examples will be given to illustrate the possibilities of the model in Eq. (4). The first example concerns the validation of a questionnaire measuring aspects of the quality of life of severe asthmatic patients. A sample of 145 patients filled in a test battery containing, amongst others, a subscale of 10 dichotomous items constructed to measure respiration complaints. The fit of the Rasch model according to Glas' R-tests (Glas, 1988) was satisfactory ($R_0 = 2.6$, $df = 8$, $p = 0.96$; $R_1 = 16.7$, $df = 26$, $p = 0.92$; $R_2 = 75.0$, $df = 52$, $p = 0.02$). The Rasch Scaling Program was used to estimate and test the goodness of fit of the Rasch model (Glas and Ellis, 1993). The standard deviation of the ability (θ) underlying the items was estimated to be 1.62 (SE = 0.15), so that the reliability was estimated as 0.49 (SE = 0.05).

Also observed were (1) the number of visits to the general practitioner; (2) the number of days on sick leave in the last six months; (3) the number of asthma attacks in the last 14 days; (4) the subjective severity of asthma; and (5) the dyspnea degree. The correlations of each of these five covariates separately and their multiple correlation with θ was estimated according to Eq. (4). These were estimated using the EGRET package (1985), and are reported in Table 1,[1] and for the sake of comparison, the correlations of the covariates with the estimated person parameters are also reported. These latter correlations were substantially smaller than the former which

[1]Note to Table 1: $\hat{\beta}$ (SE) is the estimated regression parameters according to Eq. (4) and its associated standard error. $\hat{\sigma}_\varepsilon$ (SE) is the estimated standard deviation of ε according to Eq. (4), and its associated standard error. The first r is the estimated correlation between the covariate and θ. The second r is the estimated correlation between the covariates and the estimated person parameters according to Eq. (1).

TABLE 1. Correlations Between the Ability Measured by the Items Referring to Respiration Complaints and Some Patients Characteristics.

Variable	$\hat{\beta}$ (SE)		$\hat{\sigma}_\varepsilon$ (SE)		r	r
Number of visits to the general practitioner	−0.358	(1.390)	1.53	(0.17)	−0.33	−0.01
Number of days on sick leave	0.068	(0.017)	1.37	(0.16)	0.53	0.40
Number of asthma attacks	0.040	(0.017)	1.48	(0.16)	0.41	0.25
Dyspnea degree	0.473	(0.150)	1.44	(0.16)	0.46	0.32
Multiple					0.65	0.52

illustrates to what extent errors attenuate the validity of tests and questionnaires.

The second example concerns the evaluation of the effects of neurosurgery on some aspects of the quality of life of patients with a solitary brain metastasis. A sample of 63 patients was randomized between neurosurgery and radiation therapy ($n = 32$) and radiation therapy alone ($n = 31$). The general condition of the patients was measured with the Independence Scale of the World Health Organization (WHO). This scale consists of one item with five ordered categories: 0 = "the patient is completely independent" to 4 = "the patient is completely bedridden." The WHO scale was used by the physician immediately after diagnosis (month 0), every month after for the first six months, and bimonthly after that. The maximum follow up time was 70 months. Neurosurgery appeared to extend survival; median survival was 12 months (95% confidence interval 5–19) for the surgery group and 7 months (95% confidence interval 4–8) for the radiation alone group ($p = 0.06$). However, the question was whether this extension of survival by surgery was at the expense of the quality of life.

The occurrence of a (brain) metastasis with cancer is an indication of a very bad prognosis. Therefore, the general condition of patients deteriorates with time, and, consequently, the probability of scoring in the higher categories of the WHO scale was expected to increase with time. When this increase is larger for patients receiving neurosurgery than for patients only receiving radiation therapy, then the life extension obtained by surgery is at the expense of the life quality of patients. This hypothesis was investigated using the model in Eq. (4).

Let U_{jt} be the rating of patient j at time t with probability

$$\log\left(\frac{p(U_{jt}=h \mid \theta_j)}{p(U_{jt}=h-1 \mid \theta_j)}\right) = (\psi_h - \psi_{h-1}) + (\theta_j + \alpha_t), \tag{10}$$

where θ_j is the latent general condition of j, and α_t denoted the effect of month t. In order to investigate the effect of surgery, θ and α were modeled as

$$\theta_j = \beta_1 X_j + \varepsilon_j, \tag{11}$$

where X_j is 1 if j receives surgery and 0 if not, and

$$\alpha_t = \beta_2 t + \beta_3 t^2 + \beta_4 t^3 + \beta_5 t \star X_j + \beta_6 t^2 \star X_j + \beta_7 t^3 \star X_j. \tag{12}$$

The parameters for each different month (α_t) were modeled according to a cubic polynomial to allow for the beneficial effect of treatment in the early stages of the investigation. Note that the normalization that is required for identification of α is done by equating α_0 to zero.

The latter three interaction terms in Eq. (12) were used to test the hypothesis that the change of the probabilities of the scoring of the WHO scale was different for the two patient groups. This was done using a likelihood ratio test of models including and excluding those three interaction terms: a small significant different effect was found (deviances were 900.38 and 907.76: $p = 0.02$). The estimated change of θ over time for both patient groups is displayed in Fig. 1. It appeared that there was little difference in general condition between the two treatment groups up to seven months, but the quality of life for the group who received surgery dropped dramatically in relation to the group who received radiation only after about seven months.

The above application of Eq. (4) to model repeated observations is similar to Fischer's LLRA model (Fischer, 1983, this volume; Fischer and Parzer, 1991), but a word of caution is necessary here. As was argued before, the implicit assumption of local stochastic independence is that the marginal correlation structure has the form of compound symmetry. However, a constant correlation is highly unlikely for follow up studies with a long follow up; one would favor a model in which the correlation decreases with the distance between the responses in time. However, such models are hard to apply in practice since multidimensional integrals have to be evaluated. These problems do not occur with marginal models for the response probabilities (e.g., Liang et al., 1992), but in these models the mechanism causing missing data (for instance, the fact that patients die) is not ignorable (Little and Rubin, 1987). Using the model in Eq. (4), the missing data may usually be treated as missing at random [see Diggle and Kenward (1994) for a general discussion].

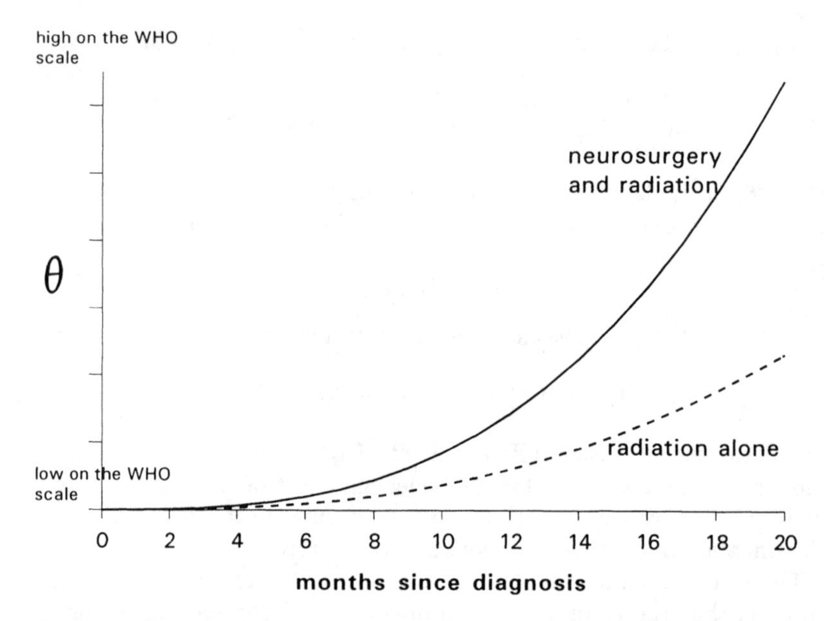

FIGURE 1. Estimated change patterns over time of the quality of life variable measured by the WHO scale for patients receiving neurosurgery and radiation and patients receiving radiation therapy alone.

Discussion

The general model in Eq. (4), known as the logistic regression model with random effects in the statistical literature, may be generalized in several aspects. A limiting assumption is that of homogeneity of the variance of ε for all covariate patterns. It is quite straightforward to relax this assumption [see also Hoijtink (1993)], and this is already done in, for instance, the RSP program (Glas and Ellis, 1993) for some special cases of Eq. (4). In the same way multilevel models may be developed. Another limiting assumption is the equidistant scoring of the categories. Theoretically, it is possible to develop models with category scoring parameters (Andersen, 1973; Anderson, 1984), but as yet little is known about their statistical properties. Finally, it seems obvious to generalize the model in Eq. (4) to polytomous items without ordered categories. However, this means that multidimensional abilities have to be included in the model. Although CML estimation still is possible in some cases (Andersen, 1973), MML estimation will be virtually impossible because multidimensional integrals appear in the likelihoods.

References

Abramowitz, M. and Stegun, I.A. (1965). *Handbook of Mathematical Functions.* New York: Dover Publications.

Albert, A. and Anderson, J.A. (1984). On the existence of maximum likelihood estimates in logistic regression models. *Biometrika* **71**, 1–10.

Andersen, E.B. (1973). Conditional inference for multiple choice questionnaires. *British Journal of Mathematical and Statistical Psychology* **26**, 31–44.

Anderson, J.A. (1984). Regression and ordered categorical variables. *Journal of the Royal Statistical Society, Series B* **46**, 1–30.

Diggle, P. and Kenward, M.G. (1994). Informative drop-out in longitudinal data analysis. *Applied Statistics* **43**, 49–94.

Dixon, W.J., Brown, M.B., Engelman, L., and Jennrich, R.I. (1990). *BMDP Statistical Software Manual,* Vol. 2. Berkeley: University of California Press.

Egret (1985). *Egret Reference Manual.* Seattle: Statistics and Epidemiology Research Corporation and Cytel Software Corporation.

Fischer, G.H. (1981). On the existence and uniqueness of maximum likelihood estimates in the Rasch model. *Psychometrika* **46**, 59–77.

Fischer, G.H. (1983). Logistic latent trait models with linear constraints. *Psychometrika* **48**, 3–26.

Fischer, G.H. (1990, September). On the existence and uniqueness of a CML solution in the polytomous Rasch model. Paper presented at the 21st Meeting of the European Mathematical Psychology Group, Bristol.

Fischer, G.H. and Parzer, P. (1991). An extension of the rating scale model with an application to the measurement of change. *Psychometrika* **56**, 637–651.

Glas, C.A.W. (1988). The derivation of some tests for the Rasch model from the multinomial distribution. *Psychometrika* **53**, 525–546.

Glas, C.A.W. (1989). *Contributions to Estimating and Testing Rasch Models.* Unpublished doctoral dissertation, University of Twente, Enschede.

Glas, C.A.W. and Verhelst, N.D. (1989). Extensions of the partial credit model. *Psychometrika* **54**, 635–659.

Glas, C. and Ellis, J. (1993). *RSP User's Manual.* Groningen, the Netherlands: I.E.C. Progamma.

Hoijtink, H. (1993). *Linear Models with a Latent Dependent Variable: Non-Parametric Error Term Density Functions.* Manuscript submitted for publication.

Isaacson, E. and Keller, H.B. (1966). *Analysis of Numerical Methods.* New York: Wiley.

Liang, K.-Y., Zeger, S.L., and Qaqish, B. (1992). Multivariate regression analyses for categorical data. *Journal of the Royal Statistical Society, Series B* **54**, 3–40.

Little, R.J.A. and Rubin, D.B. (1987). *Statistical Analysis with Missing Data*. New York: Wiley.

Mislevy, R.J. (1987). Exploiting auxiliary information about examinees in the estimation of item parameters. *Applied Psychological Measurement* **11**, 81–91.

Molenaar, I.W. and Verhelst, N.D. (1988). Logit based parameter estimation in the Rasch model. *Statistica Neerlandica* **42**, 273–296.

Prentice, R.L. (1988). Correlated binary regression with covariates specific to each binary observation. *Biometrics* **44**, 1033–1048.

Rao, C.R. (1973). *Linear Statistical Inference and Its Applications*. New York: Wiley.

van Houwelingen, J.C., le Cessie, S., and Zwinderman, A.H. (1991, July). Modelling Dependency for binary random variables. Paper presented at the Sixth Workshop on Statistical Modelling, Utrecht, The Netherlands.

Verhelst, N.D. and Eggen, T.J.H.M. (1989). *Psychometrische en Statistische Aspecten van Peilingsonderzoek* (PPON rapport 4) (in Dutch). Arnhem: Cito.

Verhelst, N.D. and Glas, C.A.W. (1993). A dynamic generalization of the Rasch model. *Psychometrika* **58**, 395–416.

Zeger, S.L. and Liang, K.-Y. (1986). Longitudinal data analysis for discrete and continuous outcomes. *Biometrics* **42**, 121–130.

Zeger, S.L., Liang, K.-Y., and Albert, P.S. (1988). Models for longitudinal data: a generalized estimation equation approach. *Biometrics* **44**, 1049–1060.

Zwinderman, A.H. (1991). A generalized Rasch model for manifest predictors. *Psychometrika* **56**, 589–600.

15

Normal-Ogive Multidimensional Model

Roderick P. McDonald

Introduction

In an attempt to provide a unified foundation for common factor analysis, true score theory, and latent trait (item response) theory, McDonald (1962a, 1962b, 1967) defined a general strong principle of local independence and described a general latent trait model, as follows: Let $\mathbf{U}$ be a $n \times 1$ random vector of manifest variables—test or possibly binary item scores—and θ a $k \times 1$ random vector of latent traits—not yet defined. The strong principle of local independence, which defines θ and the dimension k of the vector $\mathbf{U}$, states that

$$g\{\mathbf{U} \mid \theta\} = \prod_{i=1}^{k} g_i\{U_i \mid \theta\} \tag{1}$$

where $g\{\ \}$ is the conditional density of $\mathbf{U}$ and $g_i\{\ \}$ is the conditional density of the ith component. (Note that θ is not necessarily continuous and may consist of a dummy variable defining a latent class model.)

The strong principle of local independence implies the weak principle, which may be defined by writing

$$E\{\mathbf{U} \mid \theta\} = \phi(\theta) \tag{2}$$

where ϕ is a vector of functions, defining a vector of residuals

$$\mathbf{e} = \mathbf{U} - E\{\mathbf{U} \mid \theta\} \tag{3}$$

(whence, axiomatically, $\text{Cov}\{\phi, \mathbf{e}\} = \mathbf{0}$) and

$$\text{Cov}\{\mathbf{e}\} = \Delta$$

diagonal, positive definite. It follows without further assumptions that the covariance structure of $\mathbf{U}$ is given by

$$\text{Cov}\{\mathbf{U}\} = \sum = \text{Cov}\{\phi\} + \Delta. \tag{4}$$

The k components of θ account for all dependencies in probability of $U_1, \ldots, U_n$, under the strong principle of local independence, and for all their covariances under the weak principle. This fact justifies speaking of $\theta_1, \ldots, \theta_k$ indifferently as latent traits or common factors, and interpreting them in applications as those traits or states of the examinees that $U_1, \ldots, U_n$ serve to indicate or, we may say, define. In applications of latent trait theory to cognitive tests or items it is reasonable to refer to the latent traits as "abilities." Especially in multidimensional IRT it is very important to recognize that they are equally applicable to any social science data—e.g., personality inventories and attitude scales. (The problematic identification of a latent trait as a "true score" and the residuals as "errors of measurement" must rest upon extra mathematical considerations, if not on mere habits of thought.) From the manner in which latent traits are interpreted, it seems reasonable to say that when a structural model is fitted to data and tested on the basis of univariate and bivariate information only, and thus invoking only the weak form of the principle of local independence, it is unlikely that the investigator seriously imagines that the conditional covariances vanish while the variables still possess higher-order mutual statistical dependencies. Of course such higher-order dependencies are logically possible, and would account for any systematic differences between results obtained from bivariate information and results from the full information in the data.

McDonald (1982) suggested a fundamental classification of the family of latent trait models into: (1) *strictly linear models* in which the functions $\phi(\theta)$ are linear both in the coefficients of the regressions on the latent traits and in the latent traits themselves; (2) *wide-sense linear models* in which the functions are linear in the coefficients but not in the latent traits; and (3) *strictly nonlinear models* which cannot be expressed as a wide-sense linear model with a finite number of terms. The linear common factor model and the latent class model are examples of a strictly linear model. The polynomial factor model (McDonald, 1967; Etezadi-Amoli and McDonald, 1983) is wide-sense linear. The logistic and normal-ogive models for binary data are strictly nonlinear.

A central result of the early work on the general latent trait model is the demonstration (McDonald, 1967) that if a wide-sense linear model contains r functions of the k latent traits, then the covariance structure of the manifest variables can be expressed as

$$\sum = \Lambda\Lambda' + \Delta \tag{5}$$

where Λ is a $n \times r$ matrix, and Δ is as defined above. It follows that such a model cannot be distinguished from a strictly linear latent trait model with r latent traits on the basis of bivariate information alone. Exploratory methods were developed to enable such distinctions on the basis of the distribution of the latent traits in the latent space. The work described below takes a different direction, dealing with cases in which we may treat the functions $\phi_1(\theta), \ldots, \phi_r(\theta)$ as known.

We shortly focus on the problem of fitting a multidimensional normal ogive model. The first effective treatment of the (unidimensional) normal ogive model is Lord's (1952) demonstration that if a set of binary items fits the normal ogive model (and θ, with $k = 1$, has a normal density), then the tetrachoric correlations of the items can be accounted for by the Spearman single factor model. It is an open question whether the "heuristic" method based on this result, of estimating the model by factor analyzing sample tetrachorics, has been or can be substantially improved on, in terms of actual numerical results. It is well known but commonly forgotten that Pearson's derivation of a method for estimating the tetrachoric correlation, defined as the correlation "underlying" the fourfold table of two dichotomized variables, rests on the construction of tetrachoric series, which are defined as functions of Hermite-Tchebycheff orthogonal polynomials and of normal density and distribution functions. Christoffersson (1975) treated the multidimensional normal ogive model as the common factor analysis of dichotomized variables, using Pearson's tetrachoric series. Muthen (1978) suggested that Christoffersson's method could be made numerically more efficient by the use of sample tetrachoric correlations—an approach that generalizes readily to structural equation models for binary variables. It will come as no surprise when we see below that the method based on McDonald's (1967) harmonic analysis of the normal ogive in terms of Hermite-Tchebycheff polynomials and of normal density and distribution functions is closely related to Lord's, Christoffersson's, and Muthen's treatments. Nevertheless, there are enough differences to provide justification for this account and for applications of the NOHARM (Normal Ogive Harmonic Analysis Robust Method) program.

McDonald (1967) showed that a (strictly) nonlinear latent trait model such as the normal ogive and latent distance models can be approximated as closely as desired by a polynomial series (a wide-sense linear model) on the basis of harmonic analysis (Fourier analysis), a traditional device in the physical sciences for reducing a nonlinear model to a linear model. The coefficients of the polynomial series are so chosen that any finite segment of it is a least squares approximation to the desired strictly nonlinear model, weighted by the density function of the latent trait.

The main application of this method was to the (unidimensional) normal ogive model, under the assumption that the latent trait is a random variable with a normal distribution. In this case, McDonald (1967) showed that if the normal-ogive model is written as

$$P\{U_j = 1 \mid \theta\} = N(\beta_{j0} + \beta_{j1}\theta) \tag{6}$$

where $N(\cdot)$ is the (unit) cumulative normal distribution function, then a weighted least-square approximation to the model is given for any choice of r by

$$\phi_j^{(r)} = \sum_{p=0}^{r} \gamma_{jp} h_p(\theta) \tag{7}$$

where $h_p(\theta)$ is the normalized Hermite-Tchebycheff polynomial of degree p, given by

$$h_p(\theta) = [1/(p!)^{-1/2}] \sum (-)^t \theta^{p-2t} [2^t t!p - 2t!]^{-1} \tag{8}$$

with $q = s$ if either $p = 2s$ or $p = 2s + 1$,

$$\gamma_{j0} = N\{\beta_{j0}/(1 + \beta_{j1}^2)^{1/2}\} \tag{9}$$

and

$$\gamma_{jp} = p^{-1/2}[\beta_{j1}/(1 + \beta_{j1}^2)^{1/2}]^p h_{p-1}[\beta_{j0}/(1 + \beta_{j1}^2)^{1/2}] \cdot n[\beta_{j0}/(1 + \beta_{j1}^2)^{1/2}] \tag{10}$$

where $n(\cdot)$ is the (unit) normal density function. In particular,

$$\gamma_{j1} = [\beta_{j1}/(1 + \beta_{j1}^2)^{1/2} n[\beta_{j0}/(1 + \beta_{j1}^2]^{1/2}]. \tag{11}$$

By well known theory, the graph of the normal ogive $N(\cdot)$ is virtually indistinguishable from the logistic function, but unlike the latter allows fairly straightforward development of the desired harmonic series, and was therefore preferred for this purpose. McDonald (1982) showed that the normal ogive is well approximated by the cubic polynomial obtained by terminating the series in Eq. (7) at $p = 3$.

Presentation of the Model

A multidimensional normal ogive model with a linear combination rule for the latent traits—the NOHARM model (Normal-Ogive Harmonic Analysis Robust Method)—is defined as

$$P\{U_j = 1 \mid \theta\} = N\{\beta_{j0} + \beta_j'\theta\} = N\{\beta_{j0} + \beta_{j1}\theta_1 + \cdots + \beta_{jk}\theta_k \tag{12}$$

where, as before, $N(\cdot)$ is the cumulative normal distribution function. It is assumed that θ is random with a k-variate normal distribution, and a metric is chosen such that each component of θ has mean zero and variance unity. We write $\mathbf{P}$ for the $k \times k$ covariance (correlation) matrix of θ and

$$\mathbf{B} = [\beta_{jk}], \quad n \times k.$$

In some applications, a pattern may be prescribed for $\mathbf{B}$, with elements constrained to be zero (to define a "simple structure") or subject to other desired constraints, as in the counterpart factor-loading matrix in multiple factor analysis. In particular, by constraining the nonzero elements in each column to be equal (while choosing a pattern such that they are linearly independent), a multidimensional counterpart of the Rasch model is obtained. For each item score U_j, the item characteristic function $N(\beta_{j0}+\beta_j'\theta)$ is constant on planes of dimension $k-1$ orthogonal to the vector β_j. McDonald (1985) showed that Eq. (12) may be represented by the infinite polynomial series

$$P\{U_j \mid \theta\} = \phi_j^{(\infty)}(\theta) = \sum_{p=0}^{\infty} \gamma_{jp} h_p[\beta_j'\theta/d_j] \tag{13}$$

where γ_{j0}, γ_{jp} are obtained by substituting

$$d_j = (\beta_j'\mathbf{P}\beta_j) \tag{14}$$

for β_{j1}^2 in Eqs. (9) and (10), and $h_p(\cdot)$ is given by Eq. (8) as before. The first r terms of the series in Eq. (13), which will be denoted by $\phi_j^{(r)}(\cdot)$, yield a polynomial of degree r, which, like the multidimensional normal-ogive in Eq. (12), is constant on planes of dimension $k-1$ orthogonal to the vector β_j and yields a weighted least square approximation to it, as in the unidimensional case treated by McDonald (1967). It further follows that the proportion of examinees passing an item is given by

$$\pi_j = \gamma_{j0} \tag{15}$$

and the proportion passing two items j and k is given by

$$\pi_{jk}^{(\infty)} = \sum_{p=0}^{\infty} \gamma_{jp}\gamma_{kp}[\beta_j'\mathbf{P}\beta_k/(d_j d_k)]^p, \quad j \neq k = 1,\ldots,n. \tag{16}$$

In practice, the first r terms of Eq. (16) may be substituted, denoted by $\pi_{jk}(r)$, as a finite approximation to it.

Constructed data studies of the unidimensional case have shown that the precision of estimation of the item parameters does not depend upon the number of terms retained in the polynomial approximation. On the other hand, the residuals tend, of course, to reduce in absolute value as r is increased, though convergence is very rapid, and the contribution to fit from terms beyond the cubic in general seem negligible.

However, at this point it should be noted that the theory just described is much closer to that of Christoffersson (1975) than might be obvious at first sight. Indeed, Eq. (16) is identical with Eq. (21) below, given by Christoffersson, except for a reparameterization. Christoffersson defined a set of unobservable variables, $\mathbf{v}$, that follow the multiple common factor model, say,

$$v_j = \lambda_j'\mathbf{f} + \delta_j \tag{17}$$

where $\Lambda' = [\lambda_1, \ldots, \lambda_n]$, a matrix of common factor loadings, $\mathbf{f}$ is a vector of common factors, and δ_j is the jth unique factor. He then supposed that

$$\begin{aligned} U_j &= 1 \text{ if } v_j \geq t_j \\ &= 0 \text{ if } v_j < t_j. \end{aligned}$$

It then follows that the proportion of examinees passing item j is given by

$$\pi_j = N(t_j) \tag{18}$$

and the joint proportion of examinees passing items j and k is given by

$$\pi_{jk} = \sum_{p=0}^{\infty} \tau_p(t_j)\tau_p(t_k)(\lambda_j' \mathbf{P} \lambda_k)^p, \tag{19}$$

where $\tau_p(\cdot)$ is the tetrachoric function defined by

$$\begin{aligned} \tau_0(t_j) &= N(t_j) \\ \tau_p(t_j) &= (p^{-1/2})h_{p-1}(t_j)n(t_j), \quad p = 1, \ldots, \end{aligned} \tag{20}$$

and $h_p(\cdot)$ is given by Eq. (8). Using Eq. (20), we may rewrite the result (16) obtained by harmonic analysis of the model in Eq. (12) as

$$\pi_{jk}^{(\infty)} = \sum_{p=0}^{\infty} \tau_p[\beta_{j0}/(1+d_j^2)^{1/2}]\tau_p[\beta_{k0}/(1+d_k^2)^{1/2}]$$

$$\cdot[\beta_j' \mathbf{P} \beta_k (1+d_j^2)^{-1/2}(1+d_k^2)^{-1/2}]. \tag{21}$$

It is then immediately evident that Eqs. (16) and (21) are identical except for a choice of parameterization. Each is obtained from the other by writing

$$\beta_{j0} = t_j \psi_{jj}^{-1/2}; \quad \beta_j = \lambda_j \psi_{jj}^{-1/2} \tag{22}$$

where

$$\psi_{jj} = 1 - \lambda_j' \mathbf{P} \lambda_j, \tag{23}$$

the item uniqueness, i.e., the variance of δ_j or, conversely,

$$t_j = \beta_{j0}(1 + \beta_j' \mathbf{P} \beta_j)^{-1/2}; \quad \lambda_j = \beta_j (1 + \beta_j' \mathbf{P} \beta_j)^{-1/2}. \tag{24}$$

To put this another way, Christoffersson's work implies writing the multidimensional normal-ogive model as

$$P\{U_j = 1 \mid \theta\} = N\{(t_j + \lambda_j' \theta)\psi_{jj}^{-1/2}\} \tag{25}$$

in place of Eq. (12).

The equivalence of Christoffersson's (1975) tetrachoric series to McDonald's (1967) harmonic analysis has both theoretical and practical consequences, apart from the possibility that a few research workers interested in IRT but not in factor analysis may even yet have missed the point that Christoffersson's (1975) "factor analysis of dichotomized variables" is indeed the multidimensional normal ogive model with a distinct parameterization. Purely in terms of theory it is pleasing to find that the same result can be obtained either as the solution to the problem of evaluating a double integral connected with the normal distribution or as a solution to the problem of approximating a strictly nonlinear regression function by a wide-sense linear regression function. The main practical implication of the result is that it gives grounds for reducing numerical work by using what at first sight would appear to be unacceptably crude approximations, such as the simple linear approximation in Eq. (16). That is, fitting an approximation to the model may be considered instead of fitting the model itself, thereby estimating the parameters reasonably precisely, where there might not have been an expectation of obtaining reasonably precise estimates of the parameters using very crude approximations to the integrals required by the model itself.

The existence of the alternative parameterizations in Eqs. (11) and (25) for the multidimensional normal ogive requires some comment. First, it should be noted that in the well studied unidimensional case there are three distinct parameterizations in common use, and the meaning of all three and the relationships between them do not seem widely understood.

Given the seminal work of Lord, it is natural that much work on the unidimensional case has employed Lord's parameterization, namely

$$P\{U_j \mid \theta\} = N\{a_j(\theta - b_j)\}, \tag{26}$$

where b_j, a_j range over the real numbers. (After fitting the model it is possible to rescore items with negative a_j so that a_j ranges over the positive numbers.) Since the location of the point of inflection of the curve is b_j and its slope at that point is a_j, these parameters are correctly described as location and slope parameters. In the special case of cognitive items, where θ is an "ability," it is reasonable to call b_j a "difficulty" parameter. Unfortunately, Lord's parameterization does not possess a multidimensional counterpart.

In the second parameterization, in Eq. (6), β_{j1} has the same value and meaning as a_j. However, $\beta_{j0} = -a_j b_j$ is no longer a location parameter. It is still possible to say that the point of inflection is given by the solution of $\beta_{j0} + \beta_{j1}\theta = 0$, thus indirectly giving an interpretation to β_{j0}.

In the common factor parameterization in Eq. (24), the unidimensional (Spearman) case is

$$P\{U_j = 1 \mid \theta\} = N\{(t_j + \lambda_j \theta)\psi_{jj}^{-1/2}\}. \tag{27}$$

By Eq. (18), the threshold parameter $t_j = N^{-1}(\pi_j)$, a convenient transform of the classical difficulty parameter, and thus is directly interpretable. The quantities λ_j and ψ_{jj} are factor loadings and residual variances (uniquenesses) interpretable by the usual factor-analytic standards. We note that as $\lambda_j \to 1$ and $\psi_{jj} \to 0$, $\beta_{j1} \to \infty$ and we have an improper solution or Heywood case.

In the multidimensional case, Lord's parameterization is no longer directly available. Since terminology has not yet settled, it is recommended that the parameterization in Eq. (11) be referred to as the IRT parameterization and the one in Eq. (24) as the common factor parameterization of the multidimensional normal ogive model. As Reckase (1985) points out, in the former, since $P\{U_j = 1\} = .5$ at points on the $(k-1)$-dimensional plane

$$\beta_{j0} + \beta_j'\theta = 0, \tag{28}$$

to which β_j is orthogonal, it follows immediately that the minimum distance from the origin to the plane defined by Eq. (28) is along the direction-vector β_j and is given by

$$d_j = (\beta_j'\beta_j)^{1/2}, \tag{29}$$

thus generalizing Lord's location parameter. As in the unidimensional case the components of β_j range over the real numbers, but it is no longer possible in general to score the items so that they are all positive (as will be seen in the examples below). In the common factor parameterization, once again there is a simple interpretation, by (18), of t_j as the inverse-normal transformation of classical item "difficulty," which is somewhat more transparent than β_j in (11), and the loading matrix

$$\Lambda' = [\lambda_1, \ldots, \lambda_n]$$

contains numbers that can be interpreted as (standardized) item factor loadings, with the classical criteria for salient versus negligible values. The NOHARM program, as described below, allows rotation of the factor loading matrix and the corresponding matrix of direction-vectors

$$\mathbf{B} = [\beta_1, \ldots, \beta_n]$$

to approximate simple structure, or to fit a prescribed pattern of zero, nonzero, or equated coefficients, including prescribed simple structure, independent clusters or *basis items* (items chosen to measure just one latent trait). The position taken here is that these devices are virtually essential for the substantive application of a multidimensional model, as without them the structure of the data cannot be understood.

Parameter Estimation

Let p_j be the proportion of examinees passing item j, and p_{jk} be the proportion passing items j and k, in a sample of size N. In program NOHARM

(Normal Ogive Harmonic Analysis Robust Method), the threshold or position parameter is estimated in closed form by solving the sample analogue of Eq. (18), and reparameterizing it if desired, and the parameters β_j are obtained by unweighted least squares, minimizing

$$q = \sum_{j \neq k} (p_{jk} - \pi_{jk}^{(r)})^2 \tag{30}$$

where $\pi_{jk}^{(r)}$ is the r-term approximation to $\pi_{jk}^{(\infty)}$ in Eq. (16), by a quasi-Newton algorithm. The combination of the random-regressors model and the weak principle of local independence with the use of unweighted least squares makes it possible to analyze quite large numbers of items with unlimited sample size. The program allows users to read in "guessing" parameters for multiple choice cognitive items, setting the lower asymptote of the expression in Eq. (13) to a prescribed constant. (An attempt to estimate these parameters in an early version of the program suffered the usual difficulties for models with such parameters.)

The decision to employ ULS rather than the obvious choice of GLS was primarily determined by a desire to handle large data sets. The use of GLS by Christoffersson (1975) and Muthen (1978) asymptotically yields, like ML, SEs and a chi-squared test of significance, but limits applications to rather small data sets. It was also conjectured that the weight matrix for GLS would be poorly estimated until the sample size becomes extremely large. Unpublished studies show that the method gives satisfactory estimates of the parameters with sample sizes down to one hundred, and that it is reasonably robust against violations of normality of the latent trait distribution. (With an extreme distribution created by truncating the standard normal at zero, the location parameters were correctly ordered but somewhat underestimated at one end.)

Goodness of Fit

An obvious lacuna, following from the use of ULS, is the lack of a statistical test of significance of the model. One way to rationalize away this defect of the NOHARM approach is to refer to Bollen and Scott (1993) for a general recognition that all of these models are at best approximations and any restrictive model will be rejected at one's favorite level of statistical significance, given a sufficiently large sample size. Following Tanaka (1993) we can conveniently define a goodness-of-fit index

$$\gamma_{\text{ULS}} = 1 - \text{Tr}\{\mathbf{R}^2\}/\text{Tr}\{\mathbf{S}^2\} \tag{31}$$

where $\mathbf{S}$ is the item sample covariance matrix and $\mathbf{R}$ the residual covariance matrix. The application of this criterion is illustrated below. Perhaps equally important, we can use an old principle from the practice of factor

TABLE 1. Sample Raw Product-Moments and Sample Covariances for LSAT-7

Item	1	2	3	4	5
1	.828	.0222	.0248	.0302	.0200
2	.567	.658	.0520	.0293	.0123
3	.664	.560	.772	.0332	.0212
4	.532	.428	.501	.606	.0151
5	.718	.567	.672	.526	.843
Variances	.142	.225	.176	.239	.132

analysis that a model is a sufficiently close approximation to the data if we cannot find a more complex model that is identified and interpretable. For this purpose, inspection of the item residual covariance matrix is at least as useful as a goodness-of-fit index and possibly more so, since it is difficult to set criterion values for the application of such indices. A heuristic device for taking account of sample size is to recognize that, by standard sampling theory, the SEs of the parameters are in the order of $N^{-1/2}$ where N is the sample size.

Example

Data from sections of the Law School Admissions Test (LSAT) have been used by a number of writers to illustrate IRT. In particular, LSAT7 has been treated by Christoffersson (1975) as a two-dimensional case of the normal ogive model. The sample raw product-moment matrix (the product of the raw-score matrix and its transpose) for five items from LSAT7, with $N = 1{,}000$, is given in Table 1,[1] together with the sample covariances. Program NOHARM (Fraser, 1988) was used to fit three models to the data. Table 2 gives the results of fitting a unidimensional model, with Lord's parameterization, the IRT parameterization, and the common factor parameterization in Table 2a, and the item residuals in Table 2b. Tanaka's Index (25) is .99924, but the residuals can be said to be large relative to the item covariances in Table 1.

Table 3 gives the results of an exploratory two-dimensional analysis, with oblique solutions in Table 3a in the IRT and common factor parameterizations. Residuals are shown in Table 3b. The Tanaka Index becomes .999967 and the residuals are correspondingly reduced compared with the unidimensional solution. The oblique common factor solution suggests fairly clearly that item 1 measures the first dimension well, while items 2 and 3 primarily measure the second dimension, with items 4 and 5 dimensionally complex

[1] *Note to Table 1:* Product-moments in lower triangle, including the diagonal; covariances in upper triangle.

TABLE 2. Parameter Estimates: Unidimensional.

Table 2a

Item	b_j	a_j	β_{j0}	β_{j1}	t_j	λ_{j1}	ψ_j
1	−1.922	.566	1.087	.566	.946	.492	.757
2	−.759	.635	.482	.635	.407	.536	.713
3	−1.038	1.033	1.072	1.033	.745	.718	.484
4	−.644	.460	.296	.460	.269	.418	.825
5	−2.723	.398	1.084	.398	1.007	.370	.863

Table 2b

	1	2	3	4
2	.004			
3	.006	−.006		
4	−.010	.003	.003	
5	−.008	.006	.000	.001

TABLE 3. Parameter Estimates: Two-Dimensional Exploratory

Table 3a

Item	β_{j0}	β_{j1}	β_{j2}	t_j	λ_{j1}	λ_{j2}	ψ_j
1	1.684	1.603	−.231	.946	.901	−.130	.316
2	.480	−.007	.630	.407	−.006	.534	.719
3	1.317	−.191	1.568	.745	−.108	.887	.320
4	.296	.278	.231	.269	.253	.210	.826
5	1.089	.290	.164	1.007	.268	.152	.855

Table 3b

	1	2	3	4
2	−.000			
3	.000	−.000		
4	.000	−.001	.001	
5	−.000	.003	.002	−.000

and not measuring either dimension very well. The correlation between the item factors is .621. For completeness of illustration, Table 4 gives results from a confirmatory solution based simply on the apparent pattern of the exploratory results, not on substantive grounds. (This practice is, of course, not recomended.) The Tanaka Index is .999966, and the residuals remain reasonably small, suggesting an acceptable fit.

Along with extensive constructed-data studies, the example serves to show that NOHARM yields reasonable parameter estimates both in exploratory and confirmatory multidimensional models. Perhaps the most important feature illustrated, which arises from its initial conception as a nonlinear common factor model, is the provision either from a confirmatory or an exploratory simple structure, of a basis in the latent trait space, yielding interpretations by the familiar criteria of common factor theory.

TABLE 4. Parameter Estimates: Two-Dimensional Confirmatory

Table 4a

Item	β_{j0}	β_{j1}	β_{j2}	t_j	λ_{j1}	λ_{j2}	ψ_j
1	1.650	1.428		.946	.819		.329
2	.489		.667	.407		.555	.692
3	1.200		1.262	.745		.784	.386
4	.296	.274	.266	.269	.248	.241	.824
5	1.090	.289	.193	1.007	.267	.178	.853

Table 4b

	1	2	3	4
2	−.001			
3	.001	−.000		
4	.000	−.001	.000	
5	−.000	.003	−.002	.000

References

Bollen, K.A. and Long, J.S. (Eds.) (1993). *Testing Structural Equation Models.* Newbury Park, CA: Sage.

Christoffersson, A. (1975). Factor analysis of dichotomized variables. *Psychometrika* **40**, 5–22.

Etezadi-Amoli, J. and McDonald, R.P. (1983). A second generation nonlinear factor analysis. *Psychometrika* **48**, 315–342.

Fraser, C. (1988). *NOHARM: A Computer Program for Fitting Both Unidimensional and Multidimensional Normal Ogive Models of Latent Trait Theory.* NSW: Univ. of New England.

Lord, F.M. (1950). A theory of test scores. *Psychometric Monographs*, No. 7.

McDonald, R.P. (1962a). A note on the derivation of the general latent class model. *Psychometrika* **27**, 203–206.

McDonald, R.P. (1962b). A general approach to nonlinear factor analysis. *Psychometrika* **27**, 397–415.

McDonald, R.P. (1967). Nonlinear factor analysis. *Psychometric Monographs*, No. 15.

McDonald, R.P. (1982). Linear versus nonlinear models in latent trait theory. *Applied Psychological Measurement* **6**, 379–396.

McDonald, R.P. (1984). Confirmatory models for nonlinear structural analysis. In E. Diday et al., (Eds), *Data Analysis and Informatics, III.* North Holland: Elsevier.

McDonald, R.P. (1985). Unidimensional and multidimensional models for item response theory. In D.J. Weiss, (Ed), *Proceedings of the 1982 Item*

Response Theory and Computer Adaptive Testing Conference, Minneapolis: University of Minnesota.

Muthen, B.O. (1978). Contributions to factor analysis of dichotomous variables. *Psychometrika* **43**, 551–560.

Tanaka, J.S. (1993). Multifaceted conceptions of fit in structural equation models. In K.A. Bollen and J.S. Long (Eds), *Testing Structural Equation Models.* Newbury Park, CA: Sage.

16

A Linear Logistic Multidimensional Model for Dichotomous Item Response Data

Mark D. Reckase

Introduction

Since the implementation of large-scale achievement and ability testing in the early 1900s, cognitive test tasks, or test items, that are scored as either incorrect (0) or correct (1) have been quite commonly used (DuBois, 1970). Even though performance on these test tasks is frequently summarized by a single total score, often a sum of item scores, it is also widely acknowledged that multiple skills or abilities are required to determine the correct answers to these tasks. Snow (1993) states

> "The general conclusion seems to be that complex cognitive processing is involved in performance even on simple tasks. In addition to multiple processes, it is clear that performers differ in strategies. . . ."

For example, even the simplest of mathematics story problems requires both reading and mathematical skills to determine the correct answer, and multiple strategies might be used as well. Performance on such test tasks can be said to be sensitive to differences in both reading and mathematics skills. However, the test task is probably insensitive to differences in many other skills, such as mechanical comprehension, in that high or low levels of those skills do not change the likelihood of determining the correct answer for the task.

Examinees bring a wide variety of cognitive skills to the testing situation, some of which are relevant to the task at hand and some which are not. In addition, some test tasks are sensitive to certain types of skill differences, while others are not. The number of skill dimensions needed to model the item scores from a sample of individuals for a set of test tasks is dependent upon both the number of skill dimensions and level on those dimensions exhibited by the examinees, and the number of cognitive dimensions to which the test tasks are sensitive.

The mathematical formulation presented in this chapter is designed to model the results of the interactions of a sample of examinees with a set of test tasks as represented by the matrix of 0, 1 item scores for the examinees on the tasks. A linear function of skill dimensions and item characteristics describing the sensitivity of the items to skill dimensions is used as the basis for this model. The result of this linear combination is mapped to the probability metric using the logistic distribution function. While person skill dimensions are included in the model, it is a matter of construct validation as to whether the statistical dimensions derived from the response matrix directly relate to any psychological dimensions.

The formulation presented was influenced by earlier work done using the normal ogive model to represent the interaction of the examinees and items (Lord and Novick, 1968, Chap. 16; Samejima, 1974). Lord and Novick (1968) developed the relationship between the unidimensional normal-ogive model and dimensions as defined by factor analysis, and Samejima (1974) derived a multidimensional normal-ogive model that used continuously scored items rather than those scored 0 or 1.

Presentation of the Model

Form of the Model

The data that are the focus of the model is the matrix of item scores, either 0 or 1, corresponding to either incorrect or correct answers to cognitive tasks. This matrix of data is usually oriented so that the rows (N) refer to persons and the columns (n) refer to test tasks, or items. Thus, a row by column entry refers to the score received by person j ($j = 1, N$) on item i ($i = 1, n$).

Several assumptions are made about the mechanism that creates this data matrix:

1. With an increase in the value of the hypothetical constructs that are assessed, the probability of obtaining a correct response to a test item is nondecreasing. This is usually called the monotonicity assumption.

2. The function relating the probability of correct response to the underlying hypothetical constructs is "smooth" in the sense that derivatives of the function are defined. This assumption eliminates undesirable degenerate cases.

3. The probability of combinations of responses can be determined from the product of the probabilities of the individual responses when the probabilities are computed conditional on a point in the space defined by the hypothetical constructs. This is usually called the local independence assumption.

These assumptions are consistent with many different models relating examinee characteristics and the characteristics of test items. After reviewing many possible models that include vector parameters for both examinee and item characteristics [see McKinley and Reckase (1982) for a summary], the model given below was selected for further development because it was reasonable given what is known about item response data, consistent with simpler, unidimensional item response theory models, and estimable with commonly attainable numbers of examinees and test items.

The basic form of the model is a direct generalization of the three-parameter logistic model (Lord, 1980) to the case where examinees are described by a vector of parameters rather than a single scalar value. The model is given by

$$P(U_{ij} = 1 \mid \mathbf{a}_i, d_i, c_i, \theta_j) = c_i + (1 - c_i)\frac{e^{(a_i'\theta_j + d_i)}}{1 + e^{(a_i'\theta_j + d_i)}},$$

where

$P(U_{ij} = 1 \mid \mathbf{a}_i, d_i, c_i, \theta_j)$ is the probability of a correct response (score of 1) for person j on test item i;

U_{ij} represents the item response for person j on item i;

$\mathbf{a}_i$ is a vector of parameters related to the discriminating power of the test item (the rate of change of the probability of correct response to changes in trait levels for the examinees);

d_i is a parameter related to the difficulty of the test item;

c_i is the probability of correct response that is approached when the abilities assessed by the item are very low (approach $-\infty$) (usually called the lower asymptote, or less correctly, the guessing parameter); and

θ_j is the vector of abilities for examinee j.

The definitions of model parameters are necessarily brief at this point. They will be given more complete conceptual definitions later in this chapter.

Graphic Display of the Model

The equation for the model defines a surface that gives the probability of correct response for a test item as a function of the location of examinees in the ability space specified by the θ-vector. The elements of this vector are statistical constructs that may or may not correspond to particular psychological traits or educational achievement domains. When there are only two statistical constructs, the form of the probability surface can be represented graphically. Figures 1 and 2 show the probability surface for

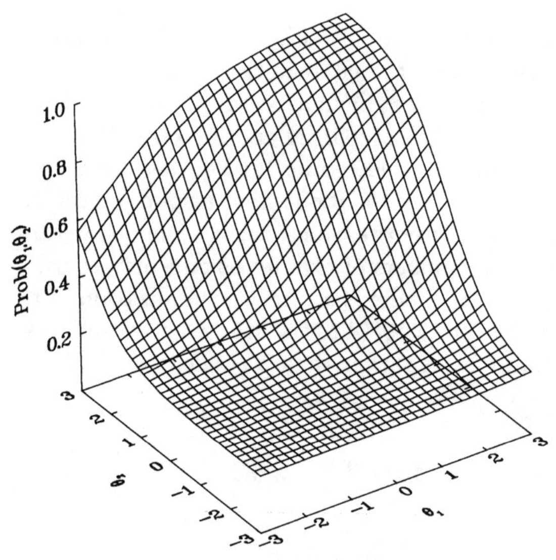

FIGURE 1. Item response surface for an item with parameters $a_1 = 0.8$, $a_2 = 1.4$, $d = -2.0$, and $c = 0.2$.

the same item ($a_1 = 0.8$, $a_2 = 1.4$, $d = -2.0$, $c = 0.2$) using two different methods of representation. Figure 1 uses a three-dimensional surface that emphasizes the monotonically increasing nature of the surface and the lower asymptote.

Figure 2 shows the surface as a contour plot of the lines of equal probability of correct response. This representation emphasizes that the equiprobable lines are straight lines and that they are all parallel to each other. This feature of the model is a result of the linear form of the exponent of e in the model equation.

Interpretation of Model Parameters

The mathematical expression for the model contains parameters for both the examinees and the test items. These parameters can be interpreted as follows.

(1) *Person parameters.* The person parameters in the model are the elements of the vector θ_j. The number of elements required to adequately model the data matrix is open to some debate. The research experience to date (Reckase and Hirsch, 1991) suggests that the number of dimensions is often underestimated and that overestimating the number of dimensions does little harm. Therefore, the order of the θ-vector should be taken to be the maximum interpretable value rather than stressing the data reduction capabilities of the methodology. Of course, the number of dimensions used to model the item-examinee interaction will depend on the purpose of the

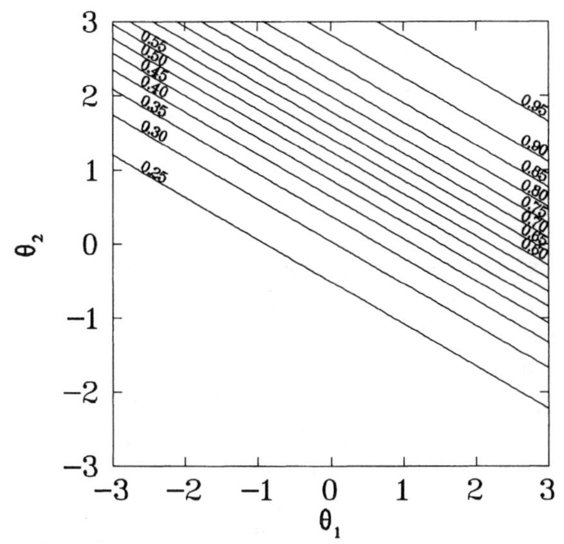

FIGURE 2. Contour plot for the item response surface given in Figure 1.

analysis.

The θ-dimensions are statistical constructs that are derived to provide adequate fit to the binary $N \times n$ data matrix. These dimensions may not have psychological or educational meaning. Whether they do or not is a matter of construct validation. Of course, the space can be rotated in a number of ways to align the θ-axes with meaningful points in the space. These rotations may or may not retain the initial covariance structure of the θ-dimensions. There is nothing in the model that requires that the dimensions be orthogonal. If the correlations among the θ-dimensions are constrained to be 0.0, then the observed correlations among the item scores will be accounted for solely by the a-parameters. Alternatively, certain items or clusters of items can be constrained to define orthogonal dimensions. Then the observed correlations among the item scores will be reflected both in the a-parameters and in correlated θ-dimensions.

(2) *Item discrimination.* The discrimination parameters for the model are given by the elements of the **a**-vector. These elements can be interpreted in much the same way as the a-parameters in unidimensional IRT models (Lord, 1980). The elements of the vector are related to the slope of the item response surface in the direction of the corresponding θ-axis. The elements therefore indicate the sensitivity of the item to differences in ability along that θ-axis. However, the discriminating power of an item differs depending on the direction that is being measured in the θ-space. This can easily be seen from Fig. 1. If the direction of interest in the space is parallel to the surface, the slope will be zero, and the item is not discriminating.

Unless an item is a pure measure of a particular dimension, it will be more discriminating for combinations of dimensions than for single dimensions. The discriminating power of the item for the most discriminating combinations of dimensions is given by

$$\mathrm{MDISC}_i = \sqrt{\sum_{k=1}^{p} a_{ik}^2},$$

where MDISC_i is the discrimination of the item i for the best combination of abilities; p is the number of dimensions in the θ-space; and a_{ik} is an element of the $\mathbf{a}_i$ vector. For more detailed information about multidimensional discrimination, see Reckase and McKinley (1991).

(3) *Item difficulty.* The d_i parameter in the model is related to the difficulty of the test item. However, the value of this parameter cannot be interpreted in the same way as the b-parameter of unidimensional IRT models because the model given here is in slope/intercept form. The usual way to represent the exponent of a unidimensional IRT model is $a(\theta - b)$, which is equivalent to $a\theta + (-ab)$. The term $-ab$ in the unidimensional model corresponds to d_i. A value that is equivalent in interpretation to the unidimensional b-parameter is given by

$$\mathrm{MDIFF}_i = \frac{-d_i}{\mathrm{MDISC}_i},$$

where the symbols are defined as above. The value of MDIFF_i indicates the distance from the origin of the θ-space to the point of steepest slope in a direction from the origin. This is an analogous meaning to the b-parameter in unidimensional IRT.

The direction of greatest slope from the origin is given by

$$\alpha_{ik} = \arccos \frac{a_{ik}}{\mathrm{MDISC}_i},$$

where α_{ik} is the angle that the line from the origin of the space to the point of steepest slope makes with the kth axis for item i; and the other symbols have been defined previously. More information can be obtained about multidimensional difficulty from Reckase (1985).

(4) *Lower asymptote.* The c_i-parameter has the same meaning as for the three-parameter logistic model. The value of the parameter indicates the probability of correct response for examinees that are very low on all dimensions being modeled.

Derived Descriptive Statistics

Along with the parameters described above, the test characteristic curves and item and test information functions (Lord, 1980) have been generalized for use with this model. The test characteristic curve generalizes to a test characteristic surface. That surface is defined by

$$\zeta(\theta) = \frac{1}{n} \sum_{i=1}^{n} P_i(\theta),$$

where $\zeta(\theta)$ is the expected proportion correct score at the point defined by the θ-vector; and $P_i(\theta)$ is shorthand notation for the probability of correct response to item i given by the model.

Item information is given by

$$I_{i\alpha}(\theta) = \frac{[\nabla_a P_i(\theta)]^2}{P_i(\theta)[1 - P_i(\theta)]},$$

where $I_{i\alpha}(\theta)$ is the information provided by item i in direction α in the space and ∇_α is the operator defining the directional derivative in direction α. The test information surface is given by the sum of the item information surfaces computed assuming the same direction. For more information about multidimensional information, see Reckase and McKinley (1991).

Parameter Estimation

Parameters for the model were originally estimated using joint maximum likelihood procedures based on the algorithms operationalized in LOGIST (Wingersky et al., 1982). The goal of the estimation procedure was to find the set of item- and person-parameters that would maximize the likelihood of the observed item responses. The basic form of the likelihood equation is given by

$$L = \prod_{j=1}^{N} \prod_{i=1}^{n} P(u_{ij} \mid \mathbf{a}_i, d_i, c_i, \theta_j),$$

where u_{ij} is the response to item i by person j, either a 0 or a 1. For mathematical convenience, the computer programs minimize the negative logarithm of L, $F = -\ln(L)$, rather than maximize L. Since the function, F, cannot be minimized directly, an interative Newton–Raphson procedure is used, first fixing the item parameters and estimating the person parameters, and then fixing the person parameters and estimating the item parameters. These procedures were implemented in both the MAXLOG (McKinley and Reckase, 1983) and MIRTE (Carlson, 1987) computer programs. McKinley (1987) has also developed a procedure based on marginal maximum likelihood (MULTIDIM).

Although the above computer programs were used for a number of applications of model, other programs have been found to be more efficient and to yield some stable parameter estimates (Ackerman, 1988; Miller, 1991). Most of our current work is done using NOHARM (Fraser, 1986; McDonald, this volume), rather than the original estimation algorithms.

Goodness of Fit

The goal of the model is to accurately explain the interaction between persons and items. To the extent that this goal is attained, the model will be found useful for a particular application. Since all IRT models are simplifications of the complex interactions of persons and test tasks, any of the models, including the one presented here, will be rejected if the sample size is large enough. The question is not whether the model fits the data, but rather, whether the model fits well enough to support the application. Detailed analysis of the skills assessed by a set of items may require more dimensions than an analysis that is designed to show that most of the variance in a set of responses can be accounted for by a single dimension. Because the importance of goodness of fit varies with the application, and because goodness-of-fit tests tend to be based on total group performance rather than focused on the item/person interaction, significance tests, as such, are not recommended. However, it is important to determine whether the model fits the data well enough to support the application.

The approach recommended here is to review carefully the inter-item residual covariance matrix to determine whether there is evidence that the use of the model is suspect for the particular application. The entries in this $n \times n$ matrix are computed using the following equation:

$$\text{cov}_{ik} = \frac{\sum_{j=1}^{N}(u_{ij} - P_i(\theta_j))(u_{kj} - P_k(\theta_j))}{N}, \quad i, k = 1, \ldots, n,$$

where i and k represent items on the test. Large residuals may indicate failure of the estimation procedure to converge, too few dimensions in the model, or an inappropriate model. The evaluation of such residuals will require informed judgment and experience. No significance testing procedure will simplify the process of evaluating the fit of the model to a set of data.

In addition to the analysis of residuals, it is recommended that, whenever possible, the results of an analysis should be replicated either on parallel forms of a test, or on equivalent samples of examinees. Experience with multidimensional IRT analyses has shown that many small effects are replicable over many test forms and may, therefore, be considered real (Ackerman, 1990). Others, however, do not replicate. The only way to discover the full nuances of the relationships in the interactions of a test and examinee population is to screen out idiosyncratic effects through careful replication.

Example

Most, if not all tests of academic achievement require multiple skills to demonstrate proficiency. The items used on these tests will likely be differentially sensitive to these multiple skills. For example some mathematics items may require the manipulation of algebraic symbols while others may require spatial skills. Often the skills required by an item may be related to the difficulty of the item. Reckase (1989) showed that the combination of multiple skills and variations in the difficulty of the items measuring those skills can result in different meanings for different points on a score scale.

To guarantee common meaning at all points on the score scale used for reporting, the relationship between the skills being measured and the difficulty of the test items must be maintained for all test forms. Multidimensional IRT analysis gives a means for identifying the dimensional structure of a test for a specified population of examinees and for comparing that structure across test forms.

The example presented here uses data from a test designed to assess the mathematics achievement of 10th grade students in the United States. The test consists of 40 multiple-choice items covering the areas of pre-algebra, elementary algebra, coordinate geometry, and plane geometry. Test forms were produced to match a content and cognitive level specifications matrix, and specifications for difficulty and discrimination. However, there are no specifications that call for items in a specific content area to be at a specific level of difficulty. The data analyzed here consisted of item scores from 1635 students who were selected to be representative of the usual examinee population. The purposes for presenting this example are to demonstrate a typical analysis of test structure using multidimensional item response theory, to show the effects of confounding the difficulty of test items with the content that they assess, and to show the effect of using too few dimensions in analyzing the data matrix. The data were first analyzed using the BILOG program (Mislevy and Bock, 1989) for the purpose of estimating the c-parameters. Those estimates were input to NOHARM, which does not estimate c, and both two-dimensional and six-dimensional solutions were obtained. The two-dimensional solution was obtained so that the results could be plotted and so the effect of underestimation of the dimensionality could be determined. The six-dimensional solution is the highest-dimensional solution that is supported by NOHARM.

The item parameter estimates and the estimates of MDISC, MDIFF, and the angles with the coordinate axes for the two-dimensional solution are presented in Table 1. The orientation of the solution in the θ-space was set by aligning Item 1 with the θ_1-axis, therefore its a_2-value is 0.0. The information in Table 1 is also presented graphically in Fig. 3. In that figure, each item is represented by a vector. The initiating point of the vector is MDIFF units from the origin of the space, the length of the vector is equal to MDISC, and the direction of the vector is specified by the angles of the item with the θ-axes. This graphic representation has been found to be helpful for visualizing the structure of the test.

A pattern in the vectors that has been found quite commonly in the analysis of achievement tests is that the easy items on the test (those at the lower left) tend to measure one dimension, in this case θ_1, while some

TABLE 1. Model and Item Parameter Estimates: Two Dimensions.

	Item Parameter Estimates				Derived Item Statistics		
Item	d	a_1	a_2	MDISC	MDIF	α_1	α_2
1	2.49	2.37	0.00	2.37	−1.05	0.00	90.00
2	1.00	0.58	0.38	0.69	−1.44	33.44	56.56
3	0.66	0.63	0.27	0.69	−0.96	22.75	67.25
4	0.76	0.99	0.47	1.10	−0.70	25.44	64.57
5	0.29	0.60	0.18	0.62	−0.46	17.04	72.96
6	−0.01	0.78	0.64	1.00	0.01	39.86	50.14
7	0.57	0.75	0.41	0.86	−0.66	28.51	61.49
8	1.24	1.64	0.15	1.65	−0.76	5.12	84.88
9	0.61	1.04	0.52	1.16	−0.53	26.39	63.61
10	0.23	1.26	0.51	1.36	−0.17	22.26	67.74
11	1.11	1.17	0.20	1.19	−0.94	9.60	80.40
12	0.92	1.26	0.39	1.32	−0.70	17.17	72.83
13	0.24	1.71	0.48	1.78	−0.13	15.58	74.42
14	−0.68	0.69	0.91	1.15	0.59	52.87	37.13
15	−0.44	0.57	0.72	0.92	0.47	51.62	38.28
16	−0.28	0.33	0.43	0.54	0.51	52.22	37.78
17	0.59	2.10	0.69	2.21	−0.27	18.31	71.69
18	−0.99	1.19	1.16	1.66	0.60	44.15	45.86
19	−0.21	0.63	0.40	0.75	0.28	32.30	57.80
20	−0.69	1.11	1.31	1.72	0.40	49.57	40.44
21	−0.04	1.02	1.18	1.56	0.02	49.06	40.94
22	−0.49	0.96	1.26	1.58	0.31	52.81	37.19
23	−0.60	0.60	0.87	1.06	0.56	55.66	34.34
24	−0.15	1.01	0.47	1.11	0.13	52.81	37.19
25	−1.47	0.83	0.79	1.15	1.28	43.52	46.48
26	−1.08	0.81	0.77	1.12	0.96	43.56	46.44
27	−0.97	0.87	0.89	1.24	0.78	45.56	44.45
28	−0.07	1.71	1.76	2.45	0.03	45.79	44.21
29	−0.84	1.12	1.16	1.61	0.52	46.13	43.87
30	−1.20	0.93	1.38	1.66	0.72	56.02	33.98
31	−0.91	0.79	1.36	1.57	0.57	59.67	30.33
32	−1.35	1.87	1.52	2.41	0.56	39.21	50.79
33	−0.62	0.60	0.48	0.77	0.80	38.39	51.61
34	−0.96	0.44	0.41	0.60	1.60	42.50	47.50
35	−1.89	1.15	2.15	2.44	0.78	61.77	28.23
36	−0.87	0.63	0.78	1.00	0.87	51.26	38.74
37	−1.31	0.56	0.97	1.12	1.17	59.81	30.19
38	−1.53	0.31	0.99	1.03	1.48	72.79	17.21
39	−3.77	0.57	2.27	2.34	1.61	75.88	14.12
40	−0.82	0.56	0.46	0.73	1.13	39.08	50.92

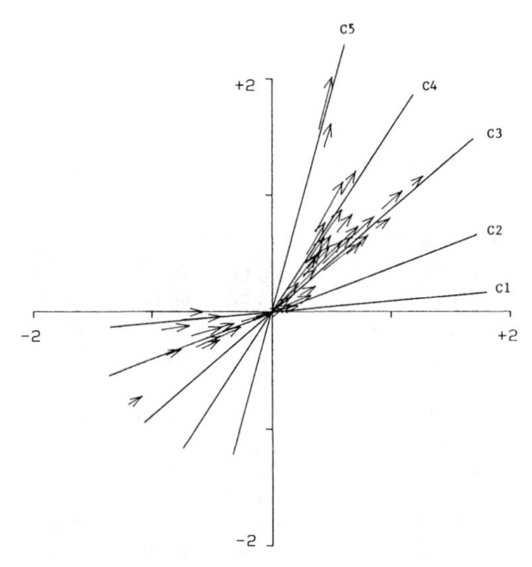

FIGURE 3. Item vectors and primary directions for content clusters from a two-dimensional analysis of a 40 item, 10th grade mathematics test.

of the more difficult items (those to the upper right) tend to measure a different dimension, in this case θ_2. To get a better sense of the substantive meaning of this solution, the angles between the item vectors were cluster analyzed to determine which sets of items tended to be discriminating in the same direction in the θ-space. The main direction in the space for each of the clusters is indicated by the lines labeled C1 to C5 in Fig. 3.

The items closest to the line marked C5 are the geometry items on the test. Those closest to C1 are the algebra items. Since the geometry items are the most difficult items on the test, those examinees who get the top score on the test must function well on the geometry items as well as the rest of the content. Differences in the number correct scores in the range from 38 to 40 are mainly differences in geometry skill, while scores at the lower end of the score scale are mainly differentiated on algebra skill. Clusters 3 and 4 are less well defined in this solution.

The values of MDISC, MDIFF, and the angles with the θ-axes for the six-dimensional NOHARM solution are given in Table 2. Note that the orientation of the solution in the space is fixed by aligning each of the first five items with an axis. The cluster analysis solution based on the angles between items in the six-dimensional space is given in Figure 4. Seven clusters are indicated in this figure. Next to the item number is a code that tells the content area of the item: PA – pre-algebra; EA – elementary algebra; PG – plane geometry; and CG – coordinate geometry.

The six-dimensional solution given in Fig. 4 represents a fairly fine grained structural analysis of the test as responded to by the sample of tenth grade students. Cluster 5 for example contains items that require computation to

TABLE 2. Item Parameter Estimates: Six Dimensions.

Item	MDISC	MDIFF	α_1	α_2	α_3	α_4	α_5	α_6
1	3.86	−1.00	0.00	90.00	90.00	90.00	90.00	90.00
2	1.44	−1.00	53.01	36.99	90.00	90.00	90.00	90.00
3	0.88	−0.82	42.61	68.48	55.32	90.00	90.00	90.00
4	1.40	−0.63	38.83	74.47	60.96	72.97	90.00	90.00
5	0.65	−0.45	39.85	79.93	64.12	81.63	65.78	90.00
6	1.12	0.01	46.47	70.67	61.84	85.55	78.05	67.66
7	0.98	−0.62	35.59	71.76	65.40	89.47	85.37	75.73
8	1.93	−0.73	7.93	85.31	86.95	85.96	86.14	89.73
9	1.22	−0.51	33.78	73.13	67.21	82.20	79.93	80.73
10	1.36	−0.17	31.28	80.16	74.53	75.67	72.20	83.10
11	1.21	−0.93	17.52	85.01	79.49	87.34	77.79	86.91
12	1.40	−0.69	23.74	83.51	80.69	72.21	81.07	85.73
13	2.28	−0.13	36.39	84.20	79.51	77.15	59.51	92.38
14	1.84	0.51	56.43	72.16	63.91	94.93	82.40	51.81
15	1.03	0.45	59.55	50.62	73.00	76.19	71.54	71.77
16	1.50	0.29	69.90	34.42	99.97	101.34	72.69	77.84
17	2.70	−0.26	35.37	80.48	80.02	76.66	61.72	89.45
18	2.23	0.56	54.87	69.03	68.79	86.92	59.06	67.82
19	0.99	0.24	39.66	89.48	66.48	91.39	85.07	60.66
20	1.90	0.39	56.34	65.47	61.25	73.63	73.23	67.64
21	2.35	0.02	50.76	68.17	78.23	60.33	92.03	65.38
22	2.13	0.29	55.80	61.01	84.03	58.61	81.94	67.42
23	1.51	0.49	59.71	59.01	88.40	89.28	65.46	56.35
24	1.37	0.12	49.77	80.09	66.46	68.45	59.56	62.87
25	1.68	1.12	60.01	79.62	75.84	82.15	43.15	70.92
26	1.26	0.91	51.09	76.19	74.40	83.08	59.76	62.87
27	1.65	0.71	55.99	80.84	79.33	80.17	52.34	61.68
28	3.60	0.03	46.93	66.52	79.99	62.98	85.65	68.64
29	1.95	0.50	56.51	65.87	61.28	65.29	76.49	74.85
30	2.07	0.69	66.29	65.66	55.77	72.99	70.48	66.84
31	1.63	0.57	61.94	64.46	79.85	63.64	70.67	59.68
32	3.22	0.54	52.45	76.21	75.53	69.96	55.61	73.34
33	1.13	0.65	53.08	100.11	78.86	51.29	75.70	69.82
34	0.87	1.26	72.19	76.77	57.91	55.38	60.14	91.84
35	2.64	0.77	67.44	73.89	67.63	64.09	67.04	57.55
36	1.19	0.81	53.07	73.30	84.71	57.51	83.17	60.31
37	1.34	1.09	66.47	84.55	62.15	71.93	70.16	50.66
38	1.46	1.29	85.34	81.71	62.10	69.90	51.46	60.18
39	2.09	1.64	78.77	81.50	69.18	64.92	51.36	60.38
40	1.19	0.87	57.03	105.06	85.55	58.85	64.03	65.58

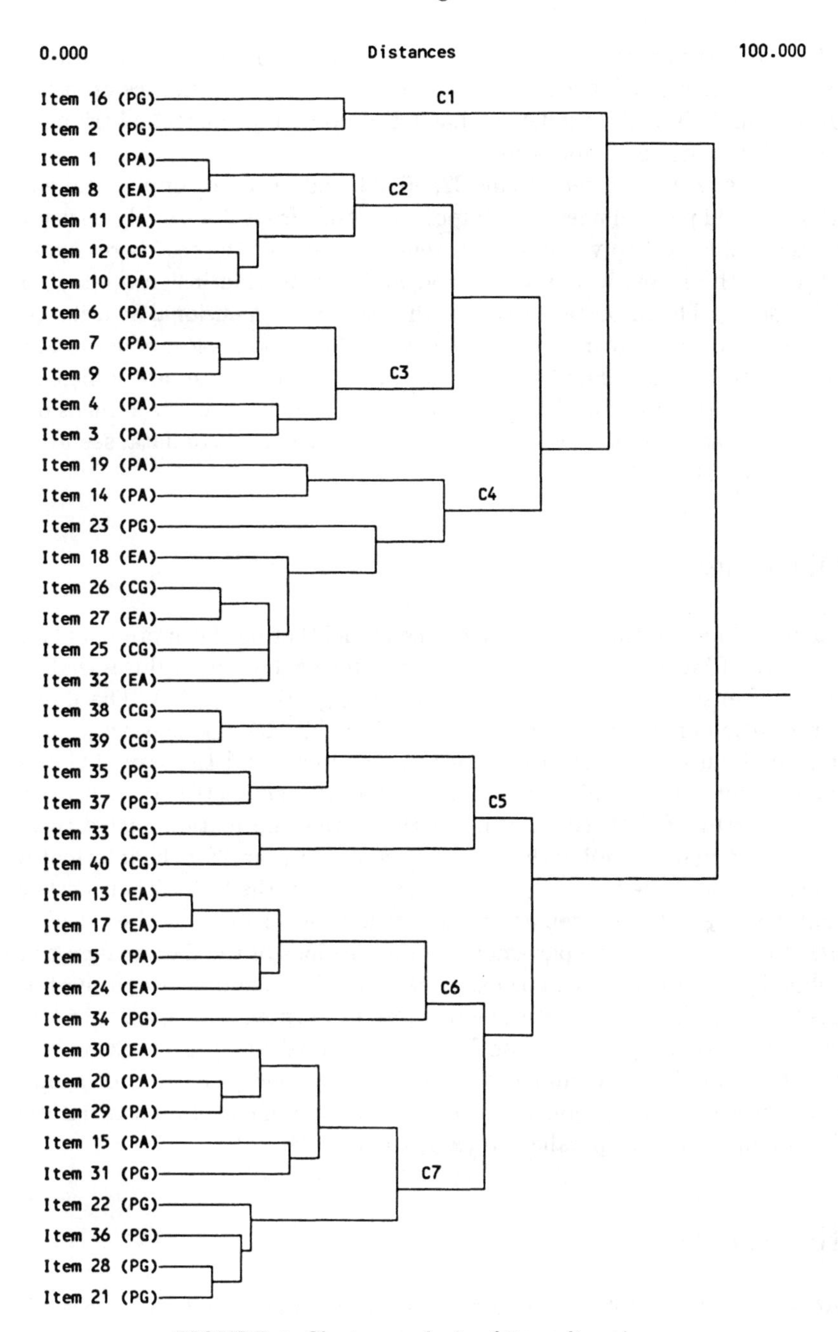

FIGURE 4. Cluster analysis of item directions.

solve geometry problems. Items 33, 38, 39, and 40 all deal with coordinates in a two-dimensional space. Item 35 has to do with coordinates on a line. Only Item 37 is slightly different, having to do with proportional triangles, but it does require computation.

Other geometry clusters, Items 22, 36, 28, and 21, for example, deal with triangles and parallel lines. The important result from these analyses is not, however, the level to which the content structure of the test is recovered, although the recovery was very good and did provide insights into item functioning. The important result is that the two-dimensional solution is a projection of the higher-level solution and information is lost when too few dimensions are used. Furthermore, the parameter estimates are sufficiently accurate with 1635 cases to support detailed analyses in six dimensions. For more details about the analysis of this particular set of data, see Miller and Hirsch (1990, 1992).

Discussion

There are many similarities between the model that has been presented and the work of McDonald (1985) and other factor analytic procedures that operate on unstandardized matrices of data (e.g., Horst, 1965). The unique contribution of the formulation presented in this chapter, however, is that it focuses on the characteristics of the test items and the way that they interact with the examinee population. Item characteristics are considered to be worthy of detailed scrutiny, both for the information that scrutiny can give to understanding the functioning of a test, and for the information provided about the meaning of scores reported on the test. Other methods that have a similar mathematical basis tend to focus more on the use of the mathematics to achieve parismonious descriptions of the data matrix or to define hypothetical psychological variables. Thus the model and methods described in this chapter are unique more in purpose and philosophy than in computational procedure or form. This model has proven useful for a variety of applications and has helped in the conceptualizing of a number of psychometric problems including the assessment of differential item functioning and test parallelism (Ackerman, 1990, 1992).

References

Ackerman, T.A. (1988). *Comparison of multidimensional IRT estimation procedures using benchmark data.* Paper presented at the ONR Contractors' Meeting, Iowa City, IA.

Ackerman, T.A. (1990). *An evaluation of the multidimensional parallelism of the EAAP Mathematics Test.* Paper presented at the Meeting of the

American Educational Research Association, Boston, MA.

Ackerman, T.A. (1992). A didactic explanation of item bias, item impact, and item validity from a multidimensional perspective. *Journal of Educational Measurement* **29**(1), 67–91.

Carlson, J.E. (1987). *Multidimensional item response theory estimation: A computer program* (Research Report ONR 87-2). Iowa City, IA: American College Testing.

DuBois, P.H. (1970). *A History of Psychological Testing.* Boston: Allyn and Bacon.

Fraser, C. (1986). *NOHARM: An IBM PC Computer Program for Fitting Both Unidimensional and Multidimensional Normal Ogive Models of Latent Trait Theory.* Armidale, Australia: The University of New England.

Horst, P. (1965). *Factor Analysis of Data Matrices.* New York: Holt, Rinehart and Winston.

Lord, F.M. (1980). *Application of Item Response Theory to Practical Testing Problems.* Hillsdale, NJ: Lawrence Erlbaum Associates.

Lord, F.M. and Novick, M.R. (1968). *Statistical Theories of Mental Test Scores.* Reading, MA: Addison Wesley.

McDonald, R.P. (1985). Unidimensional and multidimensional models for item response theory. In D.J. Weiss (Ed), *Proceedings of the 1982 Item Response Theory and Computerized Adaptive Testing Conference* (pp. 127–148). Minneapolis, MN: University of Minnesota.

McKinley, R.L. (1987). *User's Guide to MULTIDIM.* Princeton, NJ: Educational Testing Service.

McKinley, R.L. and Reckase, M.D. (1982). *The Use of the General Rasch Model with Multidimensional Item Response Data.* Iowa City, IA: American College Testing.

McKinley, R.L. and Reckase, M.D. (1983). MAXLOG: A computer program for the estimation of the parameters of a multidimensional logistic model. *Behavior Research Methods and Instrumentation* **15**, 389–390.

Miller, T.R. (1991). *Empirical Estimation of Standard Errors of Compensatory MIRT Model Parameters Obtained from the NOHARM Estimation Program* (Research Report ONR91-2). Iowa City, IA: American College Testing.

Miller, T.R. and Hirsch, T.M. (1990). *Cluster Analysis of Angular Data in Applications of Multidimensional Item Response Theory.* Paper presented at the Meeting of the Psychometric Society, Princeton, NJ.

Miller, T.R. and Hirsch, T.M. (1992). Cluster analysis of angular data in applications of multidimensional item-response theory. *Applied Measurement in Education* **5**(3), 193–211.

Mislevy, R.J. and Bock, R.D. (1989). *BILOG: Item Analysis and Test Scoring with Binary Logistic Models.* Chicago: Scientific Software.

Reckase, M.D. (1985). The difficulty of test items that measure more than one ability. *Applied Psychological Measurement* **9**(4), 401–412.

Reckase, M.D. (1989). *Controlling the Psychometric Snake: Or, How I Learned to Love Multimensionality.* Invited address at the Meeting of the American Psychological Association, New Orleans.

Reckase, M.D. and Hirsch, T.M. (1991). *Interpretation of Number Correct Scores When the True Number of Dimensions Assessed by a Test is Greater Than Two.* Paper presented at the Meeting of the National Council on Measurement in Education, Chicago.

Reckase, M.D. and McKinley, R.L. (1991). The discriminating power of items that measure more than one dimension. *Applied Psychological Measurement* **14**(4), 361–373.

Samejima, F. (1974). Normal ogive model for the continuous response level in the multidimensional latent space. *Psychometrika* **39**, 111–121.

Snow, R.E. (1993). Construct validity and constructed-response tests. In R.E. Bennett and W.C. Ward (Eds), *Construction Versus Choice in Cognitive Measurement: Issues in Constructed Response, Performance Testing, and Portfolio Assessment* (pp. 45–60). Hillsdale, NJ: Lawrence Erlbaum Associates.

Wingersky, M.S., Barton, M.A., and Lord, F.M. (1982). *LOGIST User's Guide.* Princeton, NJ: Educational Testing Service.

17

Loglinear Multidimensional Item Response Models for Polytomously Scored Items

Henk Kelderman

Introduction

Over the last decade, there has been increasing interest in analyzing mental test data with loglinear models. Several authors have shown that the Rasch model for dichotomously scored items can be formulated as a loglinear model (Cressie and Holland, 1983; de Leeuw and Verhelst, 1986; Kelderman, 1984; Thissen and Mooney, 1989; Tjur, 1982). Because there are good procedures for estimating and testing Rasch models, this result was initially only of theoretical interest. However, the flexibility of loglinear models facilitates the specification of many other types of item response models. In fact, they give the test analyst the opportunity to specify a unique model tailored to a specific test. Kelderman (1989) formulated loglinear Rasch models for the analysis of item bias and presented a gamut of statistical tests sensitive to different types of item bias. Duncan and Stenbeck (1987) formulated a loglinear model specifying a multidimensional model for Likert type items. Agresti (1993) and Kelderman and Rijkes (1994) formulated a loglinear model specifying a general multidimensional response model for polytomously scored items.

At first, the application of loglinear models to the analyses of test data was limited by the sheer size of the cross table of the item responses. Computer programs such as GLIM (Baker and Nelder, 1978), ECTA (Goodman and Fay, 1974), and SPSS LOGLINEAR (SPSS, 1988) require the internal storage of this table. However, numerical procedures have emerged that compute maximum likelihood estimates of loglinear models from their minimal sufficient statistics (Kelderman, 1992). These procedures require much less computer storage. The computer program LOGIMO (Kelderman and Steen, 1993), implementing these methods, has been specially designed to analyze test data.

It is the purpose of this chapter to introduce a general multidimensional polytomous item response model. The model is developed, starting from a saturated loglinear model for the item responses of a fixed individual. It is shown that, making the assumption of conditional (or local) independence and imposing certain homogeneity restrictions on the relation between item response and person, a general class of item response models emerges.

Item response theory (IRT) models with fixed person parameters do not yield consistent parameter estimates. Several authors have proposed loglinear IRT models that consider the person as randomly drawn from some population. These models are estimable with standard methods for loglinear or loglinear-latent-class analysis. A review of these ideas, as well as an example of their application to polytomous test data is given below. In the example several multidimensional IRT models are estimated and tested, and the best model is chosen.

Presentation of the Models

Loglinear models describe the probability of the joint realization of a set of random categorical variables, given the values of a set of fixed categorical variables. The models are called *loglinear* because the natural logarithms of these (conditional) probabilities are described by a linear model. Some useful textbooks introducing these models are Fienberg (1980), Agresti (1984), and Bishop et al. (1975). For more details on loglinear models the reader is referred to these sources. To introduce the ability parameter, loglinear models for a fixed person are considered first. Fixed-person models are the models of interest but cannot be estimated directly. Therefore, random-person models are introduced; these models are slightly more general than fixed-person models but they have the advantage of being estimable with standard loglinear theory models.

Fixed-Person Loglinear IRT Models

Let $\mathbf{Y} = (Y_1, \ldots, Y_i, \ldots, Y_n)$ be the random variable for the responses on n items and let $\mathbf{y} = (y_1, \ldots, y_i, \ldots, y_n)$ be a typical realization. The responses can be polytomous, where $y_i = 0$ usually denotes an incorrect response and $y_i = 1, \ldots, m_i$ denote correct or partially correct responses. Furthermore, let j $(= 1, \ldots, N)$ denote the person. The probability of a person's response pattern can be described by a loglinear model. The model has parameter $\lambda_{\mathbf{y}}^{\bar{\mathbf{Y}}}$ for the main effect of response pattern $\mathbf{y}$, and an interaction parameter $\lambda_{\mathbf{y}j}^{\bar{\mathbf{Y}}J}$ describing the effect of the combination of response pattern $\mathbf{y}$ and person j. Superscripts are symbolic notation showing the variables whose effect is to be described. Subscripts denote the values that these variable take. The bar over the superscript means that the variable is considered as a random variable in the model. If no ambiguity arises, superscripts will be omitted.

A general loglinear model for the probability of a random response pattern given a fixed person, can be written as

$$\log P_j(\mathbf{Y} = \mathbf{y}) = \mu_j + \lambda_{\mathbf{y}}^{\bar{\mathbf{Y}}} + \lambda_{\mathbf{y}j}^{\bar{\mathbf{Y}}J}, \quad \mu_j = -\log \sum_{z} \exp(\lambda_{\mathbf{z}}^{\bar{\mathbf{Y}}_i} + \lambda_{\mathbf{z}j}^{\bar{\mathbf{Y}}_i J}), \tag{1}$$

where the parameter μ_j is a proportionality constant that ensures that the sum of the conditional probabilities over all response patterns is equal to one. Parameters are *random* parameters if they involve random variables, and *fixed* parameters otherwise.

Equation (1) has indeterminacies in its parameterization. For example, adding a constant c to $\lambda_{\mathbf{y}}^{\bar{\mathbf{Y}}}$ and subtracting it from μ_j does not change the model. To obtain a unique parameterization one linear constraint must be imposed on the parameters. The simplest type of constraint contrasts the response patterns $\mathbf{y}$ with the zero pattern $\mathbf{y} = \mathbf{0}$. This *simple contrast* (Bock, 1975, pp. 50, 239) corresponds to the linear constraint $\lambda_{\mathbf{0}}^{\bar{\mathbf{Y}}} = 0$. In general, the parameters are constrained such that they are zero if one or more of their subscripts takes its lowest value. In the model shown in Eq. (1) these constraints are $\lambda_{\mathbf{0}}^{\bar{\mathbf{Y}}} = 0$ and $\lambda_{\mathbf{0}j}^{\bar{\mathbf{Y}}J} = \lambda_{\mathbf{y}1}^{\bar{\mathbf{Y}}J} = 0$, where $\mathbf{0} = (0, \ldots, 0)$ is a vector of zeros. An alternative way to remove the indeterminacies is to constrain the sum of the parameters over one or more subscripts to zero. For Eq. (1) these so-called *deviation contrasts* (Bock, 1975, pp. 50, 239) are $\sum_{\mathbf{y}} \lambda_{\mathbf{y}}^{\bar{\mathbf{Y}}} = 0$ and $\sum_{\mathbf{y}} \lambda_{\mathbf{y}j}^{\bar{\mathbf{Y}}J} = \sum_j \lambda_{\mathbf{y}j}^{\bar{\mathbf{Y}}J} = 0$.

In Eq. (1), all characteristics of the responses common to all persons are described by the term $\lambda_{\mathbf{y}}^{\bar{\mathbf{Y}}}$, and all characteristics of the responses that are unique to the person are described by the term $\lambda_{\mathbf{y}j}^{\bar{\mathbf{Y}}J}$. To obtain a model with an ability parameter, two additional restrictions must be imposed on the random parameters in the model shown in Eq. (1).

The first restriction on the parameters of the loglinear model is the *conditional independence* restriction (Lord and Novick, 1968). This restriction means no interactions between the person's item responses. The parameters for the joint response pattern $\mathbf{y}$ can then be written as a sum of parameters for each single y_i:

$$\lambda_{\mathbf{y}} = \lambda_{y_1} + \lambda_{y_2} + \lambda_{y_3} + \cdots \tag{2}$$

and

$$\lambda_{\mathbf{y}j} = \lambda_{y_1j} + \lambda_{y_2j} + \lambda_{y_3j} + \cdots . \tag{3}$$

Conditional independence restrictions imply (Goodman, 1970) that Eq. (1) can be written as a product of marginal probabilities,

$$P_j(\mathbf{Y} = \mathbf{y}) = \prod_{i=1}^{n} P_j(Y_i = y_i), \tag{4}$$

each with loglinear model,

$$\log P_j(Y_i = y_i) = \mu_{ij} + \lambda_{y_i}^{\bar{Y}_i} + \lambda_{y_ij}^{\bar{Y}_iJ},$$

$$\mu_{ij} = -\log \sum_{z=0}^{m_i} \exp(\lambda_z^{\bar{Y}_i} + \lambda_{zj}^{\bar{Y}_i J}). \tag{5}$$

To obtain an IRT model, the interaction between person and response is constrained to be a linear combination of k *person ability parameters* θ_{jq} ($j = 1, \ldots, N$; $q = 1, \ldots, k$):

$$\lambda_{yj}^{\bar{Y}_i J} = w_{1y}^{Y_i}\theta_{j1} + \cdots + w_{ky}^{Y_i}\theta_{jk}, \tag{6}$$

where $w_{qy}^{Y_i}$ are fixed integer-valued weights of response category y of item i with respect to ability q. To ensure that the constraint $\lambda_{0j}^{\bar{Y}_i J} = 0$ is satisfied, the convention is adopted that $w_{q0}^{Y_i} = 0$ for all $i = 1, \ldots, n$ and $q = 1, \ldots, k$. In cognitive terms, the score $y = 0$ usually corresponds to a completely incorrect response. The category weights may be further specified to define a particular IRT model. Before considering some meaningful specifications, the formulation of the model is completed first.

In applications of IRT, it is important that the difficulty of the item response is measured on the same scale as the person ability (Fischer, 1987). To accomplish this, the item main-effect parameters are written as a linear combination of more basic *response difficulty parameters:*

$$\lambda_y^{\bar{Y}_i} = -w_{1y}^{Y_i}\beta_{i1y} - \cdots - w_{ky}^{Y_i}\beta_{iky}, \tag{7}$$

where β_{iqy} is the difficulty of the yth response of item i with respect to ability q. To use Eq. (7) in applications it is necessary that the parameters β_{iqy} have empirical interpretation, and that it does not restrict the values of $\lambda_y^{\bar{Y}_i}$ ($y > 0$) in any way. Furthermore, the β_{iqy} parameters will often be set equal to zero to ensure that the estimated β_{iqy} parameters are unique. Thus $\{\beta_{iqy}, y > 0\}$ can be considered as a reparameterization of $\{\lambda_y^{\bar{Y}_i}, y > 0\}$.

Substituting Eqs. (6) and (7) into Eq. (5) yields the multidimensional polytomous item response model formulation,

$$P_j(Y_i = y) = \frac{\exp \sum_{q=1}^{k} w_{qy}^{Y_i}(\theta_{jq} - \beta_{iqy})}{\sum_{z=0}^{m_i} \exp \sum_{q=1}^{k} w_{qz}^{Y_i}(\theta_{jq} - \beta_{iqz})}. \tag{8}$$

This model is a generalization of Stegelmann's (1982) multidimensional Rasch model for dichotomously scored items. Kelderman and Rijkes (1994) have discussed it in its general polytomous form and called it the MPLT (multidimensional polytomous latent trait) model. This acronym will be used henceforth. It is easily seen that by specifying certain category weights, several well-known item response models emerge. In Table 1, specifications of category weights are given for some of these models. For example, in the dichotomous ($m_i = 1$) Rasch model a, there is only one person ability parameter ($k = 1$), and the weights are equal to the responses ($w_{1y}^{Y_i} =$

TABLE 1. Some Multidimensional Polytomous Item Response Models.

Model	Number of Abilities	Number of Response Categories	Category Weight
a Dichotomous Rasch (Rasch, 1960/1980)	1	2	$w_{11}^{Y_i} = 1$
b Partial Credit (Masters, 1982)	1	$m_i + 1$	$w_{1y}^{Y_i} = y$, $y = 1, \ldots, m_i$
c Multidimensional Rasch (Andersen, 1973)	m_i	$m_i + 1$	$w_{yy}^{Y_i} = 1$, $y = 1, \ldots, m_i$
d Multidimensional Partial Credit	m_i	$m_i + 1$	$w_{qy}^{Y_i} = 1$, $y \geq q = 1, \ldots, m_i$
e Rasch Model With Several Correct Responses (Kelderman & Rijkes, 1994)	1	$m_i + 1$	$w_{1y}^{Y_i} = 1$, $y = 1, \ldots, m_i$ $w_{21}^{Y_i} = 1, w_{23}^{Y_i} = 1$
f Duncan and Stenbeck's (1987) Multitrait Rasch Model	3	4	$w_{32}^{Y_i} = 1, w_{34}^{Y_i} = 1$ $w_{1y}^{Y_i} = y - 1$
g Partial Credit Model With Several Null Categories (Wilson & Masters, 1993)	1	$m_i + 1$ no. of null categories	$w_{1y}^{Y_i} = y$, credit

y). This restriction is equivalent to the restriction that in the loglinear model in Eq. (5), each correct response shows the same interaction with the person ($\lambda_{1j}^{\bar{Y}_1 J} = \cdots = \lambda_{1j}^{\bar{Y}_n J} = \theta_{j1}$). That is, the parameters describing the interactions between the persons and the item responses are equal across items. If this common interaction parameter is high (low) for a certain person, his or her probability of getting the items correct is also high (low). Thus, the parameter provides an indication of the persons ability.

The well-known partial credit model (PCM) (Masters, 1982, this volume) arises if the category weights are set equal to the scores. In the PCM, there is one incorrect response ($y = 0$), one correct response ($y = m_i$), and one or more partially correct responses ($y = 1, \ldots, m_i - 1$). Wilson and Adams (1993) discuss a partial credit model for ordered partition of response vectors, where every response vector corresponds to a *level* $w_{1y}^{Y_i}$.

Wilson and Masters (1993) also discuss models where one or more of the possible response categories are not observed in the data. The PCM is then changed such that $\exp(-\beta_{i1y}) \equiv 0$ and $w_{1y}^{Y_i} \equiv 0$ if y is a null category. This measure has the effect of removing the elements from the sample space with the particular null category and keeping the response framework intact (see Model g in Table 1).

Models b through h in Table 1 are models for polytomously scored items. Models b, e, and g specify one ability parameter but Models c, d, and f have several ability parameters. In Model e there is one incorrect response ($y = 0$) but several correct responses ($y > 0$). Each of these correct responses is related in the same way to the person, both within ($\lambda_{1j}^{\bar{Y}_{ij}} = \cdots = \lambda_{m_i j}^{\bar{Y}_i J} = \theta_{j1}$) and across items ($\lambda_{yj}^{\bar{Y}_1 J} = \cdots = \lambda_{yj}^{\bar{Y}_n J} = \theta_{j1}$). If the ability parameters take higher values, the probability of a correct response becomes higher too. Note, however, that different correct responses may have different response probabilities because their difficulty parameters (β_{i1y}) may have different values.

Model b has one person ability parameter, whereas it gives a response a higher category weight ($w_{1y}^{Y_i}$) as a function of its level of correctness. Model d has m_i ability parameters, where each level of correctness involves a distinct ability parameter. To ensure that the response-difficulty parameters are estimable, the restriction $\beta_{jqy} = 0$ if $q \neq y$ must be imposed on this model. Model c is a multidimensional Rasch model in which, except for the zero category, each response category has its own person parameter. It is easily verified in Eq. (8) that Model c is in fact a reparameterization of Model d where $\theta_{jq} \rightarrow \theta_{j1} + \cdots + \theta_{jq}$ and $\beta_{jqq} \rightarrow \beta_{j11} + \cdots + \beta_{jqq}$. Duncan and Stenbeck (1987) have proposed a multidimensional model for the analysis of Likert-type items.

A further restriction on a unidimensional ($k = -1$) version of the model in Eq. (8) is discussed in Adams and Wilson (1991). They impose a linear structure $\beta_{i1y} = \mathbf{a}'_{iy}\xi$ on the item parameters so that LLTM-type models can be specified for polytomous data. Following this strategy, for example, rating scale models (Andersen, this volume; Andrich, 1978) for polytomous items can be formulated.

The advantage of the MPLT model, however, lies not only in the models of Table 1. One can also go beyond these models, and specify one's own IRT model. In the Example, such an application of MPLT is described.

Random-Person IRT Models

In the previous section, all models were formulated as loglinear models for fixed persons. Each of these persons was described by one or more person parameters. A well-known problem in estimating the parameters of these models is that the number of person parameters increases as the number of persons increases. The result is that the usual asymptotic arguments for obtaining maximum likelihood estimates of the parameters do not hold so that the estimates become inconsistent (Andersen, 1973; Neyman and Scott, 1948). In this section, some new models are discussed that do have consistent maximum likelihood estimates. These models can also be formulated as loglinear models, but now for persons randomly drawn from some population.

Inserting Eq. (8) into (4) gives the probability of response vector $\mathbf{y}$ of person j:

$$\log P_j(\mathbf{Y} = \mathbf{y}) = \mu_j + \sum_{q=1}^{k} \sum_{j=1}^{n} w_{qy_j}^{Y_j} (\theta_{qj} - \beta_{iqy_j})$$

$$= \mu_j + \sum_{q=1}^{k} t_q \theta_{qj} + \sum_{i=1}^{n} \lambda_{y_i}^{\bar{Y}_i}, \tag{9}$$

$$\mu_j = -\log \sum_{\mathbf{y}} \exp\left(\sum_{q=1}^{k} t_q \theta_{qj} + \sum_{i=1}^{n} \lambda_{y_i}^{\bar{Y}_i} \right),$$

where $t_q = w_{qy_1}^{Y_1} + \cdots + w_{qy_n}^{Y_n}$ is the sum of the weights corresponding to θ_{qj}. Because $\{\beta_{iqy}, y > 0\}$ is a reparameterization of $\{\lambda_y^{\bar{Y}_i}, y > 0\}$, $\lambda_y^{\bar{Y}_i}$ will be used for simplicity.

There are two ways to eliminate the person parameters from IRT models: (1) conditioning on their sufficient statistics and (2) integrating them out. Both approaches yield new loglinear models in which persons have to be considered as randomly drawn from a population.

The joint MPLT model in Eq. (9) is an exponential-family model (Cox and Hinkley, 1974, p. 28), where the statistics t_q $(q = 1, \ldots, k)$ are jointly sufficient for the person parameters θ_{qj} $(q = 1, \ldots, k)$. A convenient property of exponential-family models is that, upon conditioning on a jointly sufficient statistic, inference about the item parameters no longer depends on the person parameters (Andersen, 1970, 1980). To see this feature, let $\mathbf{t} = (t_1, \ldots, t_k)$ be the vector of sums of category weights and let $\mathbf{T} = (T_1, \ldots, T_k)$ be the corresponding random vector. The probability of person j's sum of category weights $\mathbf{t}$ can be obtained by summing the log probabilities in Eq. (9) over all possible response patterns with the same sum of category weights:

$$P_j(\mathbf{T} = \mathbf{t}) = \exp\left(\mu_j + \sum_{q=1}^{k} t_q \theta_{qj} \right) \sum_{\mathbf{x}|\mathbf{t}} \exp\left(\sum_{i=1}^{n} \lambda_{y_i}^{\bar{Y}_i} \right). \tag{10}$$

Elimination of the item parameters by conditioning is achieved by subtracting the logarithm of Eq. (10) from (9):

$$\log P_j(\mathbf{Y} = \mathbf{y} \mid \mathbf{T} = \mathbf{t}) = \mu_t^T + \sum_{i=1}^{n} \lambda_{y_i}^{\bar{Y}_i}, \; \mu_t^T = -\log \sum_{\mathbf{y}|\mathbf{t}} \exp\left(\sum_{i=1}^{n} \lambda_{y_i}^{\bar{Y}_i} \right). \tag{11}$$

This result is a loglinear model that contains only random parameters for the item responses and a fixed parameter for the sum of category weights.

Note that the person parameters have vanished. Therefore, the same model holds for all persons with the same sum of category weights $\mathbf{t}$. Consequently, the same model holds also for the probability $P(\mathbf{Y} = \mathbf{y} \mid \mathbf{T} = \mathbf{t})$ of the responses $\mathbf{y}$ of a *randomly sampled* person with sum of category weights $\mathbf{t}$:

$$\log P(\mathbf{Y} = \mathbf{y} \mid \mathbf{T} = \mathbf{t}) = \mu_t^T + \sum_{i=1}^{n} \lambda_{y_i}^{\bar{Y}_i}. \tag{12}$$

In the terminology of loglinear modeling (Bishop et al., 1975, Sec. 5.4; Haberman, 1979, Sec. 7.3), the model in Eq. (12) can be viewed as a quasi-loglinear model for the incomplete item 1 × item 2 × ... × item k × sum-of-category-weights contingency table with structurally zero cells if the sum of category weights is not consistent with the response pattern (Kelderman, 1984; Kelderman and Rijkes, 1994). For example, Rasch (1960/1980), Andersen (1973), and Fischer (1974) discuss the estimation of item parameters after conditioning on the sufficient statistics of the person parameters in the dichotomous Rasch model.

The second approach also assumes that the persons are randomly drawn from some population and respond independently to one another. Furthermore, it is assumed that the sums of category weights $\mathbf{T}$ have a *multinomial* distribution with number parameter N and with $n-1$ unrestricted parameters for the probabilities. The probability of the person's response pattern can then be written as the following loglinear model:

$$\begin{aligned} \log P(\mathbf{Y} = \mathbf{y}) &= \log(P(\mathbf{Y} = \mathbf{y} \mid \mathbf{T} = \mathbf{t})P(\mathbf{T} = \mathbf{t})) \\ &= \mu + \lambda_{\mathbf{t}}^{\bar{\mathbf{T}}} + \sum_{i=1}^{n} \lambda_{y_i}^{\bar{Y}_i}, \\ \lambda_{\mathbf{t}}^{\bar{\mathbf{T}}} &= \log P(\mathbf{T} = \mathbf{t}) - \log P(\mathbf{T} = \mathbf{0}), \\ \mu &= -\log \sum_{\mathbf{y}} \exp\left(\lambda_{\mathbf{t}}^{\bar{\mathbf{T}}} + \sum_{i=1}^{n} \lambda_{y_i}^{\bar{Y}_i}\right). \end{aligned} \tag{13}$$

For the case of the dichotomous Rasch model, this approach was proposed by Tjur (1982), Duncan (1984), and Kelderman (1984). The results can readily be generalized to the MPLT.

The models in Eqs. (12) and (13) differ in the sampling scheme that is assumed for the data. The former model assumes *product-multinomial* sampling, whereas the latter assumes *multinomial* sampling. Bishop et al. (1975, Sec. 3.3) showed that, for both models, the kernel of the likelihood is identical. As a result, both models have the same set of likelihood equations for estimating the parameters and the same statistics for testing their goodness of fit.

Both models also disregard the proper sum-of-category-weights distribution in Eq. (10). The model in Eq. (12) does this by considering the sum of category weights as fixed and concentrating only on the conditional distribution. The model in Eq. (13) does so by replacing the sum-of-category-weights distribution for each person by an unrestricted *multinomial* sum-of-category-weights distribution for the population. Tjur (1982) calls this model an "extended random model." Obviously, the extended random model and the original model in Eq. (9) are not the same. Note that the individual sum-of-category-weights distribution has a quite restrictive form. This restriction is not respected in the extended random model.

Another derivation of the loglinear Rasch model, has shed more light on the difference between both models. Cressie and Holland (1983) arrive at the loglinear Rasch model in Eq. (13) by integrating out the person parameters. They call this model the "extended Rasch model." Introducing more general notation here, let the persons again be randomly drawn from a population and let $\mathbf{\Theta} = (\Theta_1, \ldots, \Theta_q, \ldots, \Theta_k)$ be the vector random variable for the person parameters with realization $\boldsymbol{\theta} = (\theta_1, \ldots, \theta_q, \ldots, \theta_k)$ and a distribution $f(\boldsymbol{\theta})$. Integrating the MPLT model in Eq. (9) over this distribution, the probability of a response pattern $\mathbf{y}$ becomes

$$P(\mathbf{Y} = \mathbf{y}) = \exp\left(\sum_{i=1}^{n} \lambda_{y_i}^{\bar{Y}_i}\right) \int \frac{\exp \sum_{q=1}^{k} t_q \theta_q}{\sum_y \exp\left(\sum_{q=1}^{k} t_q \theta_q + \sum_{i=1}^{n} \lambda_{y_i}^{\bar{Y}_i}\right)} f(\boldsymbol{\theta})\, d\boldsymbol{\theta}, \tag{14}$$

where $\lambda_y^{\bar{Y}}$ satisfies the constraints imposed by the chosen model. For the case of the dichotomous Rasch model, Cressie and Holland (1983) then replaced the logarithm of the integral by an unrestricted parameter σ_t $(= \mu + \lambda_t^{\bar{T}})$ that depends only on the sum of category weights. They showed that the sum-of-category-weights parameters must satisfy complicated constraints, which can be checked (see also Hout et al., 1987; Lindsay et al., 1991) but under which estimation is hard to pursue. If these constraints are ignored, Cressie and Holland's extended Rasch model is obtained. This model is the same loglinear model as Tjur's extended random model in Eq. (13).

The extended Rasch model is less restrictive than the original model in Eq. (14) but de Leeuw and Verhelst (1986) and Follmann (1988) proved that, for the case of the dichotomous Rasch model, under certain mild conditions on the distribution f, both models have estimators that are asymptotically equivalent.

Parameter Estimation

For the case of the MPLT, an extended loglinear formulation can be used to estimate the item parameters. These parameter estimates correspond to conditional maximum likelihood estimates. The log-likelihood of the model in Eq. (13) is

$$l = \log \prod_{\mathbf{y}} P(\mathbf{Y} = \mathbf{y})^{f_{\mathbf{y}}} = N\mu + \sum_{\mathbf{t}} f_{\mathbf{t}}^{T} \lambda_{\mathbf{t}}^{\bar{T}} + \sum_{i=1}^{n} \sum_{y_i} (f_{y_i}^{Y_i} \lambda_{y_i}^{\bar{Y}_i}), \tag{15}$$

where $f_{\mathbf{y}}$ is the observed sample frequency of vector $\mathbf{y}$, f_t^T the frequency of sum of category weights $\mathbf{t}$, and $f_{y_i}^{Y_i}$, the frequency of response y_i. Setting the derivatives with respect to the parameters to zero, the following likelihood equations are obtained:

$$f_{\mathbf{t}}^{\mathbf{T}} = F_t^{\mathbf{T}} \qquad f_{y_i}^{Y_i} = F_{y_i}^{Y_i} \tag{16}$$

for all $\mathbf{t}$ and $y_i = 0, \ldots, m_i$ $(i = 1, \ldots, n)$, where $F = E(f)$ denotes the expected frequency under Eq. (13) [see Haberman (1979), p. 448)]. Equations (16) can be solved by iterative methods, such as iterative proportional fitting (IPF) or Newton–Raphson. In IPF, the (unrestricted) parameters are updated until convergence by

$$\lambda_{\mathbf{t}}^{(\text{new})} = \lambda_{\mathbf{t}}^{(\text{old})} \frac{f_{\mathbf{t}}}{F_t^{(\text{old})}}; \quad \lambda_{y_i}^{(\text{new})} = \lambda_{y_i}^{(\text{old})} \frac{f_{y_i}}{F_{y_i}^{(\text{old})}}, \tag{17}$$

for all $\mathbf{t}$ and $y_i = 0, \ldots, m_i$ $(i = 1, \ldots, n)$, where $F^{(\text{old})}$ is the expected frequency computed from the previous parameter values $\lambda^{(\text{old})}$. Note that this algorithm does no longer require the full contingency table $\{f_{\mathbf{y}}\}$ or $\{F_{\mathbf{y}}\}$. For a description of a Newton–Raphson algorithm that operates on the sufficient statistics, see Kelderman (1992).

Both algorithms still have the following two practical difficulties left to be solved. First, the marginal expected frequencies $\{F_{\mathbf{t}}\}$ and $\{F_{y_i}\}$ require summation over all remaining variables. This problem can be solved by writing the model in a multiplicative form and, using the distributive law of multiplication over summation, reducing the number of summations. The reduction is achieved because the summations are only over parameters whose indices contain the summation variable. Second, for an arbitrary MPLT model, marginal frequencies $\{F_{\mathbf{t}}\}$ may be hard to compute because the response vectors $\mathbf{x}$ over which summation has to take place to obtain $\{F_{\mathbf{t}}\}$ from $\{F_{\mathbf{x}}\}$ must be consistent with the vector of sums of category weights $\mathbf{t}$. This problem can be solved by keeping track of the sum of the category weights $\mathbf{t}$ while summing over the x_i variables. For example, suppose there are four items and an MPLT model with multiplicative parameters $\psi = \exp(\mu)$, $\phi_t = \exp(\lambda_t)$, $\phi_{y_1} = \exp(\lambda_{y_1})$, $\phi_{y_2} = \exp(\lambda_{y_2})$, $\phi_{y_3} = \exp(\lambda_{y_3})$, and $\phi_{y_4} = \exp(\lambda_{y_4})$. Furthermore, let $t_q^{(i)} = w_{qy_1}^{Y_1} + \cdots + w_{qy_i}^{Y_i}$ be the sum of category weights computed over the first i variables and let $\mathbf{t}^{(i)} = (t_1^{(i)}, \ldots, t_k^{(i)})$ be the vector of these partial sums of category weights. The expected marginal frequency for the sums of category weights can now be computed as

$$F_{\mathbf{t}} = N\psi\phi_t \sum_{\mathbf{t}^{(3)},y_4;\mathbf{t}} \phi_{y_4} \sum_{\mathbf{t}^{(2)},y_3;\mathbf{t}}^{(3)} \phi_{y_3} \sum_{y_1,y_2;\mathbf{t}^{(2)}} \phi_{y_2}\phi_{y_1}, \tag{18}$$

where $\sum_{a,b;c}$ means summation over all values of a and b that are consistent with c. The summation can be obtained in two steps. First, the products in the summand as well as their partial sums of category weights, e.g., $\{(\phi_{y_1}\phi_{y_2}),\ \mathbf{t}^{(2)};\ y_1 = 1,\ldots,m_1;\ y_2 = 1,\ldots,m_2\}$, are computed. Second, these products $(\phi_{y_1}\phi_{y_2})$ are summed only if the partial sums of category weights $(\mathbf{t}^{(2)})$ are identical. This step yields a sum for each distinct value of the sum of category weights. If the model is the dichotomous Rasch model (Table 1, Model a), this method to compute marginal expected frequencies is identical to the so-called summation algorithm for the computation of elementary symmetric functions (Andersen, 1980). See Verhelst et al. (1984) for a thorough discussion of the accuracy of the computation of elementary symmetric functions.

In the program LOGIMO (LOglinear Irt MOdeling, Kelderman and Steen, 1993), the above method is used to compute the marginal frequencies $\{F_{\mathbf{z}}\}$, where $\mathbf{z}$ may be any vector of item or sum-of-category-weights variables. LOGIMO solves the likelihood equations of any loglinear model with sum-of-category-weights variables using iterative proportional fitting or Newton-Raphson methods. It is written in Pascal and runs on a 386 PC/MS-DOS system or higher and can be obtained from iec *Pro*GAMMA, Box 841, 9700 AV Groningen, The Netherlands.

The program OPLM (Verhelst et al., 1993) estimates the parameters in Eq. (8) for the unidimensional case ($k = 1$). It can be obtained from the authors at Cito, Box 1034, 6801 MG, Arnhem, The Netherlands.

Goodness of Fit

The overall fit of MPLT models can be tested by customary statistics for loglinear models, such as Pearson's statistic (X^2) and the likelihood-ratio statistic (G^2) (Bishop et al., 1975; Haberman, 1979). However, the usual asymptotic properties of these statistics break down if the number of items is large (Haberman, 1977; Koehler, 1977; Lancaster, 1961), albeit that X^2 seems to be more robust than G^2 (Cox and Placket, 1980; Larnz, 1978). In this case, the following two alternative test statistics can be used.

One approach is to compare the model of interest (M) with a less restrictive model (M*) using the likelihood-ratio statistic $-2[(l(\text{M}) - l(\text{M}^*)]$ with degrees of freedom equal to the difference in numbers of estimable parameters of both models (Rao, 1973, pp. 418–420). If one model is not a special case of the other, Akaike's (1977) information criterion (AIC), (2[(number of parameters) $-l$]), can be compared for both models. The model with the

TABLE 2. Specification of Cognitive Processes Involved in the Responses on the Items of the ACSP Medical Laboratory Test.

Item	I Applies Knowledge				II Calculates				III Correlates Data				IV Correct			
	a	b	c	d	a	b	c	d	a	b	c	d	a	b	c	d
1			2	1											1	
2	1		2												1	
3	2	1	1										1			
4		1	1			2	1							1		
5	2	1	1		1								1			
6	1		1	1			1								1	
7	1	1	1						1	2	1			1		
8	1	1								1				1		
9	1	1	2	1							1				1	
10	1	1			2	1			1				1			
11	1		1		1		1				1				1	

smallest AIC is chosen as the best fitting model.

The second approach is to consider the Pearson X^2 statistics for marginal contingency tables rather than the full contingency table. For example, for the dichotomous Rasch model, one could calculate a Pearson statistic for each combination of an item i and a sum of category weights q (van den Wollenberg, 1979, 1982). In the next section, an example will be presented in which both approaches are used to check model fit.

Example

The American Society of Clinical Pathologists (ASCP) produces tests for the certification of paramedical personnel. In this section the responses of 3331 examinees to 11 four-choice items from a secure data base were re-analyzed. The items measure the ability to perform medical laboratory tests. The composite test score used was equal to the number of correct responses given by the examinee.

Although each item had one correct alternative and three incorrect alternatives, it was hypothesized by content experts that incorrect responses might often have been chosen after cognitive activities similar to those necessary to arrive at the correct response. Therefore, it was felt that the incorrect responses might also contain valid information about the examinee. It was hypothesized that three cognitive processes had been involved in answering the items: "Applying Knowledge" (I), "Calculating" (II), and "Correlating Data" (III). Table 2 provides the weights that content experts assigned to each of the item responses for each cognitive process. For example, the correct response in Item 4 involved two calculations, whereas

TABLE 3. AIC Statistics for Eleven-Item and Nine-Item Data Sets.

		Eleven-Item Data Set		Nine-Item Data Set	
Model	Ability	NPAR	AIC-18000	NPAR	AIC-18000
Independence	None	34	704	28	1223
A	I, II, III	262	265	219	1088
B	IV	43	104	36	854
C	I, II, III, IV	645	124	446	996
D	I, III, IV			191	942

Response c involved only one. The 11 items were selected from the data base such that a balanced representation of the three cognitive processes was obtained. The correct responses (IV) are also given. It was hypothesized that giving the correct response required an additional metacognitive activity that went beyond Cognitive Processes I, II, and III. Finally, it was assumed that for each examinee distinct parameters were needed to describe the ability to perform each of the Cognitive Processes I, II, III, and IV.

To study whether the items provided information about the hypothesized abilities I, II, and III, several MPLT models from Eq. (9) were specified. Item responses were described by λ rather than β parameters so that responses with zero scoring weights could have different probabilities.

To obtain an interpretable and unique set of parameters, two restrictions had to be imposed on the λ parameters. First, to make the parameters of the incorrect responses comparable, a reparameterization was done to guarantee that their sum was equal to zero in each item. In an item i, this result was achieved by subtracting their mean from all parameters of item i and adding it to the general mean parameter μ. Second, to fix the origin of the ability scale, the sum of the item parameters corresponding to the correct responses was set equal to zero. This was done by subtracting their mean from the correct response parameters and next subtracting t_4 times this value from λ_t^T.

The second column of Table 3 shows which ability parameters were specified in each model. The weights for each of these ability parameters are given in Table 2. In the complete independence model, no traits were specified. The corresponding loglinear model had main effects of Items 1 through 11 only. Model C contained all ability parameters, Model A only the ability parameters for the correct response. Model D had all ability parameters except the one for "Calculating." The model will be discussed later on.

From the AIC values in Table 3, it is seen that the complete independence model did not explain the data as well as the other models. Furthermore, Models B and C, which also contained an ability for Cognitive Process

TABLE 4. Goodness-of-Fit Statistics for Grouped Item × Sum-of-Category Weights IV (Model B; 11-Item Data Set).

	Item										
	1	2	3	4	5	6	7	8	9	10	11
Chi-Square	44	45	63	30	33	27	116	34	31	34	42
DF	25	26	26	25	26	26	26	25	25	25	25

IV, had better fit to the data than Model A, which contained only ability parameters for Cognitive Processes I, II, and III. Surprisingly, the more restrictive model (Model B) provided a slightly better fit than the most inclusive model (Model C). This result suggests that the contribution of Cognitive Processes I, II, and III to explaining test behavior in this situation is quite small—in fact, probably smaller than the errors associated with the model parameter estimates. In this situation, Model B, which was based on the number-correct scoring, probably described the response behavior to a sufficient degree.

To test whether the items fitted Model B, Pearson statistics were computed for each of the grouped item-response × sum-of-category-weights IV contingency tables. Because the sum of category weights is a sufficient statistic for the ability parameter, Pearson fit statistics are sensitive to lack of fit of the responses of an item with respect to the particular ability parameter. Note that the overall goodness-of-fit statistics X^2 of G^2 could not be used in this case because the contingency table had too many cells (4^{11}) relative to the number of examinees (3331).

It is seen from Table 4 that Item 3 and 7 did not fit the model very well. Therefore, it was decided to set these items aside in the analysis and analyze the remaining nine-item data set. Models A, B, and C were fitted again. Table 3 shows that the nine-item data set had the same pattern of fit as the 11-item data set: Model B fitted better than Models A or C. In this case, again, the data could not identify any of the cognitive-process abilities.

To consider one more alternative model, Model D was suggested. It was conjectured that too many cognitive processes were specified in Models A and C. In particular, the "Calculation" process (II) could have been too easy to discriminate between examinees. Therefore, in Model D, this ability was removed. Although this model fitted better than Model C, it does not fit better than Model B, indicating that the remaining abilities I and III could not be detected in the data.

In Table 5, grouped-Pearson X^2 statistics and parameter estimates are given for Model B for the nine-item data set. It is seen that the fit of the individual items to the model was reasonable. The estimates of the

TABLE 5. Parameter Estimates and Goodness of Fit Statistics of Model B in Nine-Item Data Set. (Asterisk Denotes a Correct Response.)

	Item								
	1	2	4	5	6	8	9	10	11
Chi-Square	33	38	40	32	21	16	21	22	28
DF	21	22	22	22	23	20	23	20	21
Response a	0.54	0.88	0.37	0.01*	0.14	−1.13	0.30	0.46*	−0.97*
Response b	0.95	−0.02	0.66*	−0.07	0.93	0.07*	−0.60	−1.05	1.29
Response c	−0.92*	−0.50*	−1.00	0.48	0.47*	0.58	−0.21*	−0.16	−0.05*
Response d	−1.50	−0.85	0.63	−0.41	−1.07	0.54	0.30	0.90	−0.31

λ parameters are also given in Table 5. Items 1 and 2 turned out to be difficult but Items 4, 6, and 10 were relatively easy. Parameter estimates for the incorrect alternatives showed, for example, that Alternative d of Item 1 was more attractive than Alternatives a or b.

References

Adams, R.J. and Wilson, M. (1991). The random coefficients multinomial logit model: A general approach to fitting Rasch models. Paper presented at the Annual Meeting of the American Educational Research Association, Chicago, April.

Agresti, A. (1984). *Analysis of Ordinal Categorical Data.* New York: Wiley.

Agresti, A. (1993). Computing conditional maximum likelihood estimates for generalized Rasch models using simple loglinear models with diagonals parameters. *Scandinavian Journal of Statistics* **20**, 63–71.

Akaike, H. (1977). On entropy maximization principle. In P.R. Krisschnaiah (Ed), *Applications of Statistics* (pp. 27–41). Amsterdam: North Holland.

Andersen, E.B. (1970). Asymptotic properties of conditional maximum likelihood estimators. *Journal of the Royal Statistical Society B* **32**, 283–301.

Andersen, E.B. (1973). Conditional inference and multiple choice questionnaires. *British Journal of Mathematical and Statistical Psychology* **26**, 31–44.

Andersen, E.B. (1980). *Discrete Statistical Models with Social Science Applications.* Amsterdam: North Holland.

Andrich, D. (1978). A rating scale formulation for ordered response categories. *Psychometrika* **43**, 561–573.

Baker, R.J. and Nelder, J.A. (1978). *The GLIM System: Generalized Linear Interactive Modeling.* Oxford: The Numerical Algorithms Group.

Bishop, Y.M.M., Fienberg, S.E., and Holland, P.W. (1975). *Discrete Multivariate Analysis.* Cambridge, MA: MIT Press.

Bock, R.D. (1975). *Multivariate Statistical Methods in Behavioral Research.* New York: McGraw Hill.

Cox, M.A.A. and Hinkley, D.V. (1974). *Theoretical Statistics.* London: Chapman and Hall.

Cox, M.A.A. and Placket, R.L. (1980). Small samples in contingency tables. *Biometrika* **67**, 1–13.

Cressie, N. and Holland, P.W. (1983). Characterizing the manifest probabilities of latent trait models. *Psychometrika* **48**, 129–142.

de Leeuw, J. and Verhelst, N.D. (1986). Maximum likelihood estimation in generalized Rasch models. *Journal of Educational Statistics* **11**, 183–196.

Duncan, O.D. (1984). Rasch measurement: Further examples and discussion. In C.F. Turner and E. Martin (Eds), *Surveying Subjective Phenomena* (Vol. 2, pp. 367–403). New York: Russell Sage Foundation.

Duncan, O.D. and Stenbeck, M. (1987). Are Likert scales unidimensional? *Social Science Research* **16**, 245–259.

Fienberg, S.E. (1980). *The Analysis of Cross-Classified Categorical Data.* Cambridge, MA: MIT Press.

Fischer, G.H. (1974). *Einführung in die Theorie psychologischer Tests* [*Introduction to the Theory of Psychological Tests*]. Bern: Huber. (In German.)

Fischer, G.H. (1987). Applying the principles of specific objectivity and generalizability to the measurement of change. *Psychometrika* **52**, 565–587.

Follmann, D.A. (1988). Consistent estimation in the Rasch model based on nonparametric margins. *Psychometrika* **53**, 553–562.

Goodman, L.A. (1970). Multivariate analysis of qualitative data. *Journal of the American Statistical Association* **65**, 226–256.

Goodman, L.A. and Fay, R. (1974). *ECTA Program, Description for Users.* Chicago: Department of Statistics University of Chicago.

Haberman, S.J. (1977). Log-linear models and frequency tables with small cell counts, *Annals of Statistics* **5**, 1124–1147.

Haberman, S.J. (1979). *Analysis of Qualitative Data: New Developments* (Vol. 2). New York: Academic Press.

Hout, M., Duncan, O.D., and Sobel, M.E. (1987). Association and heterogeneity: Structural models of similarities and differences. *Sociological Methodology* **17**, 145–184.

Kelderman, H. (1984). Loglinear Rasch model tests. *Psychometrika* **49**, 223–245.

Kelderman, H. (1989). Item bias detection using loglinear IRT. *Psychometrika* **54**, 681–697.

Kelderman, H. (1992). Computing maximum likelihood estimates of loglinear IRT models from marginal sums. *Psychometrika* **57**, 437–450.

Kelderman, H. and Rijkes, C.P.M. (1994). Loglinear multidimensional IRT models for polytomously scored items. *Psychometrika* **59**, 147–177.

Kelderman, H. and Steen, R. (1993). *LOGIMO: Loglinear Item Response Modeling* [computer manual]. Groningen, The Netherlands: iec ProGAMMA.

Koehler, K.J. (1977). *Goodness-of-Fit Statistics for Large Sparse Multinomials.* Unpublished doctoral dissertation, School of Statistics, University of Minnesota.

Lancaster, H.O. (1961). Significance tests in discrete distributions. *Journal of the American Statistical Association* **56**, 223–234.

Larnz, K. (1978). Small-sample comparisons of exact levels for chi-square statistics. *Journal of the American Statistical Association* **73**, 412–419.

Lord, F.M. and Novick, M.R. (1968). *Statistical Theories of Mental Test Scores.* Reading, MA: Addison Wesley.

Lindsay, B., Clogg, C.C., and Grego, J. (1991). Semiparametric estimation in the Rasch model and related exponential response models, including a simple latent class model for item analysis. *Journal of the American Statistical Association* **86**, 96–107.

Masters, G.N. (1982). A Rasch model for partial credit scoring. *Psychometrika* **47**, 149–174.

Neyman, J. and Scott, E.L. (1948). Consistent estimates based on partially consistent observations. *Econometrica* **16**, 1–32.

Rao, C.R. (1973). *Linear Statistical Inference and Its Applications* (2nd ed.). New York: Wiley.

Rasch, G. (1960/1980). *Probabilistic Models for Some Intelligence and Attainment Tests.* Chicago: The University of Chicago Press.

SPSS (1988). *SPSS User's Guide* (2 ed.). Chicago, IL: Author.

Stegelmann, W. (1983). Expanding the Rasch model to a general model having more than one dimension. *Psychometrika* **48**, 257–267.

Thissen, D. and Mooney, J.A. (1989). Loglinear item response theory, with applications to data from social surveys. *Sociological Methodology* **19**, 299–330.

Tjur, T. (1982). A connection between Rasch's item analysis model and a multiplicative Poisson model. *Scandinavian Journal of Statistics* **9**, 23–30.

van den Wollenberg, A.L. (1979). *The Rasch Model and Time Limit Tests.* Unpublished doctoral dissertation, Katholieke Universiteit Nijmegen, The Netherlands.

van den Wollenberg, A.L. (1982). Two new test statistics for the Rasch model. *Psychometrika* **47**, 123–140.

Verhelst, N.D., Glas, C.A.W., and van der Sluis, A. (1984). Estimation problems in the Rasch model. *Computational Statistics Quarterly* **1**, 245–262.

Verhelst, N.D., Glas, C.A.W., and Verstralen, H.H.F.M. (1993). *OPLM: Computer Program and Manual.* Arnhem, The Netherlands: Cito.

Wilson, M. and Adams, R.J. (1993). Marginal maximum likelihood estimation for the ordered partition model. *Journal of Educational Statistics* **18**, 69–90.

Wilson, M. and Masters, G.N. (1993). The partial credit model and null categories. *Psychometrika* **58**, 87–99.

18
Multicomponent Response Models

Susan E. Embretson

Introduction

Cognitive theory has made significant impact on theories of aptitude and intelligence. Cognitive tasks (including test items) are viewed as requiring multiple processing stages, strategies, and knowledge stores. Both tasks and persons vary on the processing components. That is, the primary sources of processing difficulty may vary between tasks, even when the tasks are the same item type.

Processing components have been studied on many tasks that are commonly found on aptitude tests. For example, cognitive components have been studied on analogies (Mulholland et al., 1980; Sternberg, 1977), progressive matrices (Carpenter et al., 1990), spatial tasks (Pellegrino et al., 1985), mathematical problems (Embretson, 1995a; Mayer et al., 1984) and many others.

These studies have several implications for measurement since persons also vary in performing the various processing components. First, item response theory (IRT) models that assume unidimensionality are often inappropriate. Since tasks depend on multiple scores of difficulty, each of which may define a source of person differences, multidimensional models are theoretically more plausible. Although unidimensional models can be made to fit multidimensional tasks, the resulting dimension is a confounded composite. Second, the same composite ability estimate may arise from different patterns of processing abilities, thus creating problems for interpretation. Third, a noncompensatory or conjunctive multidimensional IRT model is theoretically more plausible than a compensatory model for multicomponent tasks. That is, solving an item depends on the conjunction of successful outcomes on several aspects of processing.

The Multicomponent Latent Trait Model (MLTM) (Whitely, 1980) was developed to measure individual differences in underlying processing components on complex aptitude tasks. MLTM is a conjunctive multidimensional model in which task performance depends on component task difficulties and component person abilities. A generalization of MLTM, the General Component Latent Trait Model [GLTM; Embretson (1984)]; permits the stimulus features of tasks to be linked to component task difficulties.

Such stimulus features are typically manipulated in experimental cognitive studies to control the difficulty of specific processes. Thus, GLTM permits a more complete linkage to cognitive theory than the original MLTM.

MLTM and GLTM have many research applications, especially if the sources of performance differences is a foremost concern. Perhaps the most extensive application is for construct validation research. The fit of alternative MLTM or GLTM models and the component parameter estimates provide data that are directly relevant to the theoretical processing that underlies test performance. Furthermore, MLTM and GLTM are also quite useful for test design, including both item development and item selection. The model parameters can be used to develop tests with specified sources of processing difficulty. Additionally, applications of MLTM and GLTM to research on individual and group differences provide greater explanatory power. That is, the sources of performance differences, in terms of underlying processes, can be pinpointed. These applications will be illustrated or discussed in this chapter.

Presentation of the Model

MLTM specifies the relationship between the response to the item and responses to underlying processing components as conjunctive. That is, the underlying components must be executed successfully for the task to be solved. Thus, the probability of solving the task is given by the product of the probabilities of solving the individual tasks, as follows:

$$P(U_{ijT} = 1 \mid \underline{\theta}_j, \underline{b}_i) = (s - g) \prod_k P(U_{ijk} = 1 \mid \theta_{jk}, b_{ik}) + g, \tag{1}$$

where θ_{jk} is the ability for person j on component k, b_{ik} is the difficulty of item i on component k, U_{ijk} is the response for person j on the kth component of item i, U_{ijT} is the response for person j on the total task T for item i, g is the probability of solving the item by guessing and s is the probability of applying the component outcomes to solve the task.

In turn, the processing components are governed by the ability of the person and the task difficulty. The person and item parameters of MLTM are included in a logistic model that contains the component ability θ_{jk} and component difficulty b_{ik} such that the full MLTM model may be written as follows:

$$P(U_{ijT} = 1 \mid \underline{\theta}_j, \underline{\xi}_i) = (s - g) \prod_k \frac{\exp(\theta_{jk} - b_{ik})}{1 + \exp(\theta_{jk} - b_{ik})} + g, \tag{2}$$

where θ_{jk} and b_{ik} are defined as in Eq. (1). An inspection of Eq. (2) shows that the component probabilities are specified by a Rasch model.

For example, verbal analogies have been supported as involving two general components, rule construction and response evaluation (see Whitely,

1981). In a three-term analogy, the task is to complete the analogy with a term that relates to the third term in the same way as the second term relates to the first term. For example,

Event : Memory :: Fire : ___________

1) Matches 2) Ashes* 3) Camera 4) Heat

would require: (1) determining the analogy rule "something that remains afterwards"; and (2) evaluating the four alternatives as remainders of "Fire." MLTM would give the probability of solving the task as the probability of constructing the rule correctly times the probability of response evaluation by the rule. (Handling data with sequential outcomes will be discussed below.)

The item response curves show the relationships between components. The degree to which solving the item depends on a given component (e.g., θ_1) depends on the logit ($d_{ijk} = \theta_{jk} - b_{ik}$) of the other components. Figure 1 presents some item response curves for an item with two components, for simplicity assuming that $s = 1.0$ and $g = 0.0$. Note that when d_{ijk} is high, such that the item is very easy or the person's ability is high, the probability of passing the item is well approximated by the probability of passing the first component. However, when d_{ijk} is low, then the regression on θ_1 decreases sharply. Furthermore, the asymptotic value is not 1.0; it is the second component probability, as specified by the logit.

A variant of MLTM is appropriate for sequentially dependent strategies (Embretson, 1985), each of which may contain one or more components. In this case, the alternative strategies are attempted, in turn, only if the primary strategy fails. Thus, the probability of solving the item is represented as the sum of the conditional strategy probabilities. For example, a multiple strategy theory of verbal analogy solving could assume that the main strategy is the rule-oriented as described above. If that strategy fails, then an associated strategy, finding an alternative that has high associative strength to the third term to the alternatives, is attempted. If that fails, then random guessing is attempted. The following strategy model represents this example:

$$P_T = (s_r - g)P_1P_2 + (s_a - g)P_a(1 - P_1P_2) + g, \tag{3}$$

where P_T, P_1, P_2, and P_a are probabilities that depend on persons and items, as in Eq. (1), but for brevity omitting the full notation. P_T is the total-item probability, P_1 and P_2 are component probabilities for the rule-oriented strategy, P_a is a component probability for the associational strategy, s_r is the probability of applying the rule-oriented strategy, s_a is the conditional probability of applying the associational strategy and g is the conditional probability of guessing correctly.

GLTM, a generalization of MLTM, permits constraints to be placed on item difficulty, similar to the Linear Logistic Latent Trait Model (LLTM)

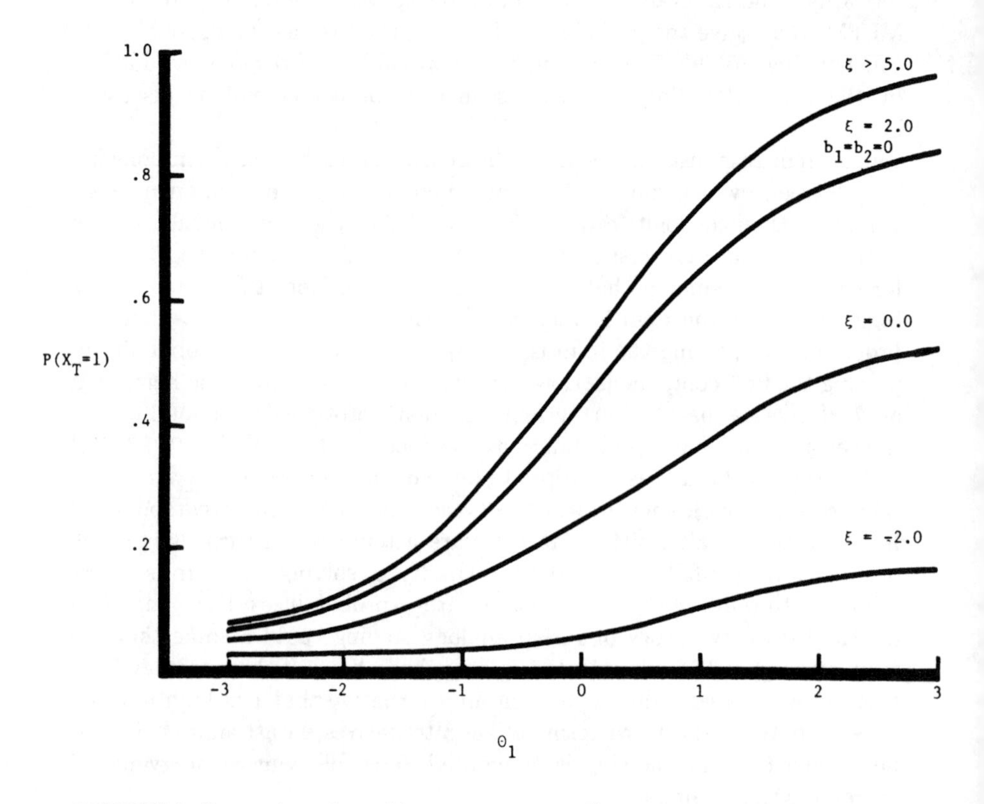

FIGURE 1. Regression of total item response on Component 1 ability as a function of Component 2 logit.

(Fischer, 1983; this volume). Unlike LLTM, in which only the total item response is modeled, GLTM sets constraints within components. These constraints permit a cognitive model of task difficulty, based on the item stimulus features, to be embedded in the measurement model.

The full GLTM may be written as follows:

$$P(U_{ijT} = 1 \mid \underline{\theta}_j, \underline{\alpha}_k, \underline{\beta}_k) = (s-g) \prod_k \frac{\exp(\theta_{jk} - \sum_m \beta_{mk} v_{imk} + \alpha_g)}{1 + \exp(\theta_{jk} - \sum_{mk} \beta_{mk} v_{imk} + \alpha_k)} + g, \tag{4}$$

where θ_{jk} is defined as in Eq. (2), v_{imk} is a score representing the difficulty of item 1 on stimulus factor m in component k, β_{mk} is the weight of stimulus complexity factor m in item difficulty on component k, α_k is the normalization constant for component k, s is the probability of applying the component outcomes.

Parameter Estimation

The original MLTM and GLTM estimation method (Embretson, 1984; Whitely, 1980) required subtasks to identify the component parameters. The subtasks operationalize a theory of task processing. For example, the rule-oriented process for solving the verbal analogy presented above would be operationalized as follows: (1) the total task, with standard instructions, (2) the rule construction subtask, in which the stem (Event:Memory::Fire:?) is presented, with instructions to give the rule in the analogy, and (3) the response evaluation subtask, the total task plus the correct rule, with instructions to select the alternative that fulfills the rule.

There are 2^{K+1} possible responses patterns for an item, where K is the number of postulated components. For example, Table 1 presents a sample space for two components and a total task, with eight possible response patterns. MLTM, from Eq. (2), would give the probabilities of the response pattern as shown in the last column. Now, if $\underline{U}_p$ is the vector of responses U_{ij1}, U_{ij2}, U_{ijT} to the two components and total task for person j on item i, s, P_1, and P_2 are defined as in Eqs. (1) and (2) and Q_1 and Q_2 are $(1 - P_1)$ and $(1 - P_2)$, respectively, the probability of any response pattern can be given as

$$P(\underline{u}_p) = [g^{u_T}(1-g)^{1-u_T}]^{1-\Pi u_k}[s^{u_T}(1-s)^{1-u_T}]^{\Pi u_k} \prod_k [P_k^{u_k} Q_k^{1-u_k}], \tag{5a}$$

where the subscripts i and j are omitted in this expression, for brevity.

Note that s, the probability of applying component outcomes, enters into the probability only if the components are passed ($\prod u_k = 1$), while g enters only if the components are failed ($1 - \prod u_k = 1$). Furthermore, the status of the total task determines if s and g or their compliments enter into the equation. Assuming local independence, the probabilities given in Eq. (5)

TABLE 1. Response Patterns, MLTM Probabilities and Observed Frequencies for a Two-Component Verbal Analogy Task.

C_1	C_2	T	MLTM	Probabilities	Observed Frequencies
0	0	0	$(1-g)$	$Q_1\ Q_2$	202
0	1	0	$(1-g)$	$Q_1\ P_2$	539
1	0	0	$(1-g)$	$P_1\ Q_2$	97
1	1	0	$(1-s)$	$P_1\ P_2$	352
0	0	1	g	$Q_1\ Q_2$	64
0	1	1	g	$Q_1\ P_2$	539
1	0	1	g	$P_1\ Q_2$	57
1	1	1	s	$P_1\ P_2$	1789

can be multiplied over items and persons to obtain the joint likelihood of the data, L, as follows:

$$L = \prod_j \prod_i [g^{u_T}(1-g)^{1-u_T}]^{1-\Pi u_k}[s^{u_T}(1-s)^{1-u_T}]^{\Pi u_k} \prod_k [P_k^{u_k} Q_k^{1-u_k}]. \quad (5b)$$

Since neither s nor g vary over items or persons, well-known theorems on the binomial distribution (e.g., Andersen, 1980) can be applied to give the maximum likelihood estimators as their relative frequencies, as follows:

$$s = \sum_j \sum_i \left(\prod_k u_k \right) u_T \Big/ \sum_j \sum_i \prod_k u_k \quad (6a)$$

and

$$g = \sum_j \sum_i \left(1 - \prod_k u_k \right) u_T \Big/ \sum_j \sum_i \left(1 - \prod_k u_k \right). \quad (6b)$$

Taking the partial derivative of L with respect to b_{ik}, yields the following estimation equation for items:

$$\partial \ln L / \partial b_{ik} = \sum_j (u_{ijk} - (1 + \exp(b_{ik} - \theta_{jk}))^{-1}). \quad (7)$$

Setting the derivatives to zero gives the I estimation equations for item difficulties of the K components. Note that the estimation equations for each component involves only data from the corresponding subtask. Thus, the joint maximum likelihood estimates may be obtained independently from the subtasks. If a CML procedure is applied, the conditions for the existence and uniqueness of the estimates are well established (Fischer, 1983; this volume). Similarly, the person component parameters can be estimated, given the item component difficulties, by maximum likelihood. Program MULTICOMP (Embretson, 1984) may be used to provide the estimates for both MLTM and GLTM.

The original maximum likelihood estimation algorithm for MLTM and GLTM (Embretson, 1984), as described above, is feasible if subtasks can be used to identify the components. However, the algorithm is limited if: (1) subtask data are impractical or (2) metacomponent abilities are involved in task performance. Metacomponents are not readily represented by subtasks, because they involve guiding the problem solving process across items to assure that effective strategies are applied. The population parameter s does represent metacomponent functioning, but it is constant over persons and items.

Recently, Maris (1992) has developed a program for estimating latent item responses which is based on the Dempster et al. (1977) EM algorithm. The EM algorithm is appropriate for all kinds of missing data problems. In the Maris (1992) implementation of the EM algorithm for conjunctive models, the probabilities for components in MLTM, $P(U_{ijk} = 1 \mid \theta_{jk}, b_{ik})$, are treated as missing data. Thus, component parameters can be estimated directly from the total task, without subtask data. Maris (1992) has operationalized both maximum likelihood and modal a posteriori (Bayesian) estimators for conjunctive models, such as MLTM, in his program COLORA (Maris, 1993). Although only a partial proof for finite parameter estimates in conjunctive models is available, simulation data do support the convergence of the estimates. The current version of COLORA, however, is somewhat limited in handling large data sets, since person parameters must be estimated jointly with item parameters. A planned MML estimation procedure will greatly expand data handling capacity.

It should be noted that the Maris (1992) program for conjunctive models, if applied without subtask data, estimates components that are empirically-driven to provide fit. The components do not necessarily correspond to any specified theoretical component unless appropriate restrictions are placed on the solution. Although Maris (1992) recommends using subtask data to place the appropriate restrictions, another method is to place certain restrictions on the parameters, in accordance with prior theory. This will be shown below in the Examples section.

Goodness of Fit

Goodness of fit for items in MLTM or GLTM may be tested by either a Pearsonian or likelihood ratio chi-square. The 2^{K+1} response patterns for each item, including the total task and K components, can be treated as multinomial responses. To obtain a sufficient number of observations in each group, persons must be grouped by ability estimates, jointly on the basis of K component abilities. The number of intervals for each component depends on the ability distributions and the sample size. In general, for the goodness-of-fit statistic to be distributed as χ^2, no fewer than five observations should be expected for any group. The Pearsonian goodness-of-fit statistic for items can be given as follows:

$$G_p^2 = \sum_g \sum_p (r_{igp} - N_{ig}P(\underline{U}_{ig}))^2 / N_{ig}P(\underline{U}_{igp}), \tag{8}$$

where $P(\underline{U}_{igp})$ is the probability of the response pattern from Eq. (5), r_{igp} is the number of observations on pattern p in score group g for item i, N_{ig} is the number of observations in score group g on item i.

Alternatively, the likelihood ratio goodness-of-fit test can be given as follows:

$$G_L^2 = 2\sum_g \sum_p r_{igp}(In(r_{igp}/N_{ig}P(\underline{U}_{igp}))). \tag{9}$$

Bock (1975) notes that small sample simulations show that G_L^2 is more powerful than G_P^2. If G is the number of groups and P is the number of item categories, the degrees of freedom for Eqs. (8) or (9) can be given the number of cells minus the number of constraints from the expected values. Following Bock and Mislevy (1990) in assuming no constraints for score groups, the degrees of freedom are $G(P-1)$. These values can be summed over items for a global test of fit.

In the case of GLTM, alternative models of component item difficulty (from the stimulus complexity factors v_{ikm}) can be compared by a likelihood ratio χ^2, based on the estimation algorithm, if the models are hierarchially nested. If L_1 and L_2 are the likelihoods of two models, such that L_1 is nested within L_2, a chi-square goodness-of-fit test can be given as follows:

$$G_N^2 = -2(\ln L_1 - \ln L_2), \tag{10}$$

which can be assumed to be asymptotically distributed as χ with degrees of freedom equal to the difference in the number of parameters between the two models.

Since likelihood ratio comparison tests, like Eq. (10), are sensitive to sample size, a fit index is useful to guide interpretations. Fit indices have often been proposed in the context of structural equation modeling (e.g., Bentler and Bonnett, 1980). Embretson (1983a) developed a fit index for LLTM and GLTM that utilized comparisons to a null model (in which all items are postulated to be equally difficult) and a saturated model (in which separate difficulties are estimated for each item). Thus, within a component, the null model, L_0, would be specified as a constant value for item difficulties, while the saturated model, L_s, would be the Rasch model. The model to be evaluated, L_m, contains at least one less parameter than the saturated model. The fit index, Δ^2, is given as follows:

$$\Delta^2 = (\ln L_0 - \ln L_m)/(\ln L_0 - \ln L_s). \tag{11}$$

Roughly, the denominator of Eq. (11) indicates the amount of information that could be modeled, since the saturated model is compared with the null model. The numerator compares the information in the proposed model with the null model. Alternatively, the fit index in Eq. (11) may also be formulated as a ratio of G_N^2 the goodness-of-fit statistics, from various pairs of models, as follows:

$$\Delta^2 = (G^2_{n/s} - G^2_{m/s})/G^2_{n/s}. \tag{12}$$

Embretson (1983a) finds that Δ^2 is very close in magnitude to the squared product moment correlation of the Rasch model item difficulties with the estimated value for item difficulty from the complexity factor model [obtained by evaluating the logistic function for items in Eq. (4)].

Examples

Component Processes in Verbal Analogies

Historically, verbal analogies have been often considered the best item type for measuring "g" (Spearman, 1927). More recently, they have been studied intensively by cognitive component analysis (e.g., Sternberg, 1977). Understanding the processing components that are involved in solving verbal analogies contributes to construct representation aspect of construct validity [see Embretson (1983b)].

Whitely and Schneider (1980) present several studies on the components of verbal analogy items. In these studies, both the rule construction and the response evaluation subtask are used to identify components. Additionally, however, subtasks are also used to identify alternative processing strategies. For example, the success of an associative strategy is measured by presenting the third term (Fire:) and the response alternatives. The person attempts to find the alternative that has the highest associative relationship. In the analogy above, this strategy would not be very successful since two distractors (Matches, Heat) have strong associative relationships to Fire. Furthermore, a working backwards strategy has been measured with a subtask for rule construction after the person has viewed the response alternatives.

MLTM and its variants, such as Eq. (5) can be compared by examining their fit, using the chi-square tests described above, plots of observed and predicted values, and the fit of the subtasks to the Rasch model (implicit in MLTM and GLTM). In one study, Whitely and Schneider (1980) fit the original MLTM (Whitely, 1980), which is Eq. (3) without the s or g parameters. They found that fit was substantially increased by adding a guessing parameter to the model, while adding the working backwards strategy resulted in only some improvement in fit. However, this study preceded the development of the full MLTM and GLTM models that contain both the s and g parameters.

Table 1 shows the probabilities for the various response patterns in a reanalysis of the Whitely and Schneider (1980) data, which contained 35 items and 104 subjects. Response patterns that are inconsistent in the original Whitely (1980) model are quite frequent. That is, the item is often solved when the components are failed, and the item is sometimes failed when the components are solved. Thus, both g and s, to represent guessing and strategy application, respectively, are appropriate for the data. MLTM, from Eq. (3) was fit to the data. The s parameter was found to be 0.84, while the g parameter was 0.39. The latter is higher than the expected 0.25 from random guessing in the multiple choice items. However, the two components were relatively independent sources of item difficulty as indicated by a moderately low correlation of 0.44.

Model fit was examined by a Pearson chi-square, as described above. Since the sample size was small, the data were collapsed into two response patterns, on the basis of the total item outcome. Subjects were categorized into four groups, by splitting jointly on the two components. G_P^2 was computed for each item and then summed over items. The observed value of G_P^2 was 200.64, which with 140 degrees of freedom is significant at the 0.05 level.

Although the model failed to fit, useful predictions were made by the model. The total item probabilities correlated 0.70 with the MLTM predictions. Furthermore, the person's accuracy on the total item correlated 0.73 with MLTM predictions. It should be noted that five items failed to fit the model. By eliminating these items, and reanalyzing the data, G_P^2 was 107.81, which did not exceed χ_{120}^2 at the 0.05 level. Thus, the poor overall fit was due only to a few items.

GLTM was estimated since stimulus complexity factor scores were available for 18 of the 35 analogy items. The available scores represent aspects of rule construction. Embretson and Schneider (1989) find substantial evidence for a contextualized inference process, in which inferences are modified by the third analogy term, but not by the response alternatives. Table 2[1] shows the GLTM parameter estimates for the stimulus complexity factor estimates for the rule construction component. It can be seen that difficult items are more likely to involve new inferences on the additional of the full stem context (i.e., the third term). Easy items, in contrast, are more likely to have many inferences available initially and to involve the selection of an inference from those initially available. The loglikelihood of the GLTM model, with these stimulus complexity factors, was -1065.91. The loglikelihoods of the null model (constant values for the first component only) and the saturated model were -1375.99 and -1003.13, respectively. Thus, compared to the null model, the model with five stimulus complexity factors fit significantly better ($\chi_5^2 = 620.16$, $p < 0.001$), but did not fit as well

[1] *Note to Table 2:* ** means $p < 0.01$.

TABLE 2. Stimulus Complexity Factor Weights for Rule Construction Component.

Variable	β	σ_β
Number of initial inferences	-0.871^{**} $p < .01$	0.273
Probability correct inference in stem context	-1.298^{**} $p < .01$	0.376
New inferences in stem context	4.708^{**} $p < .01$	1.084
Select inferences in stem context	-6.435^{**} $p < .01$	1.785
Modify inferences in stem context	-2.069	1.369

as the saturated Rasch model ($\chi^2_{12} = 62.78$, $p < 0.001$). However, the fit index Δ^2 of 0.83 was relatively high, showing the usefulness of the stimulus complexity factor model in explaining rule construction difficulty.

The various results on model fitting indicate that the rule-oriented strategy accounts fairly well for solving verbal analogies, thus supporting the task as measuring inductive reasoning. However, some items involve different strategies, such as association (Embretson 1985). Eliminating such items will improve the construct representation of the test.

The component person parameters from verbal analogies have also been used in several studies on nomothetic span (e.g., Embretson et al., 1986). These will not be illustrated here because the next empirical application focuses on nomothetic span.

Working Memory versus General Control Processes

Another empirical application (Embretson, 1995b) uses the Maris (1992) EM algorithm to distinguish between two competing explanations of fluid intelligence. Many theories (Brown, 1978; Sternberg, 1985) suggest that general control processes, or metacomponents, are the most important source of individual differences. These control processes are used by the examinee to select, maintain and evaluate a strategy for item solving. Alternatively, other theories emphasize the role of working memory capacity in inference processes. For example, both Carpenter et al. and Kyllonen and Christal (1990) suggest that working memory capacity is the primary basis of individual differences in fluid intelligence.

Working memory can be distinguished from general control processing on a measuring task for general intelligence by GLTM if some constraints are set to identify the hypothesized components. A bank of progressive matrices items, which are well established measures of fluid intelligence, had been specially constructed to represent the Carpenter et al. (1990) theory. Thus, the memory load of each item, according to the theory, was known. Several forms of the Abstract Reasoning Test were administered to 577 Air Force recruits. Additionally, subtest scores from the Armed Services Vocational

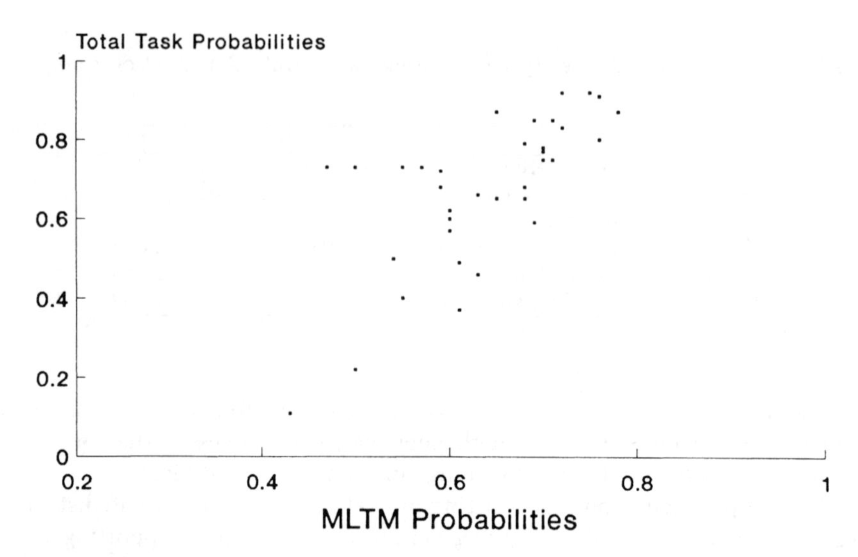

FIGURE 2. Scatterplot of total task probabilities by predicted values from MLTM model for items.

Aptitude Battery (ASVAB) were available to examine the impact of the two components on nomothetic span.

To distinguish general control progressing from working memory capacity, a model with two latent (i.e., covert) response variables was postulated. The first latent response variable, U_{ij1}, is strategy application. This variable reflects the implementation of the rule strategy in task processing. The second latent response variable, U_{ij2}, is the success of the inference strategy. The following model may be postulated for the total task, U_{ijT}:

$$P(U_{ijT} = 1) = P(U_{ij1})P(U_{ij2}). \tag{13}$$

To identify working memory capacity in Eq. (13), indices of memory load are required for each item. No item information is required for general control processes since items are assumed to have a constant value. Thus, the full model, with the person and item parameters that govern the latent response variables is the following:

$$P(U_{ijT} = 1 \mid \underline{\theta}_j, \underline{\alpha}, \underline{\beta}) = \frac{\exp(\theta_{j1} - \alpha_1)}{1 + \exp(\theta_{j1} - \alpha_1)} \frac{\exp(\theta_{j2} - \beta_2 v_{i2} - \alpha_2)}{1 + \exp(\theta_{j2} - \beta_2 v_{i2} - \alpha_2)}, \tag{14}$$

where θ_{j1} is the ability for person j on general control processes, α_1 is an intercept which expresses the (constant) difficulty of items on strategy application, θ_{j2} is working memory capacity for person j, v_{i2} is the score for item i on memory load, β_2 is the weight of memory load in rule inference difficulty, and α_2 is an intercept for rule inference difficulty.

The parameters for the model in Eq. (14) were estimated with the COLORA program (Maris, 1993). A Pearsonian chi-square test indicated that

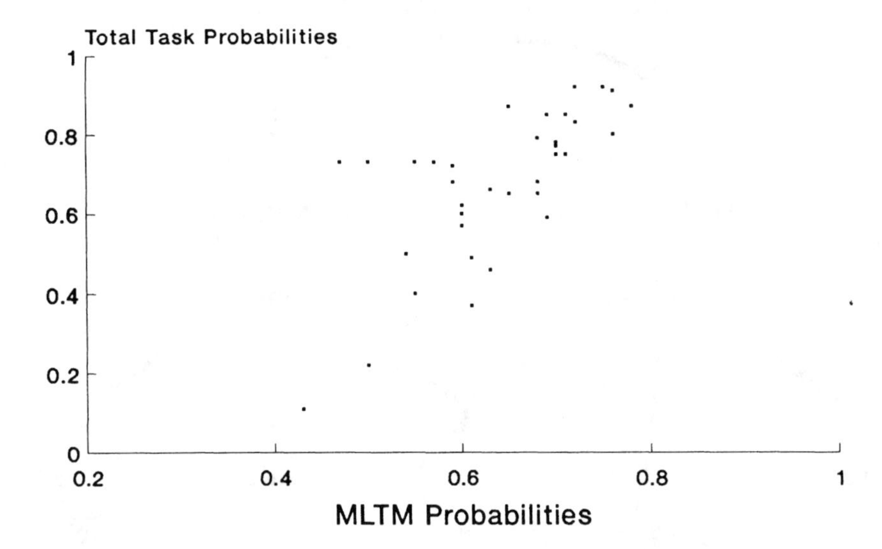

FIGURE 3. Scatterplot of total task probabilities by predicted values from MLTM model for persons.

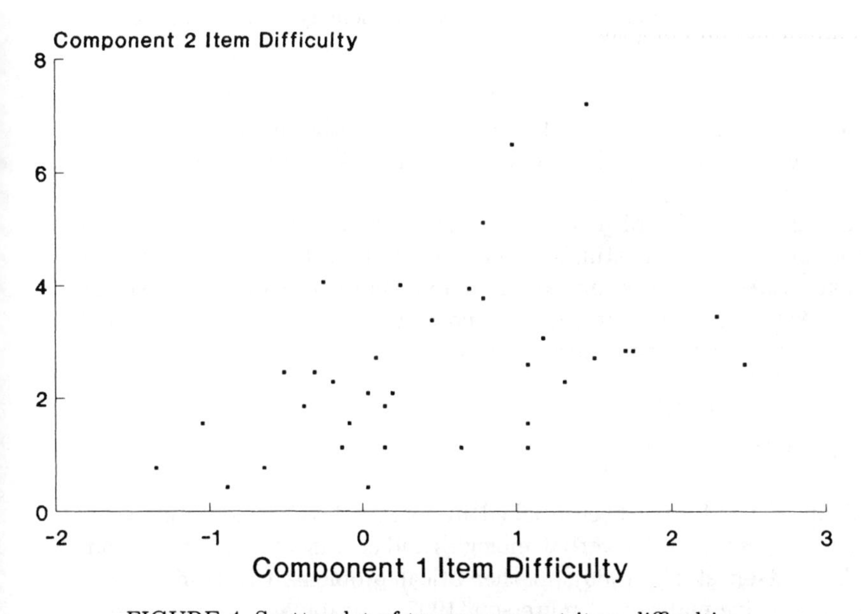

FIGURE 4. Scatterplot of two component item difficulties.

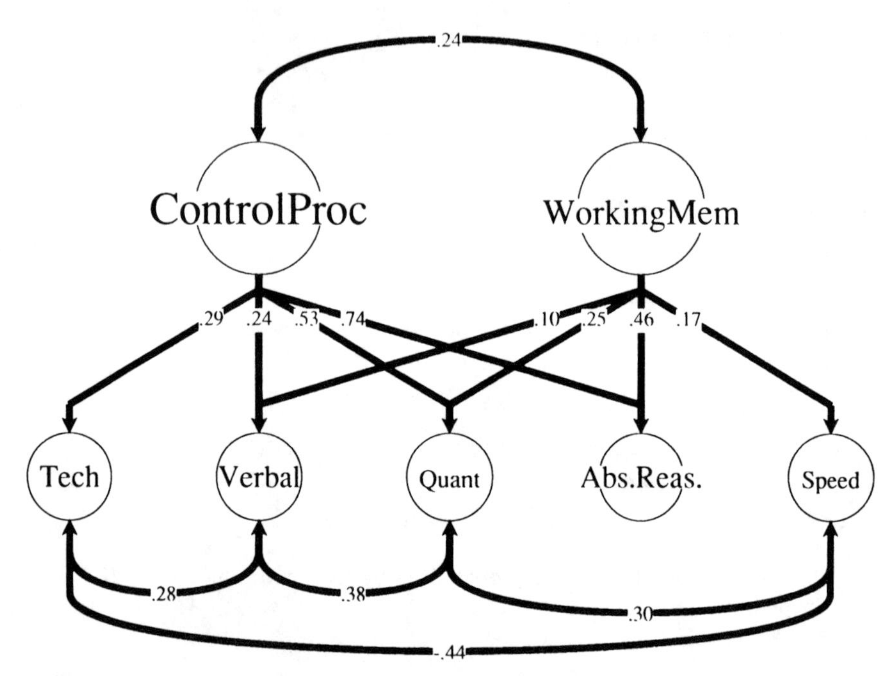

FIGURE 5. Structural equation model of working memory and general control processes and reference tests.

the data fit the model ($p > 0.05$). Furthermore, the average prediction residuals were small (0.06), for predicting total task probabilities from the model.

In summary, the MLTM model with latent response variables separated the contribution of two postulated components to abstract reasoning. The results suggested that although both components had a role in construct validity, general control processes are a more important source of individual differences than working memory capacity.

Discussion

MLTM and GLTM have been applied in construct validation studies on many item types, including verbal analogies and classifications (Embretson, 1985; Embretson et al., 1986), mathematical problems (Bertrand et al., 1993), progressive matrices (Embretson, 1993), vocabulary items (Janssen et al., 1991) and spatial tasks (McCollam and Embretson, 1993).

MLTM and GLTM have special advantages in contemporary construct validation studies, as illustrated in the two examples above, because they provide a complete set of parameters to represent both person and task differences in processing. The cognitive processing paradigm in aptitude research permits two aspects of construct validity, construct representation and nomothetic span (Embretson, 1983b), to be separated. Construct representation research concerns what is measured by identifying the underlying processes, knowledge structures and strategies that are involved in task performance. Mathematical modeling is a primary technique in such research. Nomothetic span research concerns the utility of tests, through correlations with other measures.

Another application is test design to measure specified cognitive components. If only one component is to be measured, the item difficulties on the other components must be well below the level of the target population. Ideally, the other component probabilities should approach 1.0. This can be accomplished in two ways. First, items with low b_{ik}'s on the other components can be eliminated during item selection. Second, and perhaps more efficient, the stimulus complexity factors in GLTM can be used to guide item writing. That is, items can be constructed to vary on those features that predict the b_{ik} on the target component but not on the other component. Thus, inappropriate items can be readily eliminated before item tryout.

Furthermore, MLTM and GLTM are useful in studies on individual differences. For example, sex differences are often found in mathematical problem solving. Bertrand et al. (1993) measured two underlying components of mathematical problem solving so as to pinpoint the source of sex differences, if any. Although no sex differences were observed on the computational component (involving strategic and algorithmic knowledge to solve systems of equations), boys did show higher abilities on the mathematization component (involving factual, linguistic and schematic knowledge to set up the equations). Bertrand et al. (1993) also examined the impact of lifestyle differences between students (number of hours spent watching television, reading, and so on) on the two components and on the total task.

It should be noted that research applications of MLTM and GLTM are especially active now, due to advances in the algorithm and the development of new computerized tests. Thus, continued activity can be expected both in aspects of the estimation algorithm and in applications.

Note to References: Susan E. Embretson has also published as Susan E. Whitely.

References

Andersen, E.B. (1980). *Discrete Statistical Models with Social Science Applications.* Amsterdam: North Holland.

Bentler, P.M. and Bonnett, D.G. (1980). Significance tests and goodness of fit in the analysis of covariance structures. *Psychological Bulletin* **88**,

588–606.

Bertrand, R., Dupuis, F.A., and Garneau, M. (1993). Effets des caracteristiques des items sur le role des composantes impliquees dans la performance enresolution de problemes mathematiques ecrits: une etude de validite de construit. *Rapport Final Presente au Fonds pour la Formation de Chercheurs et l'Aide a la Recherche.* Universite Laval, Santa-Foy, Quebec, Canada: Mars.

Bock, R.D. (1975). *Multivariate Statistical Methods in Behavioral Research.* New York, NY: McGraw-Hill.

Brown, A.L. (1978). Knowing when, where, and how to remember. In R. Glaser (Ed), *Advances in Instructional Psychology* (Vol. 1). Hillsdale, NJ: Erlbaum.

Carpenter, P.A., Just, M.A., and Shell, P. (1990). What one intelligence test measures: A theoretical account of processing in the Raven's Progressive Matrices Test. *Psychological Review*, 97.

Dempster, A.P., Laird, N.M., and Rubin, D.B. (1977). Maximum likelihood estimating with incomplete data via the EM algorithm. *Journal of the Royal Statistical Society, Series B*, **39**, 1–38.

Embretson, S.E. (1983a). *An incremental fix index for the linear logistic latent trait model.* Paper presented at the Annual Meeting of the Psychometric Society, Los Angeles, CA.

Embretson, S.E. (1983b). Construct validity: Construct representation versus nomothetic span. *Psychological Bulletin* **93**, 179–197.

Embretson, S.E. (1984). A general multicomponent latent trait model for response processes. *Psychometrika* **49**, 175–186.

Embretson, S.E. (1985). Multicomponent latent trait models for test design. In S. Embretson (Ed), *Test Design: Developments in Psychology and Psychometrics* (pp. 195–218). New York, NY: Academic Press.

Embretson, S.E. (1994). Applications to cognitive design systems to test development. In C. Reynolds (Ed), *Advances in Cognitive Assessment: An Interdisciplinary Perspective* (pp. 107–135). Plenum.

Embretson, S.E. (1995a). A measurement model for linking individual learning to processes and knowledge: Application and mathematical reasoning. *Journal of Educational Measurement* **32**, 277–294.

Embretson, S.E. (1995b). Working memory capacity versus general control processes in abstract reasoning. *Intelligence* **20**, 169–189.

Embretson, S.E. and Schneider, L.M. (1989). Cognitive models of analogical reasoning for psychometric tasks. *Learning and Individual Differences* **1**, 155–178.

Embretson, S.E., Schneider, L.M., and Roth, D.L. (1986). Multiple processing strategies and the construct validity of verbal reasoning tests. *Journal of Educational Measurement* **23**, 13–32.

Fischer, G.H. (1983). Logistic latent trait models with linear constraints. *Psychometrika* **48**, 3–26.

Janssen, R., Hoskens, M., and DeBoeck, P. (1991). A test of Embretson's multicomponent model on vocabulary items. In R. Steyer and K. Widaman (Eds), *Psychometric Methodology* (pp. 187–190). Stuttgart, Germany: Springer-Verlag.

Kyllonen, P. and Christal, R. (1990). Reasoning ability is (little more than) working memory capacity? *Intelligence* **14**, 389–434.

Maris, E.M. (1992). *Psychometric models for psychological processes and structures.* Invited paper presented at the European Meeting of the Psychometric Society. Barcelona, Spain: Pompeau Fabre University.

Mayer, R., Larkin, J., and Kadane, P. (1984). A cognitive analysis of mathematical problem solving. In R. Sternberg (Ed), *Advances in the Psychology of Human Intelligence*, Vol. 2 (pp. 231–273). Hillsdale, NJ: Erlbaum Publishers.

McCollam, K. and Embretson, S.E. (1993). Components or strategies? The basis of individual differences in spatial processing. Unpublished paper. Lawrence, Kansas: University of Kansas.

Mislevy, R.J. and Bock, R.D. (1990). BILOG 3: *Item Analysis and Test Scoring with Binary Logistic Models.* In: Scientific Software.

Mulholland, T., Pellegrino, J.W., and Glaser, R. (1980). Components of geometric analogy solution. *Cognitive Psychology* **12**, 252–284.

Pellegrino, J.W., Mumaw, R., and Shute, V. (1985). Analyses of spatial aptitude and expertise. In S. Embretson (Ed), *Test Design: Developments in Psychology and Psychometrics* (pp. 45–76). New York, NY: Academic Press.

Spearman, C. (1927). *The Abilities of Man.* New York: Macmillan.

Sternberg, R.J. (1977). *Intelligence, Information Processing and Analogical Reasoning: The Componential Analysis of Human Abilities.* Hillsdale, NJ: Erlbaum.

Whitely, S.E. (1980). Multicomponent latent trait models for ability tests. *Psychometrika* **45**, 479–494.

Whitely, S.E. (1981). Measuring aptitude processes with multicomponent latent trait models. *Journal of Educational Measurement* **18**, 67–84.

Whitely, S.E. and Schneider, L.M. (1980). *Process Outcome Models for Verbal Aptitude.* (Technical Report NIE-80-1). Lawrence, Kansas: University of Kansas.

19

Multidimensional Linear Logistic Models for Change

Gerhard H. Fischer and Elisabeth Seliger[1]

Introduction

The chapter presents a family of multidimensional logistic models for change, which are based on the Rasch model (RM) and on the linear logistic test model (LLTM; see Fischer, this volume), but unlike these models do not require unidimensionality of the items. As will be seen, to abandon the unidimensionality requirement becomes possible under the assumption that the same items are presented to the testees on two or more occasions. This relaxation of the usual unidimensionality axiom of IRT is of great advantage especially in typical research problems of educational, applied, or clinical psychology, where items or symptoms often are heterogeneous. [See Stout (1987, 1990) for a quite different approach to weakening the strict unidimensionality assumption.] Consider, for example, the problem of monitoring cognitive growth in children: A set of items appropriate for assessing intellectual development will necessarily contain items that address a number of different intelligence factors. If we knew what factors there are, and which of the items measure what factor, we might construct several unidimensional scales. This is unrealistic, however, because the factor structures in males and females, above- and below-average children, etc., generally differ, so that there is little hope of arriving at sufficiently unidimensional scales applicable to *all* children. Therefore, a model of change that makes no assumption about the latent dimensionality of the items is a very valuable tool for applied research.

The family of models to be treated in this chapter comprises models for two or more time points and for both dichotomous and polytomous items. The common element in all of them is that repeated measurement designs

[1]This research was supported in part by the Fonds zur Förderung der Wissenschaftlichen Forschung, Vienna, under Grant No. P19118-HIS.

are posited and that testees are characterized by parameter vectors $\boldsymbol{\theta}_j = (\theta_{1j}, \ldots, \theta_{nj})$ rather than by scalar person parameters θ_j; the components of $\boldsymbol{\theta}_j$ are associated with the items $I_1, \ldots, I_n$, and thus a separate latent dimension is assigned to each and every item in the test. It should be stressed from the beginning, however, that no assumptions are made about the mutual dependence or independence of these latent dimensions, which means that they can be conceived, for instance, as functions of a smaller number of ability factors, or even of a single factor. The models are therefore very flexible and applicable to various areas of research.

Fischer (this volume) shows how the (unidimensional dichotomous) LLTM can be used for measuring change: The same item I_i presented on different occasions is considered as a set of "virtual items" I_{it}^*, $t = 1, 2, \ldots, z$, characterized by "virtual item parameters" β_{it}^*. These β_{it}^* are then decomposed, e.g., as

$$\beta_{it}^* = \beta_i + \sum_l q_{jlt}\eta_l, \tag{1}$$

where β_i is the difficulty parameter of item I_i in a Rasch model, q_{jlt} is the dosage of treatment B_l given to persons S_j up to time point T_t (with $q_{il1} = 0$ for all S_j and all B_l), and η_l is the effect of one unit of treatment B_j. (The latter can be educational treatments, trainings, instruction, clinical therapies, psychotherapies, or any experimental conditions that influence the response behavior of the testees.) The probabilistic item response model, as in any LLTM, is

$$\text{logit } P(+ \mid S_j, I_i, T_t) = \theta_j - \beta_{it}^*, \tag{2}$$

that is, the difference between the person parameter and the (virtual) item parameter is the argument in a logistic IRF.

We shall now relax the unidimensionality of the θ-dimension by assuming that each person S_j may have n different abilities θ_{ij}, $i = 1, \ldots, n$, corresponding to the items $I_1, \ldots, I_n$ of the test. For time point T_1, $q_{jl1} = 0$ implies $\beta_{i1}^* = \beta_i$, so that the β_{i1}^* equal the difficulty parameters of the items. Inserting θ_{ij} instead of θ_j in Eq. (2), we get for T_1 that

$$\text{logit } P(+ \mid S_j, I_i, T_1) = \theta_{ij} - \beta_i, \tag{3}$$

which obviously is overparameterized: The item parameters β_i can immediately be absorbed into the θ_{ij}, giving new person parameters $\tilde{\theta}_{ij} = \theta_{ij} - \beta_i$; for simplicity, however, we shall drop the tildes and write

$$\text{logit } P(+ \mid S_j, I_i, T_1) = \theta_{ij}, \tag{4}$$

which is equivalent to setting $\beta_i = 0$ for all items I_i for normalization. Note that this is admissible because there are n such normalization conditions for the n independent latent scales. Similarly, for time point T_2 we get

$$\text{logit } P(+ \mid S_j, I_i, T_2) = \theta_{ij} - \sum_l q_{jl2}\eta_l. \tag{5}$$

The model defined by Eqs. (4) and (5) has been denoted the "linear logistic model with relaxed assumptions" [LLRA; Fischer (1977b)], which expresses that the assumption of the unidimensionality of the items has been abandoned.

Presentation of the Models

The LLRA for Two Time Points

Equations (4) and (5) are equivalent with

$$P(+ \mid S_j, I_i, T_1) = \frac{\exp(\theta_{ij})}{1 + \exp(\theta_{ij})}, \tag{6}$$

$$P(+ \mid S_j, I_i, T_2) = \frac{\exp(\theta_{ij} - \delta_j)}{1 + \exp(\theta_{ij} - \delta_j)}, \tag{7}$$

$$\delta_j = \sum_l q_{jl} \eta_l, \tag{8}$$

where q_{jl} is used for simplicity as an abbreviation of q_{jl2} if only two time points, T_1 and T_2, are considered. This is the form in which the LLRA usually appeared in the literature (Fischer, 1976, 1977a, 1977b, 1983a, 1983b, 1995b; Fischer and Formann, 1982). For convenience, we summarize the notation as follows:

θ_{ij} is person S_j's position on latent dimension D_i measured by item I_i at time point T_1,

δ_j is the amount of change in S_j between T_1 and T_2,

q_{jl} is the dosage of treatment B_j given to S_j between T_1 and T_2,

η_l is the effect of one unit of treatment B_l, $l = 1, \ldots, m$.

Equation (8) is often specified more explicitly as

$$\delta_j = \sum_l q_{jl} \eta_l + \sum_{l<k} q_{jl} q_{jk} \rho_{lk} + \tau, \tag{9}$$

where (in addition to the "main effects" η_e)

ρ_{lk} are interaction effects between treatments, $B_l \times B_k$, and

τ is a "trend effect," which comprises all causes of change that are unrelated to the treatments (e.g., general maturation of children and/or effects of repeated use of the same items).

Note that, upon appropriate redefinition of the q_{jl}, Eq. (9) always can be written in the simpler form of Eq. (8), because Eq. (9) is linear in all effect parameters η_l, ρ_{lk}, and τ. Equation (8) is therefore the more general decomposition of the change parameters δ_j, and it is more convenient for mathematical manipulations.

The LLRA for measuring change might on first sight seem rather arbitrary, because no justification for the choice of the logistic IRF and for the additivity of the effect parameters was given. Both can be derived, however, from the postulate that "specifically objective" comparisons of treatments via their effect parameters η_l be feasible, where specifically objective is synonymous with "generalizable over subjects with arbitrary parameters $\boldsymbol{\theta}_j$." [Some technical assumptions are also required, though, that cannot be discussed here. The model derivable from these assumptions essentially is of the form of Eqs. (6) and (7), however, the argument of the logistic IRF in Eqs. (6) and (7) is multiplied by an unspecified (discrimination) parameter $\alpha > 0$, which here has been equated to $\alpha = 1$.] Hence, if a researcher is inclined to consider the person parameters $\boldsymbol{\theta}_j$ as incidental nuisance parameters and desires to free his results about the treatments of interest of uncontrollable influences of these $\boldsymbol{\theta}_j$, then the LLRA is the model of choice. For a formal treatment of this justification of the LLRA, the interested reader must be referred to Fischer (1987a), see also Fischer (1995b).

Environmental Effects

The LLRA describes changes of reaction probabilities between two occasions, T_1 and T_2, and hence makes use of *pairs* of related observations, u_{ij1} and u_{ij2}. It is obvious that this model can also be employed, for instance, for describing environmental effects on the probabilities of solving items, based on the test data of pairs of twins reared apart (Fischer, 1987b, 1993; Fischer and Formann, 1981). The LLRA therefore is an interesting alternative to the common heritability approach to the nature–nurture discussion.

Let θ_{ij} be a parameter describing, for one pair of monozygotic twins (denoted M_j), the genotypic part of that ability that is required for solving item I_i, and let η_l be a generalized effect of enviroment E_l (or of an environmental factor E_l) on all latent abilities measured by a set of items, together representing "intelligence." Then the LLRA for measuring environmental effects on intelligence assumes that

$$P(+ \mid M_j, I_i, T_{j1}) = \frac{\exp(\theta_{ij} + \sum_l q_{jl1}\eta_l)}{1 + \exp(\theta_{ij} + \sum_l q_{jl1}\eta_l)} = \frac{\exp(\mu_{ij})}{1 + \exp(\mu_{ij})}, \tag{10}$$

where $P(+ \mid M_j, I_i, T_{j1})$ is the probability that twin T_{j1} of pair M_j solves item I_i, given that T_{j1} has received the dosages $q_{j11}, \ldots, q_{jm1}$ of environments (or environmental factors) E_l, and μ_{ij} is the argument of the exponential function in Eq. (10). Similarly,

$$P(+ \mid M_j, I_i, T_{j2}) = \frac{\exp[\theta_{ij} + \sum_l q_{jl2}\eta_l]}{1 + \exp[\theta_{ij} + \sum_l q_{jl2}\eta_l]}$$

$$= \frac{\exp[\mu_{ij} + \sum_l (q_{jl2} - q_{jl1})\eta_l]}{1 + \exp[\mu_{ij} + \sum_l (q_{jl2} - q_{jl1})\eta_l]} \tag{11}$$

is the probability that twin T_{j2} of pair M_j solves item I_i, where T_{j2} has received dosages $q_{j12}, \ldots, q_{jm2}$ of environments (or environmental factors) E_l. Comparing Eqs. (10) and (11) with (6) and (7), it is seen that, if the model is interpreted as an LLRA, in a purely formal sense the parameters $\mu_{ij} = \theta_{ij} + \sum_l q_{jl1}\eta_l$ play the role of "person parameters," and the *differences* $q_{jl2} - q_{jl1}$ that of the treatment "dosages." [Note that it is completely irrelevant which of the two twins of M_j is denoted T_{j1} and which T_{j2}, because interchanging them automatically changes the sign in all differences $q_{jl2} - q_{jl1}$, $l = 1, \ldots, m$, and also adapts the definition of μ_{ij} accordingly. Alternatively, the model can be understood as an LBTL for paired comparisons of different combinations of environmental conditions, see Fischer and Tanzer (1994).]

That the differences $q_{jl2} - q_{jl1}$ are now interpreted as dosages in an LLRA has an important consequence: If the sums $\sum_l (q_{jl2} - q_{jl1})$ are constant across pairs of twins, for instance, if each twin has grown up in just one environment, so that $\sum_l (q_{jl2} - q_{jl1}) = 0$ for all M_j, the η_l are no longer measured on a ratio scale, but only on an *interval scale* [see Fischer (1993)]. Therefore, one environment (or environmental condition) E_a has to be taken as the reference point for the measurement of environmental effects, e.g., $\eta_a = 0$, and all other η_l are calibrated with respect to η_a. This is a logical, even a necessary, consequence, because both genotypic ability and environmental effects on ability can never be determined relative to an absolute zero point. We cannot observe the genetic component of an ability without an environmental influence, and no environmental effect without the presence of a genetic component. Hence, the measurement of environmental effects must be carried out relative to some standard environment.

The present LLRA for environmental effects has many more interesting properties which, however, cannot be further discussed here. The interested reader is referred to Fischer (1993, 1995b). We only mention that the uniqueness conditions for the CML equations of this model imply that even small samples (as are common for data of twins reared apart) suffice for at least a rough estimate of the effects of interest and, especially, for testing hypotheses about such effects. These tests are essentially those described below in the section on hypothesis testing.

The LLRA for Several Time Points

The advantageous properties of the LLRA (see the sections on estimation and hypothesis testing below) encouraged to generalize this model to designs with any number of time points (Fischer, 1989). Assume that the same items are presented repeatedly to the persons at time points $T_1, \ldots, T_t, \ldots, T_z$, while treatments are given in the time intervals; and let the respective item score matrices be denoted by $\mathbf{U}_t$, with elements u_{ijt}.

Assuming that the item set is heterogeneous (multidimensional), as in the LLRA for two time points, individual differences are described again in terms of an n-vector of person parameters $\boldsymbol{\theta}_j = (\theta_{1j}, \ldots, \theta_{nj})$ per person S_j. Change of the persons is modeled via the item parameters, that is, to item I_i there corresponds a sequence of "virtual items," I_{it}^*, with item parameters depending on the treatments given to the person up to time point T_t. Assuming that the persons are grouped by same treatment combinations and same dosages, the virtual item parameters may be written β_{igt}^*, for $i = 1, \ldots, n$ items, $g = 1, \ldots, w$ treatment groups G_g, and $t = 1, \ldots, z$ time points. Now let these item parameters be decomposed, for instance, as

$$\beta_{igt}^* = \beta_i + \sum_l q_{glt}\eta_l + (T_t - T_1)\tau, \tag{12}$$

where the β_i are item difficulty parameters, q_{glt} is the dosage of treatment B_l given to persons of group G_g up to time point T_t, η_l is the effect of one unit of treatment B_l, and τ is the trend. Inserting the θ_{ij} and β_{igt}^* in the logistic IRF, absorbing the β_i in the θ_{ij}-parameters as before, denoting the new person parameters again θ_{ij} for simplicity, and writing $\sum_l q_{glt}\eta_l$ for the sum of effects for short, we obtain as generalization of Eq. (5)

$$\text{logit}\, P(+ \mid S_j, I_i, T_t) = \theta_{ij} - \sum_l q_{glt}\eta_l; \tag{13}$$

equivalently, we may write the probability of a positive response as

$$P(+ \mid S_j, I_i, T_t) = \frac{\exp(\theta_{ij} - \sum_l q_{glt}\eta_l)}{1 + \exp(\theta_{ij} - \sum_l q_{glt}\eta_l)}, \tag{14}$$

for $i = 1, \ldots, n$ items, $j = 1, \ldots, N$ persons, and $t = 1, \ldots, z$ time points. Formally, Eq. (14) can be interpreted as an LLTM, where there are Nn "virtual persons" S_{ij}^* with person parameters θ_{ij}, and $w(z-1)+1$ "virtual items" I_{gt}^* with parameters $\beta_{gt}^* = \sum_e q_{glt}\eta_e$. (Remember that $q_{gl1} = 0$ for all g and l, so that $\beta_{g1}^* = 0$ for all groups G_g.)

Parameter Estimation

LLRA for Two Time Points

It is an easy matter to show that the LLRA for two time points is a special case of an LLTM with a structurally incomplete design and $n_j = 2$ items per person. [Alternatively, the LLRA can be seen as a "Linear Bradley–Terry–Luce" model, LBTL, for the comparison of virtual items, see Fischer and Tanzer (1994)]. The CML estimation equations [see Fischer, this volume, Eq. (7)] can therefore be used for estimating the effect parameters. Nevertheless, it pays to look at the conditional likelihood function of the LLRA separately, because the present special case of only two time points leads to a considerable simplification of the estimation equations. Let the item score matrices for time points T_1 and T_2 be $\mathbf{U}_1 = ((u_{ij1}))$ and $\mathbf{U}_2 = ((u_{ij2}))$, respectively. The likelihood function, conditional on all marginal sums $u_{ij+} = u_{ij1} + u_{ij2}$, is

$$L = P(\mathbf{U}_1, \mathbf{U}_2 \mid \mathbf{U}_1 + \mathbf{U}_2 = \mathbf{U}_+) = \prod_i \prod_j \left(\frac{\exp(u_{ij2}\delta_j)}{1 + \exp(\delta_j)} \right)^{(u_{ij1} - u_{ij2})^2}, \tag{15}$$

where δ_j is subject to Eq. (8). This is easily recognized as the likelihood function of a logit model (Cox, 1970) for a subset of the data; the term $(u_{ij1} - u_{ij2})^2$ acts as a filter eliminating all pairs of responses with $u_{ij1} = u_{ij2}$, which are uninformative with respect to measuring change (measuring treatment effects).

Taking logarithms of the likelihood in Eq. (15) and differentiating with respect to η_l yields the CML estimation equations,

$$\sum_j q_{jl} \sum_i (u_{ij1} - u_{ij2})^2 \left(u_{ij2} - \frac{\exp(\delta_j)}{1 + \exp(\delta_j)} \right) = 0, \tag{16}$$

for $l = 1, \ldots, m$. Equations (16) are *unconditional* estimation equations of a logit model (for a subset of the data as mentioned above); they are very easy to solve—much easier than those of the more general LLTM, see Fischer, this volume—using the well-known Newton–Raphson method. The latter requires the second-order partial derivatives,

$$\frac{\partial^2 \ln L}{\partial \eta_l \partial \eta_k} = -\sum_j q_{jl} q_{jk} \sum_i (u_{ij1} - u_{ij2})^2 \frac{\exp(\delta_j)}{[1 + \exp(\delta_j)]^2}, \tag{17}$$

for $l, k = 1, \ldots, m$. These derivatives are the negative elements of the information matrix $\mathbf{I}$.

Equations (15) through (17) were given in different, but equivalent, form in some earlier publications (Fischer, 1976, 1977b, 1983b). The estimation Eqs. (16) illustrate the central property of the LLRA: They contain only the parameters δ_j (weighted sums of the effect parameters η_l), but are independent of the person parameters θ_{ij}, which have been eliminated via the conditions $u_{ij1} + u_{ij2} = u_{ij+}$. Hence, whatever the endowment of the subjects in terms of person parameters $\boldsymbol{\theta}_j = (\theta_{1j}, \ldots, \theta_{nj})$—for instance, whatever the intellectual abilities of the children or the proneness of the patients to particular patterns of symptoms—the η_l will be estimated consistently under mild regularity conditions (cf. Fischer, 1983, 1995b).

Two questions regarding the CML approach in the LLRA are of practical interest:

(i) What are the minimum conditions for Eqs. (16) to have a unique solution $\hat{\boldsymbol{\eta}}$?

(ii) What are the asymptotic properties of $\hat{\boldsymbol{\eta}}$ under regularity conditions?

Both questions are easily and satisfactorily answered by the following results:

(i) There exists a unique solution $\hat{\boldsymbol{\eta}} = (\hat{\eta}_1, \ldots, \hat{\eta}_m)$ of the CML Eqs. (16) under the restrictions in Eq. (8) if

  (a) the design comprises at least m treatment groups G_g, $g = 1, \ldots,$ m, with linearly independent dosage vectors, $\mathbf{q}_g = (q_{g1}, \ldots, g_{gm})$, and

  (b) for each of these treatment groups G_g, there exists at least one item I_i and one person $S_j \in G_g$, such that $u_{ij1} = 1$ and $u_{ij2} = 0$, and one item I_h and one person $S_k \in G_g$, such that $u_{hk1} = 0$ and $u_{hk2} = 1$.

This result is a special case of a more general, but much more complicated necessary and sufficient condition for logit models (Fischer, 1983a; Haberman, 1974; Schumacher, 1980). The present sufficient condition is indeed easily satisfied: The linear independence (a) of the dosage vectors is an obvious requirement analogous to a well-known necessary condition in regression analysis and experimental design; and (b) means that, within each treatment group, there is at least one change from a positive to a negative response to some item, and one change from a negative to a positive response to some item (which may be the same or a different item). Hence, we may expect that the CML equations will possess a unique solution even in most small-sample applications.

(ii) If the design comprises at least m treatment groups G_g, $g = 1, \ldots, m$, with linearly independent dosage vectors $\mathbf{q}_g$, and the group sizes $N_g \to \infty$, such that the sequence of person parameters θ_{ij} within each group satisfies the condition

$$\sum_i \sum_j \exp(-|\theta_{ij}|) = \infty, \tag{18}$$

then $\hat{\boldsymbol{\eta}}$ is asymptotically multivariate normal around $\boldsymbol{\eta}$ with asymptotic covariance matrix $\mathbf{I}^{-1}$ (where $\mathbf{I}$ is the information matrix).

The formulation of the condition in Eq. (18) is due to Hillgruber (1990; referenced in Pfanzagl, 1994) and prevents that, within some treatment group G_g, almost all $|\theta_{ij}|$ become infinitely large, which would render the data uninformative. Condition (ii) again is a requirement that is well approximated in most realistic applications.

Although we cannot go into the details of deeper uniqueness results here, one important aspect has to be mentioned: The above statements (i) might mislead the reader to think that the effect parameters η_l are measured on an absolute scale. Such a conclusion is not justified because, as was mentioned above, the derivation of the LLRA from a set of meaningful and testable assumptions leads to a more general logistic model with an unspecified discrimination parameter α, so that the scale for the δ-parameters is a ratio scale. If, as is often the case in applications, $q_{jl} \in \{0,1\}$, that is, subjects receive a treatment, undergo a training, take a course, etc., or do not do so, then it can be concluded that the respective η_l are also measured on a ratio scale; in such cases statements like "treatment B_l is 1.5 times as effective as treatment B_k" do make sense. If, however, the q_{jl} are dosage measures like "psychotherapy sessions per month," "milligrams of a medicine," or the like, the quotients $\eta_l : \eta_k$ are not invariant under changes of the dosage units and can be interpreted only in relation to the latter.

LLRA for Several Time Points

The task of estimating the model in Eq. (14) via CML is not as formidable as it may appear at first sight, because each virtual person S^*_{ij} responds only to z of the $w(z-1)+1$ virtual items I^*_{gt}, so that the person parameters θ_{ij} can be eliminated only by conditioning on the raw scores $\sum_t u_{ijt} = u_{ij+}$. The resulting CML equations are basically the same as those of the LLTM [Fischer (1989); see also Fischer, this volume, CML Eq. (15)]; adapted to the present notation, they are

$$\sum_{i=1}^{n}\sum_{g=1}^{w}\sum_{t=1}^{z} q_{glt}\left(s_{igt} - \sum_{r=1}^{z} n_{igr}\frac{\varepsilon_{igt}\gamma^{(t)}_{ig,r-1}}{\gamma_{igr}}\right) = 0, \tag{19}$$

where q_{glt} is defined as before; moreover,

$s_{igt} = \sum_{S_j \in G_g} u_{ijt}$ is the total number of correct responses to (real) item I_i given by persons $S_j \in G_g$ at time point T_t,

n_{igr} is the number of persons $S_j \in G_g$ who respond correctly to (real) item I_i at exactly r time points,

$\varepsilon_{igt} = -\ln(\beta^*_{igt})$,

$\gamma_{igr} = \gamma_r(\varepsilon_{ig1}, \ldots, \varepsilon_{igz})$ is the elementary symmetric function of order r of the (virtual) item parameters $\varepsilon_{ig1}, \ldots, \varepsilon_{igz}$ within group G_g, corresponding to (real) item I_i, and

$\gamma_{ig,r-1}^{(t)} = \gamma_{r-1}(\varepsilon_{ig1}, \ldots, \varepsilon_{ig,t-1}, \varepsilon_{ig,t+1}, \ldots, \varepsilon_{igz})$ is the elementary symmetric function of order $r-1$ of the same (virtual) item parameters, excluding, however, ε_{igt}.

The summation over r in Eqs. (19) runs from 1 to z for the following reasons: Cases with $r = 0$ can be ignored, because $\gamma_{ig,0}^{(t)} = 0$ for all i, g, t; cases with $r = z$ are statistically uninformative but need not be removed from the data, because they add 1 to each s_{igt}, for $t = 1, \ldots, z$, and symmetrically, $\varepsilon_{igt}\gamma_{ig,r-1}^{(t)}/\gamma_{igr} = 1$ for all t.

The numerical methods developed for CML estimation (see Fischer, this volume) can be used here again, indeed it suffices to rearrange the data accordingly. The basic idea is that the z responses of one (real) person S_j to one (real) item I_i, and those of the same person to another (real) item I_k, are considered as responses of different virtual persons S_{ij}^* and S_{kj}^*, with parameters θ_{ij} and θ_{kj}, to the same virtual items I_t^*, $t = 1, \ldots, z$, respectively, such that all person parameters θ_{ij} are projected on the same continuum. This means that LLTM programs allowing for incomplete data can be used for estimating the present model. [For further details, see Fischer (1989, 1995a).]

The generalizability of the present model to several heterogeneous subsets of unidimensional items and to designs where different items are administered at different time points, is obvious, but cannot be discussed within the scope of this chapter. Such extensions lead to nontrivial uniqueness problems, which have been solved satisfactorily at least for typical cases (cf. Fischer, 1989).

Goodness of Fit

Testing Hypotheses in the LLRA

The objective of LLRA applications is not just to estimate treatment effects, but also to test hypotheses about these effects. Conditional likelihood ratio tests turn out to be very general and convenient tools for that purpose.

Let an LLRA for two time points be defined by Eqs. (6), (7), and (8), comprising m effect parameters; this model which is believed to be true will be referred to as hypothesis H_1. Most null-hypotheses relevant in practical research can be formulated as linear constraints imposed on the effect parameters in Eq. (8), $\mu_a(\eta_1, \ldots, \eta_m) = 0$, $a = 1, \ldots, r$. Let H_0 be a null-hypothesis so defined, comprising $m_0 = m - r$ independent parameters, then

$$-2\ln\lambda = -2\ln\left\{\frac{L(\mathbf{U}_1, \mathbf{U}_2 \mid \mathbf{U}_1 + \mathbf{U}_2 = \mathbf{U}_+; H_0)}{L(\mathbf{U}_1, \mathbf{U}_2 \mid \mathbf{U}_1 + \mathbf{U}_2 = \mathbf{U}_+; H_1)}\right\} \overset{as.}{\sim} \chi^2, \tag{20}$$

with $df = m - m_0 = r$, see Fischer (1995b). Some typical hypotheses testable in this way are listed in the following [for the sake of concretization, the notation of Eq. (9) is used here again]:

(i) *No change*; $H_0: \eta_l = \tau = \rho = 0$ for all treatments B_l.

(ii) *No trend effect*; $H_0: \tau = 0$. (This test with $df = 1$ is very powerful, as it combines all the information in the data regarding a single parameter.)

(iii) *No treatment-interaction effects*; $H_0: \rho_{lk} = 0$ for all ordered pairs (B_l, B_k).

(iv) *Ineffective treatment(s)*; $H_0: \eta_l = 0$ for some or all B_l.

(v) *Equality of treatment effects*; $H_0: \eta_l = \eta_k = \eta_h = \ldots$ for certain treatments B_l, B_k, $B_h, \ldots$.

(vi) *Generalizability of effects over items (or symptoms)*; $H_0: \eta_l^{(A)} = \eta_l^{(B)} = \eta_l^{(C)} = \ldots$ for some or all B_l, where A, B, $C, \ldots$ denote subsets of items or symptoms. (Often, these subsets are the single items or items forming subscales of the test.)

(vii) *Generalizability of effects over person groups*; $H_0: \eta_l^{(U)} = \eta_l^{(V)} = \eta_l^{(W)} = \ldots$ for some or all B_l, where U, V, $W, \ldots$ denote subgroups of persons. (If person groups are defined by levels of some variable Z, this test amounts to testing for interactions between treatments and Z.)

The conditional likelihood tests are very convenient because the likelihoods needed are part of the CML estimation, and the test statistic is so simple that it can immediately be calculated by hand. However, there exist also other test statistics that are especially practical for testing the significance of single effect parameters: The inverse of the information matrix $\mathbf{I}^{-1}$, which is needed in the Newton–Raphson method anyway, yields the asymptotic variance–covariance matrix of the estimators and can be used for assessing the significance of any parameter of interest.

Many concrete examples of applications from education, applied, and clinical psychology are mentioned in Fischer (1991). One example will be given below.

Example

To illustrate how the LLRA can be applied to designs with more than two time points, a small subset of data is selected from a study on the effects of a certain communication training (Koschier, 1993). For the present example, the responses of $N_1 = 40$ persons of a Treatment Group (TG; participants of a one-week communication training seminar) and $N_2 = 34$ persons of a Control Group (CG; participants of other one-week seminars on topics unrelated to communication training) to $n = 21$ questionnaire items from the domains "Social Anxiety" (8 items), "Cooperation" (= democratic vs. authoritarian style; 5 items), and "Nervosity" (8 items), are reanalyzed. The items were presented to the respondents at three time points, namely, before (T_1), immediately after (T_2), and one month after the seminar (T_3). The response format of all items consisted in a 4-categorical rating scale with categories "fully agree" (response 3), "rather agree" (response 2), "rather disagree" (respone 1), "fully disagree" (response 0). The complete set of data is given in Table 1. In order to apply the LLRA, the graded responses have to be dichotomized (categories 3 and 2 vs. 1 and 0); this entails some loss of information, but, as will be seen later, the main results about the effects of interest are not greatly affected.

There is no justification to consider the items as unidimensional, as they stem from three different domains. It should be mentioned at this point that the IRT models for change would allow one to consider the items from each domain as a separate unidimensional scale, where differences between items are explained by means of item difficulty parameters, and to combine the three scales in one analysis (cf. Fischer, 1989). General experience with questionnaire items, however, indicates that even items from the same domain, like "Social Anxiety," often do not satisfy strict homogeneity/unidimensionality requirements; therefore it is prudent to treat the total item set as multidimensional. As has been stressed already, the LLRA does not make any assumptions about relations between the different latent dimensions and hence is not at variance with a possible unidimensionality of the subscales.

While our model thus is quite complex and very flexible regarding interindividual differences, we make rather simple assumptions about the treatment effects: The concrete questions of the study of Koschier (1993) were whether there are specific effects of the communication training that differ from general effects of other seminars and/or of a repeated presentation of the questionnaire. Such effects, if they exist, could be specific for each and every item, or generalizable over items within domains, or generalizable over all items. These are thus the hypotheses to be formalized and tested by means of the model. Each hypothetical effect will be represented by one parameter: a communication training effect between T_1 and T_2, by η_1; a "sleeper" effect of the training producing a change of response behavior between T_2 and T_3, by η_2; and a "trend" (effect of the other seminar

Table 1: Responses of $N_1 = 40$ Testees of the Treatment Group to Items I_1 through I_{21}, at 3 Time Points, Taken from the Study of Koschier (1993).

Treatment Group

S_j	Time Point 1			Time Point 2
	Anxiety $I_1 - I_8$	Cooperation $I_9 - I_{13}$	Nervosity $I_{14} - I_{21}$	Anxiety $I_1 - I_8$
1	3 2 1 2 3 1 2 2	2 2 2 1 1	2 1 1 2 2 1 2 1	1 0 0 1 0 1 2 2
2*	2 3 1 0 1 0 2 2	1 1 1 1 3	1 1 1 0 0 0 0 3	3 3 1 0 1 0 1 1
3	3 3 2 1 2 1 1 0	1 1 1 1 1	1 1 1 1 2 1 2 2	3 2 2 1 2 2 2 2
4	2 2 3 1 0 3 1 3	3 3 2 2 1	2 1 2 0 1 2 2 1	3 2 2 2 3 2 1 2
5	1 1 0 1 1 1 1 2	2 3 1 1 2	1 1 1 0 1 0 1 2	1 1 0 1 1 1 1 1
6	3 2 0 1 2 0 2 2	2 2 1 1 3	0 1 0 1 0 0 0 2	2 2 1 2 2 0 1 1
7	3 3 0 0 0 1 1 2	2 3 1 1 3	0 0 1 1 1 1 0 3	1 0 1 1 1 1 1 1
8*	3 3 1 1 2 1 1 1	2 2 1 1 2	1 1 1 2 1 1 1 2	3 3 1 1 2 1 1 1
9*	3 3 3 3 3 0 3 3	2 3 2 1 3	3 0 1 3 2 3 0 1	3 3 3 1 3 0 2 2
10	2 3 2 2 2 2 2 2	2 2 1 1 2	0 1 2 3 2 1 1 1	2 2 2 2 2 1 2 2
11*	1 2 2 1 2 1 1 3	3 3 1 1 1	1 0 2 1 0 0 2 2	1 3 1 1 3 1 0 3
12*	2 3 1 1 1 1 0 1	0 3 1 1 3	0 0 1 2 1 0 0 3	1 2 2 2 1 1 1 2
13	3 3 3 3 2 3 2 2	3 1 1 0 1	2 0 3 1 2 1 2 1	3 3 3 3 3 3 2 3
14*	3 3 2 2 3 3 3 3	2 2 2 2 0	3 2 2 3 2 2 3 1	3 2 2 2 2 2 3 0
15	3 3 2 2 3 3 3 2	1 1 2 2 0	1 1 2 1 1 1 3 1	3 3 2 1 3 2 2 2
16	3 3 2 1 2 1 1 2	1 2 1 1 3	2 2 1 2 1 0 0 2	3 1 2 1 2 1 1 1
17	3 3 3 3 3 0 2 3	3 3 0 1 3	1 1 1 2 1 0 0 1	3 3 0 3 3 0 3 3
18*	2 1 1 0 2 2 2 1	2 1 1 1 2	1 2 2 0 2 1 1 2	2 0 2 1 2 2 2 2
19	2 2 2 2 2 1 2 2	2 1 1 1 1	1 1 1 1 2 1 2 2	2 2 2 2 2 1 1 2
20	2 2 2 2 3 1 2 2	2 2 1 1 1	1 1 1 1 2 1 2 2	2 2 2 2 2 1 2 2
21	3 2 2 1 1 3 2 2	1 2 1 2 2	1 1 2 3 2 1 1 2	2 2 1 1 1 3 1 2
22*	2 3 2 1 2 2 1 2	1 2 1 1 2	1 1 1 0 1 2 1 2	3 2 1 2 2 1 1 1
23	3 3 1 1 2 2 2 1	1 2 1 1 2	1 0 1 1 1 1 1 2	2 2 1 1 2 2 1 1
24*	3 3 3 1 3 2 2 2	3 3 2 2 3	1 1 1 0 2 1 0 1	3 2 3 1 3 2 2 2
25	3 3 1 2 1 1 2 2	3 3 0 0 2	1 1 1 3 2 1 1 2	3 3 1 3 3 0 1 2
26	3 3 1 1 2 2 2 2	3 3 2 2 2	1 1 1 2 1 1 1 2	3 3 1 1 2 2 1 1
27	2 3 1 3 3 1 2 1	2 1 2 1 1	1 2 2 1 2 1 2 3	2 3 1 2 3 0 2 3
28	2 0 1 2 1 0 1 1	2 1 1 0 1	3 2 1 0 2 1 2 3	1 3 1 1 1 0 2 1
29	2 3 0 1 2 0 1 1	3 3 1 1 3	1 0 1 0 0 0 0 3	1 2 0 1 0 0 1 1
30*	3 3 1 1 2 2 3 2	0 1 2 3 0	3 2 1 3 2 3 3 3	3 3 1 1 2 1 3 1
31	2 2 3 2 1 1 2 2	2 2 1 1 3	1 1 2 2 2 1 0 3	2 2 1 1 1 1 1 2
32	3 3 1 1 3 1 3 2	2 2 2 2 1	1 1 2 1 2 1 2 2	3 3 1 1 2 1 2 2
33*	1 1 2 1 1 1 1 2	2 2 1 1 2	1 1 1 2 1 0 1 3	3 2 1 1 1 1 1 2
34*	2 2 2 2 2 2 2 2	2 2 1 2 1	1 1 1 1 2 1 2 1	2 2 2 2 2 2 2 2
35*	3 2 1 1 2 1 1 2	2 2 1 1 1	1 1 1 2 1 1 2 2	3 2 1 2 2 1 1 2
36	3 3 2 1 3 2 2 2	2 2 1 1 1	1 1 1 1 2 2 2 2	3 3 2 1 3 1 2 3
37	2 3 1 0 2 2 3 2	0 1 2 1 1	3 1 3 1 1 3 2 3	2 2 1 2 1 2 1 2
38*	2 2 1 2 2 1 2 1	2 1 2 2 1	2 1 1 1 2 3 2 1	2 3 1 1 1 1 1 0
39	3 3 2 1 2 1 2 3	2 1 1 2 2	1 2 1 0 1 1 1 3	3 3 2 1 2 1 2 2
40	3 3 1 2 3 0 0 2	3 3 1 0 2	1 0 0 0 0 0 1 2	3 3 2 2 2 0 0 2

Note: Responses 3 denote "fully agree", responses 2 "rather agree", responses 1 "rather disagree", and responses 0 "fully disagree"; asterisks denote female sex.

Continued on following page

Table 1 (continued) Treatment Group

Time Point 2		Time Point 3		
Cooperation $I_9 - I_{13}$	Nervosity $I_{14} - I_{21}$	Anxiety $I_1 - I_8$	Cooperation $I_9 - I_{13}$	Nervosity $I_{14} - I_{21}$
2 1 2 1 1	2 1 1 2 2 2 2 1	1 0 0 1 0 1 2 2	2 1 2 1 1	2 1 1 1 2 1 2 2
1 1 1 1 3	1 1 1 0 0 0 0 3	3 3 0 0 0 0 0 1	0 1 2 0 3	0 1 0 0 0 0 0 3
1 1 1 1 2	2 1 2 1 2 1 1 2	2 2 2 2 2 1 2 2	1 1 1 1 1	1 1 2 2 2 1 2 1
3 2 0 2 2	2 1 2 1 2 2 1 1	3 2 2 2 2 2 1 2	3 2 1 2 2	2 1 2 0 1 1 1 1
2 3 1 1 0	1 1 1 0 0 1 3 3	1 0 0 1 1 0 0 2	2 2 1 0 3	0 1 1 0 1 0 0 3
2 2 1 1 2	1 1 0 1 1 1 1 2	2 2 0 1 1 0 1 2	2 2 1 1 3	1 1 0 0 0 0 0 2
2 3 2 1 2	1 0 1 0 1 1 1 2	2 2 1 1 2 1 1 2	2 2 1 1 2	1 1 1 1 1 1 1 2
2 2 2 1 2	1 1 1 1 1 1 1 2	3 3 2 1 3 2 2 3	2 2 3 1 3	1 0 0 0 2 0 0 2
2 3 2 1 2	3 0 2 3 1 2 1 2	3 3 3 3 3 0 3 3	2 2 2 1 3	3 0 1 3 2 1 0 0
2 2 1 1 2	1 1 2 2 2 2 1 1	2 2 2 2 1 2 2 1	2 2 1 1 2	1 1 2 2 1 2 1 1
3 3 1 0 0	2 1 1 3 0 0 3 3	2 2 2 1 2 2 2 3	3 3 1 0 1	1 1 1 3 1 1 2 3
3 3 1 1 3	0 0 1 1 1 0 0 3	2 2 0 1 1 1 2 2	3 3 1 1 2	0 1 1 1 0 0 1 3
3 1 0 0 0	2 2 3 1 2 1 3 1	2 1 2 3 2 3 3 3	3 3 1 0 1	1 0 3 0 1 1 2 1
2 2 2 2 1	2 2 2 3 3 2 2 2	3 0 2 2 2 2 2 2	2 2 1 1 1	2 2 2 3 2 2 2 2
2 1 2 2 1	1 1 1 1 1 1 2 1	3 2 1 2 2 2 1 2	1 1 2 2 1	1 1 1 1 2 1 2 1
2 2 1 1 3	2 2 2 1 1 1 0 3	2 3 1 1 1 0 0 1	2 3 1 1 3	1 1 2 1 0 0 0 2
3 3 0 1 2	2 1 1 2 1 1 1 1	2 1 3 3 3 0 1 1	3 3 0 1 2	1 0 1 1 1 0 1 1
2 1 1 1 2	1 2 2 0 2 1 1 2	3 1 2 1 2 1 1 2	2 2 1 1 2	2 1 2 1 1 2 1 2
2 2 1 1 2	1 1 1 2 2 1 1 2	3 3 2 2 2 1 2 2	2 2 1 1 2	2 1 1 1 1 1 1 2
2 2 1 2 1	2 1 2 1 2 1 2 2	2 2 3 2 3 1 2 2	2 2 1 2 1	2 2 2 0 1 1 2 2
2 2 1 3 1	1 1 1 1 1 0 2 1	3 2 2 1 2 3 2 2	2 1 1 2 1	1 1 2 1 1 1 2 1
1 2 1 1 2	1 1 1 1 1 1 1 2	2 0 2 2 2 1 1 1	1 2 1 1 2	1 1 1 1 1 1 1 2
2 1 1 1 2	1 1 1 1 1 1 1 2	2 2 1 1 2 2 1 1	2 2 1 1 2	1 0 1 1 1 1 1 2
3 2 2 2 2	1 1 1 0 2 1 1 0	3 2 3 1 3 3 2 2	3 2 2 1 2	1 2 1 1 2 1 1 1
3 3 0 0 2	1 0 1 3 2 1 1 2	3 3 1 3 3 1 2 2	3 3 1 0 3	1 0 0 3 1 0 0 2
3 0 2 1 2	1 1 1 0 1 0 1 3	3 3 2 1 1 1 1 2	3 2 2 1 2	1 1 1 1 1 1 1 3
1 1 1 1 1	1 2 1 1 2 0 2 0	2 3 1 2 2 1 2 3	2 1 2 2 1	1 2 2 1 2 0 2 0
2 2 1 0 2	2 1 1 0 2 2 1 3	1 2 0 1 1 1 2 1	2 2 1 1 2	2 1 2 0 2 2 1 2
3 3 0 0 3	1 0 0 0 0 1 0 3	2 2 0 0 1 0 1 2	3 3 1 1 3	1 0 0 1 1 0 0 3
0 1 2 2 1	2 2 1 2 2 2 2 2	3 3 1 1 2 1 3 3	0 1 2 2 1	2 1 1 2 1 2 2 2
2 3 1 1 2	2 1 1 1 2 1 1 2	1 2 0 0 1 0 1 1	2 3 1 1 2	2 1 1 1 1 0 1 3
2 2 1 2 1	1 1 2 1 2 1 2 2	3 3 1 2 2 1 3 3	2 3 1 1 1	1 0 2 2 2 0 2 3
2 2 1 1 2	1 1 1 2 1 1 1 2	2 2 1 1 2 1 2 2	2 2 1 2 2	1 1 1 2 2 0 1 3
2 2 1 2 2	2 1 1 1 1 1 1 1	2 2 2 2 2 1 2 2	1 2 1 2 1	2 1 1 1 1 1 2 2
2 2 1 1 2	1 1 1 1 1 1 1 2	2 2 1 1 2 1 1 2	2 2 1 1 2	1 1 1 1 1 1 1 2
1 2 1 1 1	1 1 2 2 2 2 2 2	3 3 3 1 3 2 3 3	2 2 1 2 2	2 1 1 2 2 2 1 2
0 0 2 2 1	2 2 2 1 1 2 2 2	2 3 0 1 1 2 2 2	1 3 2 2 1	2 2 1 2 1 1 2 2
2 2 2 2 1	2 1 1 1 2 2 2 1	3 3 1 0 1 0 1 1	2 2 2 2 3	3 1 1 0 2 2 0 1
2 1 1 2 2	1 1 1 1 2 1 1 3	3 3 3 1 2 1 2 2	2 1 1 2 3	1 1 1 0 1 0 0 3
3 2 1 0 1	1 1 1 1 1 1 2 1	2 3 1 1 2 1 0 2	3 3 1 0 2	1 0 0 3 0 1 1 2

Table 1 (continued): Responses of $N_2 = 34$ Testees of the Treatment Group to Items I_1 through I_{21}, at 3 Time Points, Taken from the Study of Koschier (1993).

Control Group

S_j	Time Point 1			Time Point 2
	Anxiety $I_1 - I_8$	Cooperation $I_9 - I_{13}$	Nervosity $I_{14} - I_{21}$	Anxiety $I_1 - I_8$
1*	3 3 2 2 3 1 3 1	1 2 2 1 2	1 3 1 0 1 0 1 3	3 2 2 1 2 1 2 2
2	2 2 1 2 0 1 2 2	1 1 1 2 1	2 2 2 2 2 2 2 2	2 3 0 1 1 0 2 2
3*	2 3 2 2 2 2 1 2	1 1 2 2 2	2 2 2 1 2 2 1 2	2 2 2 2 2 2 2 2
4*	3 3 2 2 2 2 2 2	2 2 1 2 1	2 1 1 1 1 1 2 2	2 2 2 2 2 2 2 2
5	1 2 1 0 1 0 1 3	2 3 2 1 2	1 1 1 2 0 0 1 2	0 1 0 0 1 0 1 0
6*	1 1 2 1 0 0 2 3	1 2 1 1 1	2 1 1 2 2 1 2 2	3 2 1 1 2 1 1 1
7	0 0 0 1 2 0 3 2	3 3 2 1 2	1 3 2 2 0 0 1 2	1 3 2 2 2 0 2 2
8*	3 3 1 1 3 2 1 3	3 1 2 0 0	1 1 1 2 2 2 3 2	3 3 3 2 3 2 1 3
9*	3 2 1 1 2 2 1 2	1 3 2 1 1	1 0 2 1 1 1 2 2	3 2 1 1 2 1 2 2
10	3 2 1 1 1 0 2 3	3 3 1 0 3	1 1 1 1 1 0 0 3	2 2 1 0 2 0 1 2
11	3 3 3 0 3 0 2 2	2 2 1 1 2	2 2 2 3 2 1 1 3	3 3 3 0 3 2 2 3
12	2 1 1 1 2 1 0 2	1 2 1 2 2	1 1 1 2 1 1 1 2	1 1 1 1 2 2 1 2
13	1 1 1 1 1 2 1 1	1 2 1 1 2	2 1 0 2 1 2 1 1	1 2 1 1 1 2 1 1
14	3 3 2 0 1 0 2 2	2 3 2 2 2	1 0 2 0 2 1 1 3	3 3 2 0 2 0 3 2
15	3 0 1 1 1 0 1 2	3 3 1 1 3	2 1 0 3 1 1 0 3	2 1 1 0 1 0 0 1
16	2 3 1 1 1 1 1 2	3 2 0 0 3	1 1 1 0 1 0 0 3	2 1 1 1 1 1 1 1
17	2 2 1 1 2 0 1 2	2 3 1 0 2	1 0 1 1 1 1 1 3	2 2 1 0 1 0 1 2
18	1 1 2 1 1 0 1 2	2 2 1 1 2	2 1 1 1 1 1 1 3	1 3 1 0 1 0 2 1
19	3 3 2 1 2 1 0 3	2 1 2 2 2	2 1 1 1 1 1 1 2	2 2 2 1 2 1 1 1
20	2 3 0 0 1 0 0 3	2 3 1 0 3	2 1 2 3 0 2 0 2	2 2 2 0 1 0 0 2
21*	2 3 0 0 3 1 2 3	2 1 2 2 1	2 0 2 0 2 0 2 3	2 3 3 0 3 2 2 2
22	3 3 2 2 2 3 1 2	1 1 3 1 0	3 2 2 2 2 2 3 2	2 2 1 1 2 2 2 1
23	2 2 2 1 2 1 2 2	2 2 1 1 1	2 1 2 1 1 1 2 1	3 3 0 2 0 1 2 2
24*	1 2 1 2 1 1 2 2	0 0 1 2 1	2 1 1 1 2 1 2 2	2 2 1 1 2 1 2 2
25	3 3 0 1 3 0 2 3	2 3 0 0 2	1 1 3 0 2 2 1 3	3 3 1 2 2 1 2 3
26	2 2 1 1 2 2 1 2	2 1 2 2 2	2 2 1 1 2 2 1 2	2 2 2 1 2 1 1 2
27	1 1 1 1 1 1 1 1	1 1 1 2 1	1 1 1 2 1 1 2 2	1 2 1 1 1 1 1 1
28*	2 1 3 3 3 0 2 3	2 2 1 1 0	3 3 3 3 2 2 3 1	3 2 3 3 3 0 3 2
29	3 2 3 1 3 1 3 1	1 1 2 2 2	2 0 0 2 2 1 1 1	3 2 3 1 3 2 2 2
30	3 3 2 1 2 1 1 2	1 3 2 3 1	2 1 3 1 2 1 2 3	2 3 2 1 1 1 2 2
31*	3 3 2 2 3 2 3 2	2 2 1 1 2	1 1 1 2 1 1 1 1	3 3 2 2 3 2 3 2
32	3 3 2 1 2 1 1 2	3 3 1 1 2	1 1 1 1 1 1 1 1	3 3 2 1 2 1 2 2
33*	2 3 0 2 2 2 2 3	1 0 2 2 1	1 1 2 2 1 2 2 2	2 2 1 2 2 2 2 2
34*	3 3 3 3 3 0 1 2	2 3 1 0 2	0 1 1 0 1 0 1 1	3 3 2 3 3 0 2 2

Continued on following page

Table 1 (continued) Control Group

Time Point 2		Time Point 3		
Cooperation $I_9 - I_{13}$	Nervosity $I_{14} - I_{21}$	Anxiety $I_1 - I_8$	Cooperation $I_9 - I_{13}$	Nervosity $I_{14} - I_{21}$
1 1 2 2 3	1 3 0 0 0 1 0 3	3 3 2 2 2 2 1 2	1 1 2 1 2	1 3 1 0 2 0 1 2
1 1 2 3 3	2 1 0 1 1 1 0 1	2 2 1 1 2 2 2 2	1 1 2 2 1	2 2 1 1 2 1 2 1
1 1 2 2 1	2 2 2 2 2 2 2 2	2 2 2 2 2 1 2 2	1 1 1 2 1	2 2 2 1 2 2 2 2
2 2 1 1 1	1 1 1 1 1 1 2 2	2 2 2 2 2 1 2 2	2 1 2 1 2	2 1 1 1 1 1 1 2
3 3 1 1 2	0 1 0 0 1 1 1 3	2 3 0 3 3 0 0 3	3 3 1 2 3	0 0 0 0 0 0 0 3
1 2 2 2 1	2 1 1 2 1 1 2 2	3 2 2 1 2 1 1 2	2 1 1 1 2	2 2 1 2 1 1 1 2
2 3 1 1 1	2 1 2 2 1 0 2 3	3 1 3 0 2 0 3 2	2 2 1 1 2	3 1 2 1 1 1 1 3
2 1 1 0 1	2 1 0 2 1 3 2 2	3 3 2 2 3 1 0 3	3 1 1 1 3	1 1 1 2 2 1 0 1
1 2 1 1 2	1 1 2 2 1 1 1 2	3 2 2 2 2 2 2 2	2 2 1 1 1	2 1 2 2 1 1 2 1
3 3 1 1 3	1 0 1 1 1 0 0 2	2 2 2 2 2 1 2 2	2 2 1 2 2	1 1 1 2 2 1 1 2
1 2 1 1 1	2 2 1 3 3 1 2 2	3 3 2 3 3 3 2 2	2 1 1 1 1	3 3 1 1 2 2 2 1
1 2 1 2 2	1 1 1 2 1 1 1 2	1 3 1 2 2 2 1 1	1 2 2 2 2	2 1 1 2 1 1 1 2
2 2 2 1 2	2 1 0 2 1 1 1 2	1 1 1 1 1 2 1 1	1 2 2 1 2	2 1 1 1 1 1 1 1
1 3 1 3 1	1 1 2 0 2 0 2 3	3 3 2 0 2 0 2 2	1 1 2 2 1	1 1 2 0 2 1 2 3
2 2 1 1 3	2 1 0 3 0 1 0 2	2 2 1 1 1 0 2 2	2 2 1 1 2	2 1 0 3 0 1 1 0
3 3 0 0 2	1 1 1 1 0 0 1 1	2 2 1 1 2 1 1 1	3 3 0 0 2	0 1 2 0 1 0 1 2
2 3 1 1 2	1 0 1 1 1 1 1 3	2 2 1 2 1 0 1 2	3 3 1 0 2	1 1 1 1 0 1 1 3
2 1 2 2 1	0 1 1 1 2 1 2 3	1 1 1 1 1 1 1 1	2 2 1 2 2	1 1 1 1 1 1 1 2
1 1 2 2 2	1 1 1 1 1 1 1 2	2 3 1 1 2 1 1 1	1 1 2 2 2	2 1 1 1 1 1 1 2
1 3 1 0 3	2 1 1 3 0 1 0 2	3 3 0 3 3 1 1 2	2 2 1 1 3	1 1 1 1 0 1 0 3
2 1 2 2 1	1 1 1 0 2 1 2 2	3 3 3 0 3 1 2 3	2 2 2 1 2	2 1 1 1 2 1 1 1
1 2 2 2 2	2 3 1 2 1 1 1 2	3 2 2 2 3 2 3 2	1 1 2 2 0	2 2 2 2 2 2 3 2
2 2 1 1 2	2 1 2 1 2 1 1 1	3 3 2 2 2 1 2 2	2 2 1 0 2	2 1 2 1 1 1 1 1
1 1 2 2 2	2 2 2 1 2 2 1 1	3 3 2 2 3 1 2 2	0 2 2 2 2	2 2 1 1 2 1 1 0
2 3 1 1 2	1 1 1 0 2 0 1 3	3 3 1 2 2 2 2 2	3 2 1 1 2	1 1 1 0 1 1 1 2
1 1 2 2 2	2 2 1 1 1 1 1 1	2 2 2 1 2 2 1 2	1 1 1 2 2	2 2 1 1 1 2 1 2
2 1 2 2 1	1 1 1 2 2 1 2 2	2 2 1 1 1 1 1 1	1 1 2 2 2	1 1 1 1 1 1 1 2
1 1 1 1 0	3 2 2 3 2 3 3 2	3 1 3 3 3 1 3 2	1 2 1 1 0	3 2 3 3 3 3 3 1
1 3 2 2 3	1 0 0 2 1 0 0 1	3 2 3 2 3 2 2 2	1 1 2 2 1	0 0 0 0 2 0 2 1
2 2 2 2 2	2 1 3 2 2 1 1 2	2 3 1 1 2 1 2 2	2 2 2 2 1	2 2 2 1 2 1 2 2
1 2 1 1 2	1 1 1 1 1 1 1 2	2 3 2 2 2 2 3 2	1 2 1 1 2	1 1 1 1 1 1 1 1
2 3 1 1 2	1 1 1 1 1 1 1 1	3 3 2 1 2 1 1 2	3 3 1 1 3	0 0 1 1 1 1 0 2
1 1 3 3 1	1 2 2 1 2 2 2 2	2 3 1 1 1 0 3 3	1 0 3 2 1	1 2 2 1 2 2 2 2
2 2 1 1 3	0 0 1 0 1 0 0 3	3 2 3 1 3 0 2 2	2 2 1 0 2	1 0 1 0 1 1 1 3

TABLE 2. Matrices $\mathbf{Q}_{TG}$ and $\mathbf{Q}_{CG}$ of Weights for η_1, η_2, and τ, for 3 Time Points (T_1, T_2, T_3).

Time Point	*TG*			*CG*		
	η_1	η_2	τ	η_1	η_2	τ
T_1	0	0	0	0	0	0
T_2	1	0	1	0	0	1
T_3	1	1	2	0	0	2

plus the effect of repeatedly responding to the questions), by τ.

As a basis of all tests, a "saturated" model is required that is (trivially) true. In our case, a saturated model would have to comprise individual effects for all persons and would therefore hardly be manageable. We therefore use a "quasi-saturated" model that assumes generalizability of effects over individuals, but provides parameters for differential effects with regard to each item. Estimating this model is easily done by fitting one separate model to each item I_i, with three effect parameters, η_{i1}, η_{i2}, τ_i. The matrices $\mathbf{Q}_{TG}$ and $\mathbf{Q}_{CG}$ of weights q_{gl1}, q_{gl2}, and q_{gl3}, for $S_j \in TG$ and $S_j \in CG$, respectively, are given in Table 2. This model will be denoted Model 1.

We refrain from giving the $21 \times 3 = 63$ parameter estimates; they obviously have very little statistical precision (each triplet of estimates being based on a single item), and they will not be needed later. The log-likelihood at the point of the CML solution of Model 1 is $\ln L_1 = -491.84$, which will be used as a yardstick for the assessment of other hypotheses.

First we test the hypothesis of no change, setting all effects to zero, $\eta_{i1} = \eta_{i2} = \tau_i = 0$ for all I_i. This null-hypothesis is denoted Model 0. The log-likelihood results as $\ln L_0 = -537.22$, and the likelihood ratio test statistic is

$$-2\ln\lambda = -2(\ln L_0 - \ln L_1) = -2(491.84 - 537.22) = 90.76,$$

with $df = 21 \times 3 = 63$, which is significant ($\chi^2_{.95} = 82.53$). Hence, Model 0 is rejected, and it is concluded that some change does occur in the responses of the testees.

In a next step, we test the hypothesis that effects generalize over items within domains, assuming effects η_{A1}, η_{A2}, τ_A for all Social Anxiety items, η_{C1}, η_{C2}, τ_C for all Cooperation items, and η_{N1}, η_{N2}, τ_N for all Nervosity items. This amounts to applying the LLRA with the matrices $\mathbf{Q}_{TG}$ and $\mathbf{Q}_{CG}$ separately to the items from each domain, denoted Model 2. The estimates so obtained are given in Table 3,[2] the log-likelihood is $\ln L_2 =$

[2]Note to Table 3: Positive parameters reflect an increase, negative ones a decrease in the respective behavior; asterisks denote one-sided significance at $\alpha = 0.05$.

TABLE 3. Results of the Estimation of Model 2 (Dichotomous LLRA).

Domains	Parameter Estimates & Standard Deviations			Significance
Social Anxiety	η_{A1}	-1.26	0.28	$p = 0.00^*$
	η_{A2}	-0.18	0.28	$p = 0.25$
	τ_A	0.50	0.13	$p = 0.00^*$
Cooperation	η_{C1}	0.39	0.40	$p = 0.16$
	η_{C2}	0.43	0.41	$p = 0.15$
	τ_C	0.00	0.15	$p = 0.50$
Nervosity	η_{N1}	0.32	0.29	$p = 0.13$
	η_{N2}	-0.08	0.29	$p = 0.39$
	τ_N	-0.35	0.13	$p = 0.00^*$

-516.82. To test Model 2 against Model 1, we consider

$$-2\ln\lambda = -2(\ln L_2 - \ln L_1) = -2(491.84 - 516.82) = 49.96,$$

with $df = 21 \times 3 - 3 \times 3 = 54$, which clearly is nonsignificant ($\chi^2_{.95} = 72.15$). Hence it is concluded that the effects generalize over items within domains.

Now we test the hypothesis that effects generalize over all items of all domains. This hypothesis provides only three effect parameters, η_1, η_2, τ, and is denoted Model 3; since the sign of the effects on Cooperation are opposite to those on Social Anxiety and Nervosity, we have the restrictions $\eta_{C1} = -\eta_1$, $\eta_{A1} = \eta_{N1} = \eta_1$, $\eta_{C2} = -\eta_2$, $\eta_{A2} = \eta_{N2} = \eta_2$, $\tau_C = -\tau$, $\tau_A = \tau_N = \tau$. The log-likelihood results as $\ln L_3 = -531.07$, and the test statistic as

$$-2\ln\lambda = -2(\ln L_3 - \ln L_1) = -2(491.84 - 531.07) = 78.46,$$

with $df = 21 \times 3 - 3 = 60$, which is nonsignificant ($\chi^2_{.95} = 79.08$), if only by a narrow margin. Hence, Model 3 can be retained. The parameter estimates under this model are

$$\begin{aligned}
\hat{\eta}_1 &= -0.47, & \hat{\sigma}(\hat{\eta}_1) &= 0.18,\\
\hat{\eta}_2 &= -0.16, & \hat{\sigma}(\hat{\eta}_2) &= 0.18,\\
\hat{\tau} &= 0.05, & \hat{\sigma}(\hat{\tau}) &= 0.08.
\end{aligned}$$

The only significant effect is that of the communication seminar at time point T_2, which has the expected direction. However, we still remain somewhat skeptical about Model 3, because it just failed to depart significantly from Model 1, so that probably it would have to be rejected if the samples had been somewhat larger. We therefore view Model 2 more closely, see the parameter estimates in Table 3. At least two of the three significant effects are readily interpretable: As expected, the communication training immediately reduces Social Anxiety (time point T_2), but there is no after-

(or "sleeper"-)effect (time point T_3). For both groups, there is a trend for Nervosity to decrease over time (significant τ_N). Somewhat unexpectedly, there is a similar trend for Social Anxiety to increase over time (significant τ_A); this might be due to a growth of consciousness of social relations in both groups.

For the sake of completeness, Model 2 is finally tested for fit by splitting the sample of testees by gender and re-estimating the model separately in each group; this yields $\ln L_2^{(f)} = -182.67$ (for females) and $\ln L_2^{(m)} = -330.11$ (for males). The likelihood ratio statistic for testing whether the effect parameters generalize over the two gender groups is

$$\begin{aligned} -2\ln\lambda &= -2(\ln L_2 - \ln L_2^{(f)} - \ln L_2^{(m)}) \\ &= -2(-516.82 + 182.67 + 330.11) = 8.08, \end{aligned}$$

with $df = 2 \times 9 - 9 = 9$, which clearly is nonsignificant ($\chi^2_{.95} = 16.92$). We conclude that the effects generalize over the two gender-groups and take this as an indication of fit of Model 2.

A final word about the asymptotics of the conditional likelihood ratio statistics in this example seems to be indicated: The asymptotics rest on condition (ii) in the section on parameter estimation for the LLRA, that is, each of the two treatment groups should be "large." In our case, what counts is the number of "virtual" persons, N_g^*, per group G_g. Since there are $n = 21$ items, we have $N_{TG}^* = 21 \times 40 = 840$ for the Treatment Group, and $N_{CG}^* = 21 \times 34 = 714$ for the Control Group; these numbers should be sufficient for justifying the application of asymptotic results.

Discussion

This chapter has shown the usefulness of the dichotomous LLRA for two or more time points for measuring treatment effects and testing hypotheses about such effects. A polytomous extension of this model (for items with more than two response categories and two time points) was suggested already in Fischer (1972) and further developed in Fischer (1974, 1976, 1977a, 1977b, 1983b). This extension is a straightforward generalization of Eqs. (6) and (8), namely,

$$P(h \mid S_j, I_i, T_1) = \frac{\exp(\theta_{ijh})}{\sum_k \exp(\theta_{ijk})}, \tag{21}$$

$$P(h \mid S_j, I_i, T_2) = \frac{\exp(\theta_{ijh} + \delta_{jh})}{\sum_k \exp(\theta_{ijk} + \delta_{jk})}, \tag{22}$$

$$\delta_{jh} = \sum_l q_{jl}\eta_{lh} + \tau_h, \tag{23}$$

where $h = 0, 1, \ldots, d$ denotes the response categories C_h of the items. The parameterization in Eqs. (21) through (23) was inspired by that of the so-called "polytomous multidimensional Rasch model" (Rasch, 1961, 1965; Fischer, 1974), which assigns a separate latent dimension to each response category C_h. In this model, multidimensionality has a meaning different from that in the LLRA (above), because latent dimensions are assigned to response categories rather than to items. The model in Eqs. (21)–(23), on the other hand, combines both notions of multidimensionality and describes individual differences in terms of a separate *vector* of trait parameters for each person $\times$ item combination. Similarly, the model assigns a separate treatment effect η_{lh} to each treatment B_l per category C_h, and one trend effect τ_h per category. (Owing to necessary normalization conditions, however, the true dimensionality of these vectors is one less than the number of response categories.)

The LLRA extension in Eqs. (21)–(23) was used in just a few applications (e.g., Hammer, 1978; Kropiunigg, 1979a, 1979b), but the treatment effects turned out to be of little stability and interpretability, probably caused by the too generous parameterization of the model. Therefore this line of development was not pursued further.

More recent promising ways of dealing with multidimensionality of polytomous items are reinterpretations of the (unidimensional) "linear rating scale model" [LRMS; Fischer and Parzer (1991); see Fischer, this volume] or of the "linear partial credit model" [LPCM; Fischer and Ponocny (1994); see Fischer, this volume]. Again, the unidimensional person parameters θ_j of these models can be replaced by vectors $\boldsymbol{\theta}_j = (\theta_{1j}, \ldots, \theta_{nj})$ of different parameters for each item, and the responses of one person S_j to the n items of a test can be considered as responses of n "virtual persons" S^*_{ij}.

The multidimensional extension of the LRSM for change then becomes

$$P(h \mid S_j, I_i, T_t, G_g) = \frac{\exp\left[h\left(\theta_{ij} + \sum_l q_{glt}\eta_l\right) + \omega_h\right]}{\sum_{k=0}^{d} \exp\left[k\left(\theta_{ij} + \sum_l q_{glt}\eta_l\right) + \omega_k\right]}, \tag{24}$$

with

θ_{ij} for the position of person S_j, at time point T_1, on the latent dimension D_i measured by item I_i,

q_{glt} the dosage of treatment B_l given to persons S_j of group G_g up to time point T_t,

η_l the effect of one unit of treatment B_l,

$\omega_h = \sum_{l=1}^{h} \kappa_l$, for $h = 2, \ldots, d$, where κ_l, $l = 1, \ldots, d$, are threshold parameters measuring the difficulty of a transition from category C_{l-1} to C_l, with $\omega_0 = \omega_1 = \kappa_1 = 0$ for normalization (cf. Andrich, 1978), and

d the number of response categories C_h (the ω_h and d are assumed to be the same in all items).

The estimation in this model is technically more complicated than that of the dichotomous LLRA versions and thus cannot be treated within the scope of this chapter. The same goes for multidimensional extensions of the LPCM. [The interested reader finds all details of the algorithms in Fischer and Parzer (1991) and Fischer and Ponocny (1994, 1995), respectively. A computer program for PCs under DOS can be obtained from the authors. It is capable of estimating all the models discussed in this chapter.]

Hypothesis testing via conditional likelihood ratio tests, however, is as simple as in the dichotomous LLRA; the procedures are in fact identical to those outlined above in the section on hypothesis testing.

For the sake of illustration, we give some selected results from the 4-categorical analysis of the data in Table 1. The likelihood of Model 1 (see above) resulted as $\ln L_1 = -1407.51$, that of Model 2 as $\ln L_2 = -1511.55$. When estimating Model 1 from the 4-categorical data, different attractiveness parameters ω_{ih} are assumed for each item; for Model 2, parameters ω_h are assumed constant across item domains. The parameter estimates under Model 2 are given in Table 4. Model 2 is tested against Model 1 by means of the statistic

$$-2 \ln \lambda = -2(\ln L_2 - \ln L_1) = -2(-1511.55 + 1407.51) = 208.08,$$

with $df = 21 \times 5 - (3 \times 3 + 2) = 94$, which is significant ($\chi^2_{.95} = 117.63$). This comes as a surprise because Model 2 was retained under the dichotomous analysis. The reasons for this discrepancy are that (a) now differences of the attractiveness parameters ω_{ih} between items (which seem to be quite considerable) contribute to the significance, and (b) the 4-categorical analysis is based on more statistical information than the dichotomous one.

Even if Model 2 has now to be rejected, it is interesting to look at the parameter estimates in Table 4: All effects that had been significant in the dichotomous analysis are again significant, and two of the formerly nonsignificant ones (η_{A2}, η_{C2}) have become significant owing to the increase in statistical information. All these five parameter estimates have the same sign as those in Table 2. The two analyses can therefore be considered reasonably concurrent. The estimates of the two parameters ω_2 and ω_3 show that the transitions from category C_0 to C_1 is relatively easy compared to a transition from C_1 to C_2, and that the latter is much easier than that from C_2 to C_3.

Finally, a word of warning is in order: Firstly, it is known that dichotomous and categorical models can fit the same data only under very artificial conditions (Jansen and Roskam, 1986; Roskam and Jansen, 1989). The 4-categorical analysis is mentioned here, however, only for demonstration, even if the LRSM does not fit. Second, while the polytomous analysis exploits more information, nontrivial problems arise through the attractiveness parameters ω_h: If the items show different ω_{ih}, a response like "rather

TABLE 4. Results of the Estimation of Model 2 (Under the Polytomous LLRA).

Domains	Parameter Estimates & Standard Deviations			Significance (one-sided)
Social Anxiety	η_{A1}	−0.91	0.18	$p = 0.00^*$
	η_{A2}	−0.29	0.18	$p = 0.05^*$
	τ_A	0.33	0.09	$p = 0.00^*$
Cooperation	η_{C1}	−0.13	0.22	$p = 0.28$
	η_{C2}	0.50	0.23	$p = 0.01^*$
	τ_C	−0.03	0.10	$p = 0.38$
Nervosity	η_{N1}	0.26	0.17	$p = 0.06$
	η_{N2}	−0.25	0.17	$p = 0.07$
	τ_N	−0.22	0.08	$p = 0.00^*$
	ω_2	−3.33	0.13	$p = 0.00^*$
	ω_3	−9.68	0.28	$p = 0.00^*$

agree" no longer has the same meaning across items—so that there remains hardly any meaningful use of the data, except maybe in very large samples. Therefore, one should not be overly optimistic about the advantages of polytomous response data.

References

Andrich, D. (1978). A rating formulation for ordered response categories. *Psychometrika* **43**, 561–573.

Cox, D.R. (1970). *The Analysis of Binary Data.* London: Methuen.

Fischer, G.H. (1972). A measurement model for the effect of mass-media. *Acta Psychologica* **36**, 207–220.

Fischer, G.H. (1974). *Einführung in die Theorie psychologischer Tests.* [Introduction to Mental Test Theory. In German.] Berne: Huber.

Fischer, G.H. (1976). Some probabilistic models for measuring change. In D.N.M. de Gruijter and L.J. Th. van der Kamp (Eds), *Advances in Psychological and Educational Measurement* (pp. 97–110). New York: Wiley.

Fischer, G.H. (1977a). Some probabilistic models for the description of attitudinal and behavioral changes under the influence of mass communication. In W.F. Kempf and B. Repp (Eds), *Mathematical Models for Social Psychology* (pp. 102–151). Berne: Huber, and New York: Wiley.

Fischer, G.H. (1977b). Linear logistic latent trait models: Theory and applications. In H. Spada and W.F. Kempf (Eds), *Structural Models of Thinking and Learning* (pp. 203–225). Berne: Huber.

Fischer, G.H. (1983a). Logistic latent trait models with linear constraints.

Psychometrika **48**, 3–26.

Fischer, G.H. (1983b). Some latent trait models for measuring change in qualitative observations. In D.J. Weiss (Ed), *New Horizons in Testing* (pp. 309–329). New York: Academic Press.

Fischer, G.H. (1987a). Applying the principles of specific objectivity and generalizability to the measurement of change. *Psychometrika* **52**, 565–587.

Fischer, G.H. (1987b). Heritabilität oder Umwelteffekte? Zwei verschiedene Ansätze zur Analyse von Daten getrennt aufgewachsener eineiiger Zwillinge. [Heritability of environmental effects? Two attempts at analyzing data of monozygotic twins reared apart. In German.] In E. Raab and G. Schulter (Eds), *Perspektiven Psychologischer Forschung.* Vienna: Deuticke.

Fischer, G.H. (1989). An IRT-based model for dichotomous longitudinal data. *Psychometrika* **54**, 599–624.

Fischer, G.H. (1991). A new methodology for the assessment of treatment effects. *Evaluación Psicológica — Psychological Assessment* **7**, 117–147.

Fischer, G.H. (1993). The measurement of environmental effects. An alternative to the estimation of heritability in twin data. *Methodika* **7**, 20–43.

Fischer, G.H. and Formann, A.K. (1981). Zur Schätzung der Erblichkeit quantitativer Merkmale. [Estimating heritability of quantitative trait variables. In German.] *Zeitschrift für Differentielle und Diagnostische Psychologie* **3**, 189–197.

Fischer, G.H. and Formann, A.K. (1982). Veränderungsmessung mittels linear-logistischer Modelle. [Measurement of change using linear logistic models. In German.] *Zeitschrift für Differentielle und Diagnostische Psychologie* **3**, 75–99.

Fischer, G.H. and Parzer, P. (1991). An extension of the rating scale model with an application to the measurement of change. *Psychometrika* **56**, 637–651.

Fischer, G.H. and Ponocny, I. (1994). An extension of the partial credit model with an application to the measurement of change. *Psychometrika* **59**, 177–192.

Fischer, G.H. and Tanzer, N. (1994). Some LBTL and LLTM relationships. In G.H. Fischer and D. Laming (Eds), *Contributions to Mathematical Psychology, Psychometrics, and Methodology* (pp. 277–303). New York: Springer-Verlag.

Haberman, S.J. (1974). *The Analysis of Frequency Data.* Chicago: The University of Chicago Press.

Hammer, H. (1978). *Informationsgewinn und Motivationseffekt einer Tonbildschau und eines verbalen Lehrvortrages.* [Information gain and motivation by video show and a verbal teacher presentation. In German.] Unpublished doctoral dissertation. University of Vienna, Vienna.

Hillgruber, G. (1990). *Schätzung von Parametern in psychologischen Testmodellen.* [Parameter estimation in psychological test models. In German.] Unpublished master's thesis. University of Cologne, Cologne.

Jansen, P.G.W. and Roskam, E.E. (1986). Latent trait models and dichotomization of graded responses. *Psychometrika* **51**, 69–91.

Koschier, A. (1993). *Wirksamkeit von Kommunikationstrainings.* [The efficacy of communication training seminars. In German.] Unpublshed master's thesis. University of Vienna, Vienna.

Kropiunigg, U. (1979a). *Wirkungen einer sozialpolitischen Medienkampagne.* [Effects of a sociopolitical media campaign. In German.] Unpublished doctoral dissertation, University of Vienna, Vienna.

Kropiunigg, U. (1979b). Einstellungswandel durch Massenkommunikation. [Attitude change via mass communication. In German.] *Österreichische Zeitschrift für Soziologie* **4**, 67–71.

Pfanzagl, J. (1994). On item parameter estimation in certain latent trait models. In G.H. Fischer and D. Laming (Eds), *Contributions to Mathematical Psychology, Psychometrics, and Methodology* (pp. 249–263). New York: Springer-Verlag.

Rasch, G. (1961). On general laws and the meaning of measurement in psychology. *Proceedings of the IV Berkeley Symposium on Mathematical Statistics and Probability* (Vol. 4). Berkeley: University of California Press.

Rasch, G. (1965). *Statistisk Seminar.* [Statistical Seminar.] University of Copenhagen, Department of Mathematical Statistics, Copenhagen. (Notes taken by J. Stene.)

Roskam, E.E. and Jansen, P.G.W. (1989). Conditions for Rasch-dichotomizability of the unidimensional polytomous Rasch model. *Psychometrika* **54**, 317–332.

Schumacher, M. (1980). Point estimation in quantal response models. *Biometrical Journal* **22**, 315–334.

Stout, W. (1987). A nonparametric approach for assessing latent trait dimensionality. *Psychometrika* **52**, 589–617.

Stout, W. (1990). A new item response theory modeling approach with applications to unidimensionality assessment and ability estimation. *Psychometrika* **55**, 293–325.

Part IV. Nonparametric Models

The origins of nonparametric IRT are found in Guttman's (1947, 1950a, 1950b) early papers on scalogram analysis published before any interest existed in parametric IRT. In scalogram analysis, the response functions of test items (or statements in the case of attitude measurements) are modeled to have the shape of a step curve. Such curves assume that the relation between success on an item and the underlying ability is deterministic; that is, they assume that, with probability one, up to a certain unknown threshold on the scale examinees will be unsuccessful (disagree) with the item (statement). At and beyond the threshold, examinees with probability one will be successful on the item (agree with the statement). The technical problem is to locate items (statements) on the scale along with examinees to maximize the fit between the model and the data.

Guttman's model is refuted as soon as *one* response pattern with a wrong response is met on either side of the threshold. If this decision rule is followed strictly, and each item for which a wrong response is found is labeled as "unscalable," it is an empirical fact that hardly any items (statements) can be maintained if a sample of examinees of realistic size is used to analyze a test. Of course, in practice, some tolerance for misfit is allowed. From the beginning of scalogram analysis, it was felt that a stochastic model with a continuous response function would be more realistic for many applications, and several attempts were made to formulate such functions in a nonparametric fashion. These attempts culminated in the work by Mokken (1971), who not only gave a nonparametric representation of item response functions in the form of a basic set of formal properties they should satisfy, but also provided the statistical theory needed to test whether these properties would hold in empirical data.

Though interest in nonparametric IRT has existed for almost 50 years, in particular in applications where sets of behavior or choices have to be shown to follow a linear order, parametric IRT models have been applied to nonparametric IRT models. Logistic models for response functions were introduced, and these models offered solutions to such practical problems as test equating, item banking, and test bias. In addition, they offered the technology needed to implement computerized adaptive testing. In light of such powerful models and applications, it seemed as if the utility of nonparametric IRT was very limited.

In the early 1980s, however, mainly through the pioneering work of Holland (1981), Holland and Rosenbaum (1986), and Rosenbaum (1984, 1987a, 1987b), the topic of nonparametric IRT was re-introduced into psychometric theory. The idea was no longer to provide nonparametric models as an alternative to parametric models but to study the minimum assumptions that have to be met by any response model, albeit nonparametric or parametric. Interest in the basic assumptions of IRT has a theoretical purpose but serves diagnostic purposes as well. Since for each assumption the observable consequences are clearly specified, aberrancies in response data can be better interpreted. A search for such aberrancies should be a standard procedure to precede the formal statistical goodness-of-fit tests in use in parametric IRT [see, for example, Hambleton (1989)]. In the same vein, nonparametric statistical techniques can be used to describe the probabilities of success on test items as monotonic functions of the underlying ability. As such functions are based on minimum assumptions, they can be assumed to be closer to the "true response functions" than those provided by any parametric model. Therefore, they are useful, for example, as a first check on whether a certain parametric form of response function would be reasonable.

This section offers three chapters on nonparametric IRT. The chapter by Mokken summarizes the early results in nonparametric IRT for dichotomous items and relates them to the concepts developed in the recent approaches to nonparametric IRT. Molenaar generalizes the theory of dichotomous items to polytomous items. Ramsay discusses techniques to estimate response functions for dichotomous items based on ordinal assumptions. Plots of these estimated response functions can be used as graphical checks on the behavior of response functions.

Additional reading on nonparametric IRT is found in Cliff (1989) who proposed an ordinal test theory based on the study of rank correlations between observed and true test scores. A nonparametric treatment of various concepts of the dimensionality of the abilities underlying a test is given by Junker (1991, 1993) and Stout (1987, 1990).

References

Cliff, N. (1989). Ordinal consistency and ordinal true scores. *Psychometrika* **54**, 75–92.

Guttman, L. (1947). The Cornell technique for scale and intensity analysis. *Educational and Psychological Measurement* **7**, 247–280.

Guttman, L. (1950a). The basis for scalogram analysis. In S.A. Stouffer, L. Guttman, E.A. Suchman, P.F. Lazarsfeld, S.A. Star,and J.A. Clausen (Eds), *Measurement and Prediction: Studies in Social Psychology in World War II* (Vol. 4). Princeton, NJ: Princeton University Press.

Guttman, L. (1950b). Relation of scalogram analysis to other techniques.

In S.A. Stouffer, L. Guttman, E.A. Suchman, P.F. Lazarsfeld, S.A. Star, and J.A. Clausen (Eds), *Measurement and Prediction: Studies in Social Psychology in World War II* (Vol. 4). Princeton, NJ: Princeton University Press.

Hambleton, R.K. (1989). Principles and selected applications of item response theory. In R.L. Linn (Ed), *Educational Measurement* (pp. 147–200). New York: Macmillan.

Holland, P.W. (1981). When are item response models consistent with observed data? *Psychometrika* **46**, 79–92.

Holland, P.W. and Rosenbaum, P.R. (1986). Conditional association and unidimensionality in monotone latent variable models. *Annals of Statistics* **14**, 1523–1543.

Junker, B.W. (1991). Essential independence and likelihood-based ability estimation for polytomous items. *Psychometrika* **56**, 255–278.

Junker, B.W. (1993). Conditional association, essential independence and monotone unidimensional item response models. *Annals of Statistics* **21**, 1359–1378.

Mokken, R.J. (1971). *A Theory and Procedure of Scale Analysis, with Applications in Political Research.* New York/Berlin: Walter de Gruyter - Mouton.

Rosenbaum, P.R. (1984). Testing the conditional independence and monotonicity assumptions of item response theory. *Psychometrika* **49**, 425–435.

Rosenbaum, P.R. (1987a). Probability inequalities for latent scales. *British Journal of Mathematical and Statistical Psychology* **40**, 157–168.

Rosenbaum, P.R. (1987b). Comparing item characteristic curves. *Psychometrika* **52**, 217–233.

Stout, W.F. (1987). A nonparametric approach for assessing latent trait unidimensionality. *Psychometrika* **52**, 589–617.

Stout, W.F. (1990). A new item response theory modeling approach with applications to unidimensionality assessment and ability estimation. *Psychometrika* **55**, 293–325.

20
Nonparametric Models for Dichotomous Responses

Robert J. Mokken

Introduction

The development of nonparametric approaches to psychometric and sociometric measurement dates back to the days before the establishment of regular item response theory (IRT). It has its roots in the early manifestations of scalogram analysis (Guttman, 1950), latent structure analysis (Lazarsfeld, 1950), and latent trait theory (Lord, 1953).

In many situations, such as attitude scaling, the analysis of voting behavior in legislative bodies, and market research, items and indicators are either difficult or scarce to obtain, or the level of information concerning item quality is not sufficiently high to warrant the use of specified parametric models. Researchers then have to assess attitudes, abilities, and associated item difficulties at the more lenient ordinal level, instead of the interval or ratio representations required by more demanding parametric models. The primary reference to this approach was Mokken (1971). Later sources are Henning (1976), Niemöller and van Schuur (1983), Mokken and Lewis (1982), Sijtsma (1988), and Giampaglia (1990).

The probabilistic models in this chapter are nonparametric alternatives to most of the current parametric ability models for responses to dichotomous items. A generalization of the initial model and procedures to polytomous items was developed by Molenaar and will be treated elsewhere (Molenaar, this volume).

Presentation of the Models

A set J of N persons $\{j = 1, \ldots, N\}$ is related to a set I of n items $\{i = 1, \ldots, n\}$ by some observed response behavior. Each set may be considered as a selection by some sampling procedure from some (sub)population of persons or (more rarely) of items. Each person j responds to each item i in the item set. Responses are supposed to be dichotomous, and, hence, can be scored as $(0, 1)$ variables. The responses and scores, represented by

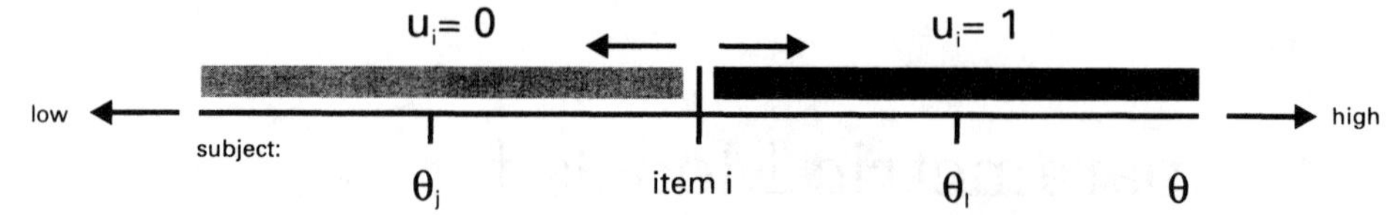

FIGURE 1. Deterministic model (Guttman scalogram).

variates U_{ij} with values u_{ij}, respectively, for each person j and item i in sets J and I,[1] are supposed to be related in the same way to an underlying, not observable or latent ability, which "triggers" the positive response.

An illustration for the deterministic model is given in Figure 1. For a dichotomous item i, there is only one step separating response "0" from response "1." For the deterministic case, this step marks a boundary on the ability variable θ: Persons with ability θ_j to the left of the boundary are not sufficiently high on θ to pass item i, and score 0, whereas persons with θ_l, to the right of the boundary, dominate item i in the required amount of θ, and score 1. In actual applications, scoring items uniformly with respect to the direction of θ is important.

In probabilistic ability models, responses U_{ij} of person j to item i are assumed to be generated by probabilities, depending on the values of persons and items on the ability θ. For the simple deterministic case of Fig. 1, these probabilities can be given as:

$$P\{U_{ij} = 1; \theta_j\} = 0;$$
$$P\{U_{ij} = 0; \theta_l\} = 1.$$

More generally the probabilities are given by functions depending on the item and the value θ of the ability of a given person j:

$$\pi_i(\theta_j) = P\{U_{ij} = 1; \theta_j\}, \quad \text{and}$$
$$1 - \pi_i(\theta_j) = P\{U_{ij} = 0; \theta_j\}.$$

The functions $\pi_i(\theta)$ are called *item response functions* (IRF's). For an example, see Fig. 2. Other well-known names are "trace lines" or "trace functions" in latent structure analysis and "item characteristic curves" (ICC) in IRT.

The values of $\pi_i(\theta)$ may be considered as local difficulties, measuring the difficulty of item i for a person located at point θ along the ability continuum. Sometimes an item difficulty parameter b is added, such as in $\pi_i(\theta, b_i)$, to denote the point on θ where the probability of passing the item is equal to 0.50, that is, where $\pi_i(b_i, b_i) = 0.50$.

---

[1]According to the conventions for this Handbook, indices correspond to the transposed person-by-items data matrix.

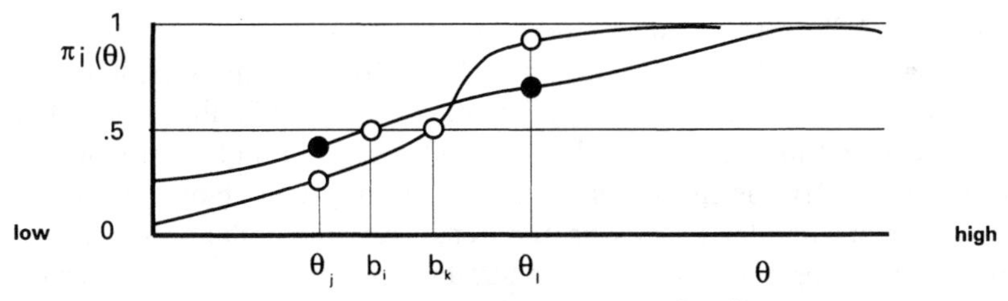

FIGURE 2. Two singly monotonic (MH) IRF's.

Two related nonparametric models for dichotomous cumulative items can be used. The basic elements of these models are treated next.[2]

Monotonic Homogeneity

Some requirements or assumptions concerning the form of the item probabilities $\pi(\theta)$ imply certain types of homogeneity between the items. A first requirement is the following one of *monotonic homogeneity* (MH):

> For all items $i \in I$, $\pi_i(\theta)$ should be monotonically nondecreasing in θ, that is, for all items $i \in I$ and for all values (θ_j, θ_l) it should hold that
>
> $$\theta_j \leq \theta_l \Leftrightarrow \pi_i(\theta_j) \leq \pi_i(\theta_l)$$

A related requirement is the one of *similar ordering* (SO) of the persons in J by the items in I in terms of their IRF's:

> A set of items or IRF's is similarly ordering a set of persons $\theta_1, \theta_2, \ldots, \theta_N$ if, whenever $\pi_i(\theta_1) \leq \pi_i(\theta_2) \leq \cdots \leq \pi_i(\theta_N)$ for *some* $i \in I$, then $\pi_k(\theta_1) \leq \pi_k(\theta_2) \leq \cdots \leq \pi_k(\theta_N)$ for *all* $k \in I$.

The SO property of a set of items with respect to a set of persons reflects the possibility of a unidimensional representation of the persons in terms of an ability supposed to underlie their response behavior. It can be shown that SO and MH are equivalent properties. MH sets of IRF's correspond to the cumulative or monotonic trace lines familiar in ability analysis (see Fig. 2). The SO property emphasizes their particular appropriateness for unidimensional representation.

Double Monotonicity

A set of SO or MH items suffices for the purpose of a joint ordering of persons on an ability. However, it is not sufficient for a uniform ordering of

---

[2]In the sequel, the main results and properties will be given without derivations, for which we may refer to Mokken (1971, Chap. 4).

(local) item difficulties, $\pi_i(\theta)$ for persons as they vary in ability θ. Again, this can be seen for the two MH IRF's in Fig. 2. Item k is more difficult than item i, but as their IRF's are intersecting, the local difficulty order of the items is reversed for persons on different sides of the point of intersection.

So although MH has the items similarly ordering the persons, it does not warrant persons similarly ordering the items. An additional or stronger requirement is necessary to ensure also similar ordering of items by persons. This is the requirement of *double monotonicity* (DM) or *strong monotonicity homogeneity* (Mokken, 1971)[3]:

> A MH set of items, I, satisfies the condition of double monotonicity (DM) with respect to an ability θ (or a set of persons, J) if for all pairs of items $(i, k) \in I$ it holds that, if for some θ_0: $\pi_i(\theta_0) \leq \pi_k(\theta_0)$, then for all θ and $j \in J$: $\pi_i(\theta_j) \leq \pi_k(\theta_j)$, where item i is assumed to be the more difficult item.

Figure 3 gives an illustration for a set of three DM items. The item difficulty parameters b_1, b_2, b_3, reflect the order of the local item difficulties (with item 1 being most difficult), which is the same for all persons, that is,

$$b_1 > b_2 > b_3 \Leftrightarrow \text{for all } \theta\text{: } \pi(\theta, b_1) < \pi(\theta, b_2) < \pi(\theta, b_3).$$

Sets of two-parameter logistic items with different discrimination parameter are examples of MH sets (Birnbaum, 1968). Sets of two-parameter logistic items with equal discrimination parameter are examples of DM sets. These are equivalent to models based on the single item parameter logistic IRF associated with the Rasch (1960) model.

Two Types of Independence Assumptions

In IRT two types of independence assumptions are basic for the models:

1. Local or conditional independence or independence of responses within persons. This condition assumes that for every single person from J (i.e., for any fixed value of θ) the response to any item from I is independent of the responses to any other item in I. This assumption is basic to most probabilistic theories of measurement, implying that all systematic variation in the responses of persons to items is solely due to the variation of persons over θ. All variation in a single point θ is random and residual, as the sole source of systematic variation is then kept constant.

[3]Rosenbaum (1987b) introduced an equivalent concept where one item is *uniformly more difficult* than another when its IRF lies on or above the surface of the other one.

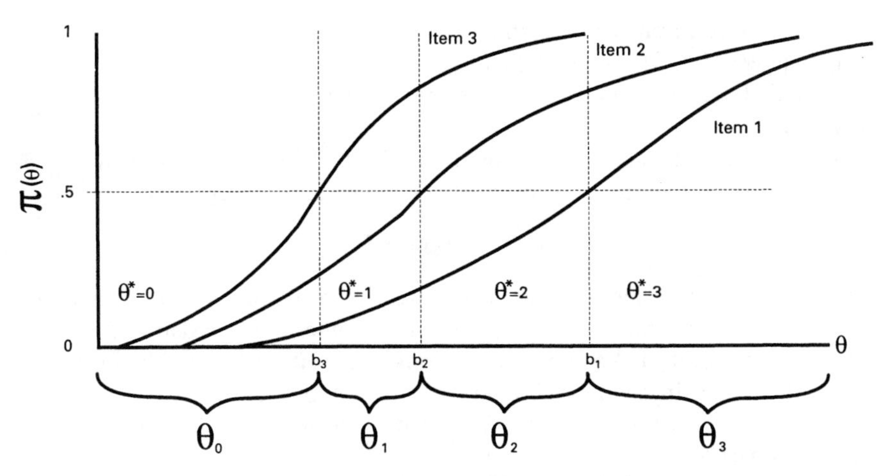

FIGURE 3. Double monotony: Classes and class scores.

2. Sampling independence or independence of responses between persons. This condition assumes that the selection of respondents, as well as the procedure of test administration, imply that the responses of any person from set J to the items in set I are not related to responses to I of any other person in J.

These two basic assumptions determine the mathematical expression of the joint probability of persons responding to items.

Let $\mathbf{u}_j = (u_{1j}, \ldots, u_{nj})$, $u_{ij} = 0, 1$, denote the response vector of person j (with value θ_j) for n items. Obviously, $\mathbf{u}_j$ can take 2^n possible values. Assumption 1 implies that for any person j the probability of a response pattern $\mathbf{u}_j$ is given by the product of the probabilities of the individual item responses in the pattern. Also, Assumption 2 can be used to calculate the probability of a matrix with response data for N persons as the product of the probabilities of the response vectors of the individual persons.

Let π_{ik} denote the joint probability of a correct response on items i and k. In addition, the simple score t_υ of a response pattern $\mathbf{u}_\upsilon$ is defined as the number of items correct in that pattern: $t_\upsilon = \sum_i u_{i\upsilon}$. This notation is used to discuss the following properties.

Simple Monotonicity (MH). An early result (Mokken, 1971) states that for MH sets of items, under the assumption of local independence, all item pairs are nonnegatively correlated for all subgroups of subjects and all subsets of items:

> MH1: for an MH set of items, I, it holds for every distribution $F(\theta)$ that $\pi_{ik} \geq \pi_i \pi_k$, for all $(i, k) \in I$.

An immediate implication is that the expected value of the Guttman error $\pi_{ik}(1,0)$ ($i \leq k$; i more difficult than k) is smaller than expected under conditional marginal (or posterior) independence, given the manifest marginals.

Rosenbaum (1984) [see also Holland and Rosenbaum (1986)] proved the following more general result from the same set of assumptions:

$$\text{Cov}\{f(\mathbf{U}_1), g(\mathbf{U}_1) \mid \mathbf{h}(\mathbf{U}_2)\} \geq 0,$$

where $\mathbf{u} = (\mathbf{u}_1, \mathbf{u}_2)$ denote a partition of response vector $\mathbf{u}$ in two subsets $\mathbf{u}_1$ and $\mathbf{u}_2$ and $f(\mathbf{u})$ and $g(\mathbf{u})$ denote any monotonic nondecreasing functions of $\mathbf{u}$. This property is known as conditional association (CA). The property MH1 then is an immediate corollary of this CA-property.

Other properties which are useful for diagnosing the behavior of sets of items are the following:

> MH2: every pair of items $(i, k) \in I$ is CA in every subgroup of persons with a particular subscore t on the remaining set of items;
>
> MH3: for every item i the proportion correct π_i is nondecreasing over increasing score groups t, where score t is taken over the remaining $n-1$ items.
>
> MH4 (ordering of persons): the simple score $t(\mathbf{u};\theta)$ has a monotonic nondecreasing regression on ability θ (Lord and Novick, 1968).

Moreover, for all θ, $t(\mathbf{u};\theta)$ is more discriminating than scores on single items (Mokken, 1971). The score $t(\mathbf{u}_j)$ of persons j thus reflects stochastically the ordering of the persons according to that ability.

> MH5: the simple score $t(\mathbf{u};\theta)$ has monotone likelihood ratio, that is,
>
> $$\frac{P\{t(\mathbf{u};\theta) = t\}}{P\{t(\mathbf{u};\theta) = s\}}, \quad n \geq t > s \geq 0$$
>
> is nondecreasing in θ (Grayson, 1988).

This result implies that $t(\mathbf{u};\theta)$ is an optimal statistic for binary (two-group) classification procedures.

Double Monotonicity (DM). Only for sets of items which are DM, the difficulty order of the items is the same for all persons. An immediate consequence is:

> DM1: for a DM set of items for every pair of items (i, k) the order of their manifest (population) difficulties (π_i, π_k) is the same irrespective of the distribution $F(\theta)$ of θ. Hence, if $i < k$ (that is, if item i is more difficult than item k), then $\pi_i \leq \pi_k$ for all groups of persons (Mokken, 1971).

The order of the manifest probabilities π_i reflects the uniform difficulty ordering of the items for every (sub)group of persons. This is not always so for just single monotonicity (MH) because then the IRF's of the two items can intersect. For two groups of persons with an ability distribution $F(\theta)$ on different sides of the intersection point the manifest probabilities (π_i, π_k) will indicate different difficulty orders.

Another DM property concerns the joint probabilities of pairs of manifest responses for triples of items (i, k, l). Let $\pi_{ik}(1,1)$ and $\pi_{ik}(0,0)$ denote the probabilities of items i and k both correct and items failed, respectively. Let $k < l$ denote the item ordering for k more difficult than l. Then

DM2: for all $i \in I$, and all pairs $(k,l) \in I$, $k < l$:

$$\begin{array}{ll} (1) & \pi_{ik}(1,1) \leq \pi_{il}(1,1) \text{ and} \\ (2) & \pi_{ik}(0,0) \geq \pi_{il}(0,0). \end{array} \tag{1}$$

(Mokken, 1971). The two inequalities can be visualized by means of two matrices.

Let $\Pi = [\pi_{ik}(1,1)]$ of order $n \times n$ $(i, k = 1, \ldots, n$ and $i < k)$ be the symmetric matrix of manifest joint probabilities of scoring both correct, π_{ik}. According to the first part of Eq. (1), for any row i of Π its row elements will increase with k. By symmetry, the elements of column k will increase with i. Note that the diagonal elements, π_{ii}, are based on replicated administrations of the item, and generally cannot be observed directly.

Let $\Pi^{(0)} = [\pi_{ik}(0,0)]$ of order $n \times n$ be the symmetric matrix, with diagonal elements not specified, containing the manifest probabilities of both items failed, then the second relation in Eq. (1) implies a reverse trend in rows and columns: The elements in row i will decrease with k and, by symmetry, the elements in any column will decrease with i. As the two matrices Π and $\Pi^{(0)}$ can be estimated from samples of persons, these results allow for empirically checking for DM.

Rosenbaum (1987b) derived related results, considering for item pairs the event that exactly one of the two items is answered correctly. The corresponding probabilities are considered as conditional probabilities given some value of an arbitrary function $h(\mathbf{u}_2)$ of the response pattern $\mathbf{u}_2$ of the remaining $n-2$ items. It is convenient to take the simple score $t(\mathbf{u}_2)$ or score groups based on $t(\mathbf{u}_2)$ (Rosenbaum, 1987b).

DM3: If item i is more difficult than k $(i < k)$, then

$$P\{U_i = 1 \mid U_i + U_k = 1;\ t(\mathbf{u}_2)\} \leq 0.50$$

or equivalently

$$P\{U_i = 1 \mid t(\mathbf{u}_2)\} \leq P\{U_k = 1 \mid t(\mathbf{u}_2)\}, \tag{2}$$

that is, item i will be answered correctly by fewer persons than k in any score group $t(\mathbf{u}_2)$ on the remaining $n-2$ items $\mathbf{u}_2$.

Parameter Estimation

Once it has been established that a set of items can be used as a unidimensional (MH or DM) scale or test, the major purpose of its application is to estimate the θ values of the persons. In parametric models, this can be done by direct estimation of θ in the model in which it figures as a parameter. As nonparametric models do not contain these parameters, more indirect methods are needed to infer positions or orderings of respondents along the ability continuum.

One simple method is to use the simple score $t(\mathbf{u})$. According to MH4, the score is correlated positively with θ, and according to MH5 it is an optimal statistic for various types of classification.

Schriever (1985) advocated optimal score methods derived from multiple correspondence analysis (MCA), where the first principal component Y_1 of the correlation matrix of the items $\mathbf{U} = [U_1, \ldots, U_n]$ optimally fits the ability θ. This first principal component can be written as

$$Y_1 = \sum_{i=1}^{k} \alpha_{i1}\phi_{i1}(u_i), \tag{3}$$

where a correct and an incorrect response score are recoded as

$$\phi_{i1}(1) = \left(\frac{1-\pi_i}{\pi_i}\right)^{1/2},$$

$$\phi_{i1}(0) = -\left(\frac{\pi_i}{1-\pi_i}\right)^{1/2},$$

respectively, and $\alpha_1 = [\alpha_{11}, \ldots, \alpha_{n1}]$, with $\alpha_1^T\alpha_1 = 1$, is an eigenvector for the largest eigenvalue of the correlation matrix of the items.

Even stronger order conditions are valid for a special case of DM.[4] Let a rescored correct response be denoted by γ_{i1} and a rescored incorrect response by ω_{i1}. Let I_n be a MH set of n items. Finally, let I_m be a DM subset of m items (i,k), with $i < k$, satisfying the following monotone likelihood ratio type of conditions: $\pi_k(\theta)/\pi_i(\theta)$ and $(1-\pi_k(\theta))/(1-\pi_i(\theta))$ are nonincreasing in θ. Then, assuming the $(i,k) \in I_m$ to be ordered according to difficulty (that is, item 1 is the most difficult item, etc.), the following result holds:

> DM4: the scores γ_{i1} and ω_{i1} reflect the order of the DM items in the set of items:
>
> $$\gamma_{11} > \cdots > \gamma_{m1} > 0; \quad \text{and}$$
> $$0 > \omega_{11} > \cdots > \omega_{m1}$$

[4] More precisely, the IRF's of $(i,k) \in I_m$ are required to be DM and to demonstrate total positivity of order two (TP_2) (Karlin, 1968; Schriever, 1985).

(Schriever, 1985).

This type of scoring seems intuitively satisfactory: Answering a difficult item correctly contributes heavily to the total score, whereas an incorrect response is not penalized too much. Moreover, together with DM1–DM3, this property can be used for testing a set of items for DM. The method of optimal scoring can be generalized to polytomous item responses.

Lewis (Lewis, 1983; Mokken and Lewis, 1982), using the ordering assumptions of the DM model, introduced prior knowledge for use with a Bayesian method of allocating persons to $n+1$ ordered ability classes θ_i^* (i: $0,\ldots,n$; see Fig. 3 for three items and four score classes) on the basis of their observed response patterns. Working directly with posterior distributions and using exact, small sample results, this method enables one: (1) to obtain interval estimates for θ; (2) to make classification decisions based on utilities associated with different mastery levels; and (3) to analyze responses obtained in tailored adaptive testing situations.

Goodness of Fit

Parametric models are formulated in terms of fully specified response functions defined on a parameter structure. Suitable methods for estimation and testing their goodness of fit to the data at hand are necessary for their effective application. Nonparametric models are more general, hence less specific with respect to estimation and testing. Different statistical methods have to be applied to make inferences. In this section, some statistics will be considered which are pertinent to a set of items as a scale (MH or DM).

Scalability: H-Coefficient

For MH sets of items to exist, positive association is a necessary condition (MH1). For dichotomous items, coefficient H of Loevinger (1947, 1948) was adapted by Mokken (1971) to define a family of coefficients indicating MH scalability for pairs of items within a set, a single item with respect to the other items of a set and, the set of items as a whole.[5]

One intuitive way to define coefficient H is in terms of Guttman error probabilities $\pi_{ik}(1,0)$ ($i<k$; $\pi_i<\pi_k$). For any pair of items (i,k), let the

[5]The H coefficient is due to Loevinger (1947, 1948). However, she did not devise an item coefficient H_i of this type but proposed another instead.

Guttman error probabilities be defined by

$$
\begin{aligned}
e_{ik} &= \pi_{ik}(1,0); \quad e_{ik}^{(0)} = \pi_i(1-\pi_k) \text{ if } i < k; \\
e_{ik} &= \pi_{ik}(0,1); \quad e_{ik}^{(0)} = (1-\pi_i)\pi_k \text{ if } i > k;
\end{aligned}
\tag{4}
$$

where e_{ik} and $e_{ik}^{(0)}$ denote the probabilities of observed error and expected error under for marginal (bivariate) independence. Then the coefficient for an *item pair* (i,k) is defined by[6]

$$
H_{ik} = 1 - \frac{e_{ik}}{e_{ik}^{(0)}} . \tag{5}
$$

In the deterministic case $e_{ik} = 0$ and $H_{ik} = 1$, so that high values of H_{ik} correspond to steep (discriminating) IRF's. In the case of marginal independence, $e_{ik} = e_{ik}^{(0)}$ and $H_{ik} = 0$. So low values of H_{ik} are associated with at least one nondiscriminating (flat) IRF. Negative correlations ($H_{ik} < 0$) contradict MH1 because error probabilities $e_{ik}^{(0)}$ are even larger than expected for completely random responses.

In a similar way, for any single item i, coefficient H_i can be given with respect to the other $n-1$ items of I as a linear combination (weighted sum) of the H_k involved. Let $e_i = \sum_{k \neq i} e_{ik}$ and $e_i^{(0)} = \sum_{k \neq i} e_{ik}^{(0)}$, then the coefficient for *item* i is defined by:

$$
H_i = 1 - \frac{e_i}{e_i^0} = \frac{\sum_{k \neq i}^{n} \pi_{ik}^{(0)} H_{ik}}{\sum_{k \neq i}^{n} \pi_{ik}^{(0)}} . \tag{6}
$$

The H_i values can be used to evaluate the fit of item i with respect to the other items in I.

Finally, a coefficient can be defined the same way for the *full set* of items, I, in terms of an error ratio and as a linear combination of the H_i or H_{ik}. Let $e = \sum_{k<i} e_{ik}$ and $e^{(0)} = \sum_{k<i} e_{ik}^{(0)}$, then the coefficient for the scale is given by:

$$
H = 1 - \frac{e}{e^0} = \frac{\sum_{i<k}^{n} \pi_{ik}^{(0)} H_i}{\sum_{i<k}^{n} \pi_{ik}^{(0)}} = \frac{\sum_{i<k}^{n} \pi_{ik}^{(0)} H_{ik}}{\sum_{i<k}^{n} \pi_{ik}^{(0)}} . \tag{7}
$$

For MH sets of items, property MH1 implies that the coefficients are all nonnegative:

$$
0 \leq H_{ik},\ H_i, \text{ or } H \leq 1. \tag{8}
$$

Moreover, let $\min(H_i; i = 1, \ldots, n) = c$, then $H \geq c$, $0 \leq c \leq 1$, and H is at least as large as the smallest H_i, H can also be written as a normalized variance ratio of the simple score $t(\mathbf{u})$ (Mokken, 1971).

[6]It should be noted that H_{ik} is equal to $\phi/\phi_{\max}$, where ϕ and $\phi_{\max}$ denote Pearson's correlation coefficient in a 2×2-table and its maximum value, given the marginals π_i and π_k, respectively.

An MH scale is defined as a set of items which are all positively correlated (MH1) with the property that every item coefficient (H_i) is greater than or equal to a given positive constant c ($0 < c < 1$).[7] From Eq. (7) we have that H, the coefficient testing the scalability of the set of items as a whole, will then also be greater than c, which can be designated as the scale-defining constant. This suggested the following classification of scales:

$$\begin{array}{ll} 0.50 \leq H: & \text{strong scale;} \\ 0.40 \leq H < 0.50: & \text{medium scale;} \\ 0.30 \leq H < 0.40: & \text{weak scale.} \end{array}$$

Experience based on a few decades of numerous applications has shown that in practice the lower bound $c = 0.30$ performs quite satisfactorily, delivering long and useful scales. Meijer et al. (1990) compared the results for $c = 0.30$ with $c = 0$, finding that the former restriction yielded sets of items that discriminated better among persons.

Sample estimates of $\hat{H}_{ik}$, $\hat{H}_i$, and $\hat{H}$ can be obtained by inserting the usual ML estimates for $\pi(\mathbf{u})$, π_{ik}, π_i, etc., into the relevant equations. Asymptotic sampling theory for these estimates was completely developed by Mokken (1971, Chap. 4.3). Generally, coefficients of scalability satisfy the following two requirements:

1. The theoretical maximum is 1 for all scales.

2. The theoretical minimum, assuming MH, is zero for all MH-scales.

In addition, they can be used for the following goals:

1. Testing theoretically interesting hypotheses about H and H_i.

2. Constructing (population specific) confidence intervals for H and H_i.

3. Evaluating existing scales as a whole with H, as well as the scalability of individual items with the item coefficients H_i.

4. Constructing a scale from a given pool of items.

5. Multiple scaling: the construction of a number of scales from a given pool of items.

6. Extending an existing scale by adding new items from a pool of items.

For more details, see Mokken (1971), Mokken and Lewis (1982), or Molenaar et al. (1994).

---

[7]The term "scale" (or, for that matter, "test") is used here, as it is a familiar concept in social research and attitude scaling. It has no immediate connection with the basic concept of scale in axiomatic theories of measurement, where it is used to denote the triple of an empirical system, a numerical system, and a set of mapping rules.

Reliability

For the case of DM sets of items, Mokken (1971) showed a method of estimating item and test reliabilities based on using DM2 for an interpolation for the diagonal elements of the matrix Π of Eq. (1). Sijtsma and Molenaar (1987) investigated this approach further, developing improved estimates. Meijer and Sijtsma (1993) demonstrated the use of item reliability as a measure of discriminating power and slope for nonparametric IRF's in person fit analysis.

Software

In the seventies, a FORTRAN package (SCAMMO) was available on Control Data Cyber (Niemöller and van Schuur, 1980) and IBM 360 mainframes (Lippert et al., 1978). This package handled dichotomous items only. In the eighties, PC versions (MSP) were developed for use under MS DOS, incorporating the options and additional possibilities of Molenaar's generalization of the model to polytomous items (Debets et al., 1989). Recently, the latest version, MSP 3.0, distributed by ice ProGAMMA, has been totally redesigned (Molenaar, et al., 1994).

Example

An early example taken from the author's electoral studies (Mokken, 1971, Chap. 8) will give a first illustration of the method for dichotomous items. A set of items designed to measure "sense of political efficacy," a familiar attitudinal variable in electoral research, is considered. The first version of the items, referring to politics at the national level, had been proven to be scalable in the USA and the Netherlands. A new set of eight items was designed to refer to this attitude at the local level of community politics in the city of Amsterdam. There were good reasons to suppose these items would form a scalable set as well. The test of the items as well as the results of a test of their scalability ($c = 0.30$; $\alpha = 0.05$) are given in Table 1.[8] As expected, Table 1 shows the items to be reasonably (MH) scalable. The item coefficients range from 0.31 (L.6) to 0.48 (L.8), the H coefficient for the total score was .41. An analysis across various subgroups confirmed MH in the sense of positive correlation between pairs of items, although due to sampling variability, an occasional H coefficient showed values below c (0.30).

---

[8] *Note on Table 1.* Sample taken from Amsterdam electorate (n = 1,513); $\hat{H} = 0.41$ (95% confidence interval: $[0.38 \leq H \leq 0.43]$). Source: Mokken (1971, p. 259).

TABLE 1. A Local Efficacy Scale (Eight Items).

	Items	Marginals	$\hat{H}_1$
L1.	If I communicate my views to the municipal authorities, they will be taken into account (Positive alternative: "agree")	0.33	0.35
L2.	The municipal authorities don't care much about the opinions of people like me (Positive alternative: "disagree")	0.34	0.46
L3.	Members of the City Council don't care much about the opinions of people like me (Positive alternative: "disagree")	0.35	0.44
L4.	People like me don't have any say about what the city government does (Positive alternative: "disgree")	0.37	0.39
L5.	If I communicate my views to members of the City Council, they will be taken into account (Positive alternative: "agree")	0.37	0.39
L6.	Sometimes city policies and governments in Amsterdam seem so complicated that a person like me can't really understand what's going on (Positive alternative: "disagree")	0.41	0.31
L7.	In the determination of city politics, the votes of people like me are not taken into account (Positive alternative: "disagree")	0.62	0.47
L8.	Because I know so little about city politics, I shouldn't really vote in municipal elections (Positive alternative: "disagree")	0.68	0.48

Systematic inspection of the matrices Π, and $\Pi^{(0)}$ (see Tables 2–3)[9] showed the eight item set not to be doubly monotonic (DM). Removal of item L1 would likely have improved the scale in this respect. The example also shows that visual inspection, always a necessary aid of judgement, is hardly a sufficient tool in itself. In recent versions of MSP, more objective tests of DM2 and DM3 have been implemented (Molenaar; this volume).

TABLE 2. $\hat{\Pi}$ Matrix of Local Efficacy Scale (Eight Items).

Item	L_1	L_2	L_3	L_4	L_5	L_6	L_7	L_8
L_1	–	0.20	0.20	**0.17**	0.24	**0.16**	0.26	0.27
L_2	0.20	–	0.24	0.23	0.22	0.21	0.29	0.29
L_3	0.20	0.24	–	0.21	0.22	0.22	0.29	0.29
L_4	**0.17**	0.23	0.21	–	0.21	0.21	**0.32**	0.31
L_5	0.24	0.22	0.22	0.21	–	0.19	0.28	0.30
L_6	**0.16**	0.21	0.22	0.21	0.19	–	0.32	0.36
L_7	0.26	0.29	0.29	**0.32**	0.28	0.32	–	0.50
L_8	0.27	0.29	0.29	0.31	0.30	0.36	0.50	–
Sample Difficulties	0.33	0.34	0.35	0.37	0.37	0.41	0.62	0.68

TABLE 3. $\hat{\Pi}^{(0)}$ Matrix of Local Efficacy Scale (Eight Items).

Item	L_1	L_2	L_3	L_4	L_5	L_6	L_7	L_8
L_1	–	0.52	**0.51**	**0.47**	0.54	**0.41**	0.30	0.26
L_2	0.52	–	0.55	0.52	0.51	0.45	0.32	0.27
L_3	0.51	0.55	–	0.50	0.50	0.46	0.32	0.26
L_4	**0.47**	0.52	0.50	–	0.47	0.43	0.33	0.26
L_5	0.54	0.51	0.50	0.47	–	0.41	0.29	0.25
L_6	**0.41**	0.45	0.46	0.43	0.41	–	0.28	0.27
L_7	0.30	0.32	0.32	0.33	0.29	0.28	–	0.20
L_8	0.26	0.27	0.26	0.26	0.25	0.27	0.20	–
Sample Difficulties	0.33	0.34	0.35	0.37	0.37	0.41	0.62	0.68

Discussion

Over the years, the methods sketched above have proven their usefulness in numerous applications in many countries as well as such contexts as health research, electoral studies, market research, attitude studies, and

[9] Source for Tables 2 and 3 is Mokken (1971, p. 280).

labor studies (e.g., Giampaglia, 1990; Gillespie, et al., 1988; Heinz, 1981; Henning and Six, 1977; Lippert et al., 1978).

References

Birnbaum, A. (1968). Some latent trait models and their use in inferring an examinee's ability. In F.M. Lord and M.R. Novick, *Statistical Theories of Mental Test Scores* (pp. 397–479). Reading, MA: Addison-Wesley.

Debets, P., Sijtsma, K., Brouwer, E., and Molenaar, I.W. (1989). MSP: A computer program for item analysis according to a nonparametric IRT approach. *Psychometrika* **54**, 534–536.

Giampaglia, G. (1990). *Lo Scaling Unidimensionale Nella Ricerca Sociale.* Napoli: Liguori Editore.

Gillespie, M., TenVergert, E.M., and Kingma, J. (1988). Secular trends in abortion attitudes: 1975–1980–1985. *Journal of Psychology* **122**, 232–341.

Grayson, D.A. (1988). Two-group classification in latent trait theory: Scores with monotone likelihood ratio. *Psychometrika* **53**, 383–392.

Guttman, L. (1950). The basis for scalogram analysis. In S.A. Stouffer et al. (Eds.), *Measurement and Prediction* (pp. 60–90). Princeton, NJ: Princeton University Press.

Heinz, W. (1981). *Klassifikation und Latente Struktur.* Unpublished doctoral dissertation. Rheinischen Friedrich-Wilhelms-Universität, Bonn, Germany.

Henning, H.J. (1976). Die Technik der Mokken-Skalenanalyse. *Psychologische Beiträge* **18**, 410–430.

Henning, H.J. and Six, B. (1977). Konstruktion einer Machiavellismus-Skala. *Zeitschrift für Sozial Psychologie* **8**, 185–198.

Holland, P.W. and Rosenbaum, P.R. (1986). Conditional association and unidimensionality in monotone latent variable models. *Annals of Statistics* **14**, 1523–1543.

Karlin, S. (1968). *Total Positivity I.* Stanford, CA: Stanford University Press.

Lazarsfeld, P.F. (1950). The logical and mathematical foundation of latent structure analysis. In S.A. Stouffer et al. (Eds), *Measurement and Prediction* (pp. 362–412). Princeton, NJ: Princeton University Press.

Lewis, C. (1983). Bayesian inference for latent abilities. In S.B. Anderson and J.S. Helmick (Eds.), *On Educational Testing* (pp. 224–251). San Francisco: Jossey-Bass.

Lippert, E., Schneider, P., and Wakenhut, R. (1978). Die Verwendung der Skalierungsverfahren von Mokken und Rasch zur Überprüfung und Revision von Einstellungsskalen. *Diagnostica* **24**, 252–274.

Loevinger, J. (1947). A systematic approach to the construction and evaluation of tests of ability. *Psychological Monographs* **61**, No. 4.

Loevinger, J. (1948). The technic of homogeneous tests compared with some aspects of "scale analysis" and factor analysis. *Psychological Bulletin* **45**, 507–530.

Lord, F.M. (1953). An application of confidence intervals and of maximum likelihood to the estimation of an examinee's ability. *Psychometrika* **18**, 57–77.

Lord, F.M. and Novick, M.R. (1968). *Statistical Theories of Mental Test Scores.* Reading, MA: Addison-Wesley.

Meijer, R.R. and Sijtsma, K. (1993). Reliability of item scores and its use in person fit research. In R. Steyer, K.F. Wender, and K.F. Widaman (Eds.), *Psychometric Methodology: Proceedings of the 7th European Meeting of the Psychometric Society* (pp. 326–332). Stuttgart, Germany: Gustav Fischer Verlag.

Meijer, R.R., Sijtsma, K., and Smid, N.G. (1990). Theoretical and empirical comparison of the Mokken and the Rasch approach to IRT. *Applied Psychological Measurement* **11**, 283–298.

Mokken, R.J. (1971). *A Theory and Procedure of Scale Analysis with Applications in Political Research.* New York, Berlin: Walter de Gruyter, Mouton.

Mokken, R.J. and Lewis, C. (1982). A nonparametric approach to the analysis of dichotomous item responses. *Applied Psychological Measurement* **6**, 417–430.

Molenaar, I.W., Debets, P., Sijtsma, K., and Hemker, B.T. (1994). *MSP, A Program for Mokken Scale Analysis for Polytomous Items, Version 3.0, (User's Manual).* Groningen, The Netherlands: iec ProGAMMA.

Niemöller, B. and van Schuur, W.H. (1980). *Stochastic Cumulative Scaling. STAP User's Manual, Vol. 4.* Amsterdam, The Netherlands: Technisch Centrum FSW, University of Amsterdam.

Niemöller, B. and van Schuur, W.H. (1983). Stochastic models for unidimensional scaling: Mokken and Rasch. In D. McKay, N. Schofield, and P. Whiteley (Eds.), *Data Analysis and the Social Sciences* (pp. 120–170). London: Francis Pinter.

Rasch, G. (1960). *Probabilistic Models for Some Intelligence and Attainment Tests.* Copenhagen: Nielsen and Lydiche.

Rosenbaum, P.R. (1984). Testing the conditional independence and monotonicity assumptions of item response theory. *Psychometrika* **49**, 425–435.

Rosenbaum, P.R. (1987a). Probability inequalities for latent scales. *British Journal of Mathematical and Statistical Psychology* **40**, 157–168.

Rosenbaum, P.R. (1987b). Comparing item characteristic curves. *Psychometrika* **52**, 217–233.

Schriever, B.F. (1985). *Order Dependence.* Unpublished doctoral dissertation, Free University. Amsterdam, The Netherlands. Sijtsma, K. (1988).

Contributions to Mokken's Nonparametric Item Response Theory. Unpublished doctoral dissertation, Free University, Amsterdam, The Netherlands.

Sijtsma, K. and Molenaar, I.W. (1987). Reliability of test scores in nonparametric item response theory. *Psychometrika* **52**, 79–97.

Sijtsma, K. and Meijer, R.R. (1992). A method for investigating the intersection of item response functions in Mokken's nonparametric IRT model. *Applied Psychological Measurement* **16**, 149–157.

Stouffer, S.A., Guttman, L., Suchman, E.A., Lazarsfeld, P.F., Star, S.A., and Clausen, J.A. (1950). *Measurement and Prediction. Studies in Social Psychology in World War II*, vol. IV. Princeton, NJ: Princeton University Press.

21

Nonparametric Models for Polytomous Responses

Ivo W. Molenaar

Introduction

Mokken (this volume) has argued that his nonparametric IRT model for dichotomous responses can be used to order persons with respect to total score on a monotone homogeneous (MH) set of n items, such that apart from measurement error, this reflects the order of these persons on the property measured by the item set (ability, attitude, capacity, achievement, etc.). If the stronger model of double monotonicity (DM) holds, one can also order the items with respect to popularity. In a majority of cases, the respondents giving a positive reply to a difficult item will also answer positively to all more easy items. It has been explained how Loevinger's H-coefficient per item pair, per item and for the scale can be used to express the extent to which this Guttman pattern holds true, and to search for homogeneous scales from a larger pool of items.

Not only in attitude measurement but also in measuring achievement, it will often be the case that an item is scored into a limited number (say three to seven) ordered response categories, such that a response in a higher category is indicative of the possession of a larger amount of the ability being measured. The more this holds, the more one can expect to gain by using a model for polytomously scored items. For the same number of items presented, one will have a more refined and more reliable instrument than obtained from either dichotomously offered or post hoc dichotomized items. The latter also has other drawbacks (see Jansen and Roskam, 1986).

This leads naturally to the question of whether Mokken's nonparametric IRT model can be extended to cover the case of $m > 2$ ordered response categories. It will be argued here that this can be done for the most important aspects of the model.

Presentation of the Model

Just as in the case of dichotomous items (Mokken, this volume), the basic data being modeled form an N by n data matrix. In order to follow the notation of other chapters, the elements of its transpose are the responses u_{ij} of person j to item i for $j = 1, 2, \ldots, N$ and $i = 1, 2, \ldots, n$. Now, however, item i is either offered, or post hoc scored, into a set C of m_i ordered response categories, for which one mostly uses the integers $0, 1, \ldots, m_i - 1$. The number of categories will be denoted by m if it is the same across items; this is often desirable, and will be assumed here for ease of notation.

Next, each item i is decomposed into $m - 1$ dichotomous item steps denoted by V_{ijh} $(h = 1, 2, \ldots, m - 1)$:

$$\begin{array}{ll} V_{ijh} = 1 & \text{iff } U_{ij} \geq h; \\ V_{ijh} = 0 & \text{otherwise.} \end{array} \tag{1}$$

Thus the score of person j on item i equals the number of item steps passed:

$$U_{ij} = \sum_{h=1}^{m-1} V_{ijh}. \tag{2}$$

The polytomous Mokken model is essentially equal to the dichotomous Mokken model applied to the $(m-1)^*n$ item steps. It will become clear below, however, that a few modifications are required.

As a first step of the model specification, the item step response functions (ISRF's) are defined for each ability value θ by

$$\pi_{ih}(\theta) = P(V_{ijh} = 1; \theta) = P(U_{ij} \geq h; \theta). \tag{3}$$

Just as in the dichotomous case, the requirement of monotone homogeneity (MH) postulates that all ISRF's $\pi_{ih}(\theta)$ are monotonic nondecreasing functions of the ability value θ. This property is again equivalent to that of similar ordering (Mokken, this volume), now for the $(m-1)^*n$ item steps.

Note that our definition of ISRF's, if they were not only nondecreasing but even logistic, would refer to the so-called cumulative logits $\ln[P(U_{ij} \geq h)/P(U_{ij} < h)]$, as opposed to the continuation-ratio logits $\ln[P(U_{ij} = h)/P(U_{ij} < h)]$ or the adjacent-categories logits $\ln[P(U_{ij} = h)/P(U_{ij} = h-1)]$ (see Agresti, 1984, p. 113).

The requirement of double monotonicity (DM) now means that the difficulty order of all $(m-1)^*n$ item steps is the same for each ability value, or equivalently that the ISRF's may touch but may not cross: If for $i, k \in I$ and for $g, h \in \{1, 2, \ldots, m-1\}$, there exists a value θ_0 for which $\pi_{ih}(\theta_0) < \pi_{kg}(\theta_0)$, then $\pi_{ih}(\theta) \leq \pi_{kg}(\theta)$ holds for all θ. The only difference with the dichotomous case is that such a requirement is trivial for the case $i = k$ of two item steps pertaining to the same item: if $h > g$, then

$\pi_{ih}(\theta) \leq \pi_{ig}(\theta)$ for all θ by definition. Indeed it is obvious, in terms of our item step indicators V_{ijh} defined above, that

$$\begin{aligned} V_{ijh} = 1 \Rightarrow V_{ijg} = 1 \quad & \text{for all } g < h; \\ V_{ijh} = 0 \Rightarrow V_{ijg} = 0 \quad & \text{for all } g > h. \end{aligned} \tag{4}$$

So there is some deterministic dependence between item steps belonging to the same item. For item steps from different items, however, local or conditional independence is postulated, just like in the dichotomous case (Mokken, this volume), and sampling independence between responses of different persons is also assumed.

Next, consider the practical consequences of MH and DM that were listed for the dichotomous case by Mokken (this volume). His result that any item pair correlates nonnegatively for all subgroups of subjects, when MH holds, remains valid for the polytomous case: by Mokken's early result applied to just two item steps, say V_{ih} and V_{kg}, one obtains $\text{cov}(V_{ih}, V_{kg}) \geq 0$. By Eq. (2) the covariance between U_i and U_k is equal to the sum of the $(m-1)*(m-1)$ such covariances between all item steps, each of which is nonnegative, and the result follows.

Rosenbaum's (1984) more general conditional association (CA) result, however, cannot be derived from just local independence and increasing ISRF's. For a generalization of the proof of his Lemma 1, one needs the so-called order 2 total positivity (TP_2) property of $P(U_i = h \mid \theta)$, i.e., for any $\theta' > \theta$ it must hold that $P(U_i = h \mid \theta')/P(U_i = h \mid \theta)$ increases with h. This is trivial when h can only be 0 or 1, because $P(U_i = 0 \mid \theta) = 1 - P(U_i = 1 \mid \theta)$ in this case. For three categories, however, a counterexample was presented by Molenaar (1990).

This implies also that property MH2 (CA per item pair in rest score groups on the remaining $n-2$ items) cannot be demonstrated without the additional TP_2 assumption. Property MH3 would now mean that $P(U_i \geq h)$ would not decrease over increasing rest score groups on the other $n-1$ items. A proof, unpublished to date, was prepared by Snijders (1989). Property MH4 immediately follows from Eq. (2) and the dichotomous MH4 property. Property MH5 (monotone likelihood ratio of θ and total score) is proven by Grayson (1988) in a way that makes very explicit use of the dichotomous character of the item scores. In the polytomous case MLR in the total score holds in the partial credit model but can be violated in extreme cases otherwise, see Hemker et al. (1996).

Mokken's property DM1 is also valid in the polytomous case, where π_i now becomes $P(U_i \geq h)$. The same holds for Mokken's property DM2: One now has two matrices of order $(m-1)n$ by $(m-1)n$ with rows and columns corresponding to item steps. Matrix entries pertaining to the same item cannot be observed, but all other entries should, apart from sampling fluctuations, be increasing (for Π) and decreasing (for $\Pi^{(0)}$). DM3 is meaningful for polytomous items when U_i and U_k are replaced by item step indicators V_{ih} and V_{kg}.

Parameter Estimation

Scalability Coefficients

My first attempt to generalize Mokken scaling to polytomous items used the scalability coefficient H between two item step pairs. This was unsatisfactory, for two reasons. First, it follows from Eq. (4) that between any two steps belonging to the same item, say item i, the pairwise item step coefficient is identically 1: By definition, one cannot pass a difficult item step, say $U_i \geq 2$, and at the same time fail an easier one pertaining to the same item, say $U_i \geq 1$. Second, the search, test and fit procedures described by Mokken for the dichotomous case lead to decisions to admit or to remove certain items. It would make little sense to take such decisions at the item step level, say by admitting $U_i \geq 2$ but removing $U_i \geq 1$ from the scale. Although one could argue that this is permissible, and takes the form of a recoding in which categories 0 and 1 are joined, it will usually be preferable to keep or remove entire items, based on the joint scalability of all steps contained in an item.

A suitable definition of the scalability coefficient for a pair of items with m ordered answer categories is obtained by establishing the perfect Guttman patterns in their cross table. This will be briefly described in the Example section; for details see Molenaar (1991). The derivation of a coefficient H for item i, and of a coefficient H for the total scale, proceeds exactly as in the dichotomous case. The features of H listed in Mokken (this volume) continue to hold.

The reason to discuss scalability coefficients under the heading Parameter Estimation will be clear: such coefficients are initially defined for the population. When their sample counterparts are used for inference, the sampling variance should be taken into account. It refers to the conditional distribution of cell frequencies in the isomarginal family of all cross tables with the same marginals. The software package MSP (Molenaar et al., 1994) uses the mean and variance of the sample H values under the null model of independence to obtain a normal approximation for testing the hypothesis that a population H value equals zero. Space limitations prohibit details being provided here.

Ability Estimation

The sum score across the n items of a multicategory Mokken scale, which is equal to the total number of item steps passed by Eq. (2), is positively correlated with the ability θ by property MH4. The stronger monotone likelihood ratio property, by which the distribution of θ would be stochastically increasing with total score, is only proven by Grayson (1988) for the dichotomous case. Ordering of persons by total score, however, will be indicative of their ability ordering (see also the next subsection on reliability).

Note that each item contributes equally to the total score if the number m of categories is the same across items. If one item would, for example, have two categories and another item four, then one could pass only one item step on the former and three on the latter. Unless one assumes that the presence of more categories implies higher discrimination of the item, this unequal contribution of items to the sum score appears to be undesirable. It is thus recommended that the same number of categories across items be used.

Reliability

The extension of the reliability derivations by Mokken (1971) and Sijtsma and Molenaar (1987) to the polytomous case is relatively straightforward: In the matrix Π per item step one may interpolate the missing values (where row and column refer to steps of the same item) from the observed values (where they refer to different items). The procedures are described by Molenaar and Sijtsma (1988) and have been implemented in the MSP program from version 2 onward. Note that the reliability results could be misleading if double monotonicity is seriously violated. Research by Meijer et al. (1993), however, indicates that minor violations of DM tend to have little influence on the reliability results.

Goodness of Fit

The search and test procedures based on the H-coefficients have already been described by Mokken (this volume); they work exactly in the same way for polytomous items. Although it is plausible that scales obtained in this way will very often comply with the MH and DM requirements, this section will present some additional tests and diagnostics that assess the properties of the ISRF's more directly. This material is presented in more detail in Chap. 7 of the *MSP User Manual* (Molenaar et al., 1994), with examples from the MSP output regarding such tests and diagnostics.

The model of MH assumes that the item step characteristic curves are increasing functions of the latent trait value, and the model of DM also assumes that these curves do not intersect. The search and test procedures for scale construction and scale evaluation will often detect major violations of these assumptions because decreasing and/or intersecting curves will lead to far lower H-values per item or per item pair. Such detection methods are rough and global, however, and their success will depend on factors such as the proportion of respondents with latent trait values in the interval for which the curves do not follow the assumptions.

More detailed checks of model assumptions would thus be welcome, in particular when the assumptions are intimately linked to the research goal.

For validity considerations it may be important to establish that the item step curves increase over the whole range of the latent trait. For an empirical check of an item hierarchy derived from theory, it may be important that the same difficulty order of items or item steps holds for the whole range, or that it holds for subgroups like males and females. One would thus sometimes like to use a detailed goodness-of-fit analysis that produces detailed conclusions per item step or per subgroup of persons.

Such analyses, however, are difficult, for a number of reasons. The first is that the assumptions refer to certain probabilities for given latent trait values, whereas all we can do is use the ordering of subjects with respect to their observed total score T as a proxy for their ordering on the latent trait. This means that we can only obtain rough estimates of the curves for which the assumptions should hold. An additional flaw is that the observed scores have even more measurement error when they are partly based on items that violate the model assumptions. A third problem is that detailed checks of many estimated curves for many score values multiplies the risk of at least some wrong conclusions: If one inspects several hundred pairs of values for which the model assumptions predict a specific order, by pure chance several of them will exhibit the reverse order, and in a few cases, this reverse order may even show statistical significance.

Checking of Monotone Homogeneity

The check of MH (increasing item step curves) is the most important one: ordering the persons is often the main goal. Let T denote a person's total score on a Mokken scale consisting of n items which each have m ordered response categories coded as $0, 1, \ldots, m-1$; the modifications for other codings are trivial. One may subdivide the total sample into score groups containing all persons with total score $T = t$, where $t = 0, 1, \ldots, n*(m-1)$. If the scale is valid, persons with $T = t+1$ will on average have larger ability values than persons with $T = t$. Thus, if one forms the fractions of persons in each score group that pass a certain fixed item step, these fractions should increase with t if the item step response function increases with the latent trait value. Just like an item total correlation is inflated because the item itself contributes to the total score (psychometricians therefore prefer an item rest correlation), it is superior to base the above subdivision not on the total score but on the rest score (say R) on the remaining $n-1$ items. The analysis of MH is therefore based on the fraction of persons passing a fixed item step in the rest score groups $R = r$ for $r = 0, 1, \ldots, (n-1)*(m-1)$, based on the other $n-1$ items.

Unless the total number of item steps is very small, several of these rest score groups may contain only a few persons, or even no persons at all. For this reason one may first joint adjacent rest score groups until each new group contains enough persons. Here one needs a compromise between too few groups (by which a violation could be masked) and too many groups (by which the fractions per group would be very instable).

Every time an item step is passed by a larger fraction in some rest score group than in some higher rest score group, the absolute difference between such fractions is called a violation. Decisions about MH for a given item may be based on the number of violations, their sum and maximum, and their significance in the form of a z-value that would be for large group sizes normally distributed in the borderline case of exactly equal population fractions. In the 2×2 table of two rest score groups crossed by the item step result (0 or 1), the exact probability of exceedance would be found from the hypergeometric distribution. The z-value then comes from a good normal approximation to this hypergeometric distribution (Molenaar, 1970, Chap. 4, Eq. 2.37). It is clear that all such tests are one-sided; when there is no violation no test is made.

For most realistic data sets, quite a few violations of MH tend to be found by the procedure. Most of them tend to be numerically small and to have low z-values, however; they may well be due to sampling variation. Indeed some of these violations disappear when a slightly different grouping of raw rest score groups into larger clusters is applied. In simulated data in which one non-monotone item was added to a set of MH items, the procedure has been shown to correctly spot the non-monotone item in most cases.

Often, however, an item with non-monotone ISRF's is already detected because its item H-value is much lower than that of the remaining items. When either a low item H-value or the above procedure casts doubt on an item, it is obvious that substantive considerations should also be taken into account in a decision to remove or to keep it. Moreover, it is recommended to remove one item at a time: removal of an item changes the rest score, so the fit of any other item may well change (the same holds for their item H-values, which are recalculated across $n-2$ rather than $n-1$ other items).

Checking DM Via the Rest Score

The property that two-item step response functions may not intersect holds trivially for two steps belonging to the same item; therefore only pairs of item step curves belonging to two different items need to be examined. Such a pair is ordered by the sample popularity of the two item steps (the rare case of exactly equal sample popularity will require a special procedure not discussed here). The question then is whether there exist one or more intervals on the latent trait axis for which this overall order is reversed.

Like for the MH check, the present method estimates the curves by the item step popularities in rest score groups. For a fair comparison, the rest score is here defined as the sum score on the remaining $n-2$ items. There is a violation if the overall more popular item step is less popular in a certain rest score group. The z-score for each violation is now based on a McNemar test. The frequency of 10 and 01 patterns for the two item steps in each rest score group must reflect their overall popularity order. The boundary case of equal probabilities of 01 and 10 in the group considered leads to a one-sided probability of exceedance in a binomial distribution with success probability 0.5. The software package MSP uses its z-value from a very accurate normal approximation to the binomial distribution with success probability 0.5 (Molenaar, 1970, Chap. 3, Eq. 5.5).

The use of this procedure has led to similar findings as presented for the checking of MH. In this case, it is important to keep in mind that each violation of DM involves two different items. When there is one bad item, whose curves intersect with many others, the DM tables for other items will also show many violations, which will diminish or even vanish when the offending item is removed. Moreover, this item will often have a low item H-value. Again it is recommended to remove one item at a time, even when two or more items appear to have many violations of double monotonicity.

Checking DM via the Π *Matrices*

In the polytomous case, the $n \times (m-1)$ by $n \times (m-1)$ matrices Π and $\Pi^{(0)}$ contain the joint probabilities of passing (Π) and failing ($\Pi^{(0)}$) pairs of item steps. For cells referring to steps belonging to the same item no sample estimates are available. The DM assumption implies for all other cells that, apart from sampling fluctuation, their rows and columns should be nondecreasing (for Π) and nonincreasing (for $\Pi^{(0)}$).

Consider one line of the matrices, in which the order of two columns should reflect their overall popularity. When this is violated in one of the two matrices, the general procedure combines the evidence from the two matrices into one $2 \times 2 \times 2$ cross table for the three item steps involved, as required for a valid and complete analysis. Such violations can again be counted and their maximum, sum, and significance can be assessed.

Checking Equality of ISRF's Across Groups

It is an important assumption of item response theory that the response probabilities depend on a person's latent trait value, and on no other characteristics of the person. For an up-to-date and complete treatment of the mathematical implications of such a statement see Ellis and Van den Wollenberg (1993); for an alternative test procedure for the dichotomous case, see Shealy and Stout (1993). Here it suffices to mention an example. If an achievement test contains one item that is easy for boys but difficult for girls with the same ability, then one speaks of item bias or differential item functioning. It is often desirable to detect and remove such items. In our nonparametric IRT setting, we may investigate DIF by checking for equal item step order in the groups of respondents defined by a variable specified by the user. It is recommended to do this only for those grouping variables for which item bias would be both conceivable and harmful (it makes little sense to split on the basis of the first character of the respondent's name, for example). The point here is not whether one group has systematically higher scores on a scale than the other; rather, it is the question whether the scale has the same meaning and structure in subgroups of persons, in particular whether the item steps occur in the same order of popularity. When for some subgroups two item steps have the reverse ordering, this is a violation. Such violations can again be counted and summed into a summary table per item, and the significance of a violation can be expressed in a z-value.

Example

Agresti (1993) presented the responses of 475 respondents to the 1989 General Social Survey. With response format 0 = always wrong, 1 = almost always wrong, 2 = wrong only sometimes, and 3 = not wrong, their opinions were asked on teenage sex, premarital sex by adults, and extramarital sex, respectively. The three items will be denoted TEEN (teenagers of age 14–16 having sex relations before marriage); PRE (a man and a woman having sex relations before marriage), and EXTRA (a married person having sex relations with someone other than the marriage partner).

One may wonder whether a common latent trait, say sexual permissiveness, is measured, and how items and persons are positioned on that trait. It might be better to have more than three items, and possibly different ones, but for the purpose of illustrating polytomous Mokken scaling, a short test leads to easier presentation, so such objections will be ignored.

The data can be viewed as nine item steps that may be ordered from easy to difficult with the result that PRE ≥ 1 is passed by 69% of the respondents, PRE ≥ 2 by 61%, PRE ≥ 3 by 39%, TEEN ≥ 1 by 25%, EXTRA ≥ 1 by 19%, TEEN ≥ 2 by 10%, EXTRA ≥ 2 by 8%, TEEN ≥ 3 by 3%, and EXTRA ≥ 3 by 1%. The frequency count per response pattern showed 140 scores of 000 (rejecting all three kinds of sex) and only four scores of 333 (no objections at all); whereas many respondents were at least somewhat tolerant toward premarital sex by adults, a large majority strongly objected to teenage sex, and even more to extramarital sex.

The extent to which individual response patterns were in agreement with this difficulty order of the item steps in the total group can be expressed in terms of the scalability coefficients. First consider the pairwise H of the items PRE and TEEN, obtained from their cross tabulation in Table 1.[1]

There were 141 respondents with score 0 on both items. Someone with a slightly larger sexual tolerance is expected to score 1 on premarital sex

[1] *Note.* The number of Guttman errors is given in brackets below the observed frequencies.

TABLE 1. Cross Tabulation of the Items PRE and TEEN for 475 Persons.

	PRE			
TEEN	0	1	2	3
0	141 (0)	34 (0)	72 (0)	109 (0)
1	4 (3)	5 (2)	23 (1)	38 (0)
2	1 (6)	0 (4)	9 (2)	23 (0)
3	0 (9)	0 (6)	1 (3)	15 (0)

but still score 0 on teenage sex (34 persons do so), because PRE ≥ 1 is the easiest item step. For people with a still higher position on the latent trait, the expected response becomes TEEN = 0, PRE = 2 (72 persons) and then TEEN = 0, PRE = 3 (109 persons). Only then is one assumed to endorse the more difficult item step, TEEN ≥ 1 and score TEEN = 1, PRE = 3 (38 persons), next TEEN = 2, PRE = 3 and finally the most tolerant answer TEEN = 3, PRE = 3.

The seven cells of the table marked zero (0) in brackets form a path from 00 to 33 on which one never endorses a difficult item step while rejecting an easier one, and on which the total score on the two items rises from 0 to 6. There were $141 + 34 + \cdots + 15 = 432$ respondents along this path; the other 43 persons had score patterns with at least one Guttman error. Note that the 23 respondents with TEEN = 1 and PRE = 2 had just one such error (for the whole group the step PRE ≥ 3 comes just before the step TEEN ≥ 2). The one person with TEEN = 2 and PRE = 0, however, had six pairs of item steps in which the easier one was rejected and the more difficult one endorsed. As explained in more detail in Molenaar (1991) and in the MSP Manual (Molenaar et al., 1994), one may thus obtain a weighted error count of 72 for the 43 persons who were not on the path marked by zeros (0).

This number was compared to the expected weighted count in the zero cells under the null hypothesis of statistical independence of the scores on both items, which was found to be 240.56. Then, the pairwise H of the two items equaled H(TEEN,PRE) = $1 - 72/240.56 = 0.70$. This value is also equal to the observed correlation between the two item scores divided by the maximum correlation that could be obtained given the marginal frequencies for each item (Molenaar, 1991); that calculation will be skipped here. From the other cross tables not reproduced here one obtains in the same way H(EXTRA,TEEN) = 0.45 and H(EXTRA,PRE) = 0.71 (note that the path followed from 00 to 33 may have a different shape in each table, dependent on the popularities of the item steps under consideration). The item H values were found to be 0.57, 0.58, and 0.70 for EXTRA, TEEN, and PRE, respectively, and the scale of three items had estimated scalability $H = 0.62$ and estimated reliability 0.69. All these values differed significantly from zero, and under the standard settings of MSP there appeared to be no violations of single or double monotonicity.

It can be concluded that the three items form a scale for sexual tolerance on which 140 persons have the minimum score of 0 and four persons have the maximal score of 9; the mean score is 2.36 with a standard deviation of 2.06 and the distribution of scores is slightly skewed in the positive direction. From a detailed analysis of all answer patterns, it emerges that 366 persons had no Guttman errors (from their total score, their responses on the items can be inferred), 51 persons had only one Guttman inversion, and the frequency for 2 to 7 errors is 15, 28, 5, 3, 3, 3, respectively. No one had eight or more errors. Note that for an unlikely pattern like TEEN = 0, EXTRA = 3, PRE = 0 one would obtain 18 errors because the six easiest item steps would be failed and the three most difficult ones passed.

In this example both item steps and persons were successfully ordered on a latent trait that measured sexual permissiveness. Space does not permit a more detailed explanation of the example, or a full illustration of the other facets of the model and the software. The latter can be purchased from ProGAMMA, P.O. Box 841, 9700 AV Groningen, The Netherlands.

References

Agresti, A. (1984). *Analysis of Ordinal Categorical Data.* New York: Wiley.

Agresti, A. (1993). Computing conditional maximum likelihood estimates for generalized Rasch models using simple loglinear models with diagonals parameters, *Scandinavian Journal of Statistics* **20**, 63–71.

Ellis, J. and Van den Wollenberg, A.L. (1993). Local homogeneity in latent trait models: A characterization of the homogeneous monotone IRT model. *Psychometrika* **58**, 417–429.

Grayson, D.A. (1988). Two-group classification in latent trait theory: Scores with monotone likelihood ratio. *Psychometrika* **53**, 383–392.

Hemker, B.T., Sijtsma, K., Molenaar, I.W., and Junker, B.W. (1996). Polytomous IRT models and monotone likelihood ration in the total score, *Psychometrika*, accepted.

Jansen, P.G.W. and Roskam. E.E. (1986). Latent trait models and dichotomization of graded responses. *Psychometrika* **51**, 69–91.

Meijer, R.R., Sijtsma, K., and Molenaar, I.W. (1996). Reliability estimation for single dichotomous items based on Mokken's IRT model, *Applied Psychological Measurement*, in press.

Mokken, R.J. (1971). *A Theory and Procedure of Scale Analysis. With Applications in Political Research.* New York, Berlin: Walter de Gruyter, Mouton.

Molenaar, I.W. (1970). *Approximations to the Poisson, Binomial and Hypergeometric Distribution Functions* (MC Tract 31). Amsterdam: Mathematisch Centrum (now CWI).

Molenaar, I.W. (1990). Unpublished lecture for the Rasch research group. Arnhem: CITO.

Molenaar, I.W. (1991). A weighted Loevinger H-coefficient extending Mokken scaling to multicategory items. *Kwantitatieve Methoden* **12**(37), 97–117.

Molenaar, I.W., Debets, P., Sijtsma, K., and Hemker, B.T. (1994). *User's Manual MSP.* Groningen: Iec ProGAMMA.

Molenaar, I.W. and Sijtsma, K. (1988). Mokken's approach to reliability estimation extended to multicategory items. *Kwantitatieve Methoden* **9**(28), 115–126.

Rosenbaum, P.R. (1984). Testing the conditional independence and monotonicity assumptions of item response theory. *Psychometrika* **49**, 425–435.

Shealy, R. and Stout, W. (1993). A model-based standardization approach that separates true bias/DIF from group ability differences and detects test bias/DIF as well as item bias/DIF. *Psychometrika* **58**, 159–194.

Snijders, T.A.B. (1989). Unpublished notes.

Sijtsma, K. and Molenaar, I.W. (1987). Reliability of test scores in nonparametric item response theory. *Psychometrika* **52**, 79–97.

22
A Functional Approach to Modeling Test Data

J.O. Ramsay

Introduction

The central problem in psychometric data analysis using item response theory is to model the response curve linking a level θ of ability and the probability of choosing a specific option on a particular item. Most approaches to this problem have assumed that the curve to be estimated is within a restricted class of functions defined by a specific mathematical model. The Rasch model or the three-parameter logistic model for binary data are best known examples. In this chapter, however, the aim is to estimate the response curve directly, thereby escaping the restrictions imposed by what can be achieved with a particular parametric family of curves. It will also be assumed that the responses to an item are polytomous, and can involve any number of options.

First some notation. Let a test consist of n items, and be administered to N examinees. Assume that the consequence of the interaction of an examinee j and item i is one of a finite number m_i set of states. These states may or may not be ordered, and little that appears in this chapter will depend on their order or on whether the items are dichotomous. The actual option chosen will be represented by the *indicator vector* $\mathbf{y}_{ij}$ of length m_i with a 1 in the position corresponding to the option chosen and zeros elsewhere.

At the core of almost all modern procedures for the modeling of testing data is the problem of fitting the N indicator vectors $\mathbf{y}_{ij}$ for a specific item i on the basis of the covariate values θ_j. The model for these indicator vectors is a vector-valued function $\mathbf{P}_i(\theta)$ whose values are the probabilities that a candidate j with ability θ_j will choose option h, or, equivalently, will have a 1 in position h of indicator vector $\mathbf{y}_{ij}$. The general statistical problem of estimating such a smooth function on the basis of a set of indicator variables is known as the *multinomial regression problem.* The special case of two options is the *binomial regression* or *binary regression problem*, and there is a large literature available, which is surveyed in Cox and Snell (1989). McCullagh and Nelder (1989) cover the important exponential family class of models along with the highly flexible and effective generalized linear model or GLM algorithm for fitting data.

Although the value θ_j associated with examinee j is not directly observed, various techniques in effect use various types of surrogates for these values. The total number of correct items for long tests, for example, can serve. Attempts to estimate both item characteristics and the values of θ_j by maximum likelihood will alternate between an item-estimation step and an ability-estimation step, so that multinomial regression is involved in the item-estimation phase. For techniques that marginalize likelihood over a prior distribution for θ, numerical integration is almost always involved, and in this case the known values of θ are appropriately chosen quadrature points. Finally, certain nonparametric approaches to be described below will assign values of θ more or less arbitrarily to a pre-determined set of rank values. Like the quadrature procedures, these techniques, too, can bin or group the values prior to analysis to speed up calculation.

22.0.1 Parametric and Nonparametric Modeling

Some thoughts are offered next as to the relative merits of parametric versus nonparametric modeling strategies. The essential problem in multinomial regression is to estimate the vector-valued probability function $\mathbf{P}_i$. The principal challenges are to propose flexible or at least plausible classes of functions that respect the constraints that probabilities must lie within $[0, 1]$ and sum to one. A secondary but often critical issue is computational convenience since N can be in the tens or hundreds of thousands. Finally, a number of statistical considerations lead to the need for $\mathbf{P}_i$ to have reasonably smooth first derivatives, and hence to be itself smooth.

On the advantage side, parametric models are often motivated by some level of analysis of the psychological processes involved in the choice that an examinee makes when confronted with an item. The binary three-parameter logistic or 3PL model, for example, is essentially a mixture model motivated by the possibility that with a certain probability, denoted by parameter c, examinees will choose the correct of several options with certainty. Partly as a consequence of this psychological analysis, the parameter estimates can be useful descriptors of the data and thus provide numerical summaries of item characteristics that users can be taught to understand at some level. The use of a fixed and usually small number of parameters means that the machinery of classical mathematical statistics can be employed to provide interval estimates and hypothesis tests, although there is usually room for skepticism about the relevance of asymptotic theory in this context. Finally, some simple parametric models exhibit desirable statistical and mathematical properties, tempting one to wish that they were true or even to consider devising tests where they might be appropriate.

On the down side, one has the ever-present concern about whether a parametric model offers an adequate account of the data. Most parametric models fail when the sample size gets large enough. But there is a very important counter-argument that should be always kept in mind: A simple wrong model can be more useful for many statistical purposes than a complex correct model. Bias is not everything in data analysis, and the reduction in sampling variance resulting from keeping the number of parameters small can often more than offset the loss due to increased bias.

Many parametric models have been proposed for various binary regression problems, but the multinomial case, ordered or not, has proven more challenging. Existing models have tended to be within the logistic-normal class (Aitchison, 1986), to be Poisson process approximations (McCullagh and Nelder, 1989), or to be so specific in structure as to apply to only a very limited class of data. It is also not always easy to see how to extend a particular linear model to allow for new aspects of the problem, such as multidimensionality or the presence of observed covariates.

A more subtle but nonetheless important argument against parametric models is their tendency to focus attention on parameters when in fact it is the functions themselves that are required. For example, the proper interpretation of estimates of parameters a, b, and c in the 3PL model requires a fair degree of statistical and mathematical sophistication, whereas other types of data display such as graphs can speak more directly to naive users of test analysis technology.

A particular issue is the ontological status of θ. Parametric models are often motivated by appealing to the concept of a "latent trait" or something like "ability" that is imagined to underly test performance. Index θ is understood by far too many users of test analysis technology as a type of measurement on an interval scale of an examinee's latent trait, a notion much favored by the widespread use of affectively loaded terms like "measure" and "instrument" to describe tests. Although careful accounts of item response theory such as Lord and Novick (1968) caution against this misinterpretation, and affirm that θ can be monotonically transformed at will even in the context of parametric models, there are far more passages in the journal and textbook literature that tout the interval scale properties of θ as assessed in the context, for example, of the 3PL model as one of the prime motivations for using parametric item response theory.

Finally, parametric models can be problematical on the computational side. The nonlinear dependency of $\mathbf{P}_i$ on parameters in most widely used models implies iterative estimation even when θ values are fixed, and these iterations can often converge slowly. A closely related problem is that two parameter estimates can have a disastrous degree of sampling correlation, as is the case for the guessing and discrimination parameters in the 3PL model, resulting in slow convergence in computation and large marginal sampling variances for even large sample sizes.

The term "nonparametric" has undoubtably been over-used in the statistical literature, and now refers to many things besides rank- and count-based statistical techniques. Many of the approaches to be considered below do involve parameter estimation. Perhaps the defining considerations are whether the parameters themselves are considered to have substantive or interpretive significance, and whether the number of parameters is regarded as fixed rather than at the disposal of the data analyst.

The main advantages to be gained by nonparametric models are flexibility and computational convenience. The fact that the number of parameters or some other aspect of the fitting process is available for control means that the analysis can be easily adapted to considerations such as varying sample sizes and levels of error variance. Moreover, the model usually depends on the parameters, when they are used, in a linear or quasi-linear manner, and this implies that parameter estimation can involve tried-and-true methods such as least squares. An appropriate choice of nonparametric procedure can lead to noniterative or at least rapidly convergent calculations.

Nonparametric techniques often lend themselves easily to extensions in various useful directions, just as the multivariate linear model can be extended easily to a mixture of linear and principal components style bilinear analysis. They can also adapt easily to at least smooth transformations of the index θ, and have less of a tendency to encourage its over-interpretation.

The issue of how to describe the results of a nonparametric analysis can be viewed in various ways. The lack of obvious numerical summaries can be perceived as a liability, although appropriate numerical summaries of the function $\mathbf{P}$ can usually be constructed. On the other hand, nonparametric models encourage the graphical display of results, and the author's experience with the use of his graphically-oriented program TestGraf (Ramsay, 1993) by students and naive users has tended to confirm the communication advantage of the appropriate display over numerical summaries.

Presentation of the Models

This section contains an overview of nonparametric modeling strategies, and then focuses on a kernel smoothing approach. While specific examples are drawn from the author's work, there is no intention here to convey the impression that any particular approach is the best. This is a rapidly evolving field with great potential for developing new and better ideas.

Most nonparametric modeling strategies employ in some sense an expansion of the function to be modeled as a linear combination of a set of basis functions. That is, let $f(\theta)$ be the model, and let $x_k(\theta)$, $k = 1, \ldots, K$, be a set of K known functions. Then the model is proposed to have the form

$$f(\theta) = b_1 x_1(\theta) + \cdots + b_K x_K(\theta). \tag{1}$$

Familiar examples of basis functions x_k are the monomials θ^{k-1}, orthogonal polynomials, and 1, $\sin(\theta)$, $\cos(\theta)$, etc. Less familiar but very important in recent years are bases constructed from joining polynomial segments smoothly at fixed junction points, the polynomial regression splines (de

Boor, 1978), and the various special forms that these have taken. Other types of basis functions will be mentioned below. Associated with the choice of basis is the N by K matrix $\mathbf{X}$, which contains the values of each basis function at each argument value. The coefficients b_k of the linear combination are the parameters to be estimated, although the number of basis functions is to some extent also an estimable quantity. Let vector $\mathbf{b}$ contain these coefficient values. The vector $\mathbf{Xb}$ then contains the approximation values for the data being approximated.

Once the coefficients have been estimated for a particular problem, there are usually a set of Q *evaluation points* θ_q, $q = 1, \dots, Q$, often chosen to be equally spaced, at which the model function is to be evaluated for, among other reasons, plotting and display purposes. The function values are $\mathbf{Yb}$, where Q by K matrix $\mathbf{Y}$ contains the basis functions evaluated at the evaluation points. As a rule $Q << N$, so it is the size of N that dominates the computational aspects of the problem.

The following discussion of strategies for nonparametric modeling will be within this linear expansion frame of reference.

What constitutes a good basis of functions for a particular problem? All of the following features are to some extent important:

Orthogonality. Ideally, the basis functions should be orthogonal in the appropriate sense. For example, if least squares analysis is used, then modern algorithms for computing the solution to a least squares fitting problem without orthogonality require of an order of K^2N floating point operations (flops), for large N, whereas if the columns of $\mathbf{X}$ are orthogonal, only KN flops are required. Moreover, rounding error in the calculations can be an enormous problem if matrix $\mathbf{X}$ is nearly singular, a problem that orthogonality eliminates.

Local support. Because the independent variable values θ are ordered, it is highly advantageous to use basis functions which are zero everywhere except over a limited range of values. The cross-product matrix $\mathbf{X}^t\mathbf{X}$ is then band-structured, and the number of flops in the least squares problem is again of order KN. Regression splines such as B-splines and M-splines are very important tools because of this local support property (Ramsay, 1988). Local support also implies that the influence of a coefficient in the expansion is felt only over a limited range of values of θ. This can imply a great deal of more flexibility per basis function than can be achieved by non-local bases such as polynomials, and partly explains the popularity of regression splines. The importance of local support will be further highlighted below in discussing smoothing.

Appropriate behavior. Often of critical importance is the fact that the basis functions have certain behaviors that are like those of the functions being approximated. For example, we use sines and cosines in time series analysis in part because their periodic behavior is strongly characteristic of the processes being analyzed. One particularly requires that the basis functions have the right characteristics in regions where the data are sparse or nonexistent. Polynomials, for example, become increasingly unpredictable or unstable as one moves toward more extreme values of the independent variable, and are therefore undesirable bases for extrapolation or for estimating behavior near the limits of the data. This issue is of particular importance in the multinomial regression problem, especially when the functions being approximated are probability functions.

In broad terms, nonparametric techniques can be cross-classified in two ways:

1. Do we model function $\mathbf{P}$ directly, or do we model some transformation of $\mathbf{P}$, and then back-transform to get $\mathbf{P}$?

2. If we use an expansion in terms of basis functions, is the number K of basis functions fixed by the data analyst, or is it determined by the data?

If the model function f is intended to estimate a multinomial probability function $\mathbf{P}_i$, then the probability constraints can pose some tough problems. Again, things are easier in the binary case because only one function per item is required, and it is only necessary that its value be kept within the interval $[0, 1]$. In the multinomial case the m_i probability functions must also be constrained to add to one, and this complicates the procedures. On the other hand, if the constraints can be effectively dealt with, the direct modeling of probability has the advantage of not getting too far from the data. Smoothing, least squares estimation, and even maximum likelihood estimation are estimation procedures with well-developed algorithms and often well-understood characteristics. Specific examples of these direct modeling approaches will be detailed below.

The alternative strategy is to bypass the constraints by transforming the problem to an unconstrained form. In the binary case, the log-odds transformation

$$H(\theta) = \ln \frac{P(\theta)}{1 - P(\theta)} \tag{2}$$

is widely used over a large variety of data analysis problems. This transformation is also the *link function* in the exponential family representation of the Bernoulli distribution, and is used to advantage in the generalized linear model or GLM algorithm. McCullagh and Nelder (1989) detail many applications of this technique, which has proven to be generally stable, simple to implement, remarkably flexible, and to generate many useful statistical summaries and tests. Since H is unbounded, there are no constraints to worry about, and expansions of H in terms of such standard bases as polynomials can be used. O'Sullivan et al. (1986) used smoothing techniques to develop what has come to be called a *generalized additive model* (GAM) for binary regression problems, and Hastie and Tibshirani (1990) review this and other GAM models of potential interest to nonparametric modelers of psychometric data.

The log-odds transformation is not without its potential problems, however. The transformation presumes that the probabilities are bounded away from 0 and 1, and, consequently, estimates of H can become extremely unstable if the data strongly or completely favor 0 or 1 choice probabilities, which is not infrequently the case. In these cases, some form of conditioning procedure, such as the use of a prior distribution, is often used, and the computational edge over direct modeling can be rather reduced.

In the multinomial case, the counterpart of the log-odds transformation can take two forms (Aitchison, 1986). In the first, a specific category, which here will be taken for notational convenience to be the first, is chosen as a base or reference category, and the transformation is

$$H_h(\theta) = \ln \frac{P_h(\theta)}{P_1(\theta)}, \quad h = 2, \ldots, m_i. \tag{3}$$

Of course, this transformation only works if the base probability P_1 keeps well clear of 0 or 1, and in the context of testing data, this may not be easy to achieve. Alternatively, the more stable transformation

$$H_h(\theta) = \ln \frac{P_h(\theta)}{\bar{P}(\theta)}, \quad h = 1, \ldots, m_i \tag{4}$$

can be used, where the denominator is the geometric mean of the probabilities. While zero probabilities still cause problems, one can usually eliminate these before computing the mean of the remainder. However, using the geometric mean means that one more function H_h is produced than is strictly required, and some linear constraint such as fixing one function, or requiring the pointwise mean to be zero, is then needed.

The classical techniques for functional approximation have assumed that the data analyst pre-specifies the number K of basis functions on the basis of some experience or intuition about how much flexibility is required for the problem at hand. Various data-driven procedures can also be employed to guide the choice of K, and these are closely connected with the problem of variable selection in multiple regression analysis.

In recent years, an impressive variety of procedures collectively referred to as *smoothing* have found great favor with data analysis. A comparison of fixed basis versus smoothing procedures can be found in Buja et al. (1989), and the discussion associated with this paper constitutes a virtual handbook of functional approximation lore.

The simplest of smoothing techniques is *kernel smoothing*, in which the expansion is of the form

$$f(\theta) = \sum_{j}^{N} y_j z\left(\frac{\theta - \theta_j}{\lambda}\right), \tag{5}$$

where θ is an evaluation point at which the value of function f is to be estimated. A comparison of this expansion with Eq. (1) indicates that the coefficient b_k has been replaced by the observed value y_j, and the basis function value for evaluation point is now

$$x_j(\theta) = z\left(\frac{\theta - \theta_j}{\lambda}\right). \tag{6}$$

Clearly, the problem of estimating the coefficients of the expansion has been completely bypassed, although the number of basis functions is now N. How can this work? Two features are required of function z, called a *smoothing kernel:*

1. z must be strongly localized as a function of θ. This is because each y_j effectively contributes or votes for a basis function proportional to itself at θ, and only those values of y associated with values of θ_j close to θ are wanted to have any real impact on $f(\theta)$. This is because only these observations really convey useful information about the behavior of f in this region. Parameter λ plays the role of controlling how local z is.

2. The following condition is needed:

$$\sum_j^N z\left(\frac{\theta - \theta_j}{\lambda}\right) = 1. \tag{7}$$

   This condition ensures that the expansion is a type of average of the values y_j, and along with the localness condition, implies that $f(\theta)$ will be a local average of the data.

The second condition is easy to impose, once more suitable family of local functions have been identified. Kernel smoothing local bases are usually developed by beginning with some suitable single function $K(u)$, of which the uniform kernel, $K(u) = 1$, $-1 \leq u \leq 1$, and 0 otherwise, is the simplest example. Another is the Gaussian kernel, $K(u) = \exp(-u^2/2)$. The basis functions are then constructed from K by shifting and rescaling the argument, so that (a) the peak is located at θ_q, and (b) the width of the effective domain of z is proportional to λ. Finally the normalizing of z can be achieved by dividing by the sum of z values (called the Nadaraya–Watson smoothing kernel), or by other techniques (Eubank, 1988).

Using Nadaraya–Watson kernel smoothing with a Gaussian kernel, the nonparametric estimate of $\mathbf{P}_i$ is

$$\mathbf{P}_i(\theta) = \frac{\sum_j^N \mathbf{y}_{ij} \exp -[(\theta - \theta_j)/\lambda]^2/2}{\sum_j^N \exp -[(\theta - \theta_j)/\lambda]^2/2}. \tag{8}$$

But where do the values θ come from? Here, the fact that these values are in effect any strictly monotone transformation of the ranks of the examinees is relied upon. The estimation process begins, as do most item response modeling techniques, with a preliminary ranking of examinees induced by some suitable statistic. For multiple choice exams, for example, this statistic can be the number of correct items, and for psychological scales it can be the scale score. Or, it can come from a completely different test or some other test.

The ranks thus provided are replaced by the corresponding quantiles of the standard normal distribution, and it is these values that provide θ. Why the normal distribution? In part, because traditionally the distribution of latent trait values have been thought of as roughly normally distributed. But in fact any target distribution could have served as well.

Flexibility is controlled by the choice of the smoothing parameter λ: the smaller λ the smaller the bias introduced by the smoothing process, but the larger the sampling variance. Increasing λ produces smoother functions, but at the expense of missing some curvature.

The great advantages of kernel smoothing are the spectacular savings in computation time, in that each evaluation of f only requires N flops, and in the complexity of code. Other advantages will be indicated below. For example, a set of test data with 75 items and 18,500 examinees is processed by TestGraf (Ramsay, 1993) on a personal computer with a 486 processor in about 6 minutes. By contrast, commonly used parametric programs for dichotomous items take about 500 times as long, and polytomous response procedures even longer.

While the notion of using the observation itself as the coefficient in the expansion is powerful, it may be a little too simple. Kernel smoothing gets into trouble when the evaluation values θ_q are close to the extremes of θ. Local polynomial fitting is an extension of kernel smoothing that uses simple functions of the observations rather than y_j as coefficients, and Hastie and Loader (1993) lay out the procedure's virtues. Other types of smoothing, such as spline smoothing, can be more computationally intensive, but bring other advantages.

The direct modeling of probability functions by kernel smoothing developed by Ramsay (1991) and implemented in the computer software TestGraf was motivated by the need to produce a much faster algorithm for analyzing polytomous response data. A large class of potential users of test analysis software work with multiple choice exams or psychological scales in university, school, and other settings where only personal computers are available. Their sample sizes are usually modest, meaning between 100 and 1000. Moreover, their level of statistical knowledge may be limited, making it difficult for them to appreciate either the properties of parametric models or to assess parameter estimates. On the other hand, direct graphical display of option response functions may be a more convenient means of summarizing item characteristics. Finally, in many applications, including those using psychological scales, the responses cannot be meaningfully reduced to dichotomous, with one response designated as "correct."

Goodness of Fit

Various diagnostics of fit are possible to assess whether an estimated response curve gives a reasonable account of a set of data. Most procedures appropriate for parametric models are equally applicable to nonparametric fits. Ramsay (1991, 1993) discusses various possibilities. One useful technique illustrated in Ramsay (1991) is the plotting of the observed proportion of examinees passing an item among those whose total score is some fixed value x against the possible values of x. This is an empirical item-total score regression function. Each point in this plot can also be surrounded by pointwise confidence limits using standard formulas. At the same time, expected total score $E(x)$ can be computed as a function of θ, and subsequently the nonparametric estimates of probabilities plotted against expected total score. By overlaying these two plots, an evocative image of how well the estimated response curves fits the actual data is produced, and the user can judge if over-smoothing has occurred by noting whether the estimated curve falls consistently within the empirical confidence limits.

One great advantage offered by nonparametric methods is the fact that the fitting power is under user control. In the case of kernel smoothing, it is smoothing parameter λ that permits any level of flexibility required in the curve. Of course, there is an inevitable trade-off between flexibility and sampling variance of the estimate, and another positive feature of nonparametric modeling is that this trade-off is made explicit in a parameter.

There seems to be no discernible loss in mean square error of estimation of the functions $\mathbf{P}_i$ incurred by using kernel smoothing. Analysis of simulated data where the generating models were in the 3PL class produced fits which were at least as good as those resulting from using maximum likelihood estimation with the correct model. Of course, what is being fitted here is the function itself, and not parameter estimates.

With kernel smoothing approximation, in particular, it is also very simple to compute pointwise confidence regions for the true response curve. These are invaluable in communicating to the user the degree of precision that the data imply, and they are also helpful in deciding the appropriate level of smoothing. TestGraf along with an extensive manual is available on request from the author.

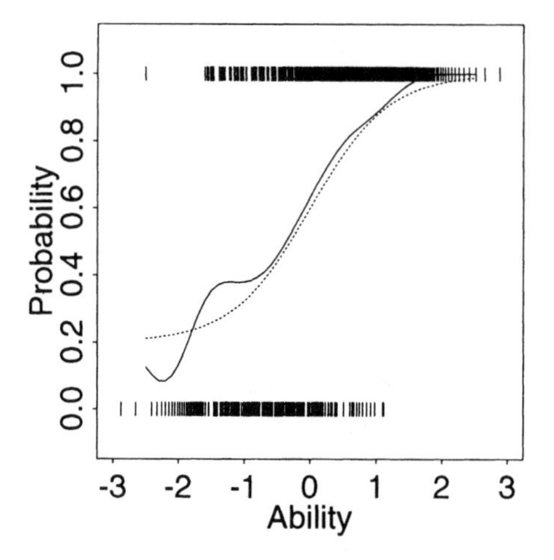

FIGURE 1. A fit by kernel smoothing to simulated data. (The solid curve indicates the smoothing estimate, and the dotted curve is the response curve which generates the data. The binary observations are indicated by the small vertical bars.)

Examples

Figure 1 gives an impression of how kernel smoothing works in practice. The smooth dashed line indicates a response curve that is to be estimated. The values of θ used for this problem were the 500 quantiles of the standard normal distribution, and for each such value, a Bernoulli 0–1 random variable was generated using the response curve value to determine the probability of generating one. The actual values of these random variables are plotted as small vertical bars. The solid line indicates the approximation resulting by smoothing these data with a Gaussian Nadaraya–Watson kernel smooth using $\lambda = 0.3$.

Figure 2 displays a test item from an administration of the Advanced Placement Chemistry Exam developed by Educational Testing Service and administered to about 18,500 candidates. The exam contained 75 multiple choice items, each with five options. The response of omitting the item was coded as a sixth option. The display was produced by TestGraf (Ramsay, 1993). The solid line is the correct option response function, and the vertical bars on this curve indicate pointwise 95% confidence regions for the true curve. It will be observed that the nearly linear behavior of this response function is not consistent with a logistic-linear parametric model such as the three-parameter logistic.

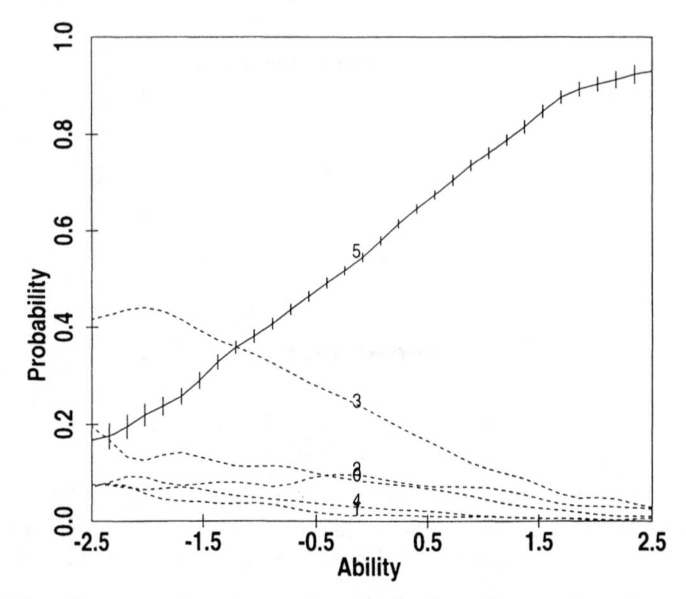

FIGURE 2. Response functions estimated by kernel smoothing for a multiple choice item. (The solid line is the response curve for the correct option and the dotted curves are for the incorrect options. The vertical bars on the solid curve indicate 95% pointwise confidence limits for the position of the true curve.)

Discussion

While the main nonparametric approach described in this chapter is based on kernel smoothing, many other approaches are possible. Monotone regression splines were investigated by Ramsay and Abrahamowicz (1989) and Ramsay and Winsberg (1991) for the modeling of dichotomous data. These curves are based on a set of basis functions called *regression splines* constructed from joining polynomial segments smoothly, and which can be designed to accommodate constraints such as monotonicity (Ramsay, 1988). Abrahamowicz and Ramsay (1991) applied regression spline modeling to polytomous response data.

A promising approach is the combination of spline smoothing with the GLM algorithm and statistical model. O'Sullivan et al. (1986) used polynomial smoothing splines to develop a nonparametric binary regression model. However, it can be very advantageous to adapt the nature of the spline to the character of the fitting problem, and Wang (1993) has developed a specialized smoothing spline which is very effective at not only estimating the response curve itself, but also its derivative and the associated information function. The increase in computation time over kernel smoothing does not seem to be prohibitive.

Response curve estimation in psychometric data analysis is typical of problems in which the essential task is to estimate a function. While parametric families can be a means to this end, they can also be too restrictive to capture features of actual data, and estimating a function via estimating parameters can bring other difficulties. By contrast, there are now a number of function estimation techniques which are fast, convenient, and arbitrarily accurate. Unless there are substantive reasons for preferring a particular parametric model, nonparametric estimation of the response curve may become the method of choice.

References

Abrahamowicz, M. and Ramsay, J.O. (1991). Multicategorical spline model for item response theory. *Psychometrika* **56**, 5–27.

Aitchison, J. (1986). *The Statistical Analysis of Compositional Data.* London: Chapman and Hall.

Buja, A., Hastie, T., and Tibshirani, R. (1989). Linear smoothers and additive models (with discussion). *The Annals of Statistics* **17**, 453–555.

Cox, D.R. and Snell, E.J. (1989). *Analysis of Binary Data* (2nd ed.). London: Chapman and Hall.

de Boor, C. (1978). *A Practical Guide to Splines.* New York: Springer-Verlag.

Eubank, R.L. (1988). *Spline Smoothing and Nonparametric Regression.* New York: Marcel Dekker, Inc.

Hastie, T. and Loader, C. (1993). Local regression: Automatic kernel carpentry (with discussion). *Statistical Science* **18**, 120–143.

Hastie, T. and Tibshirani, R. (1990). *Generalized Linear Models.* London: Chapman and Hall.

Lord, F.M. and Novick, M.R. (1968). *Statistical Theories of Mental Test Scores.* Reading, MA: Addison-Wesley.

McCullagh, P. and Nelder, J.A. (1989). *Generalized Linear Models.* London: Chapman and Hall.

O'Sullivan, F., Yandell, B., and Raynor, W. (1986). Automatic smoothing of regression functions in generalized linear models. *Journal of the American Statistical Association* **18**, 96–103.

Ramsay, J.O. (1988). Monotone regression splines in action (with discussion). *Statistical Science* **3**, 425–461.

Ramsay, J.O. (1991). Kernel smoothing approaches to nonparametric item characteristic curve estimation. *Psychometrika* **56**, 611–630.

Ramsay, J.O. (1993). *TestGraf: A Program for the Grapical Analysis of Multiple Choice Test Data.* Unpublished manuscript. McGill University, Montreal, Canada.

Ramsay, J.O. and Abrahamowicz, M. (1989). Binomial regression with monotone splines: A psychometric application. *Journal of the American Statistical Association* **84**, 906–915.

Ramsay, J.O. and Winsberg, S. (1991). Maximum marginal likelihood estimation for semiparametric item analysis. *Psychometrika* **56**, 365–379.

Wang, X. (1993). The analysis of test data using smoothing splines. Unpublished thesis, McGill University, Montreal, Canada.

Part V. Models for Nonmonotone Items

The first models in IRT were developed for responses to items in tests designed to measure such quantities as abilities, skills, knowledge, and intelligence. For these quantities, monotonicity of the response functions makes sense. Indeed, as explained in the chapters addressing nonparametric models in Section IV, one of the basic assumptions a set of dichotomous response data should meet is the one that states that the probability of a correct response is a monotonically increasing function of θ. IRT shares the assumption of monotonicity with response models in the fields of psychophysics and bioassay (see Chapter 1).

However, the behavioral and social sciences do have a domain of measurement for which the assumption of monotonicity is unlikely to hold. This is the domain of attitudes, opinions, beliefs, and values. Usually, variables in this domain, for which this introduction uses the term "attitude" as a *pars pro toto*, are measured by instruments consisting of a set of statements which persons are asked to indicate the extent to which they agree or disagree. It is a common experience that attitudes show that "extremes may meet." That is, it is not unusual to find that persons with opposite attitudes agreeing with the same statements. For example, consider the statement, "The courts usually give fair sentences to criminals." It is likely that those persons who think the courts are too lenient in sentencing and those who think the courts give overly hash sentences, would be in agreement with respect to their opposition to the statement. Of course, their reasons for disagreeing with the statement are *totally opposite* to each other. This finding is a direct violation of the assumption of monotonicity.

The first successful attempt to establish a stochastic model for attitude measurement was made by Thurstone (1927). His model was also presented under the more provocative title *Attitudes can be measured* in Thurstone (1928). Thurstone's model can only be used to infer the locations or scale values of attitude statements on an underlying unobserved scale from comparisons between pairs of statements. The model does not have any parameters for the attitudes of persons. Attitude measurement can therefore not take the form of model-based estimation but has to resort to *ad hoc* procedures for the inference of attitude measures from the scale values of statements the person agrees with.

An attempt to place persons and statement locations jointly on a scale of

Coombs' (1964) method of unfolding. This method is able to "unfold" preferential choice data into a single continuum through the use of the principle that preferences between statements are guided by the distances between their locations and the person's location. The method has the advantage of jointly scaling of persons and statements but is based on deterministic rules and does not allow for randomness in the response behavior of persons or in any other aspect of its underlying experiment. Therefore, though Coombs' paradigm was immediately recognized to expose the fundamental mechanism at work in preferential choice data, the need for a stochastic formulation of the mechanism has been felt for some time. A review of the attempts to do so is given in Bossuyt (1990, Chap. 1).

Some of these attempts have also tried to formulate these models for the experiment of direct responses of (dis)agreement to attitude statements rather than preferences between pairs of statements. Such models would make data collection more efficient because if n is the number of statements, only n responses rather than $\binom{n}{2}$ preferences are needed. At the same time, such models would have much in common with the models typically formulated in IRT. Formally, a stochastic model for direct responses to attitude statements in which the mechanism of folding is at work, takes the familiar form of a mathematical function describing the relation between the probability of a certain response and an underlying unknown variable. The only difference with IRT models is that the function cannot be monotonic.

This section offers two chapters on models for nonmonotone items which have the well-known form of a response function. The chapter by Andrich uses the fact that response functions of the nonextreme categories in polytomous models also are nonmonotonic. His model is, in fact, the result of collapsing a 3-category rating scale model (see Section I) into a 2-category model for agree-disagree responses. The PARELLA model by Hoijtink is motivated by Coombs' parallelogram analysis but specifies the response function directly as a Cauchy density function.

To date, the chapters in this section present the only two models known to specify a response function for direct responses to attitude statements. However, additional reading is found in Verhelst and Verstralen (1993) who independently presented an equivalent form of the model in the chapter by Andrich.

References

Bossuyt, P. (1990). *A Comparison of Probabilistic Unfolding Theories for Paired Comparison Data.* New York, NY: Springer-Verlag.

Coombs, C.H. (1964). *A Theory of Data.* New York, NY: Wiley.

Thurstone, L.L. (1927). A law of comparative judgement. *Psychological Review* **34**, 273–286. (Reprinted in *Psychological Review* **101**, 266–270.)

Thurstone, L.L. (1928). Attitudes can be measured. *American Journal of Sociology* **33**, 529–554.

Verhelst, N.D. and Verstralen, H.H.F.M. (1993). A stochastic unfolding model derived from the partial credit model. *Kwantitatieve Methoden* **42**, 73–92.

23

A Hyperbolic Cosine IRT Model for Unfolding Direct Responses of Persons to Items

David Andrich

Introduction

The two main mechanisms for characterizing dichotomous responses of persons to items on a single dimension are the *cumulative* and the *unfolding*. In the former, the probability of a positive response is a monotonic function of the relevant parameters; in the latter, it is single-peaked. This chapter presents a unidimensional IRT model for unfolding. Figure 1 shows the response functions (RFs) of the probabilities of the responses, including the resolution of the negative response into its two constituent components. Table 1 shows a deterministic unfolding response pattern for five items.

Presentation of the Model

Although introduced by Thurstone (1927, 1928) for the measurement of attitude, the study of unfolding is associated with Coombs (1964) who worked within a deterministic framework, and when more than four or so items are involved, the analysis is extremely complex. Probabilistic models have been introduced subsequently (e.g., Andrich, 1988; Davison, 1977; Post, 1992; van Schuur, 1984, 1989). In this chapter, a rationale that links the responses of persons to items directly to the unfolding mechanism through a graded response structure is used to construct an item response theory (IRT) model for unfolding.

In addition to the measurement of attitude, unfolding models have been applied to the study of development along a continuum, e.g., in psychological development (Coombs and Smith, 1973); development in learning goals (Volet and Chalmers, 1992); social development (Leik and Matthews, 1968); in general preference studies (Coombs and Avrunin, 1977); and in political science (van Blokland-Vogelesang, 1991; van Schuur, 1987).

The model studied here is developed from first principles using a concrete example in attitude measurement. Consider a dichotomous response

TABLE 1. Deterministic Ideal Cumulative and Unfolding Response Patterns to Five Items.

Items				
1	2	3	4	5
0	0	0	0	0
1	0	0	0	0
1	1	0	0	0
0	1	1	0	0
0	0	1	1	0
0	0	0	1	1
0	0	0	0	1
0	0	0	0	0

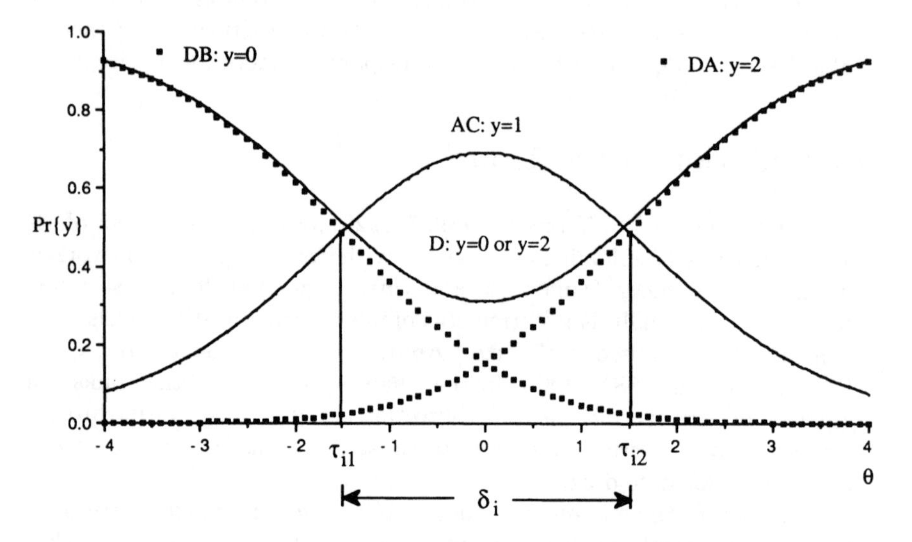

FIGURE 1. Response functions of the Agree Close (AC) and Disagree (D) responses and the resolution of the Disagree response into its constituent components: Disagree Below (DB) and Disagree Above (DA).

of Agree or Disagree of a person to the statement "I think capital punishment is necessary but I wish it were not." This statement appears in the example later in the chapter, and reflects an ambivalent attitude to capital punishment. If the person's location is also relatively ambivalent and therefore close to the location of the statement, then the person will tend to agree to the statement, and if a person's location is far from that of the statement—either very much *for* or very much *against* capital punishment, then the probability of Agree will decrease and that of Disagree will increase correspondingly. This gives the single-peaked form of the response function for the Agree response shown in Fig. 1. However, it is more instructive to consider the Disagree rather than the Agree response.

Let the locations of person j and statement i be θ_j and δ_i, respectively. Then formally, if $\theta_j << \delta_i$ or $\theta_j >> \delta_i$, the probability of a Disagree response tends to 1.0. This reveals that the Disagree response occurs for *two* latent reasons, one because the person has a much stronger attitude *against* capital punishment, the other because the person has a much stronger attitude *for* capital punishment, than reflected by the statement. The RF with broken lines in Fig. 1 show the resolution of the single Disagree response into these two constituent components. This resolution shows that there are three possible latent responses that correspond to the two possible manifest responses of Agree/Disagree: (i) Disagree because persons consider themselves below the location of the statement (disagree below –DB); (ii) Agree because the persons consider themselves close to the location of the statement (agree close –AC); and (iii) disagree because the persons consider themselves above the location of the statement (disagree above –DA). Furthermore, the probabilities of the two Disagree responses have a monotonic decreasing and increasing shape, respectively. This means that, as shown in Fig. 1, the three-responses take the form of responses to three graded responses. Accordingly, a model for graded responses can be applied to this structure. Because it is the simplest of models for graded responses, and because it can be expressed efficiently and simply in the case of three categories, the model applied is the Rasch (1961) model which can take a number of forms, all equivalent to

$$\Pr\{y_{ij}\} = \gamma_{ij}^{-1} \exp\left[-\sum_{h=1}^{x} \tau_{ih} + y(\theta_j - \delta_i)\right], \tag{1}$$

where $y_{ij} \in \{0, 1, 2, \ldots, m\}$ indicates the $m+1$ successive categories beginning with 0, τ_{ih}, $h = 1, \ldots, m$ are m thresholds on the continuum dividing the categories; and $\gamma_{ij} = \sum_{y=0}^{m} \exp\left[-\sum_{h=1}^{y} \tau_{ih} + y(\theta_j - \delta_i)\right]$ is the normalizing factor which ensures that the sum of the probabilities is 1.0 (Andersen, 1977; Andrich, 1978; Wright and Masters, 1982). Furthermore, without loss of generality (Andrich, 1978), it is taken that $\sum_{h=1}^{m} \tau_{ih} \equiv 0$.

The correspondence between the three responses in Fig. 1 and the random variable in Eq. (1), in which case $m = 2$, is as follows: $y = 0 \leftrightarrow$ DB;

$y = 1 \leftrightarrow$ AC; $y = 2 \leftrightarrow$ DA. It is evident that the RFs in Fig. 1 operate so that, when θ_j is close to δ_i, the probability of the middle score of 1 (AC) is greater than the probability of either 0 (DB) or 2 (DA). This is as required in the unfolding mechanism.

Now define the parameter λ_i according to $\lambda_i = (\tau_{i2} - \tau_{i1})/2$. Then the location parameter δ_i is in the middle of the two thresholds, and λ_i represents the distance from δ_i to each of the thresholds (Andrich, 1982). These parameters are also shown in Fig. 1. It is now instructive to write the probability of each RF explicitly in terms of the parameter λ_i:

$$\Pr\{y_{ij} = 0\} = \gamma_{ij}^{-1}, \tag{2a}$$

$$\Pr\{y_{ij} = 1\} = \gamma_{ij}^{-1} \exp[\lambda_i + (\theta_j - \delta_i)], \tag{2b}$$

$$\Pr\{y_{ij} = 2\} = \gamma_{ij}^{-1} \exp 2(\theta_j - \delta_i). \tag{2c}$$

Because the thresholds define the points where the probability of each extreme response becomes greater than the middle response, the probabilities of, respectively, AC and DB, or AC and DA are identical at $\delta_i \pm \lambda_i$. Thus, λ_i is very much like the half-unit of measurement, such as half a centimeter, about the points marking off units on a ruler. For example, any object deemed to be located within half a centimeter on either side of a particular number of say x centimeters, will be declared to be x centimeters long. Analogously, a location θ_j of person j within $\pm\lambda_i$ of δ_i gives the highest probability for the Agree response, which reflects that the person is located close to the statement. This parameter is discussed further in Andrich and Luo (1993), and consistent with the interpretation presented briefly here, it is termed the *unit* parameter—it characterizes the natural unit of measurement of the statement.

Although the model characterizes the three implied responses of a person to a statement, there are, nevertheless, only two manifest responses, and, in particular, only one manifest Disagree response. That is, $y = 0$ and $y = 2$ are not distinguished in the data. To make the model correspond to the data, define a new random variable U_{ij}, which takes the values $u_{ij} = 0$ when $y_{ij} = 0$ or $y_{ij} = 2$ and $u_{ij} = 1$ when $y_{ij} = 1$. Then

$$\Pr\{u_{ij} = 0\} = \Pr\{y_{ij} = 0\} + \Pr\{y_{ij} = 2\} \tag{3a}$$

and

$$\Pr\{u_{ij} = 1\} = \Pr\{y_{ij} = 1\}. \tag{3b}$$

Inserting the explicit expressions of Eq. (2) into Eq. (3) gives

$$\Pr\{u_{ij} = 0\} = \gamma_{ij}^{-1}[1 + \exp 2(\theta_j - \delta_i)] \tag{4a}$$

and

$$\Pr\{u_{ij} = 1\} = \gamma_{ij}^{-1} \exp[\lambda_i + (\theta_j - \delta_i)], \tag{4b}$$

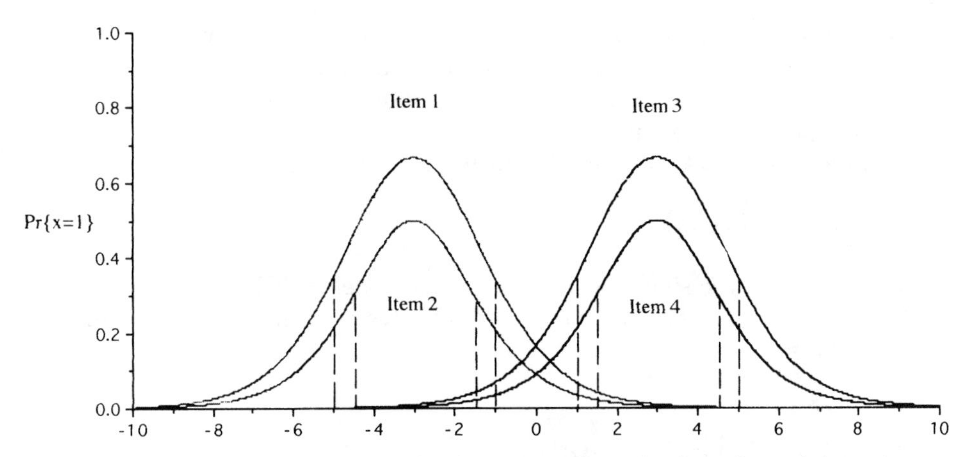

FIGURE 2. Response functions for four items: $\delta_1 = \delta_2$; $\delta_3 = \delta_4$; and $\lambda_1 = \lambda_3$; $\lambda_2 = \lambda_4$.

where $\gamma_{ij} = 1 + \exp[\lambda_i + (\theta_j - \delta_i)] + \exp 2(\theta_j - \delta_i)$.

Because the random variable U_{ij} is dichotomous, it is efficient to focus on only one of Eqs. (4a) or (4b). Focusing on Eq. (4b), and writing the normalizing factor γ_{ij} explicitly gives

$$\Pr\{u_{ij} = 1\} = \frac{\exp[\lambda_i + (\theta_j - \delta_i)]}{1 + \exp[(\lambda_i + \theta_j - \delta_i)] + \exp 2(\theta_j - \delta_i)}. \tag{5}$$

Multiplying the numerator and denominator by $\exp[-(\theta_j - \delta_i)]$, and simplifying gives

$$\Pr\{u_{ij} = 1\} = \frac{\exp \lambda_i}{\exp \lambda_i + \exp(\theta_j - \delta_i) + \exp(-\theta_j + \delta_i)}. \tag{6}$$

Recognizing that the hyperbolic cosine, $\cosh(a) \equiv [\exp(a) + \exp(-a)]/2$, gives

$$\Pr\{u_{ij} = 1\} = \frac{\exp \lambda_i}{\exp \lambda_i + 2\cosh(\theta_j - \delta_i)} \tag{7a}$$

and

$$\Pr\{u_{ij} = 0\} = 1 - \Pr\{u_{ij} = 1\} = \frac{2\cosh(\theta_j - \delta_i)}{\exp \lambda_i + 2\cosh(\theta_j - \delta_i)}. \tag{7b}$$

Equations (7a) and (7b) can be written as the single expression

$$\Pr\{u_{ij}\} = \gamma_{ij}^{-1}(\exp \lambda_i)^{u_{ij}}\left[2\cosh^{1-u_{ij}}(\theta_j - \delta_i)\right], \tag{8}$$

where $\gamma_{ij} = \exp \lambda_i + 2\cosh(\theta_j - \delta_i)$ is now the normalizing factor.

For obvious reasons, the model of Eq. (8) is termed the hyperbolic cosine model (HCM). Figure 2 shows the RFs for $u_{ij} = 1$ for four statements, two each with the same unit λ_i, but different locations δ_i, and two each with the same location δ_i but different λ_i. To consolidate the interpretation of the parameter λ_i, note that the greater its value, the greater the region in which a person is most likely to give an Agree response.

In the case that $\lambda_i = \lambda$ for all i, then Eq. (8) specializes to

$$\Pr\{u_{ij}\} = \frac{1}{\gamma_{ij}}(\exp\lambda)^{u_{ij}}\left[2\cosh^{1-u_{ij}}(\theta_j - \delta_i)\right]. \tag{9}$$

This is termed the simple hyperbolic cosine model (SHCM). Verhelst and Verstralen (1991) have presented effectively the same model but in a different form.

Parameter Estimation

Although the HCM is constructed from a Rasch model for graded responses, by combining two categories, the distinguishing feature of the Rasch models, namely the existence of sufficient statistics for the person and statement parameters (Andersen, 1977), is destroyed. Therefore, methods of estimation that involve conditioning on sufficient statistics are not available. Other methods, including the joint maximum likelihood (JML), the EM algorithm, and the marginal maximum likelihood procedures, are being investigated. The procedure described here is the simplest of these, the JML.

The likelihood of the matrix of responses persons $j = 1, J$ to statements $i = 1, I$ is given by

$$L = \prod_i \prod_j \gamma_{ij}^{-1} e^{\lambda_i u_{ij}} \left[2\cosh(\theta_j - \delta_i)\right]^{1-u_{ij}} \tag{10}$$

and provides the log-likelihood equation

$$\log L = \sum_i \sum_j u_{ij}\lambda_i + \sum_i \sum_j (1 - u_{ij}) \log 2\cosh(\theta_j - \delta_i) - \sum_i \sum_j \log \gamma_{ij}. \tag{11}$$

Differentiating Eq. (11) partially with respect to each of the parameters θ, δ, λ, and equating to 0, provides the solution equations

$$\varphi(\delta_i) = \sum_j (p_{ij} - x_{ij})\tanh(\theta_j - \delta_i) = 0, \quad i = 1, I; \tag{12a}$$

$$\varphi(\theta_j) = \sum_i (p_{ij} - x_{ij})\tanh(\theta_j - \delta_i) = 0, \quad j = 1, J; \tag{12b}$$

$$\varphi(\lambda_i) = \sum_i (p_{ij} - x_{ij}) = 0, \quad i = 1, I; \tag{12c}$$

where $p_{ij} = \Pr\{x_{ij} = 1\}$. In addition, the constraint $\sum_{i=1}^{I} \hat{\delta}_i = 0$ is imposed.

A Solution Algorithm

The Newton–Raphson algorithm is efficient in reaching an iterative solution to the implicit equations. The complete multivariate algorithm is not feasible because as N increases, the matrix of second derivatives becomes too large to invert. The alternative algorithm commonly used in such situations is to take the statement parameters as fixed while the person parameters are improved individually to the required convergence criterion; the person parameters are then fixed, and the statement parameters are improved individually until the whole set of estimates converges. In that case, the algorithm takes the form

$$[\hat{\lambda}_i]^{(q+1)} = [\hat{\lambda}_i]^{(q)} - [\psi_{\lambda\lambda}]^{-1(q)}\varphi(\lambda_i), \quad i = 1, I, \tag{13a}$$

$$[\hat{\delta}_i]^{(q+1)} = [\hat{\delta}_i]^{(q)} - [\psi_{\delta\delta}]^{-1(q)}\varphi(\delta_i), \quad i = 1, I-1, \tag{13b}$$

and

$$[\hat{\theta}_j]^{(q+1)} = [\hat{\theta}_j]^{(q)} - [\psi_{\theta\theta}]^{-1(q)}\varphi(\theta_j), \quad n = 1, N, \tag{13c}$$

where $\psi_{\lambda\lambda} = E[\partial^2 L/\partial\lambda_i^2]$; $\psi_{\delta\delta} = E[\partial^2 L/\partial\delta_i^2]$; $\psi_{\theta\theta} = E[\partial^2 L/\partial\theta_j^2]$. The hypothesis that $\lambda_i = \lambda$ for all i can be tested using the usual likelihood ratio test. The full procedure and program is described in Luo and Andrich (1993).

Initial Estimates

The initial values $\lambda_i^{(0)}$ are simply taken as log 2 because the model then simplifies to $\Pr\{x_{ij} = 1\} = 1/(1 + \cosh(\theta_j - \delta_i))$, a symmetric counterpart of the simple cumulative Rasch model (Andrich and Luo, 1993). Although no empirical case has yet been found, it is possible for an estimate of λ_i to be negative, in which case the response curve would be U-shaped (Andrich, 1982), and it would provide immediate evidence that the response process does not give a single peaked RF.

The initial location values of $\delta_i^{(0)}$ are obtained by setting all $\theta_j = 0$ and all $\lambda_i = \log 2$, giving, on simplification $\delta_i^{(0)} = \cosh^{-1}((N - s_i)/s_i)$, where $s_i = \sum_j u_{ij}$ is the total score of a statement. Because $\cosh \delta_i \geq 1$, if for some i, $(N - s_i)/s_i \leq 1$, then the minimum of these values is taken, and the difference $\alpha = 1 - \min[(N - s_i)/s_i]$ calculated to give

$$\delta_i^{(0)} = \cosh^{-1}[\alpha + (N - s_i)/s_i]. \tag{14}$$

The unfolding structure implies that statements at genuinely different locations can have the same total score statistic s_i. This difference can be taken into account by assigning a negative sign to the initial estimates of approximately half of the statements and a positive sign to the other half. There are two ways of choosing the statements that receive a negative sign, one empirical, the other theoretical, and of course, they can be used together. First, if data have an unfolding structure, then the traditional factor loadings on the first factor of a factor analysis unfolds into the positive and negative loadings (Davison, 1977). Second, a provisional ordering of the statements should be possible according to the theory governing the construction of the variable and the operationalization of the statements. The importance of the theoretical ordering will be elaborated upon in the discussion of fit between the data and the model.

The initial estimates $\theta_j^{(0)}$ are obtained from the initial estimates of the statement locations $\delta_i^{(0)}$ according to $\theta_j^{(0)} = \sum_{i=1}^{I_j} u_{ij}\delta_i^{(0)}/I_j$, where I_j is the number of items that person j has with a score $u_{ij} = 1$. These are the average values of the statements to which each person agreed.

Information and Standard Errors

According to maximum likelihood theory, large sample variances of the estimates $\hat{\lambda}_i$, $\hat{\delta}_i$, $\hat{\theta}_i$ are given by

$$\sigma^2_{\hat{\lambda}_i} = -1/E[\psi_{\lambda\lambda}] = -1/\sum_j p_{ij}(1-p_{ij}), \tag{15a}$$

$$\sigma^2_{\hat{\delta}_i} = -1/E[\psi_{\delta\delta}] = -1/\sum_j p_{ij}(1-p_{ij})\tanh^2(\theta_j-\delta_i), \tag{15b}$$

and

$$\sigma^2_{\hat{\theta}_j} = -1/E[\psi_{\theta\theta}] = -1/\sum_j p_{ij}(1-p_{ij})\tanh^2(\theta_j-\delta_i), \tag{15c}$$

respectively. Andrich and Luo (1993) show that the approximations are very good.

Inconsistency of Parameter Estimates

From the work on estimation of parameters in the Rasch models (Andersen, 1973; Wright and Douglas, 1977) it is known that the JML estimates of the HCM are not consistent in the case of a fixed number of items and an unlimited increase in the number of persons. However, no assumptions regarding the distribution of person parameters needs to be made, and this is particularly desirable in attitude measurement, where, for example, attitudes may be polarized and the empiricial study of the shape of this distribution is important.

With the number of items of the order of 15 or so, the inconsistency is noticeable (Andrich and Luo, 1993), but very small. However, in the case of the analysis of a particular sample of data, this effect is essentially a matter of scale in that the estimates are stretched relative to their real values. When the number of items is of the order of 100, the effect of the inconsistency is not noticeable. In the simple Rasch model, the estimates can be corrected effectively by multiplying them by $(I-1)/I$ (Wright and Douglas, 1977), and it may be possible to work out a correction factor for the HCM. Alternative procedures, such as the marginal maximum likelihood, may overcome the inconsistency without imposing undesirable constraints on the shape of the distribution. These possibilities are still being explored.

Goodness of Fit

In considering tests of fit between the data and a model, the perspective taken in this chapter is that the model is an explicit rendition of a theory, and that the data collection is in turn governed by the model. Therefore, to the degree that the data accord with the model, to that degree they confirm both the theory and its operationalization in the data collection, and vice versa. In the application of IRT, the model chosen is expected to summarize the responses with respect to some substantive variable in which the items reflect differences in degree on the latent continuum. Thus the aim should be to construct items at different locations on the continuum, and the relative order of the items, become an hypothesis about the data. This theoretical ordering, taken as an hypothesis, is especially significant when the model that reflects the response process is single-peaked because, as already indicated, there are always two person locations that give the same probability of a positive response.

The hypothesis that the responses take a single-peaked form can be checked by estimating the locations of the persons and the statements, dividing the persons into class intervals and checking if the proportions of persons responding positively across class intervals takes the single peaked form specified by the model. This is a common general test of fit, and can be formalized as

$$\chi^2 = \sum_{i=1}^{I}\sum_{g=1}^{G} \frac{\left(\sum_{j\in g} u_{ij} - \sum_{j\in g} E[u_{ij}]\right)^2}{\sum_{j\in g} V[u_{ij}]}$$

$$= \sum_{i=1}^{I}\sum_{g=1}^{G} \frac{\left(\sum_{j\in g} u_{ij} - \sum_{j\in g} p_{ij}\right)^2}{\sum_{j\in g} p_{ij}(1-p_{ij})}, \qquad (16)$$

where $g = 1, G$ are the class intervals. Asymptotically, as the number of persons and items increases, this statistic should approximate the χ^2 distribution on $(G-1)(I-1)$ degrees of freedom. The power of this test of fit is governed by the relative locations of the persons and the statements, where the greater the variation among these the greater the power.

Complementary to this formal procedure, a telling and simpler check is to display the responses of the persons to the statements when both are ordered according to their estimated locations. Then the empirical order of the statements should accord with the theoretical ordering, which in the case of attitude statements is according to their affective values, and the matrix of responses should show the parallelogram form shown in Table 1. The study of the fit between the data and the model using the combination of these approaches, the theoretical and the statistical, is illustrated in the example.

Example

The example involves the measurement of an attitude to capital punishment using a set of eight statements originally constructed by Thurstone's (1927, 1928) methods and subsequently studied again by Wohlwill (1963) and Andrich (1988). The data involve the responses of 41 persons in a class in Educational Measurement at Murdoch University (Australia) in 1993, and the sample will be discussed again. Table 2[1] shows the statements, their estimated affective values, and standard errors under the HCM model in which first all statements are assumed to have the same unit λ, and second, where the unit λ_i is free to vary among statements. Table 3 shows the frequencies of all observed patterns, the estimated attitudes, and their standard errors. It may be considered that the sample is small. However, it has the advantage that the analyses can be studied very closely, and perhaps even more importantly, it shows that the model can be applied successfully even in the case of small samples. In this case, there is already strong theoretical and empirical evidence that the statements do work as a scale, and so the analysis takes a confirmatory role.

In Table 2 the statements are ordered according to their estimated affective values and in Table 3 the persons are likewise ordered according to the estimate of the attitudes. This helps appreciate the definition of the variable and is a check on the fit. Table 2 shows that the ordering of the statements begins with an attitude that is strongly against capital punishment, through an ambivalent attitude, to one which is strongly for capital punishment. In addition, the likelihood ratio test confirms that the unit value is the same across statements, and this is confirmed by the closeness of the estimates of the affective values of statements when equal and unequal units are assumed and likewise for the estimates of the attitudes of the persons. The ordering of the persons shows the required feature of 1's in a parallelogram around the diagonal. Figure 3 shows the distribution of the persons, and it is evident that it is bimodal.

Even without any further checks on the fit, it should be apparent that the data are consistent with the model, and therefore this confirms the hypothesis of the ordering of the statements and their usefulness for mea-

---

[1] *Note:* Likelihood ratio χ^2 for Ho: $\lambda_i = \lambda$: $\chi^2 = 6.64$, df $= 6$, $p > 0.36$.

TABLE 2. Scale Values of Statements about Capital Punishment from Direct Responses

	Statement	Equal Unit λ_i		Estimated λ_i	
		$\hat{\delta}_i(\hat{\sigma}_{\delta_i})$	$\hat{\lambda}(\hat{\sigma}_{\lambda})$	$\hat{\delta}_i(\hat{\sigma}_{\delta_i})$	$\hat{\lambda}_i(\hat{\sigma}_{\lambda_i})$
1.	Capital punishment is one of the most hideous practices of our time.	−10.11(1.14)	6.36(0.23)	−9.80(1.10)	6.54(1.09)
2.	Capital punishment is not an effective deterrent to crime.	−7.78(1.00)	6.38(0.23)	−7.83(0.93)	6.75(0.93)
3.	The state cannot teach the sacredness of human life by destroying it.	−4.24(0.50)	6.38(0.23)	−5.11(0.52)	7.69(0.52)
4.	I don't believe in capital punishment but I am not sure it isn't necessary.	−2.45(0.47)	6.38(0.23)	−2.26(0.48)	5.78(0.98)
5.	I think capital punishment is necessary, but I wish it were not.	3.20(0.79)	6.38(0.23)	3.29(0.71)	5.21(0.71)
6.	Until we find a more civilized way to prevent crime, we must have capital punishment.	6.06(0.82)	6.38(0.23)	6.44(0.82)	6.60(0.82)
7.	Capital punishment is justified because it does act as a deterrent to crime.	6.65(0.75)	6.38(0.23)	6.79(0.73)	6.34(0.73)
8.	Capital punishment gives the criminal what he deserves.	8.67(0.58)	6.38(0.23)	8.47(0.56)	6.09(0.56)

TABLE 3. Distribution of Attitude Scale Values

Attitude Estimate $\hat{\theta}(\hat{\sigma}_\theta)$ Equal $\hat{\lambda}$		Different $\hat{\lambda}_i$		Total Score	Response Pattern								Frequency
−9.70	(1.53)	−10.31	(2.42)	3	1	1	1	0	0	0	0	0	5
−6.50	(2.27)	−5.86	(2.31)	4	1	1	1	1	0	0	0	0	7
−2.32	(1.5)	−1.75	(1.07)	2	0	0	1	1	0	0	0	0	1
−2.32	(1.5)	−1.75	(1.07)	4	0	1	1	1	1	0	0	0	1
0.04	(1.05)	0.31	(1.01)	4	0	0	1	1	1	0	1	0	1
1.15	(1.06)	1.36	(1.04)	5	0	1	0	1	1	1	0	1	1
1.15	(1.06)	1.36	(1.04)	5	0	0	1	1	1	1	1	0	2
2.31	(1.10)	2.44	(1.06)	4	0	0	1	0	1	1	1	0	1
2.31	(1.10)	2.44	(1.06)	6	0	0	1	1	1	1	1	1	2
2.31	(1.10)	2.44	(1.06)	4	0	0	0	1	1	1	1	0	1
2.31	(1.10)	2.44	(1.06)	4	0	0	1	0	1	1	0	1	1
3.67	(1.28)	3.67	(1.22)	5	0	0	1	0	1	1	1	1	1
3.67	(1.28)	3.67	(1.22)	5	0	0	0	1	1	1	1	1	3
3.67	(1.28)	3.67	(1.22)	3	0	0	0	0	1	1	1	0	2
6.88	(2.81)	6.30	(2.31)	4	0	0	0	1	0	1	1	1	1
6.89	(2.81)	6.32	(2.31)	4	0	0	0	0	1	1	1	1	10
10.69	(1.57)	10.36	(2.01)	3	0	0	0	0	0	1	1	1	1

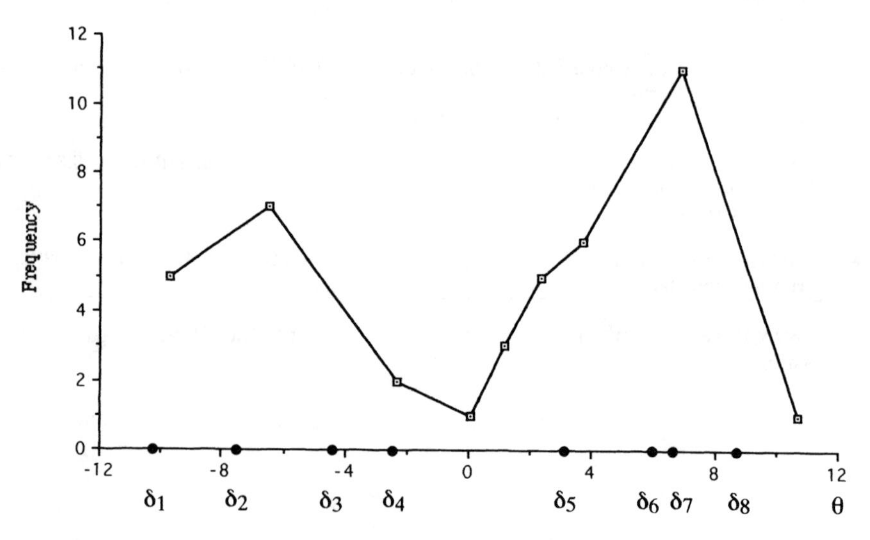

FIGURE 3. Distribution of attitudes of persons and locations of statements in the sample.

suring an attitude to capital punishment. The global test of fit according to Eq. (17), in which the sample is divided into three class intervals, has a value $\chi^2 = 18.00$, df $= 14$, $p > 0.21$, which confirms this impression. In addition to the distribution of the persons, Fig. 3 shows the locations of the statements. Given the evidence that the data conforms to the SHCM (i.e., HCM with equal units), this figure summarizes the effort to simultaneously locate statements and persons on an attitude continuum when direct responses of persons to statements subscribe to the unfolding mechanism.

The original data involved 50 persons, but the papers of two persons had no responses, and of three persons had incomplete responses. Although the models can be operationalized to cater for missing data, it was decided to use only complete data. It was surmised that, because the class had a number of students with non-English-speaking backgrounds, that the persons who did not complete their papers might have been from such backgrounds.

Lack of familiarity with the language of response is relevant in all assessment, but it has a special role in the measurement of attitude where the statements often deliberately take the form of a cliche, catch phrase, or proverb, and it is not expected that a person ponders at length to make a response. Indeed, it is required to have a relatively quick and spontaneous affective, rather than a reasoned cognitive, response, and this generally requires fluency in the vernacular.

The responses of the remaining 45 students with complete direct responses were then analyzed according to the model. The theoretical ordering was violated quite noticeably in that the statement *I don't believe in capital punishment, but I am not sure it is not necessary* was estimated to have a stronger attitude against capital punishment than the statement *Capital punishment is one of the most hideous practices of our time.* A close examination of the data showed that the responses of four persons had glaring anomalies and they seemed to agree to statements randomly. It was surmized that these four persons may also have had trouble understanding these statements or were otherwise distracted. Therefore they, too, were removed, leaving the sample shown in Table 3. Although there is no space to describe the example in detail, responses from the same persons to the same statements were obtained according to a pairwise preference design and analyzed according to a model derived from the HCM. When the responses of these four persons were eliminated from the analysis of the pairwise preference data, the test of fit between the data and the model also improved (Andrich, in press). This confirmed that those four persons had responses whose validity was doubtful in both sets of data.

The point of this discussion is that four persons in a sample of 45 were able to produce responses that provided an ordering of statements which grossly violated the theoretical ordering of two statements, and that, with a strong theoretical perspective, these four persons could be identified. Ideally, these persons, if they were known, would be interviewed regarding their responses. Then either it would be confirmed that they had trouble with the language, or if they did not, that they perhaps read the statements in some way different from the intended reading. It is by such a process of closer study that anomalies are disclosed, and in this case possible ambiguities in statements are understood.

Acknowledgments

The research on hyperbolic cosine models for unfolding was supported in part by a grant from the Australian Research Council. G. Luo worked through the estimation equations and wrote the computer programs for the analysis. Irene Styles read the chapter and made constructive comments. Tables 2 and 3 were reproduced with permission from Applied Phychological Measurement, Inc., 1995.

References

Andersen, E.B. (1973). Conditional inference for multiple choice questionnaires. *British Journal of Mathematical and Statistical Psychology* **26**, 31–44.

Andersen, E.B. (1977). Sufficient statistics and latent trait models. *Psychometrika* **42**, 69–81.

Andrich, D. (1978). A rating formulation for ordered response categories. *Psychometrika* **43**, 357–374.

Andrich, D. (1982). An extension of the Rasch model for ratings providing both location and dispersion parameters. *Psychometrika* **47**, 105–113.

Andrich, D. (1988). The application of an unfolding direct-responses and pairwise preferences (Research Report No. 4). Murdoch, Australia: Murdoch University, Social Measurement Laboratory.

Andrich, D. (in press). Hyperbolic cosine latent trait models for unfolding direct responses and pairwise preferences. *Applied Psychological Measurement.*

Andrich, D. and Luo, G. (1993). A hyperbolic cosine latent trait model for unfolding dichotomous single-stimulus responses. *Applied Psychological Measurement* **17**, 253–276.

Coombs, C.H. (1964). *A Theory of Data.* New York: Wiley.

Coombs, C.H. and Avrunin, C.S. (1977). Single-peaked functions and the theory of preference. *Psychological Review* **84**(2), 216–230.

Coombs, C.H. and Smith, J.E.K. (1973). On the detection of structure in attitudes and developmental process. *Psychological Review* **5**, **80**(5), 337–351.

Davison, M. (1977). On a metric, unidimensional unfolding model for attitudinal and developmental data. *Psychometrika* **42**, 523–548.

Leik, R.K. and Matthews, M. (1968). A scale for developmental processes. *American Sociological Review* **33**(1), 62075.

Luo, G. and Andrich, D. (1993). HCMDR: A FORTRAN Program for analyzing direct responses according to hyperbolic cosine unfolding model (Social Measurement Laboratory Report No. 5). Western Australia: School of Education, Murdoch University.

Post, W.J. (1992). *Nonparametric Unfolding Models: A Latent Structure Approach.* Leiden: DSWO Press.

Rasch, G. (1961). On general laws and the meaning of measurement in psychology. In J. Neyman (ed.), *Proceedings of the Fourth Berkeley Symposium on Mathematical Statistics and Probability IV* (pp. 321–334). Berkeley, CA: University of California Press.

Thurstone, L.L. (1927). A law of comparative judgement. *Psychological Review* **34**, 278–286.

Thurstone, L.L. (1928). Attitudes can be measured. *American Journal of Sociology* **33**, 529–554.

van Blokland-Vogelesang, R. (1991). *Unfolding and Group Consensus Ranking for Individual Preferences.* Leiden: DSWPO Press.

van Schuur, W.H. (1984). *Structure in Political Beliefs, a New Model for Stochastic Unfolding with Application to European Party Activists.* Amsterdam: CT Press.

van Schuur, W.H. (1987). Constraint in European party activists' sympathy scores for interest groups: The left-right dimension as dominant structuring principle. *European Journal of Political Research* **15**, 347–362.

van Schuur, W.H. (1989). Unfolding German political parties: A description and application of multiple unidimensional unfolding. In G. de Soete, H. Ferger, and K.C. Klauser (eds.), *New Developments in Psychological Choice Modelling*, (pp. 259–277). Amsterdam: North Holland.

Verhelst, N.D. and Verstralen, H.H.F.M. (1991). A stochastic unfolding model with inherently missing data. Unpublished manuscript, CITO, The Netherlands.

Volet, S.E. and Chalmers, D. (1992). Investigation of qualitative differences in university students' learning goals, based on an unfolding model of stage development. *British Journal of Educational Psychology* **62**, 17–34.

Wohlwill, J.F. (1963). The measurement of scalability for noncumulative items. *Educational and Psychological Measurement* **23**, 543–555.

Wright, B.D. and Douglas, G.A. (1977). Conditional versus unconditional procedures for sample-free item analysis. *Educational and Psychological Measurement* **37**, 47–60.

Wright, B.D. and Masters, G.N. (1982). *Rating Scale Analysis: Rasch Measurement.* Chicago: MESA Press.

24

PARELLA: An IRT Model for Parallelogram Analysis

Herbert Hoijtink

Introduction

Parallelogram analysis was introduced by Coombs (1964, Chap. 15). In many respects it is similar to scalogram analysis (Guttman, 1950): Both models assume the existence of a unidimensional latent trait; both models assume that this trait is operationalized via a set of items indicative of different levels of this trait; both models assume that the item responses are completely determined by the location of person and item on the latent trait; both models assume that the item responses are dichotomous, that is, assume 0/1 scoring, indicating such dichotomies as incorrect/correct, disagree/agree, or, dislike/like; and both models are designed to infer the order of the persons as well as the items along the latent trait of interest from the item-responses.

The main difference between the models is the measurement model used to relate the item responses to locations of persons and items on the latent trait. The scalogram model is based on dominance relations between person and item:

$$\begin{aligned} U_{ij} = 1 \quad & \text{if } (\theta_j - \delta_i) > 0, \\ U_{ij} = 0 \quad & \text{if } (\theta_j - \delta_i) < 0, \end{aligned} \tag{1}$$

where U_{ij} denotes the response of person j, $j = 1, \ldots, N$ to item i, $i = 1, \ldots, n$, θ_j denotes the location of person j, and δ_i denotes the location of item i. The parallelogram model is based on proximity relations between person and item:

$$\begin{aligned} U_{ij} = 1 \quad & \text{if } |\theta_j - \delta_i| > \tau, \\ U_{ij} = 0 \quad & \text{if } |\theta_j - \delta_i| < \tau, \end{aligned} \tag{2}$$

where τ is a threshold governing the maximum distance between θ and δ for which a person still renders a positive response.

A disadvantage of both the scalogram and the parallelogram model is their deterministic nature: The item responses are completely determined by the distance between person and items. As a consequence, these models are not very useful for the analysis of empirical data. What is needed are probabilistic models that take into account that item responses are explained not only by the distance between person location and item location but also by random characteristics of either the person or the item. The logistic item response models (Hambleton and Swaminathan, 1985) can be seen as the probabilistic counterpart of the scalogram model. This chapter will describe the PARELLA model (Hoijtink, 1990; 1991a; 1991b; Hoijtink and Molenaar, 1992; Hoijtink et al., 1994), which is the probabilistic counterpart of the parallelogram model.

Most applications of the PARELLA model concern the measurement of attitudes and preferences. Some examples of such applications are the attitude with respect to nuclear power; the attitude with respect to capital punishment; political attitude; and preference for different quality/price ratios of consumer goods. PARELLA analyses are usually not finished with the estimation of the locations of the persons and the items. The estimated person locations can be used to investigate different hypotheses: Did the attitude toward gypsies in Hungary change between 1987 and 1992; does the political attitude of democrats and republicans differ; did the attitude toward save sex change after an information campaign with respect to aids; and, is the attitude in the car-environment issue related to income or age?

Presentation of the Model

The PARELLA model can be characterized by four properties that will be discussed next: unidimensionality; single peaked item characteristic curves; local stochastic independence; and sample invariance of the item locations.

Unidimensionality

The PARELLA model assumes that the latent trait a researcher intends to measure is unidimensional. This implies that the items that are used to operationalize this latent trait differ only with respect to the level of the latent trait of which they are indicative. Furthermore, this implies that the only structural determinant of the item responses is a person's location on the latent trait, i.e., that there are no other person characteristics that have a structural influence on the responses.

The representation resulting from an analysis with the PARELLA model is unidimensional since both persons and items are represented on the same scale or dimension. The locations of the items constitute (the grid of) the measurement instrument for the assessment of the trait. The locations of persons constitute the measures obtained.

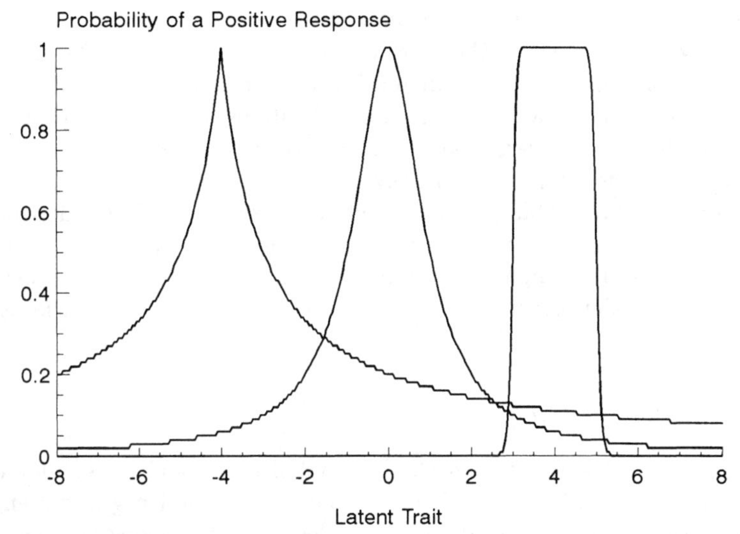

FIGURE 1. Item characteristic curves as defined by the PARELLA model for items with location and γ-parameters (from left to right) of $(-4, .5)$, $(0, 1)$, and $(4, 10)$.

Single-Peaked Item Characteristic Curves

In the PARELLA model the distribution of each item response is a function of the distance between person and item on the latent trait, and random characteristics of either the person or the item. The relative importance of these structural and random components is reflected by the parameter γ. The larger γ, the more sensitive is the probability of the response to the distance between person and item:

$$P(U_{ij} = 1 \mid \theta_j, \delta_i, \gamma) = P_{ij} = 1 - Q_{ij} = 1/(1 + |\theta_j - \delta_i|^{2\gamma}). \qquad (3)$$

In Fig. 1, the probability of a positive response in Eq. (3) (subsequently to be called item response function or IRF) is plotted as a function of θ for the following three $\delta - \gamma$-combinations: $(-4, 0.5)$, $(0, 1)$, and $(4, 10)$. It can be seen that the probability of a positive response is single peaked. It decreases in the distance between person and item location, which is as it should be in a model where proximity relations are the main determinant of an item response. Note, furthermore, that the probability of a positive response equals one if $\theta = \delta$.

Figure 1 also illustrates the function of the γ-parameter. From the IRF for $\gamma = 10$, it can be seen that a person's response is completely determined by the distance between the person and the item: If this distance is smaller than one, a person will respond 1; if this distance is larger than one, a person will respond 0. For γ-parameter values larger than 10, the PARELLA model is virtually identical to Coombs' deterministic parallelogram model.

The IRF's for $\gamma = 1$ and $\gamma = .5$ show that the item response is no longer exclusively determined by the distance between person and item. There is a non-ignorable probability (increasing with decreasing γ) that persons located at a relatively large distance from the items will response positively. Similarly, there is a non-ignorable probability that persons located closely to an item will *not* respond positively.

For $\gamma = 0$, the probability of a positive response in Eq. (3) is independent of the distance between person and item. This property implies that the item responses are completely random, and not (to at least some extent) determined by the locations of the persons and the items on the latent trait.

Local Stochastic Independence

The data typically analyzed with the PARELLA model consist for each person of a vector of 1's and 0's indicating positive and negative item responses, respectively. These data can be seen as realizations of a series of (differently distributed) Bernoulli variables. For a valid analysis of such data sets, the dependence structure between the random variables has to be taken into consideration. This can be done in two ways: Either (1) the multivariate distribution of the variables has to be specified completely; or (2) a random effects model has to be used. The latter option is followed, for example, in the logistic item response models and the PARELLA model. The rationale behind a random effects model is that the dependence between the response variables can be explained by a person-specific random component, i.e., by the location of the person on the latent trait. Within the context of item response models this principle is often identified using the label of "local stochastic independence." Local stochastic independence implies that, conditionally on the person location, the item responses are independent:

$$P(\underline{U}_j = \underline{u}_j \mid \theta_j, \delta, \gamma) = P(\underline{U}_j \mid \theta_j) = \prod_{i=1}^{n} P_{ij}^{U_{ij}} Q_{ij}^{(1-U_{ij})}, \tag{4}$$

where $\underline{U}_j$ denotes the response vector of person j.

Sample Invariance of the Item Locations

The PARELLA model contains two types of parameters: The item locations or fixed effects as well as the person locations or random effects. The model does not include an interaction between the fixed and the random effects. This has two implications that are relevant when the aim is to obtain measurements of some latent trait:

a. The absence of interaction implies that if the PARELLA model gives an adequate description of the response process, the item locations are the same for each person. In item response theory, this property is often called sample item invariance. As a consequence of this property, the estimators of the item locations do not have any (asymptotic) bias due to the sample of persons used.

b. Absence of interaction also implies that the person locations are the same for any (sub)set of items. This implies that any (sub)set of items can be used to measure a person without any bias due to the items used, provided the PARELLA model gives an adequate description of the response process for each item.

Other Parallelogram Models or Generalizations

The PARELLA model is not the only stochastic parallelogram model. Other formulations for the probability of a positive item response conditional on the locations of the person and the item have appeared in the literature. Verhelst and Verstralen (1993) and Andrich (this volume) suggests to use

$$P(U_{ij} = 1 \mid \theta_j, \delta_i, \gamma) = \exp(\theta_j - \delta_i + \gamma)/[1 + \exp(\theta_j - \delta_i + \gamma) + \exp(2(\theta_j - \delta_i))]. \tag{5}$$

In Fig. 2, the probability specified in Eq. (5) is plotted as a function of θ for the following three $\delta - \gamma$-combinations: $(-4, .5)$, $(0, 1)$, and $(4, 2)$. It can be seen that the probability of a positive response is single peaked. It decreases in the distance between person and item location, which is as it should be in a model where proximity relations are the main determinant of an item response. There are two differences between the PARELLA model and the model in Eq. (5). In the latter, the probability of a positive response is smaller than 1 for $\theta = \delta$. Furthermore, the parameter γ has a different function. In the PARELLA model the parameter represents the relative importance of the distance between person and item. As can be seen in Fig. 2, the γ-parameter in Eq. (5) jointly influences the threshold and the maximum of the item characteristic curve; i.e., the larger γ, the wider the threshold and the larger the probability of a positive response.

Still other formulations of single peaked item characteristic curves can be found in Andrich (1988), Munich and Molenaar (1990), and DeSarbo and Hoffman (1986). Others are easily constructed.

Both the PARELLA model and the model in Eq. (5) contain a location parameter for each person and item as well as a γ-parameter. One way to generalize these models would be to make the γ-parameter item specific. However, Verhelst and Verstralen (1993) show for Eq. (5) that, owing to a high correlation between the item specific γ and δ parameters, the model is not identified. For the PARELLA model no results with respect to this kind of generalizations are available yet.

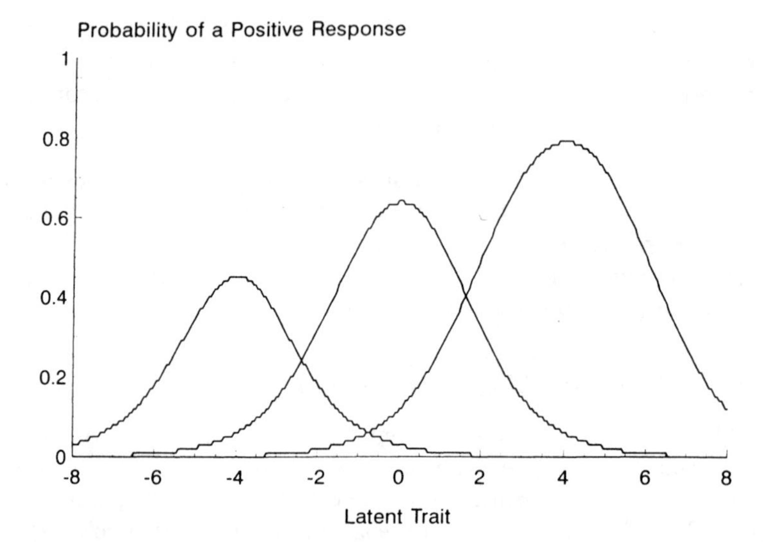

FIGURE 2. Item characteristic curves as defined by Eq. (5) for items with location and γ-parameters (from left to right) of $(-4, .5)$, $(0, 1)$, and (4.2).

Parameter Estimation

In this section, procedures for parameter estimation in the PARELLA model will be given. First, the problem of estimating the item parameters will be addressed, and, next, attention will be paid to the problem of estimating the person locations in the model.

Estimation of Item Parameters

Within item response models the basic elements in a sample are given by the response vectors $\underline{U}$ (Cressie and Holland, 1983). The marginal distribution of $\underline{U}$ can be written as follows:

$$P(\underline{U} = \underline{u}) = \int_\theta P(\underline{U} \mid \theta)\, dG(\theta), \tag{6}$$

where $g(\theta)$ denotes the density function of θ. Using the property that a continuous density function can be fairly well approximated by a step function with a finite number of steps, Eq. (6) can be rewritten as

$$P(\underline{U} = \underline{u}) = \sum_{q=1}^{Q} P(\underline{U} \mid B_q)\pi_q, \tag{7}$$

where the location and the heights of the steps (weights) are denoted by $\underline{B}$ and $\underline{\pi}$, respectively, both with index $q = 1, \ldots, Q$. An advantage of using the representation in Eq. (7) over the one in Eq. (6) is that it enables the estimation of the density function of θ without the necessity to make assumptions with respect to its shape. In other words, a nonparametric estimate of $g(\theta)$ will be obtained (Lindsay, 1983).

The likelihood function of the parameters $(\underline{\delta}, \gamma, \underline{\pi})$ conditional upon the sample of response vectors $\underline{S}$ and the step locations $\underline{B}$ is given by

$$\log L(\underline{\delta}, \gamma, \underline{\pi} \mid \underline{S}, \underline{B}) = \sum_{j=1}^{N} \log P(\underline{U}_j = \underline{u}_j)$$

$$= \sum_{j=1}^{N} \log \sum_{q=1}^{Q} P(\underline{U}_j \mid B_q)\pi_q. \tag{8}$$

Note that the locations of the steps, $\underline{B}$, do not appear among the parameters. In the software for the PARELLA model, these locations are not estimated but chosen such that the weights for the first and the last location are in the interval $\langle 0.005, 0.025 \rangle$ with the other locations equally spaced in between (Hoijtink, 1990; Hoijtink et al., 1994). In this way, at least 95% of the density function of θ is located between the first and the last location. Note further that the parameters as they appear in Eq. (8) are only identified under the restrictions that

$$\sum_{i=1}^{n} \delta_i = 0$$

and

$$\sum_{q=1}^{Q} \pi_q = 1. \tag{9}$$

If the data contain more than one sample (e.g., men and women, or pre- and post-measures), a sample structure, with samples indexed by $g = 1, \ldots, G$, can be incorporated in the model. The sum over samples of Eq. (8) under the restriction of equal item locations and equal γ parameters across samples but with sample-specific density functions of the person parameter, yields

$$\log L(\underline{\delta}, \gamma, \underline{\pi}^1, \ldots, \underline{\pi}^G \mid \underline{S}, \underline{B}) = \sum_{g=1}^{G} \left[\sum_{j=1}^{N^g} \log \sum_{q=1}^{Q} P(\underline{U}_j \mid B_q)\pi_q^g \right], \tag{10}$$

with restrictions

$$\sum_{i=1}^{n} \delta_i = 0$$

and

$$\sum_{q=1}^{Q} \pi_q^g = 1, \quad \text{for } g = 1, \ldots, G, \tag{11}$$

where N^g is the number of persons in sample g.

The estimation procedure is an application of the Expected Conditional Maximum-Likelihood (ECM) algorithm (Meng and Rubin, 1993). In an iterative sequence across three stages, subsequently the item locations, the density function of the person locations (for one or more samples), and the parameter γ are updated. Within each stage, the EM algorithm (Dempster et al., 1977) is used to update the parameters of interest.

In the M-step the values of the parameters that maximize the expected value of what Dempster et al. call the "complete data likelihood" (see below) have to be estimated. This is done conditionally upon the current estimates of the marginal posterior density function of the "missing data" (person location) for each person:

$$\pi(B_q \mid \underline{U}_j, \underline{\delta}, \gamma, \underline{\pi}^g) = \pi_{qj}^g = P(\underline{U}_j \mid B_q, \underline{\delta}, \gamma)\pi_q^g \Big/ \sum_{q=1}^{Q} P(\underline{U}_j \mid B_q, \underline{\delta}, \gamma)\pi_q^g. \tag{12}$$

Let $\{\pi_{qj}^g\}$ be the set of probabilities in Eq. (12) for $j = 1, \ldots, N$, then the expected value of the complete data likelihood is given by

$$E[\log L \mid \{\pi_{qj}^g\}] = \sum_{q=1}^{Q} \sum_{g=1}^{G} \sum_{j=1}^{N^g} \pi_{qj}^g \log[P(\underline{U}_j \mid B_q, \underline{\delta}, \gamma)]. \tag{13}$$

Within each stage, the EM-algorithm iterates between the E-step and the M-step until the estimates of the current parameters have converged. Across all three stages, the ECM-algorithm iterates until all parameter estimates have converged. Standard errors of estimation are obtained by inversion of the Hessian matrix of the likelihood functions. For further details, the reader is referred to Hoijtink and Molenaar (1992) and Hoijtink et al., (1994).

A number of simulation studies were executed to determine the accuracy of the estimators of the item locations, the γ parameter, the nonparametric estimate of $g(\theta)$, and the standard errors for each of these estimators. There was strong evidence that all parameter estimators are unbiased and consistent. Furthermore, the simulation results indicated that the standard errors of the estimators were reasonably accurate. For some simulation results, see Hoijtink (1990, 1991a).

Estimation of Person Locations

Once the item locations, the γ parameter, and the density function of the person locations for one or more samples have been estimated, an estimate of each person's location and associated standard error of estimation can be obtained. The expected a posterior estimator (EAP) (Bock and Aitkin, 1981) is the mode of the a posteriori density function of the person location conditional on the response vector $\underline{U}$:

$$EAP = \sum_{q=1}^{Q} B_q P(B_q \mid \underline{U}). \tag{14}$$

The error variance of the EAP estimate is

$$\sigma^2(EAP) = \sum_{q=1}^{Q} (B_q - EAP)^2 P(B_q \mid \underline{U}), \tag{15}$$

where, from Bayes theorem, it follows that

$$P(B_q \mid \underline{U}) = P(\underline{U} \mid B_q, \underline{\delta}, \gamma)\pi_q \Big/ \sum_{q=1}^{Q} P(\underline{U} \mid B_q, \underline{\delta}, \gamma)\pi_q. \tag{16}$$

Software for the PARELLA Model

The PARELLA software is available from ProGAMMA, P.O. Box 841, 9700 AV Groningen, The Netherlands. The software has implemented the estimation procedures described above as well as the goodness-of-fit tests that will be described in the next section. Furthermore, it contains a number of diagnostic matrices (correlation matrix, conditional adjacency matrix) and goodness-of-fit tests that were developed and studied by Post (1992) for use with nonparametric parallelogram models, i.e., models that do not have a parametric specification of the item response function. The software goes with a comprehensive manual (Hoijtink et al., 1994) describing the theory underlying both the parametric and the nonparametric parallelogram models is available. The manual describes the use of the software and the interpretation of the output. The program can handle 10,000 persons, 55 items, and 10 samples at the same time. It runs on PC's and compatibles and has a user-friendly interface to assist with the input of the data and the selection of the output options.

Goodness of Fit

As noted earlier, the PARELLA model has the four important properties of unidimensionality, single peaked item response functions, local stochastic independence, and sample invariance of item locations. In this section goodness-of-fit tests will be discussed that address the sample invariance of item locations and the single peakedness of the item response functions.

Tests for Sample Invariance of the Item Locations

Two procedures for testing the invariance of the item locations and γ are across samples $g = 1, \ldots, G$ are presented. In the first procedure the hypothesis of invariance is tested simultaneously for all parameters involved. Then, for diagnostic purposes, a separate test for each individual parameter is discussed.

The simultaneous hypotheses of sample invariance of the item and γ parameters is formulated as

$$H_0: \underline{\delta}^1 = \cdots = \underline{\delta}^G$$

and

$$H_0: \gamma^1 = \cdots = \gamma^G. \tag{17}$$

These hypotheses can be tested by a likelihood-ratio statistic consisting of the product of the unconstrained likelihood functions in Eq. (8) across the samples (L1) over this product with item and γ parameters are constrained to be equal across the samples (L2):

$$\text{LR} = -2 \log(\text{L2}/\text{L1}). \tag{18}$$

Under the hypotheses in Eq. (17), LR is asymptotically chi-squared distributed with $(G-1)n$ degrees of freedom (Hoijtink and Molenaar, 1992).

If LR is significant, the hypotheses of sample invariant item and γ parameters have to be rejected. The next step is to determine which parameter is sample dependent and to remove that item from the item set. The individual hypotheses of sample invariant locations are formulated as

$$H_0: \delta_i^1 = \cdots = \delta_i^G, \tag{19}$$

where i runs from 1 to n across the tests. In addition, the hypothesis of invariant γ parameters,

$$H_0: \gamma^1 = \cdots = \gamma^G, \tag{20}$$

has to be tested separately.

These hypotheses of invariant locations can be tested using the following Wald statistics:

$$\chi_i = \sum_{g=1}^{G} [(\hat{\delta}_i^g - \bar{\delta})^2 / (\hat{\sigma}_i^g)^2], \tag{21}$$

where $\hat{\delta}_i^g$, and $\hat{\sigma}_i^g$ denote the item parameter estimate in sample g and its standard error, respectively, and

$$\bar{\delta} = \sum_{g=1}^{G} (\hat{\delta}_i^g / (\hat{\sigma}_i^g)^2) / \sum_{g=1}^{G} (1/(\hat{\sigma}_i^g)^2). \tag{22}$$

The Wald statistic for the γ parameter is obtained substituting estimates for these parameter and its standard error.

Under the null hypothesis each Wald statistic is asymptotically chi-square distributed with $G-1$ degrees of freedom (Hoijtink and Molenaar, 1992). Since the Wald statistics are correlated, usually only the item with the largest value for the statistic is removed from the item set, after which the procedure is repeated for the reduced item set.

Test for Singled Peakedness of the Item Response Function

The adequacy of the item response function in the PARELLA model for the data at hand, can be tested for each item through a comparison of the latter with the empirical function. This is done with the ICC statistic defined below. The null distribution of the statistic is unknown but some relevant percentiles were determined via a simulation study (95th = .65, 99th = .78) (Hoijtink, Molenaar, and Post, 1994).

The ICC statistic is defined as

$$ICC_i = \left[\sum_{q=1}^{Q} |\hat{N}_{qi} - N_{qi}|\right] / \sqrt{N}, \tag{23}$$

for $i = 1, \ldots, n$, where

$$\hat{N}_{qi} = \sum_{j=1}^{N} U_{ij} P(B_q \mid \underline{U}_j), \quad \text{for } q = 1, \ldots, Q, \tag{24}$$

denotes the empirical number of persons at node q giving a positive response to item i estimated from the data, and,

$$N_{qi} = N \pi_q P_{ij}, \quad \text{for } q = 1, \ldots, Q, \tag{25}$$

is this number predicted by the PARELLA model.

If the differences in Eq. (23) are small, the PARELLA model provides an adequate description of the response process for the item at hand: the empirical choice proportions will be small at nodes located at a large distance from the item at hand, and large at nodes at a small distance.

Example

The data for this example were collected by Rappoport et al. (1986), and concern the degree of agreement with 12 political measures (see Table 1) by 697 party activists from Missouri in the United States. The original ratings of 1–5 (agree strongly to disagree strongly) were recoded to dichotomous ratings so that the data could be analyzed with the PARELLA model. In doing so, the ratings 1 and 2 were recorded as 1, whereas the ratings 3, 4, and 5 were recoded as 0. The sample consisted of the following two subsamples: Democrats (N = 317) and Republicans (N = 380).

The main question to be answered with the help of the PARELLA model is whether the 12 political measures were indicative of a latent trait ranging from a Democratic to Republican political attitude. This will only be the case if the proximity relations between the activists and the measures are primarily determined by the evaluation of the measures, that is, if being

TABLE 1. Political Measures.

Measure	Democrats			Republicans			All
	Location	Prop.	ICC	Location	Prop.	ICC	ICC
National health insurance	−2.0	0.45	0.90	−3.9	0.06	0.25	2.2
Affirmative actions program	−1.8	0.39	0.11	−1.8	0.17	0.39	0.5
Ratification of SALT II	−1.7	0.39	0.19	−3.6	0.05	0.33	1.9
Wage and price controls	−1.2	0.39	0.33	−1.4	0.17	0.36	1.3
U.S. military in Middle East	−0.5	0.48	0.94	1.4	0.67	0.20	2.1
Draft registration	0.0	0.70	0.50	1.3	0.70	0.18	1.8
Increase defense spending	0.6	0.51	0.70	0.9	0.90	0.06	1.5
Spending cuts/balancing budget	1.1	0.38	0.50	1.2	0.80	0.23	0.6
Nuclear power	1.2	0.35	0.75	1.3	0.70	0.39	1.3
Reduce inflation	1.3	0.34	0.49	1.5	0.61	0.14	1.2
Amendment banning abortion	1.3	0.35	0.53	1.7	0.52	0.78	1.7
Deregulation of oil and gas	1.6	0.28	0.71	1.4	0.67	0.21	0.7
γ parameter	0.7			1.0			
Mean of $g(\theta)$	−0.53			0.81			
Variance of $g(\theta)$	2.61			0.55			

a Democrat (Republican) tends to coincide with agreement of the political measures located on the Democratic (Republican) end of the attitude dimension.

In Table 1, the results of separate and joint analyses of the Democratic and Republican samples are presented. It is clear from the results for the test of the single peakedness of the item response function (column ICC) that within each subsample proximity relations between activists and measure are the main determinant of the evaluations of the measures since most ICC values are smaller than the critical value associated with the 99th percentile of the null distribution (0.78). However, the last column of

TABLE 2. Nonparametric Estimate of $g(\theta)$.

Step Location	Democrat Weight	Republican Weight
−3.75	0.04	0.00
−2.75	0.12	0.01
−1.75	0.14	0.00
−0.75	0.05	0.00
0.25	0.60	0.34
1.25	0.00	0.61
2.25	0.00	0.01
3.25	0.02	0.00
4.25	0.03	0.03

the table shows that the single peakedness assumption does not hold for the complete sample because most ICC values were larger than 0.78.

Such a result usually implies that the locations of the measures differ between the two samples, i.e., if both Democrats and Republicans had to order the measures from "Very Democratic" to "Very Republican" each group would give a different order. Comparing the estimates of the locations of the political measures between Democrats and Republicans (see Table 1), this result is indeed found. To be sure that the differences are not due to sample fluctuations, the likelihood ratio test for sample invariance was computed. The result leaves no room for doubt (LR = 214, DF = 12, $p =$ 0.00). It is not uncommon to find that a limited number of items/measures causes this problem. However, even after removal of 6 of the 12 measures from the analysis, the results did not improve.

Since the Democrats and the Republicans used different definitions for the political attitude dimension, their locations cannot be compared. Nevertheless, a number of interesting observations can be made. For example, in Table 1 it can be seen that the average political attitude of the Democrats equaled −0.53. This average is located toward a number of political measures of a social nature. The average of the Republicans equaled .81. This average is towards a number of political measures of a more economic nature. Thus, although these numbers cannot directly be compared, they at least suggest that the Democrats indeed were more Democratic than the Republicans.

For the variances of the distribution of the political attitudes within each sample, we found the value 2.61 for the Democrats, and .55 for the Republicans. This result implies that the Republicans constitute a much more homogeneous group with respect to the political attitude than the Democrats. In Table 2, estimates of the full density functions of the political attitudes are presented for both the Democrats and the Republicans. As can be seen, the inhomogeneity of the Democrats is mainly caused by a group of activists located around 3.75. This value actually represents a very undemocratic location. From the first column in Table 1, it can be seen that this group is located much closer to the economic measures than to the more social measures.

Discussion

Occasionally, it is found that the parametrization chosen for the PARELLA model is not flexible enough to model item response. For such cases the use of a nonparametric parallelogram model (Post, 1992; Van Schuur, 1989) is recommended. This model only assumes single peakedness of the item response function.

As a nonparametric parallelogram model only orders the persons and items along the latent trait, and does not offer a representation at interval level, they may fail to meet the demands of the researcher interested in applying parallelogram models. Currently parametrizations more flexible than Eqs. (3) and (5) are under investigation. Some of these parameterizations contain more parameters than just the person and item locations and the γ parameter.

References

Andrich, D. (1988). The application of an unfolding model of the PIRT type to the measurement of attitude. *Applied Psychological Measurement* **12**, 33–51.

Bock, R.D. and Aitkin, M. (1981). Marginal maximum likelihood estimation of item parameters: Application of an EM-algorithm. *Psychometrika* **46**, 443–459.

Coombs, C.H. (1964). *A Theory of Data.* Ann Arbor: Mathesis Press.

Cressie, N. and Holland, P.W. (1983). Characterizing the manifest probabilities of latent trait models. *Psychometrika* **48**, 129–141.

Dempster, A.P., Laird, N.M., and Rubin, D.B. (1977). Maximum likelihood estimation from incomplete data via the EM algorithm. *Journal of the Royal Statistical Society, Series B* **39**, 1–38.

DeSarbo, W.S. and Hoffman, D.L. (1986). Simple and weighted unfolding threshold models for the spatial representation of binary choice data. *Applied Psychological Measurement* **10**, 247–264.

Guttman, L. (1950). The basis for scalogram analysis. In S.A. Stouffer et al. (eds.), *Measurement and Prediction* (pp. 60–90). New York: Wiley.

Hambleton, R.K. and Swaminathan, H. (1985). *Item Response Theory. Principles and Applications.* Boston: Kluwer-Nijhoff Publishing.

Hoijtink, H. (1990). A latent trait model for dichotomous choice data. *Psychometrika* **55**, 641–656.

Hoijtink, H. (1991a). *PARELLA: Measurement of Latent Traits by Proximity Items.* Leiden: DSWO-Press.

Hoijtink, H. (1991b). The measurement of latent traits by proximity items. *Applied Psychological Measurement* **15**, 153–169.

Hoijtink, H. and Molenaar, I.W. (1992). Testing for DIF in a model with single peaked item characteristic curves: The PARELLA model. *Psychometrika* **57**, 383–397.

Hoijtink, H., Molenaar, I.W., and Post, W.J. (1994). *PARELLA User's Manual.* Groningen, The Netherlands: iecProGAMMA.

Lindsay, B.G. (1983). The geometry of mixture likelihoods a general theory. *The Annals of Statistics* **11**, 86–94.

Meng, X. and Rubin, D.B. (1993). Maximum likelihood via the ECM algorithm: A general framework. *Biometrika* **80**, 267–279.

Munich, A. and Molenaar, I.W. (1990). *A New Approach for Probabilistic Scaling* (Heymans Bulletin HB-90-999-EX). Groningen: Psychologische Instituten, Rijksuniversiteit.

Post, W.J. (1992). *Nonparametric Unfolding Models: A Latent Structure Approach.* Leiden: DSWO-Press.

Rappoport, R.B., Abramowitz, A.I., and McGlennon, J. (1986). *The Life of the Parties.* Lexington: The Kentucky University Press.

van Schuur, W.H. (1989). Unfolding the German political parties. In G. de Soete, H. Feger, and K.C. Klauer (eds.), *New Developments in Psychological Choice Modeling.* Amsterdam: North-Holland.

Verhelst, N.D. and Verstralen, H.H.F.M. (1993). A stochastic unfolding model derived from the partial credit model. *Kwantitatieve Methoden* **42**, 73–92.

Part VI. Models with Special Assumptions About the Response Process

The four models presented in this section do not fit into the other five sections and are difficult to describe as a group. At the same time, the four models have features that make them important to psychometricians in the analysis of special types of data.

First, situations often arise in practice where the IRT model of choice is to be applied to several groups. A good example is the identification of differential item functioning (DIF). The groups might consist of (1) males and females; (2) Whites, Blacks, and Hispanics; or (3) examinees from multiple nations. These comparative IRT analyses have become about as common as classical item analyses in testing agencies. Another common situation involving multiple groups arises when tests are being linked or equated to a common scale. Many more popular IRT applications involving multiple groups can be identified. It is common to analyze the results for each group separately and then link them in some way (e.g., using anchor items) for the purposes of making comparisons at the item level, ability level, or both. The model developed by Bock and Zimowski (Chap. 25) unifies many of the applications of IRT involving multiple groups and even the analysis of data when the group becomes the unit of analysis (e.g., as in program evaluation). Some of the most common applications of IRT become special cases of the multiple group IRT model. A unified treatment is valuable in its own right but may help too in formulating solutions to new IRT applications.

Rost's logistic mixture models introduced in Chap. 26 have some similar properties to the unified treatment of multiple group models of Bock and Zimowski. The main differences are that Rost's models are (1) a *mixture* of an IRT model and a latent class model (to handle multiple groups) and, to data, (2) less general (Rost has limited his work to the Rasch model only though he has considered the extension to polytomous response data). Related models by Gitomer and Yamamoto (1991) and Mislevy and Verhelst (1990) are not considered in this volume but would be excellent follow-up references.

Fundamental to every IRT model is the assumption of local independence. Unfortunately, this assumption is violated at least to some extent with many tests. For example, one violation occurs when a set of items in a test is organized around a common stimulus such as a graph or passage. In both examples, examinee responses to items may not be completely independent and this is a violation of the assumption of locally independence. It becomes a problem whenever one more ability is needed to explain test performance in excess of the abilities contained in the model of interest. Violations of the assumption of local independence complicate parameter estimation and may result in ability estimates of dubious value.

One solution to this problem is to develop IRT models which do not make the troublesome assumption. These are called locally dependent models by Jannarone (Chap. 27) and while not ready for day-to-day use, these new models do offer researchers some potential for solving a troublesome problem. More work along the same lines of Jannarone would certainly be welcome in the coming years.

One of the criticisms that has been leveled at dichotomously-scored multiple-choice items is that there is no provision for assessing partial knowledge. As both Bock, and Thissen and Steinberg have reported in their chapters, there is assumed to be partial knowledge contained in the wrong answers of multiple-choice items. Some incorrect answers reflect more partial knowledge than others and ability can be more accurately estimated if this information in partially correct answers is used. In Chap. 28, Hutchinson describes a family of models what he calls mismatch models for improving the estimation of examinee ability and gaining new information about the cognitive functioning of examinees on the test items. These models are new but deserve further exploration. Comparisons of Hutchinson's solution to the problem of assessing partial knowledge in multiple-choice items and the solutions offered in the polytomous IRT models earlier in this volume is a topic deserving of additional research.

References

Gitomer, D. and Yamamoto, (1991). Performance modeling that integrates latent trait and class theory. *Journal of Educational Statistics* **28**, 173–189.

Mislevy, R. and Verhelst, N. (1990). Modeling item responses when different subjects employ different solution strategies. *Psychometrika* **55**, 195–215.

Thissen, D. (1976). Information in wrong responses to the Raven progressive matrices. *Journal of Educational Measurement* **13**, 201–214.

25
Multiple Group IRT

R. Darrell Bock and Michele F. Zimowski

Introduction

The extension of item response theory to data from more than one group of persons offers a unified approach to such problems as *differential item functioning, item parameter drift, nonequivalent groups equating, vertical equating, two-stage testing*, and *matrix-sampled educational assessment.* The common element in these problems is the existence of persons from different populations responding to the same test or to tests containing common items. In differential item functioning, the populations typically correspond to sex or demographic groups; in item parameter drift, to annual cohorts of students; in vertical equating, to children grouped by age or grade; in nonequivalent groups equating, to normative samples from different places or times; in two-stage testing, to examinees classified by levels of performance on a pretest; and in matrix-sampled educational assessment, to students from different schools or programs administered matrix-sampled assessment instruments. In all these settings, the objective of the multiple-group analysis is to estimate jointly the item parameters and the latent distribution of a common attribute or ability of the persons in each of the populations.

In classical test theory it has long been known that the sample distribution of a fallible test score is not an unbiased estimator of the true-score distribution. For if the test score, $y = \theta + \varepsilon$, is assumed to be the sum of the true score, θ, distributed with mean μ and variance σ^2 in the population of persons, and an independent measurement error ε distributed with mean zero and variance σ_ε^2, then the mean of a sample of test scores is an unbiased estimator of μ, but the score variance estimates $\sigma^2 + \sigma_\varepsilon^2$. This fact complicates considerably the comparison of population distributions based on scores from tests with different measurement error variances, even when the tests are presumed to measure the same true score.

Andersen and Madsen (1977) were the first to show that IRT can provide direct estimation of parameters of the latent distribution without the intervening calculation of test scores. They simplified matters somewhat by assuming that the item parameters were already known from some previous large-sample calibration, but subsequent work by Sanathanan and Blumenthal (1978), de Leeuw and Verhelst (1986) and Lindsay et al. (1991) extended their results to simultaneous estimation of parameters of the items and the latent distribution, and to semi-parametric and latent-class representation of the latent distribution. All of this work was limited to the one-parameter logistic model and to one population, however, and is primarily of interest for the connections it reveals between IRT, log-linear analysis, and latent class estimation. The results are too restrictive for application to practical testing problems where items may differ in discriminating power, the effects of guessing must be accounted for, some exercises may have multiple response categories, and more than one population may be involved. A more general approach adaptable to these situations was foreshadowed in Mislevy's (1984) work on estimating latent distributions by the maximum marginal likelihood (MML) method (Bock and Aitkin, 1981; Bock and Lieberman, 1970). In this chapter, we discuss the extension of Mislevy's work to applications, such as those above, involving multiple populations.

Presentation of the Model

To be fully general, we consider data arising from person j in group k responding in category h of item i. We suppose there are g groups, N_k persons in group k, m_i response categories of item i, and a test composed of n items. A response to item i may therefore by coded as U_i, where U_i takes on any integral value 1 through m_i. Similarly, the pattern of response of person j to the n test items may be expressed as $U_j = [U_{1j}, U_{2j}, \ldots, U_{nj}]$.

We assume the existence of a twice-differentiable response function,

$$P_{ih}(\theta) = P_i(U_i = h \mid \theta), \tag{1}$$

common to all groups and persons, that describes the probability of a response in category h, given the value of a continuous and unbounded person-attribute, θ. We require the response categories to be mutually exclusive and exhaustive, so that

$$\sum_{h}^{m_i} P_{ih}(\theta) = 1.$$

We further assume conditional independence of the responses, so that the probability of pattern U_j, given θ, is

$$P(U_j \mid \theta) = \prod_{i}^{n} P_i(U_{ij} = h \mid \theta). \tag{2}$$

We also assume θ to have a continuous distribution with finite mean and variance in the population of persons corresponding to group k and write its probability density function as $g_k(\theta)$. The unconditional, or marginal, probability of pattern U_j in group k may therefore be expressed as, say,

$$\bar{P}_k(U_j) = \int_{-\infty}^{\infty} P(U_j \mid \theta) g_k(\theta) d\theta. \tag{3}$$

Following Bock (1989), we suppose that the response functions depend upon some unknown, fixed parameters, ζ, and that the population distribution functions depend on some other unknown, fixed parameters, η. In that case, Eq. (3) may be written more explicitly as

$$\bar{P}_k(U_j) = \int_{-\infty}^{\infty} P(U_j \mid \theta, \zeta) g(\theta \mid \eta_k) d\theta;$$

that is, we assume each of the response and distribution functions to be members of their respective parametric families. We address below the problem of how to estimate ζ and η simultaneously, given the observed item scores U_{kij}.

Other Representations of the Population Distributions

In educational, sociological, psychological, and medical applications of IRT, the presence of many independent sources of variation influencing the person attribute broadly justifies the assumption of normal distributions within groups. The most likely exceptions are (1) samples in which, unknown to the investigator, the respondents consist of a mixture of populations with different mean levels and (2) groups in which the respondents have been arbitrarily selected on some criterion correlated with their attribute value. Both of these exceptions, and many other situations leading to non-normal distributions of θ, are amenable to the following alternative representations treated in Mislevy (1984).

Resolution of Gaussian Components

A plausible model for distributions in mixed populations is a mixture of Gaussian components with common variance but different means and proportions. (The assumption of different variances leads to difficult estimation problems and is best avoided.) Day (1969) proposed a method of obtaining the maximum likelihood estimates of the variance, means, and proportions in manifest distributions. Mislevy (1984) subsequently adapted it to latent distributions.

Histogram

In educational testing one often encounters test data from groups of students who have been selected on complicated criteria based partly on previous measures of achievement. The effect of the selection process on the latent distribution may be too arbitrary or severe to allow parsimonious modeling. In that case, the only alternative may be a nonparametric representation of the latent density. A good choice is to estimate the density at a finite number of equally spaced points in an interval that includes almost all of the probability. If these estimates are constrained to sum to unity, they approximate the probability density in the form of a histogram.

Parameter Estimation

Fortunately, almost all practical applications of item response theory involve large samples of respondents from the population of interest. This broadly justifies maximum likelihood methods and related large-sample statistics when estimating item parameters and population distributions. Specifically, the maximum marginal likelihood (MML) method applies here.

The Likelihood Equations

When sample sizes are large in relation to the number of items, there are computational advantages in counting the occurrences of distinct response patterns in the data. Let r_{kj} be the number of occurrences of pattern j in group k, and let $s_k \leq \min(N_k, S)$, where $S = \prod_i^n m_i$, be the number of patterns with $r_{kj} > 0$. Assuming random sampling of independently responding persons, we have product-multinomial data of which the marginal likelihood is, say,

$$L_M(\zeta, \eta) = \prod_k^g \frac{N_k!}{\prod_j^{s_k} r_{kj}!} \prod_j^{s_k} [\bar{P}(U_{kj})]^{r_{kj}}.$$

The likelihood equations for the parameters of item i may be expressed as

$$\begin{aligned} \frac{\partial \log L_M}{\partial \zeta_i} &= \sum_k^g \sum_j^{s_k} \frac{r_{kj}}{\bar{P}_{kj}} \cdot \frac{\partial \bar{P}_{kj}}{\partial \zeta_i} \\ &= \sum_k^g \sum_j^{s_k} \frac{r_{kj}}{\bar{P}_{kj}} \int_{-\infty}^{\infty} \left(\frac{\partial \prod_h^{m_i} [P_{ih}(\theta)]^{u_{kijh}} / \partial \zeta_i}{\prod_h^{m_i} [P_{ih}(\theta)]^{u_{kijh}}} \right) L_{kj}(\theta) g_k(\theta) d\theta \\ &= 0, \end{aligned} \tag{4}$$

where

$$\bar{P}_{kj} = \bar{P}(U_{kj}),$$

$$u_{kijh} = \begin{cases} 1 & \text{if } U_{kij} = h \\ 0 & \text{otherwise} \end{cases},$$

and

$$L_{kj}(\theta) = P(U_{kj} \mid \theta) = \prod_{i}^{n} P_i(U_{kij} = h \mid \theta)$$

is a conditional likelihood, given θ.

Applying the differential identity

$$\frac{d\prod_h y_h^{a_h}}{\prod_h y_h^{a_h}} = \frac{1}{\prod_h y_h^{a_h}} \sum_h a_h \prod_{k \neq h} y_k dy_k = \sum_h \frac{a_h dy_h}{y_h}$$

to Eq. (4) gives

$$\sum_k^g \sum_j^{s_k} \frac{r_{kj}}{\bar{P}_{kj}} \int_{-\infty}^{\infty} \left(\sum_h^{m_i} \frac{u_{kijh} P_{ih}(\theta)}{P_{ih}(\theta)} \right) \frac{\partial P_{ih}(\theta)}{\partial \zeta_i} L_{kj}(\theta) g_k(\theta) d\theta = 0, \tag{5}$$

which must be solved under the restriction $\sum_h^{m_i} P_{ih}(\theta) = 1$.

The m-category logistic models (see Bock, this volume) give especially simple results in this context. For $m = 2$, for example, the restriction $P_{i2}(\theta) = 1 - P_{i1}(\theta)$ reduces Eq. (5) to

$$\sum_k^g \sum_j^s \frac{r_{kj}}{\bar{P}_{kj}} \int_{-\infty}^{\infty} [u_{kij1} - P_{i1}(\theta)] \frac{\partial z_i(\theta)}{\partial \begin{bmatrix} \alpha_i \\ \gamma_i \end{bmatrix}} L_{ki}(\theta) g_k(\theta) d\theta = \begin{bmatrix} 0 \\ 0 \end{bmatrix}, \tag{6}$$

where $z_i(\theta) = \alpha_i \theta + \gamma_i$ is the logit in θ, the item slope α_i, and the item intercept γ_i. Similar results for the logistic nominal categories model and ordered categories model may be deduced from derivatives given in Bock (1985).

The likelihood equations for the population parameters η_k are considerably simpler:

$$\frac{\partial \log L_M}{\partial \eta_k} = \sum_j^{s_k} \frac{r_{kj}}{\bar{P}_{kj}} \int_{-\infty}^{\infty} L_{kj}(\theta) \left(\frac{\partial g_k(\theta)}{\partial \eta_k} \right) d\theta = 0. \tag{7}$$

Suppose the distribution of θ for group k is normal with mean μ_k and variance σ_h^2. Then $g(\theta) = (1/\sqrt{2\pi}\sigma) \exp[-(\theta - \mu_k)^2/2\sigma^2]$ and

$$\frac{\partial \log L_M}{\partial \mu_k} = \sigma_k^{-2} \sum_j^{s_k} r_{kj} \int_{-\infty}^{\infty} (\theta - \mu_k) \frac{L_{kj}(\theta)}{\bar{P}_{kj}} g(\theta) d\theta = 0, \tag{8}$$

$$\frac{\partial \log L_M}{\partial \sigma_k^2} = -\frac{1}{2} \sum_j^{s_k} r_{kj} \int_{-\infty}^{\infty} [\sigma_k^2 - (\theta - \mu_k)^2] \frac{L_{kj}(\theta)}{\bar{P}_{kj}} g(\theta) d\theta = 0. \tag{9}$$

We recognize Eq. (8) as the sum of the posterior means (Bayes estimates) of θ in group k, given the response patterns U_{kj}, $j = 1, 2, \ldots, s_k$, minus the corresponding population mean. Thus, for provisional values of the item parameters, the likelihood equation for μ_k is, say,

$$\hat{\mu}_k = \frac{1}{N_k} \sum_j^{s_k} r_{kj} \bar{\theta}_{kj}, \tag{10}$$

where

$$\bar{\theta}_{kj} = \frac{1}{\bar{P}_{kj}} \int_{-\infty}^{\infty} \theta L_{kj}(\theta) g_k(\theta) d\theta$$

is the posterior mean of θ, given U_{kj}.

Similarly, making the substitution $\theta - \mu_k = (\theta - \bar{\theta}_{kj}) + (\bar{\theta}_{kj} - \mu_k)$, we see that Eq. (9) is N_k times the sample variance of the Bayes estimates of θ minus the population variance, plus the sum of the posterior variances of θ, given the observed patterns. Thus, the likelihood equation for σ^2 when the item parameters are known is

$$\hat{\sigma}^2 = \frac{1}{N_k} \sum_j^{s_k} r_{kj} [(\bar{\theta}_{kj} - \hat{\mu}_k)^2 + \sigma^2_{\theta|U_{kj}}], \tag{11}$$

where

$$\sigma^2_{\theta|U_{kj}} = \frac{1}{\bar{P}_{kj}} \int_{-\infty}^{\infty} (\theta - \bar{\theta}_{kj})^2 L_{kj}(\theta) g(\theta) d\theta$$

is the posterior variance of θ, given U_{kj}. These equations are in a form suitable for an EM solution (see Bock, 1989; Dempster et al., 1981).

In IRT applications, the integrals in Eqs. (5) and (7) do not have closed forms and must be evaluated numerically. Although Gauss–Hermite quadrature is the method of choice when the population distribution is normal, it does not generalize to other forms of distributions we will require. For general use, simple Newton–Cotes formulas involving equally-spaced ordinates are quite satisfactory, as demonstrated in the computing examples below.

Estimating θ

In IRT applications, the most prominent methods of estimating the person-attribute, θ, are maximum likelihood and Bayes. In multiple-group IRT, the Bayes estimator, which appears in Eq. (10), has the advantage of incorporating the information contained in the person's group assignment. Conveniently, it is also a quantity that is calculated in the course of estimating the item parameters by the MML method. The quadrature required to evaluate the definite integral poses no special problem, but the range and number of quadrature points must be sufficient to cover the population distributions of all groups. The square root of the corresponding posterior variance, which appears in Eq. (11), serves as the standard error of the estimate.

In some applications (achievement testing, for example), it may not be desirable to include information from group membership in the estimation of θ. In that case, the population density function in the Bayes estimator should be replaced by the sum of the group density functions normalized to unity.

Gaussian Resolution

In the present notation, the resulting likelihood equations at iteration t for the proportion and mean attributable to component ℓ, $\ell = 1, 2, \ldots, \mathcal{L}$, of the distribution in group k are

$$\hat{p}_{k\ell}^{(t+1)} = \frac{1}{N_k} \sum_{j}^{s_k} \frac{r_{kj}}{\bar{P}_{kj}} \int_{-\infty}^{\infty} L_{kj}(\theta) \hat{p}_{k\ell}^{(t)} g_{k\ell}(\theta) d\theta, \tag{12}$$

$$\hat{\mu}_{k\ell}^{(t+1)} = \frac{1}{N_k} \sum_{j}^{s_k} \frac{r_{kj}}{\bar{P}_{kj}} \int_{-\infty}^{\infty} \theta L_{kj}(\theta) \hat{p}_{k\ell}^{(t)} g_{k\ell}(\theta) d\theta, \tag{13}$$

where $g_{k\ell}(\theta) = (2\pi\sigma_k^2)^{-1/2} \exp[1 - (\theta - \hat{\mu}_{k\ell})^2 / 2\hat{\sigma}_k^2]$ and $L_{kj}(\theta)\hat{p}_{k\ell} g_{k\ell}(\theta)/\bar{P}_{kj}$ is the posterior probability that a person in group k with attribute value θ belongs to population component ℓ, given U_{kj}.

Similarly, for the common σ^2,

$$(\hat{\sigma}_k^2)^{(t+1)} = \frac{1}{N_k} \sum_{k}^{g} \sum_{j}^{s_k} \frac{r_{kj}}{\bar{P}_{kj}} \sum_{\ell}^{\mathcal{L}} (\theta - \hat{\mu}_{k\ell}^{(t)})^2 L_{kj}(\theta) \hat{p}_{k\ell}^{(t)} g_{k\ell}(\theta) d\theta. \tag{14}$$

These equations are in a form suitable for an EM solution starting from plausible provisional values $\hat{p}_{k\ell}^{(0)}$, $\hat{\mu}_{k\ell}^{(0)}$, and $(\hat{\sigma}_k^2)^{(0)}$. Typically, one starts with $\ell = 1$ and proceeds stepwise to higher numbers of components. The difference of marginal log likelihoods at each step provides a test of the hypothesis that no further components are required in group k. The difference in log likelihoods for group k is evaluated as

$$\chi_{ML}^2 = \sum_{j}^{s_k} r_{kj} \left(\log \bar{P}_{kj}^{(\ell+1)} / \log \bar{P}_{kj}^{(\ell)} \right), \tag{15}$$

where $\bar{P}_{kj}^{(\ell+1)}$ is the marginal probability of pattern j in group k after fitting the $\ell + 1$ component latent distribution, and $\bar{P}_{kj}^{(\ell)}$ is the similar probability for the ℓ component model. Under the null hypothesis, Eq. (15) is distributed in large samples as chi-square with *df* $= 2$. To be conservative, the $\ell + 1$ component should be added only if this statistic is clearly significant (say, 3 to 4 times its degrees of freedom).

Resolution of Gaussian components has interesting applications in behavioral and medical genetics, where it is used to detect major-gene effects on a quantitative trait in a background of polygenic variation (see Bock and Kolakowski, 1973; Dorus et al., 1983). It is also a tractable alternative to the computationally difficult Kiefer and Wolfowitz (1956) step-function representation of latent distributions, and it has the advantage of being analytic.

The Latent Histogram

Estimation of the latent distribution on a finite number of discrete points is especially convenient in the present context, because the density estimates are a by-product of the numerical integrations on equally-spaced ordinates employed in the MML estimation. That is, the estimated density for group k at point X_m is, say,

$$\hat{\phi}_{km} = \bar{N}_{km} \Big/ \sum_{q}^{Q} \bar{N}_{kq}, \tag{16}$$

where $\bar{N}_{kq} = \sum_{j}^{s_k} r_{kj} L_{kj}(X_q) g_k(X_q) / \bar{P}_{kj}$. These density estimates can be obtained jointly with the item parameter estimates provided the indeterminancy of location and scale is resolved by imposing on X_q the restrictions

$$\frac{1}{g} \sum_{k}^{g} \sum_{q}^{Q} X_q \hat{\phi}_{kq} = 0 \quad \text{and} \quad \frac{1}{g} \sum_{k}^{g} \sum_{q}^{Q} X_q^2 \hat{\phi}_{kq} = 1.$$

[See Mislevy (1984).] These point estimates of density may be cumulated to approximate the distribution function. Optimal kernel estimation (Gasser et al., 1985) may then be used to interpolate for specified percentiles of the latent distribution.

Example

The purpose of educational assessment is to evaluate the effectiveness of educational institutions or programs by directly testing learning outcomes. Inasmuch as only the performance of the students in aggregate is in question, there is no technical necessity of computing or reporting scores of individual students, except perhaps as a source of motivation (see Bock and Zimowski, 1989). Lord and Novick (1968, pp. 255–258) have shown that, for this type of testing, the most efficient strategy for minimizing measurement error at the group level is to sample both students and items and to present only *one* item to each student. In statistical terminology, this procedure is an example of *matrix sampling*: the students correspond to the rows of a matrix and the items correspond to the columns. If multiple content domains are measured simultaneously by presenting one item from each domain to each student, the procedure is called *multiple matrix sampling.* The original conception was that the results of a matrix sampled assessment would be reported at the school or higher level of aggregation simply as the percent of correct responses among students presented items from a given domain. Standard errors of these statistics under matrix sampling are available for that purpose (Lord and Novick, 1968; Sirotnik and Wellington, 1977).

An IRT treatment of such data is also possible, however, even though, with each student responding to only one item in each domain, matrix sampling data would not seem suitable for conventional IRT analysis. (At least two items per respondent are required for nondegenerate likelihoods of the item or person parameters.) Bock and Mislevy (1981) proposed a group-level IRT analysis of multiple matrix sampling data that retains most of the benefits of the person-level analysis. They developed the group-level model that the California Assessment Program applied successfully to binary scored multiple-choice items and multiple-category ratings of exercises in written expression. Briefly, the statistical basis of this model, as described in Mislevy (1983), is as follows.

The groups to which the model applies are students at specified grade levels of the schools in which the effectiveness of instruction is periodically evaluated. The probability that a randomly selected student j in a given grade will respond correctly to item i of a given content domain is assumed to be a function of a school parameter ν, and one or more item parameters ζ. Writing this probability for school k and item i as

$$P_{ki} = P(U_{kij} = 1 \mid \nu_k, \zeta_i),$$

and assuming that the students respond independently, we have for the probability that r_{ki} of the N_{ki} students presented item i will respond correctly:

$$P(N_{ki}, r_{ki}) = \frac{N_{ki}!}{r_{ki}!(N_{ki} - r_{ki})!} P_{ki}^{r_{ki}} (1 - P_{ki})^{N_{ki} - r_{ki}}. \tag{17}$$

Then on the condition that each student is presented only one item from the domain, the likelihood of ν and ζ, given responses to n items in N schools, is

$$L(\nu, \zeta) = \prod_k^N \prod_i^n P(N_{ki}, r_{ki}). \tag{18}$$

Assuming that a good-fitting and computationally tractable group-level response function can be found, the likelihood equations derived from Eq. (18) can be solved by standard methods for product-binomial data on the assumption that ν is either a fixed effect or a random effect. Solutions for the fixed-effect case have been given by Kolakowski and Bock (1982) and Reiser (1983). In the random-effects case, the maximum marginal likelihood method of Bock and Aitkin (1981) applies if Eq. (17) is substituted for the likelihood for person-level data on the assumption of conditional independence.

MML analysis is attractive because the substitution $N_{ki} = 1$ and $r_{ki} = U_{kii}$ in Eq. (17) specializes the computing algorithm to the person-level model for binary-scored items. It also is more stable numerically than the fixed-effects analysis when N_{ki} (the number of students in school k presented item i) is small.

Concerning the crucial question of the choice of group-level response function, there is good reason to assume, as a working hypothesis testable in the data, the normal ogive model or its logistic approximation. For if the normal-ogive model applies at the student level, and the student proficiencies within schools are distributed $N(\nu_k, \sigma^2)$—where ν_k is the school mean and σ^2 is homogeneous among schools—then the response process for item i within schools, $y = \theta + \varepsilon_i$, will be normal with mean ν_k and variance $\sigma^2 + \alpha_i^{-1}$, where α_i is the item slope. In that case, the proportion of students responding correctly to item i in school k will be

$$P_{ki} = \Phi\left(\frac{\nu_k - \beta_i}{\sqrt{\sigma^2 + \alpha_i^{-1}}}\right),$$

where Φ is the standard normal distribution function and β_i is the item threshold. This line of reasoning broadly justifies the use of the conventional person-level item-response models at the group level, and it extends as well to the model for guessing effects (see Mislevy, 1984).

The validity of the model is easy to check because, with different students presented each item, the frequencies of correct response are strictly independent and

$$\chi_k^2 = \sum_i^n \frac{(r_{ki} - N_k P_{ki})^2}{N_k P_{ki}(1 - P_{ki})} \tag{19}$$

is distributed as χ^2 on n degrees of freedom. If Eq. (19) is generally nonsignificant for most schools in the sample, there is no evidence for failure of the model. For the generally easy items of the California assessment, Bock and Mislevy (1981) found uniformly good fit of the two-parameter logistic model.

The group-level model extends readily to multiple-category data and is especially valuable in the analysis and scoring of responses to essay questions. The California Direct Writing Assessment, for example, required students to write on one matrix-sampled essay topic in a 45-minute period. The essays were graded by trained readers on a six-category scale for each of three aspects of writing proficiency. Although these ratings did not permit IRT analysis at the student level, the group-level treatment was straightforward and greatly facilitated annual refreshing of the essay topics by nonequivalent groups equating.

The example is based on data from the California Direct Writing Assessment. Eighth-grade students in a sample of 20 public schools wrote a

40-minute essay in response to a randomly assigned prompt for a particular type of writing. Each type of writing was represented by ten different prompts.

Each essay was scored on six-point scales of "Rhetorical Effectiveness" and "Conventions of Written English." The data in Table 1 summarize the scores of the former for twelveth grade students in a random sample of 20 California schools in response to ten prompts of a type of writing called "Autobiographical Incident." Because eight different types of writing were assessed, making a total of eighty distinct prompts, the data are sparse, even in large schools, as is evident in the table. Nevertheless, they are sufficient to estimate item parameters and school-level scores by the graded model or the generalized partial credit model (see Muraki, this volume).

Table 2 shows the MML estimates of the item slope and threshold parameters of the generalized rating scale model. The category parameters are shown in Table 3. A normal latent distribution with mean 0 and variance 1 was assumed in the estimation. As a consequence of the small number of schools and the few students per school responding to these prompts, the standard errors of the item parameters are relatively large.

School scale scores of the California Direct Writing Assessment were scaled to a mean of 250 and standard deviation of 50 in the first year of the program. The scale for subsequent years, with 60 percent replacement of prompts each year, was determined by nonequivalent groups equating. Table 4 represents first year maximum likelihood estimation of scale scores computed from the estimated parameters in Tables 2 and 3. The sparse data again result in relatively large standard errors. Maximum likelihood rather than Bayes estimation is necessary in this context to avoid regressions to the mean proportional to the number of students responding per school.

Discussion

With the exception of the group-level model, applications of multiple-group IRT in large-scale testing programs require substantial computing resources. They are quite amenable, however to 486 or Pentium micro computers with 8 MB of RAM and a large hard disk, and to RISC and SPARC workstations.

With the exception of the resolution of latent distributions into Gaussian components, the multiple-group procedures are implemented on these platforms in the case of binary scored items in the BILOG-MG program of Zimowski et al. (1996). Incorporation of the Gaussian resolution is in progress for the BILOG program (Mislevy and Bock, 1996) and the BILOG-MG program. Implementation of multiple-group procedures for multiple-category ratings is in progress for the PARSCALE program of Muraki and Bock (1991). The group-level model above is implemented in the BILOG, BILOG-MG, and PARSCALE programs.

TABLE 1. School Level Data from the California Direct Writing Assessment: Six-Category Ratings of Ten Essay Prompts.

School	Prompt	Categories	Prompt	Categories
1 178	1	0 1 0 1 1 0	6	0 0 1 1 0 0
	2	0 0 0 2 0 0	7	0 0 0 0 0 0
	3	0 1 0 0 1 0	8	0 0 1 2 0 0
	4	0 0 1 1 1 0	9	0 0 1 2 0 0
	5	0 1 0 1 0 0	10	0 0 0 2 0 0
2 206	1	0 0 1 2 0 0	6	0 0 1 1 0 0
	2	0 1 0 0 2 0	7	0 0 0 1 1 0
	3	0 0 1 1 1 0	8	0 0 0 1 2 0
	4	0 1 0 1 1 0	9	0 0 0 1 1 1
	5	0 0 1 0 1 0	10	0 0 0 3 0 0
3 209	1	1 0 0 0 1 0	6	0 0 3 0 0 0
	2	0 0 0 1 1 0	7	0 1 1 0 0 0
	3	0 0 1 2 0 0	8	0 0 1 2 0 0
	4	0 0 0 1 2 0	9	0 0 1 0 1 0
	5	0 0 0 2 0 0	10	0 0 1 1 1 0
4 182	1	0 0 1 1 1 0	6	0 0 1 0 2 0
	2	0 0 1 0 1 0	7	0 0 0 1 1 0
	3	0 0 1 0 0 0	8	0 0 0 1 0 1
	4	0 0 0 0 2 0	9	0 1 0 1 1 0
	5	0 0 0 1 0 1	10	0 0 2 0 0 0
5 254	1	0 0 0 1 1 1	6	1 1 0 0 0 0
	2	0 0 4 0 0 0	7	0 0 0 2 2 0
	3	0 1 2 0 0 0	8	1 0 2 0 0 0
	4	0 0 1 1 0 0	9	0 0 1 1 1 0
	5	1 2 0 0 0 0	10	0 0 1 1 1 0
6 219	1	0 0 0 1 0 1	6	0 0 1 0 1 1
	2	0 1 0 0 1 0	7	0 0 0 0 0 0
	3	1 0 1 0 0 0	8	0 0 3 0 0 0
	4	0 0 1 2 0 0	9	0 0 2 1 0 0
	5	1 0 1 0 1 0	10	0 1 2 1 0 0
7 466	1	0 0 1 1 4 0	6	0 0 1 3 1 0
	2	0 1 2 2 0 1	7	0 0 0 6 0 0
	3	0 1 1 2 3 0	8	0 0 0 3 3 0
	4	0 0 1 1 2 0	9	1 0 1 2 1 0
	5	0 2 1 2 0 0	10	0 0 1 1 2 1
8 40	1	0 0 1 0 0 0	6	0 0 1 0 0 0
	2	0 0 0 1 0 0	7	0 0 1 0 0 0
	3	0 0 0 0 0 0	8	0 0 1 0 0 0
	4	0 0 0 0 0 0	9	0 0 0 0 0 0
	5	0 0 0 0 0 0	10	0 0 1 0 0 0
9 338	1	0 2 0 2 0 0	6	0 0 1 1 2 0
	2	0 0 1 2 1 0	7	0 0 2 2 0 0
	3	0 1 5 0 0 0	8	0 0 2 2 1 0
	4	0 1 1 2 0 0	9	0 1 2 1 1 0
	5	0 0 0 1 1 0	10	0 2 0 1 0 1
10 371	1	0 1 2 1 0 0	6	0 0 1 2 0 0
	2	0 1 1 2 1 0	7	0 0 0 2 1 0
	3	0 0 0 3 2 0	8	0 0 0 4 1 0
	4	0 1 2 2 1 0	9	0 1 0 3 2 0
	5	0 0 2 1 2 0	10	0 0 1 2 0 0

TABLE 1. (Cont.)

School	Prompt	Categories	Prompt	Categories
11 363	1	0 0 0 4 0 0	6	0 1 1 0 2 0
	2	0 1 1 1 1 1	7	0 0 0 1 3 1
	3	0 1 2 0 1 0	8	0 0 2 1 0 0
	4	0 0 3 1 0 1	9	0 0 1 1 2 0
	5	0 0 2 1 1 0	10	0 0 3 0 2 0
12 347	1	0 0 2 1 1 2	6	0 0 3 1 0 0
	2	1 1 1 0 0 1	7	0 0 3 2 0 0
	3	1 2 0 1 1 0	8	0 0 3 0 0 1
	4	0 0 2 1 0 0	9	0 1 1 1 0 0
	5	0 0 1 2 1 1	10	0 1 3 1 0 0
13 423	1	0 0 2 0 2 0	6	0 0 1 3 2 0
	2	0 0 1 3 3 0	7	0 0 1 3 2 0
	3	0 1 1 1 2 0	8	0 0 2 2 1 0
	4	0 0 1 2 2 0	9	0 1 1 2 1 0
	5	0 1 1 0 1 2	10	0 0 2 2 0 0
14 245	1	0 0 0 2 2 0	6	0 0 1 1 1 0
	2	0 0 0 0 2 0	7	0 0 0 1 0 0
	3	0 1 1 0 1 0	8	0 0 3 1 0 0
	4	0 0 0 1 2 0	9	0 1 1 1 1 0
	5	0 0 1 0 1 0	10	0 0 0 3 1 0
15 227	1	0 0 1 1 0 0	6	0 1 2 1 0 0
	2	0 0 2 1 1 0	7	0 0 2 0 0 0
	3	0 1 0 0 1 1	8	0 0 2 0 0 1
	4	0 1 1 0 1 0	9	0 0 0 2 0 1
	5	0 0 0 2 0 0	10	0 0 2 0 0 0
16 199	1	0 0 1 0 0 0	6	0 1 0 0 1 0
	2	1 0 0 1 0 0	7	0 0 1 0 0 1
	3	0 1 2 0 0 0	8	0 1 2 0 1 0
	4	0 2 0 1 0 0	9	0 0 0 0 2 1
	5	0 0 2 0 0 0	10	0 1 1 0 0 0
17 204	1	0 0 1 0 0 0	6	0 0 4 0 1 0
	2	0 1 0 0 1 0	7	0 0 3 0 0 0
	3	0 0 2 1 0 0	8	0 1 1 1 0 0
	4	0 1 1 0 0 0	9	0 0 2 1 0 0
	5	0 0 1 1 0 0	10	0 1 0 2 0 0
18 285	1	0 0 2 0 1 1	6	0 0 4 0 1 0
	2	0 0 0 2 2 0	7	0 1 1 2 0 0
	3	2 0 0 1 1 0	8	2 0 0 0 0 0
	4	0 0 2 1 0 0	9	0 0 3 0 0 0
	5	0 2 1 0 1 0	10	0 0 0 2 1 0
19 20	1	0 0 0 0 0 0	6	0 0 0 0 0 0
	2	0 0 0 0 0 0	7	0 0 0 0 0 0
	3	0 0 0 0 0 0	8	0 0 0 0 0 0
	4	0 0 1 0 0 0	9	0 0 0 1 0 0
	5	0 0 0 0 0 0	10	0 0 0 0 0 0
10 371	1	0 0 1 0 0 0	6	0 0 2 1 0 0
	2	0 2 0 2 0 0	7	0 0 1 1 1 0
	3	0 1 0 2 1 0	8	0 0 1 1 2 0
	4	0 1 2 1 0 0	9	0 0 0 3 0 0
	5	0 1 1 0 0 0	10	0 1 0 2 0 0

TABLE 2. Estimated Item Parameters for Rhetorical Effectiveness in Writing an "Autobiographical Incident."

	Effectiveness	
Prompt	Slope (S.E.)	Thresholds (S.E.)
1	0.518(0.104)	0.376(0.124)
2	0.789(0.143)	0.118(0.098)
3	0.515(0.098)	0.236(0.124)
4	1.068(0.206)	0.339(0.088)
5	0.534(0.099)	−0.066(0.119)
6	0.703(0.123)	0.099(0.100)
7	0.864(0.155)	0.135(0.093)
8	0.601(0.111)	0.258(0.113)
9	0.483(0.099)	0.101(0.141)
10	0.820(0.148)	0.124(0.096)

TABLE 3. Estimated Unadjusted Category Parameters.

	1	2	3	4	5
Effectiveness	0.0	1.731	0.595	0.109	−0.901
(S.E.)	(0.0)	(0.195)	(0.094)	(0.084)	(0.124)

TABLE 4. Group-Level Scores and (SE) for the Schools (Scaled to Mean 250 and SD 50).

School	Rhetorical Effectiveness		School	Rhetorical Effectiveness	
1	236	(36)	11	210	(24)
2	175	(32)	12	284	(25)
3	242	(32)	13	193	(23)
4	164	(36)	14	190	(30)
5	291	(30)	15	259	(31)
6	273	(32)	16	290	(33)
7	187	(22)	17	325	(33)
8	341	(64)	18	295	(27)
9	267	(24)	19	289	(110)
10	217	(23)	20	268	(29)

References

Andersen, E.B. and Madsen, M. (1977). Estimating the parameters of a latent population distribution. *Psychometrika* **42**, 357–374.

Bock, R.D. (1985 reprint). *Multivariate Statistical Methods in Behavioral Research.* Chicago: Scientific Software International.

Bock, R.D. (1989). Measurement of human variation: A two-stage model. In R.D. Bock (ed.), *Multilevel Analysis of Educational Data* (pp. 319–342). New York: Academic Press.

Bock, R.D. and Aitkin, M. (1981). Marginal maximum likelihood estimation of item parameters: Application of an EM algorithm. *Psychometrika* **46**, 443–445.

Bock, R.D. and Kolakowski, D. (1973). Further evidence of sex-linked major-gene influence on human spatial visualizing ability. *American Journal of Human Genetics* **25**, 1–14.

Bock, R.D. and Lieberman, M. (1970). Fitting a response model for n dichotomously scored items. *Psychometrika* **35**, 179–197.

Bock, R.D. and Mislevy, R.J. (1981). An item response model for matrix-sampling data: The California grade-three assessment. *New Directions for Testing and Measurement* **10**, 65–90.

Bock, R.D. and Zimowski, M. (1989). *Duplex Design: Giving Students A Stake in Educational Assessment.* Chicago: Methodology Research Center, NORC.

Day, N.E. (1969). Estimating the components of a mixture of normal distributions. *Biometrika* **56**, 463–473.

de Leeuw, J. and Verhelst, N. (1986). Maximum likelihood estimation in generalized Rasch models. *Journal of Educational Statistics* **11**, 193–196.

Dempster, A.P., Rubin, D.B., and Tsutakawa, R.K. (1981). Estimation in covariance component models. *Journal of American Statistical Association* **76**, 341–353.

Dorus, E., Cox, N.J., Gibbons, R.D., Shaughnessy, R., Pandey, G.N., and Cloninger, R.C. (1983). Lithium ion transport and affective disorders within families of bipolar patients. *Archives of General Psychiatry* **401**, 945–552.

Gasser, T., Müller, H.-G., and Mammitzsch, V. (1985). Kernels for nonparametric curve estimation. *Journal of the Royal Statistical Society, Series B* **47**, 238–252.

Kiefer, J. and Wolfowitz, J. (1956). Consistency of the maximum likelihood estimator in the presence of infinitely many incidental parameters. *Annals of Mathematical Statistics* **27**, 887–906.

Kolakowski, D. and Bock, R.D. (1982). A multivariate generalization of probit analysis. *Biometrics* **37**, 541–551.

Lindsay, B., Clogg, C.C., and Grego, J. (1991). Semiparametric estimation in the Rasch model and related exponential response models, including a simple latent class model for item analysis. *Journal of the American Statistical Association* **86**, 96–107.

Lord, F.M. and Novick, M.R. (1968). *Statistical Theories of Mental Test Scores (with Contributions by A. Birnbaum)*. Reading, MA: Addison-Wesley.

Mislevy, R.J. (1983). Item response models for grouped data. *Journal of Educational Statistics* **8**, 271–288.

Mislevy, R.J. (1984). Estimating latent distributions. *Psychometrika* **49**, 359–381.

Mislevy, R.J. and Bock, R.D. (1996). *BILOG 3: Item Analysis and Test Scoring with Binary Logistic Models.* Chicago: Scientific Software International.

Muraki, E. and Bock, R.D. (1991). *PARSCALE: Parametric Scaling of Rating Data.* Chicago: Scientific Software International.

Reiser, M.R. (1983). An item response model for demographic effects. *Journal of Educational Statistics* **8**(3), 165–186.

Sanathanan, L. and Blumenthal, N. (1978). The logistic model and estimation of latent structure. *Journal of the American Statistical Association* **73**, 794–798.

Sirotnik, K. and Wellington, R. (1977). Incidence sampling: An integrated theory for "matrix-sampling." *Journal of Educational Measurement* **14**, 343–399.

Zimowski, M.F., Muraki, E., Mislevy, R.J., and Bock, R.D. (1996). *BILOG-MG: Multiple-Group IRT Analysis and Test Maintenance for Binary Items.* Chicago: IL: Scientific Software International.

26
Logistic Mixture Models

Jürgen Rost

Introduction

Discrete mixture distribution models (MDM) assume that observed data do not stem from a homogeneous population of individuals but are a mixture of data from two or more latent populations (Everitt and Hand, 1981; Titterington et al., 1985). Applied to item response data this means that a particular IRT model does not hold for the entire sample but that different sets of model parameters (item parameters, ability parameters, etc.) are valid for different subpopulations.

Whereas it has become a common procedure to compare parameter estimates between different manifest subpopulations defined, for example, by sex, age, or grade level, the subpopulations addressed by discrete MDM are latent, i.e., unknown both with respect to their number and membership of individuals. It is the aim of a mixture analysis to identify these latent populations. As an example, spatial reasoning tasks can be solved by different cognitive strategies, say, one strategy based on mental rotation of the stimulus and another based on feature comparison processes. If different individuals employ different strategies, an IRT model cannot fit the item response data because different strategies imply different item difficulties for the same items. On the other hand, the model may hold within each of the subpopulations employing the same strategy. The items, then, may have different parameter values for each subpopulation.

Hence, the task of a data analysis with a discrete MDM is twofold: First to unmix the data into homogeneous subpopulations, and second to estimate the model parameters for each of the subpopulations. However both tasks are done simultaneously by defining a discrete mixture model for the item responses and estimating all parameters by maximum likelihood methods.

Presentation of the Model

The general structure of *mixed* IRT models is as follows:

$$p(\mathbf{u}) = \sum_{g=1}^{G} \pi_g p(\mathbf{u} \mid g), \tag{1}$$

where $p(\mathbf{u})$ is the pattern probability, i.e., the probability of the response vector $\mathbf{u} = (u_1, u_2, \ldots, u_n)$, G is the number of subpopulations or classes, π_g is a probability parameter defining the size of class g with restriction

$$\sum_{g=1}^{G} \pi_g = 1, \tag{2}$$

and $p(\mathbf{u} \mid g)$ the pattern probability within class g. The parameters π_g are also called the *mixing proportions.*

In the sequel, only discrete mixtures of the one-parameter logistic model, i.e., the Rasch model, and its polytomous generalizations are treated in detail. One reason among others is that parameter estimation becomes harder when multiplicative (discrimination) parameters are involved as well.

Let U_{ij} denote the response variable of individual j on item i, then the conditional response probability of an individual being in class g is defined as

$$p(U_{ij} = 1 \mid g) = \frac{\exp(\theta_{jg} - \sigma_{ig})}{1 + \exp(\theta_{jg} - \sigma_{ig})}, \tag{3}$$

where θ_{jg} is a class-specific individual parameter, denoting the ability of individual j to solve the items, if she/he would belong to class g. Hence, each individual gets as many parameters as there are latent classes. In the same way, σ_{ig} is a class-specific item parameter describing the difficulty of item i when it is solved by individuals in class g. The marginal response probability, then, is the *mixed dichotomous Rasch model* (Rost, 1990):

$$p(U_{ij} = 1) = \sum_{g=1}^{G} \pi_g \frac{\exp(\theta_{jg} - \sigma_{ig})}{1 + \exp(\theta_{jg} - \sigma_{ig})}, \tag{4}$$

with norming conditions

$$\sum_{g=1}^{G} \pi_g = 1 \quad \text{and} \quad \sum_{i=1}^{n} \sigma_{ig} = 0 \ \text{ for all classes } g, \tag{5}$$

where n is the number of items. Here a third type of model parameter is involved, namely the mixing proportions π_g defined in Eq. (2). From the usual assumption of stochastic independent responses follows the conditional pattern probability

$$p(\mathbf{u} \mid g) = \prod_{i=1}^{n} \frac{\exp(u_i(\theta_{jg} - \sigma_{ig}))}{1 + \exp(\theta_{jg} - \sigma_{ig})}$$

$$= \frac{\exp\left(\sum_{i=1}^{n} u_i \theta_{jg}\right) \cdot \exp\left(-\sum_{i=1}^{n} u_i \sigma_{ig}\right)}{\prod_{i=1}^{n}(1 + \exp(\theta_{jg} - \sigma_{ig}))}. \quad (6)$$

The model assumes that the Rasch model holds within a number of G different subpopulations, but in each of them with a possibly different set of ability and item parameters. Whereas the mixing proportions π_g are model parameters which are estimated by maximum likelihood (ML) methods (see below), the number G of latent classes cannot be estimated directly but has to be inferred from comparing the model fit under the assumption of different numbers of latent classes.

A major application of the model in Eq. (4) is the possibility of testing the fit of the ordinary Rasch model to a set of data. Because item parameters have to be constant over different subsamples, a widely applied goodness-of-fit test, the conditional likelihood ratio (CLR) test by Andersen (1973), is based on a splitting of the sample into various subsamples, e.g., score groups. From a mixture models perspective, the CLR-test is testing the null-hypothesis of a one-class Rasch model against the alternative hypothesis of a manifest mixture Rasch model, where the score or some other criterion is the mixing variable. Testing the one-class solution against the two-class solution of the mixed Rasch model (MRM), is a more powerful test of the hypothesis of constant item parameters across all subsamples: the MRM identifies that partition of the population into two subpopulations, among which the item parameters show highest differences. As a consequence, it is not necessary to try out several splitting criteria for the sample of individuals in order to test the assumption of constant item parameters for all individuals (Rost and von Davier, 1995).

Another field of application are tests where different groups of people employ different solution strategies for solving items in a test. Because different solution strategies usually are connected with different sets of item difficulties, the analysis of these tests requires a model which takes account of different item parameters for these subpopulations (Rost and von Davier, 1993).

In order to apply the model some further assumptions have to be made regarding the ability parameters θ_{jg}. Mislevy and Verhelst (1990) have chosen a marginal likelihood approach, i.e., they specify a distribution function of θ and estimate the parameters in this function along with the item parameters. Kelderman and Macready (1990) discuss the concept of the mixed Rasch model in the framework of log-linear models. Here, the ability parameters are neither estimated directly nor eliminated using the assumption of a distribution function. The log-linear formulation of the Rasch model provides conditional item parameter estimates and some kind of score parameters reflecting the ability distribution.

Rost (1990) chose to condition out the ability parameters within the classes to estimate the score frequencies within the classes, and to provide unconditional ability estimates on the basis of the conditional estimates of item parameters. Although this topic sounds like a technical question of parameter estimation, it implies a reparameterization of the MRM with a different set of parameters and, therefore is described in this section.

The conditional pattern probability can be factorized by conditioning on the score r associated with this pattern, $r = \sum_{i=1}^{n} u_i$, i.e.,

$$p(\mathbf{u} \mid g) = p(\mathbf{u} \mid g, r) p(r \mid g). \tag{7}$$

The pattern probability under the condition of score r is, just as in the ordinary Rasch model, free of the ability parameters and can be computed by means of the symmetric functions γ_r of the item parameters:

$$p(\mathbf{u} \mid r, g) = \frac{p(\mathbf{u} \mid g)}{\sum_{\mathbf{u}|r} p(\mathbf{u} \mid g)} = \frac{\exp\left(-\sum_{i=1}^{n} u_i \sigma_i\right)}{\gamma_r(\exp(-\sigma))}. \tag{8}$$

By introducing new probability parameters $\pi_{rg} = p(r \mid g)$ for the latent score probabilities, the marginal pattern probability is

$$p(\mathbf{u}) = \sum_{g=1}^{G} \pi_g \pi_{rg} \frac{\exp\left(-\sum u_i \sigma_{ig}\right)}{\gamma_r(\exp(-\sigma))} \tag{9}$$

with normalization condition

$$\sum_{r=1}^{n-1} \pi_{rg} = 1 \quad \text{for all } g. \tag{10}$$

In the normalization of the score probabilities, those of the extreme scores $r = 0$ and $r = n$ are excluded, the reason being that these score frequencies cannot be estimated separately for each class because the patterns of only 0's or 1's have identical probabilities of one in each class g. As a consequence, the number of independent score parameters is $2 + G(n-2)$.

The norming condition for the class sizes, therefore, is

$$\sum_{g=1}^{G} \pi_g = 1 - p(r=0) - p(r=n). \tag{11}$$

It follows from this model that each individual belongs to each class with a (posterior) probability which depends on the response pattern in the following way:

$$p(g \mid \mathbf{u}) = \frac{\pi_g p(\mathbf{u} \mid g)}{\sum_{g=1}^{G} \pi_g p(\mathbf{u} \mid g)}. \tag{12}$$

According to these probabilities, each individual can be assigned to that latent population, where his or her probability is highest. The model provides two pieces of diagnostic information about each individual: First, the latent population to which the individual belongs, and second, the ability estimate. In this sense, the mixed Rasch model simultaneously classifies and quantifies on the basis of the observed response patterns.

Logistic Mixture Models for Ordinal Data

The mixed Rasch model can easily be generalized to such Rasch models for ordinal data as the partial credit model (Masters, 1982, this volume), the rating-scale model (Andrich, 1978; Andersen, this volume), the dispersion model (Andrich, 1982), or the successive interval model (Rost, 1988). In this family of models, the partial credit model is the most general one. It is defined by the following response function:

$$p(U_{ij} = h) = \frac{\exp(h\theta_j - \sigma_{ih})}{\sum_{s=0}^{m} \exp(s\theta_j - \sigma_{is})} \quad \text{for } h = 0, 1, 2, \ldots, m, \qquad (13)$$

where the item-category parameter σ_{ih} is a *cumulated threshold parameter* defined as

$$\sigma_{ih} = \sum_{s=1}^{h} \tau_{is}, \quad \sigma_{i0} = 0, \qquad (14)$$

and τ_{is} is the location of threshold s on the latent continuum. Generalized to a discrete mixture model, the marginal response probability becomes

$$p(U_{ij} = h) = \sum_{g=1}^{G} \pi_g \frac{\exp(h\theta_{jg} - \sigma_{ihg})}{\sum_{s=0}^{m} \exp(s\theta_{jg} - \sigma_{isg})} \quad \text{with } \sigma_{ihg} = \sum_{s=1}^{h} \tau_{isg} \qquad (15)$$

(Rost, 1991; von Davier and Rost, 1995). The normalization conditions are

$$\sum_{g=1}^{G} \pi_g = 1, \ \sum_{i=1}^{n} \sum_{h=1}^{m} \tau_{ihg} = 0 \ \text{ for all } g, \text{ and } \sigma_{i0g} = 0 \text{ for all } i \text{ and } g.$$

Again, the likelihood function can be defined on the basis of conditional pattern probabilities, so that the individual parameters are eliminated and score probabilities are introduced:

$$L = \prod_{j=1}^{N} \sum_{g=1}^{G} \pi_g \pi_{rg} \frac{\exp\left(-\sum_{i=1}^{n} \sigma_{ihg}\right)}{\gamma_r(\exp(-\sigma))}. \qquad (16)$$

One drawback of this kind of reparametrization is the relatively high number of score parameters, $2 + G(nm - 2)$, which, for example, lowers the power of the goodness-of-fit tests. In order to reduce this number, a *logistic two-parameter function* can be used to approximate the score distributions within the latent classes. In this function, the parameter μ is a location parameter whereas λ represents the dispersion of the score distribution in class g:

$$\hat{\pi}_{rg} = \frac{\exp\left(\frac{r}{mn}\mu_g + \frac{4r(nm-r)}{(nm)^2}\lambda_g\right)}{\sum_{s=0}^{nm} \exp\left(\frac{s}{nm}\mu_g + \frac{4r(nm-s)}{(nm)^2}\lambda_g\right)}. \tag{17}$$

This distribution function can be used to model different kinds of single peaked distributions; it even becomes u-shaped when λ is negative.

As special cases of the mixed partial credit model in Eq. (15), the following restricted ordinal Rasch models can be defined (von Davier and Rost, 1995):

(1) the *mixed rating scale model*

$$p(U_{ij} = h) = \sum_{g=1}^{G} \pi_g \frac{\exp(h\theta_{jg} - h\sigma_{ig} - \psi_{hg})}{\sum_{s=0}^{m} \exp(\cdots)} \text{ with } \psi_{hg} = \sum_{s=1}^{h} \tau_{sg} \tag{18}$$

and normalization conditions $\psi_{0g} = \psi_{mg} = \sum_{i=1}^{n} \sigma_{ig} = 0$ for all classes g;

(2) the *mixed dispersion model*

$$p(U_{ij} = h) = \sum_{g=1}^{G} \pi_g \frac{\exp(h\theta_{jg} - h\sigma_{ig} - h(h-m)\frac{1}{2}\delta_{ig})}{\sum_{s=0}^{m} \exp(\cdots)} \tag{19}$$

with normalization condition $\sum_{i=1}^{n} \sigma_{ig} = 0$ for all g; and

(3) the *mixed successive interval model*

$$p(U_{ij} = h) = \sum_{g=1}^{G} \pi_g \frac{\exp(h\theta_{jg} - h\sigma_{ig} - \psi_{hg} - h(h-m)\frac{1}{2}\delta_{ig})}{\sum_{s=0}^{m} \exp(\cdots)} \tag{20}$$

with normalization conditions $\psi_{0g} = \psi_{mg} = \sum_{i=1}^{n} \sigma_{ig} = \sum_{i=1}^{n} \delta_{ig} = 0$ for all classes g.

These models can be applied, e.g., to questionnaires for attitude measurement in order to separate groups of individuals with a different attitude structure in terms of different item parameters in different subpopulations. Moreover, subpopulations may not only differ with respect to their sets of item parameter values but also with respect to the threshold distances between the categories of the response scale. These threshold distances can be interpreted in terms of response sets common to all individuals in that particular latent class. Large distances between the thresholds of the middle category of a rating scale can be interpreted as a tendency toward the mean, whereas a low threshold parameter value for the first categories combined with a high parameter value for the last reflects a tendency toward extreme judgments. Often, a latent class with threshold parameters not showing the expected increasing order can be interpreted as a class of unscalables because ordered thresholds are a prerequisite for measuring a latent trait with rating scales.

Until now, all of these mixed ordinal Rasch models have been defined such that the same type of model is assumed in all classes. Gitomer and Yamamoto (1991) proposed a hybrid model where in one class the Rasch model is assumed to describe the item response process while in other classes the ordinary latent class model may also be defined for the models described here, so that a large number of different mixture models can be generated (von Davier and Rost, 1996). However, data analysis with these models should be theory driven in any case: The idea of mixed logistic models is not to fit all possible data sets by a colorful mixture of IRT models. Rather, the idea is to have a mixture model when there are strong reasons to assume that different things may happen in different subpopulations: different response sets, sloppy response behavior with unscalable individuals, different cognitive strategies, or different attitude structures. Last but not least, the idea is to test the basic assumption of all IRT models namely that the responses of all individuals can be described by the same model and the same set of parameters. If that is the case, the one-class solution, which is an ordinary IRT model, holds.

Parameter Estimation

The parameters in the mixed Rasch model and its generalizations to ordinal data can be estimated by means of an extended EM-algorithm with conditional maximum likelihood estimation of the item parameters in the M-step. On the basis of preliminary estimates (or starting values) of the model parameters, the pattern frequencies for each latent class are estimated in the E-step as:

$$\hat{n}(\mathbf{u}, g) = n(\mathbf{u}) \frac{\pi_g p(\mathbf{u} \mid g)}{\sum_{g=1}^{G} \pi_g p(\mathbf{u} \mid g)}, \tag{21}$$

where $n(\mathbf{u})$ denotes the observed frequency of response vector $\mathbf{u}$, and $\hat{n}(\mathbf{u}, g)$ is an estimate of the portion of that frequency in class g. The conditional pattern frequencies are defined by Eq. (6), or, as a function of the item and score parameters, by Eqs. (7) and (8). For the sake of simplicity, the estimation equations for the M-step will be given only for the dichotomous mixed Rasch model. Parameter estimation for the ordinal models can be done analogously and bears no special problems, except for the computation of the symmetric functions, where the so-called summation algorithm has to be applied (von Davier and Rost, 1995).

In the M-step, these proportions of observed pattern frequencies in Eq. (21) form the basis for calculating better estimates of the class size, item and score parameters π_{rg}. These parameters can be estimated separately for each latent class by maximizing the log-likelihood function in class g:

$$\log L_g = \sum_{\mathbf{u}} \hat{n}(\mathbf{u} \mid g) \left[\log(\pi_{rg}) - \sum_{i=1}^{n} u_i \sigma_{ig} - \log(\gamma_r(\exp(-\sigma))) \right]. \quad (22)$$

Setting the first partial derivatives with respect to σ_{ig} to zero yields the estimation equations for the item parameters within class g:

$$\hat{\sigma}_{ig} = \log \frac{n_{ig}}{\sum_{r=0}^{n} m_{rg} \frac{\gamma_{r-1,i}}{\gamma_r}}, \quad (23)$$

where n_{ig} denotes preliminary estimates of the number of individuals with a positive response on item i in class g, m_{rg} estimates the number of individuals with score r in class g [both calculated by means of $\hat{n}(\mathbf{u}, \mathbf{g})$ obtained in the previous M-step] and $\gamma_{r-1,i}$ are the elementary symmetric functions of order $r-1$ of all item parameters except item i. The elementary symmetric functions on the right-hand side of Eq. (23) are calculated by means of preliminary item parameter estimates, and new (better) estimates are obtained on the left-hand side of Eq. (23). Only one iteration of this procedure suffices because it is performed in each M-step of the EM-algorithm, and, hence, converges to maximum-likelihood-estimates in the course of the EM-procedure.

The estimates of the score probabilities and class sizes are explicit:

$$\hat{\pi}_{ig} = \frac{m_{rg}}{n_g} \quad (24)$$

and

$$\hat{\pi}_g = \frac{n_g}{N}, \quad (25)$$

where n_g denotes the number of individuals in class g, computed on the basis of $n(\mathbf{u}, g)$.

The ability parameters θ_{jg} in Eq. (4) do not appear in these equations because their sufficient statistics r_j were substituted. They can, however, be estimated using the final estimates of the item and score parameters. This is achieved by maximizing the following intra-class likelihood:

$$\log L_g = \sum_j \log p(\mathbf{u}_j \mid g) = \sum_j r_j \theta_{jg} + \sum_i n_{ig} \sigma_{ig}$$
$$- \sum_j \sum_i \log(1 + \exp(\theta_{jg} + \sigma_{ig})) \quad (26)$$

with respect to the unknown ability parameters θ_{jg}, which only depend on the score r_j of individual j. The number of individuals in class g solving item i, n_{ig}, need not to be known because this term vanishes when the first partial derivatives of (26) with respect to the trait parameters θ_{jg} are computed. The estimation equations are

$$r_j = \sum_{i=1}^{n} \frac{\exp(\theta_{jg} + \sigma_{ig})}{1 + \exp(\theta_{jg} + \sigma_{ig})}, \tag{27}$$

which can be solved iteratively. Hence, the class-dependent trait parameters of the model in Eq. (4) can be estimated in a second step of the estimation procedure, making use of the conditional item parameter estimates, σ_{ig}, obtained in the first step.

Each individual has as many trait (or ability) parameter estimates as there are latent classes. These can be interpreted as conditional trait estimates, i.e., individual j has the trait value θ_{jg} under the condition that he or she belongs to class g. However, these conditional abilities of a single individual j usually do not differ much from one class to another, because the estimates depend mainly on r_j which, of course, is the same in all classes.

On the other hand, the class membership of an individual is nearly independent of his or her total score but strongly dependent on which items have been solved. In this sense, the MRM enables one to separate the quantitative and the qualitative aspects of a response pattern: The continuous mixing variable mainly depends on *how many* items have been solved, the discrete mixing variable mainly depends on *which* items have been solved.

Software

The models described in the previous sections can be computed by means of the Windows-program WIN-MIRA [MIxed RAsch model; von Davier (1995)]. The program provides ML-estimates of the expected score frequencies and individual parameters and conditional ML-estimates of the class-specific item parameters including estimates of the standard errors based on Fisher's information function. As a separate output file for all persons, the overall ability estimates along with the number of the most likely latent class for each person, and all class membership probabilities, are provided.

Although there are no technical limitations from doing so, it usually makes little sense to apply a mixture model to more than 20 or 30 dichotomous items or 15 to 20 polytomous items, respectively. For large numbers of items the likelihood function becomes very flat, and the risk increases that there are several local maxima. Computation time strongly depends on the size of the data set and the number of classes but usually a PC-486 would not take more than a few minutes to compute the parameters of a model with reasonable accuracy.

Goodness of Fit

To test the fit of a logistic mixture model to empirical data, the usual statistics of cross-table analysis and latent class models can be applied but a selection has to be made with respect to the size of the data set. The strongest, and from a statistical point of view the most satisfying tests, are the Pearson chi-square and the likelihood ratio for comparing observed and expected pattern frequencies.

Both statistics yield, under regular conditions, similar results, and, likewise, have similar asymptotic requirements. However, these requirements are usually not fulfilled when more than 6 or 8 dichotomous items are analyzed, or even only 4 items with 4 categories: In the case of, say about 500 different possible response patterns an expectation of 1 or more for *all* pattern frequencies would require such gigantic sample sizes that these statistics are only applicable when some kind of pattern aggregation takes place.

Unfortunately, the same argument holds for testing the number of latent classes in a mixture model by means of a likelihood-ratio statistic. A likelihood-ratio statistic, which is the likelihood of a model with G classes divided by the likelihood of the mixture of $G+1$ classes, is only asymptotically chi-square distributed if all patterns have a reasonable chance to be observed (which is not possible for even 12 items).

For these reasons, information criteria like the AIC or the BIC (Bozdogan, 1987; Read and Cressie, 1988) are a useful alternative for comparing competitive models without drawing statistical inferences in the usual sense. These indices enable the conclusion that a particular model describes the data better than a specified alternative model, given the number of independent model parameters.

The information criteria are defined as:

$$\begin{aligned} \text{AIC} &= -2\,\log(L) + 2k, \\ \text{BIC} &= -2\,\log(L) + \log(N)k, \end{aligned} \tag{28}$$

where L is the maximum of the likelihood function of a given model, and k is the number of independent model parameters. The smaller the value, the better the model fits. These criteria are based on exactly the same information as the LR-chi-square statistic, i.e., the log-likelihood and the number of parameters. The crucial point, of course, is the kind of "penalty function" connecting the two aspects of model fit. In this respect, the BIC prefers simple solutions, i.e., it penalizes overparametrization more than the AIC.

The fact that the number of estimated parameters plays such an important role when comparing the fit of two models was one reason for introducing a logistic approximation to the latent score distributions with only two parameters for each class.

Software

The Windows-Software WIN-MIRA (von Davier, 1995) provides the log-likelihood of all models computed, the log-likelihood of the saturated model, the LR-statistic based upon these values as well as the AIC and BIC value. A bootstrapping procedure is optional. Furthermore, the standard errors of the ability estimates are given, and the item-Q index as a measure of item fit (Rost and von Davier, 1994) is calculated for all latent classes. The latter allows an insight into the fit of the Rasch model within each latent class.

Examples

A typical application of mixed models for dichotomous items is to spatial reasoning tasks. Here it is assumed that subpopulations of individuals either employ some kind of analytical strategy, in which feature comparison processes take place, or that they employ some kind of strategies based on an analogous cognitive representation of the stimuli, called "holistic" strategies. As a consequence, at least two latent classes with a preference to one of these strategies are to be expected (Köller et al., 1994; Mislevy et al., 1990; Mislevy et al., 1991; Rost and von Davier, 1993).

Applications of the polytomous mixed models are primarily in the field of attitude questionnaires (Rost and Georg, 1991), measurement of interests (Rost, 1991) or personality assessment. In a project on the scalability of individuals with personality questionnaires, five scales of a questionnaire assessing the so-called "big five" personality factors were analyzed (Borkenau and Ostendorf, 1991). As an example, the results for the dimension "conscientiousness" are reported next.

Twelve items with 4 response categories ("strongly disagree," "disagree," "agree," "strongly agree") were designed to measure the dimension "conscientiousness." A total number of 2112 individuals, an aggregation of different samples, were analyzed with the mixed partial credit model, using the approximation of the score distributions by means of the two parameter logistic function described earlier. Out of 16,777,216 possible patterns, 1937 different response patterns were observed, so that the chi-square statistics could not be applied without (arbitrary) grouping.

The decision on the number of latent populations was made on the basis of the BIC-index because the AIC turned out to identify so many latent classes that they were no longer interpretable. (This finding is a general experience when working with data sets of this size.) Table 1 shows the results needed for the decision on the number of classes.

According to these results, the two-class solution fits best. The two classes have an interesting interpretation which can be drawn from the graphical representation of the model parameters in Figs. 1 and 2. Figure

TABLE 1. Goodness of fit Statistics for the Conscientiousness Example.

G	$-\log L$	x	BIC	AIC
1	24300.7	37	50884.5	50675.4
2	24815.7	75	50205.4	49781.4
3	24683.8	113	50232.4	49598.6
4	24567.6	151	50290.7	49437.1

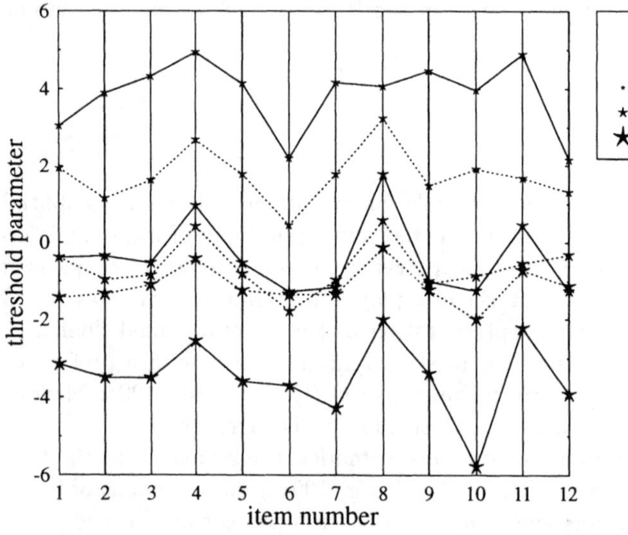

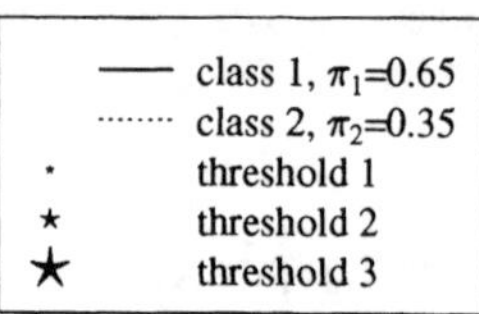

FIGURE 1. The thresholds of the 2-class solution for the scale "conscientiousness."

1 shows the threshold parameters of all 12 items in both classes.

The bigger class with 65.2 percent of the total population is characterized by ordered thresholds of all items and reasonable threshold distances. This finding is to be expected for individuals that used the rating scale in correspondence with the dimension to be measured. The smaller class with 34.8 percent of the population is characterized by small threshold distances, especially for the second and third threshold. This result may be indicative of different response sets in both classes or even of the fact that the response format is not used adequately in the second class.

Figure 2 shows the estimated distributions of the individual parameters in both classes. Each dot or each square represents a score group. It turns out that the same score groups are assigned to more extreme parameter estimates in class 1 than in class 2.

The range of the estimated conscientiousness parameter values obviously is larger in the 65% class than in the small class. This result is also indicative of the fact that the questionnaire measures the trait in both populations

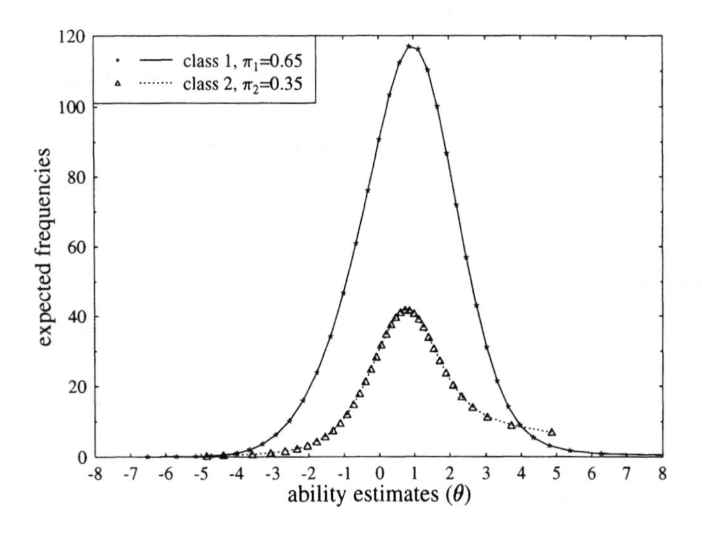

FIGURE 2. Expected frequencies of ability estimates in both classes.

in a different way.

Discussion

Mixture models for item response analysis are a relatively new development in IRT. They seem especially useful where test analysis is driven by substantial theory about qualitative differences among people. Whenever different strategies are employed to solve items, or different cognitive structures govern the responses to attitude or personality assessment items, a mixture model may help to reveal subgroups of individuals connected to one of these strategies or structures.

Further development should go into the direction of mixtures of different models, for example, models with a Rasch model in one population and some model representing guessing behavior in the other population. In general, mixture models provide an elegant way of testing an ordinary (non-mixed) IRT-model by focussing on the basic assumption of all IRT-models, which is homogeneity in the sense of constant item parameters for all individuals.

References

Andrich, D. (1978). Application of a psychometric rating model to ordered categories which are scored with successive integers. *Applied Psycholog-*

ical Measurement **2** 581–594.

Andrich, D. (1982). An extension of the Rasch model for ratings providing both location and dispersion parameters. *Psychometrika* **47**, 104–113.

Andersen, E.B. (1973). Conditional inference for multiple-choice questionnaires. *British Journal of Mathematical and Statistical Psychology* **26**, 31–44.

Borkenau, P. and Ostendorf, F. (1991). Ein Fragebogen zur Erfassung fünf robuster Persönlichkeitsfaktoren. *Diagnostica* **37**, 29–41.

Bozdogan, H. (1987). Model selection for Akaike's information criterion (AIC). *Psychometrika* **53**, 345–370.

Everitt, B.S. and Hand, D.J. (1981). *Finite Mixture Distributions.* London: Chapman and Hall.

Gitomer, D.H. and Yamamoto, K. (1991). Performance modeling that integrates latent trait and class theory. *Journal of Educational Measurement* **28**, 173–189.

Kelderman, H. and Macready, G.B. (1990). The use of loglinear models for assessing differential item functioning across manifest and latent examinee groups. *Journal of Educational Measurement* **27**, 307–327.

Köller, O., Rost, J., and Köller, M. (1994). Individuelle Unterschiede beim Lösen von Raumvorstellungsaufgaben aus dem IST-bzw. IST-70-Untertest "Wüfelaufgaben." *Zeitschrift für Psychologie* **202**, 64–85.

Masters, G.N. (1982). A Rasch model for partial credit scoring. *Psychometrika* **47**, 149–174.

Mislevy, R.J. and Verhelst, N. (1990). Modeling item responses when different subjects employ different solution strategies. *Psychometrika* **55**, 195–215.

Mislevy, R.J., Wingersky, M.S., Irvine, S.H., and Dann, P.L. (1991). Resolving mixtures of strategies in spatial visualisation tasks. *British Journal of Mathematical and Statistical Psychology* **44**, 265–288.

Read, T.R.C. and Cressie, N.A.C. (1988). *Goodness-of-Fit Statistics for Discrete Multivariate Data.* New York: Springer.

Rost, J. (1988). Measuring attitudes with a threshold model drawing on a traditional scaling concept. *Applied Psychological Measurement* **12**, 397–409.

Rost, J. (1990). Rasch models in latent classes: An integration of two approaches to item analysis. *Applied Psychological Measurement* **14**, 271–282.

Rost, J. (1991). A logistic mixture distribution model for polytomous item responses. *British Journal of Mathematical and Statistical Psychology* **44**, 75–92.

Rost, J. and von Davier, M. (1993). Measuring different traits in different populations with the same items. In R. Steyer, K.F. Wender, and K.F. Widaman (eds.), *Psychometric Methodology, Proceedings of the 7th European Meeting of the Psychometric Society* (pp. 446–450). Stuttgart/ New York: Gustav Fischer Verlag.

Rost, J. and von Davier, M. (1994). A conditional item fix index for Rasch models. *Applied Psychological Measurement* **18**, 171–182.

Rost, J. and von Davier, M. (1995). Mixture distribution Rasch models. In G. Fischer and I. Molenaar (eds.), *Rasch Models: Foundations, Recent Developments, and Applications* (pp. 257–268). Springer.

Rost, J. and Georg, W. (1991). Alternative Skalierungsmöglichkeiten zur klassischen Testtheorie am Beispiel der Skala "Jugendzentrismus." *ZA-Information* **28**, 52–75.

Titterington, D.M., Smith, A.F.M., and Makov, U.E. (1985). *Statistical Analysis of Finite Mixture Distributions.* Chichester: Wiley.

von Davier, M.V. and Rost, J. (1995). WINMIRA: A program system for analyses with the Rasch model, with the latent class analysis and with the mixed Rasch model. Kiel: Institute for Science Eduation (IPN), distributed by Iec Progamma, Groningen.

von Davier, M.V. and Rost J. (1995). Polytomous mixed Rasch models. In G. Fischer and I. Molenaar (eds.), *Rasch Models: Foundations, Recent Developments, and Applications* (pp. 371–379). Springer.

von Davier, M.V. and Rost, J. (1996). Self-monitoring—A class variable? In J. Rost and R. Langeheine (eds.), *Applications of Latent Trait and Latent Class Models in the Social Sciences.* Münster: Waxmann.

27

Models for Locally Dependent Responses: Conjunctive Item Response Theory

Robert J. Jannarone

Introduction

The last 15 years have been locally dependent IRT advances along nonparametric and parametric lines. Results include nonparametric tests for unidimensionality and response function monotonicity (Holland, 1981; Holland and Rosenbaum, 1986; Rosenbaum, 1984, 1987; Stout, 1987, 1990; Suppes and Zanotti, 1981), locally dependent models without individual difference provisions (Andrich, 1985; Embretson, 1984; Gibbons et al. 1989; Spray and Ackerman, 1986) and locally dependent models with individual differences provisions (Jannarone, 1986, 1987, 1991; Jannarone et al. 1990; Kelderman and Jannarone, 1989).

This chapter features locally dependent, conjunctive IRT (CIRT) models that the author and his colleagues have introduced and developed. CIRT models are distinguished from other IRT models by their use of nonadditive item and person sufficient statistics. They are useful for IRT study because they make up a statistically sound family, within which special cases can be compared having differing dimensionalities, local dependencies, nonadditives and response function forms.

CIRT models are also useful for extending IRT practice, because they can measure learning during testing or tutoring while conventional IRT models cannot. For example, measuring how students respond to reinforcements during interactive training and testing sessions is potentially useful for placing them in settings that suit their learning abilities. However, such measurement falls outside the realm of conventional IRT, because it violates the local independence axiom.

The IRT local independence axiom resembles the classical laws of physics and CIRT resembles modern physics in several ways (Jannarone, 1991). Just as modern physics explains particle reaction to measurement, CIRT explains human learning during measurement; just as modern physics includes classical physics as a special case, CIRT includes conventional IRT as a special case; just as modern physics extensions are essentially nonadditive, so are CIRT extensions; just as modern physics extensions are potentially useful, so are CIRT extensions and just as its usefulness has resulted in modern physics acceptance, locally dependent IRT will become accepted eventually.

IRT and CIRT are different than classical and modern physics in historical impact terms, and neither IRT nor CIRT will become household terms for some time. They figure to become increasingly important, however, as information becomes increasingly available and human abilities to learn from it become increasingly taxed.

Presentation of the Model

Conjunctive IRT Model Formulation

Although a variety of CIRT models have been proposed, this chapter emphasizes the family of conjunctive Rasch kernels because of their sound psychometric properties. (Kernels in this context correspond to IRT probability models with fixed person parameters.) To outline notation, Roman symbols are measurements and Greek symbols are parameters; upper case symbols are random variables and lower case symbols are their values; bold symbols are arrays, superscripts in braces are power labels, subscripts in parentheses are array dimensions and subscripts not in parentheses are array elements or vector labels; Greek symbols are parameters defined on $\{-\infty, \infty\}$; U and u are item response random variables and values defined on $\{0, 1\}$; i labels denote items, j labels denote subjects and k labels denote testlets.

Each member of the conjunctive Rasch family is a special case of a general Rasch kernel,

$$Pr\{\mathbf{U}_{(n)j} = \mathbf{u}_{(n)j} \mid \mathbf{\Theta}_{(2^n-1)j} = \boldsymbol{\theta}_{(2^n-1)j}; \boldsymbol{\beta}_{(2^n-1)}\}$$

$$\propto \exp\left\{\sum_{i=1}^{n}(\theta_{ij}^{[1]} - \beta_i^{[1]})u_{ij} + \sum_{i=1}^{n-1}\sum_{i'=i+1}^{n}(\theta_{ii'j}^{[2]} - \beta_{ii'}^{[2]})u_{ij}u_{i'j}\right.$$

$$\left. + \cdots + (\theta_{12\cdots nj}^{[n]} - \beta_{12\cdots n}^{[n]})u_{1j}u_{2j}\cdots u_{nj}\right\}, \quad j = 1, \ldots, N. \tag{1}$$

The θ values in Eq. (1) are person parameters usually associated with abilities and the β values in Eq. (1) are item parameters usually associated with difficulties.

Equation (1) is too general to be useful as it stands, because it is not identifiable (Bickel and Doksum, 1977). For example, adding a positive constant to β_1 and adding the same positive constant to each θ_{1j} does not change any item response probabilities based on Eq. (1). As a result, constraints must be imposed on Eq. (1) to create special cases that can identify unique parameters.

One such special case is the conventional Rasch kernel,

$$Pr\{\mathbf{U}_{(n)j} = \mathbf{u}_{(n)j} \mid \Theta_j = \theta_j; \boldsymbol{\beta}_{(n)}\} = \prod_{i=1}^{n} \frac{\exp\{(\theta_j - \beta_i)u_{ij}\}}{1 + \exp\{\theta_j - \beta_i\}}$$

$$\propto \exp\left\{\sum_{i=1}^{n}(\theta_j - \beta_i)u_{ij}\right\}, \quad j = 1, \ldots, N, \tag{2}$$

which is obtained by equating all first-order person parameters in Eq. (1) to

$$\theta_{1j}^{[1]} = \theta_{2j}^{[1]} = \cdots = \theta_{nj}^{[1]} = \theta_j, \quad j = 1, \ldots, N, \tag{3}$$

and excluding all higher order terms in Eq. (1) by setting

$$\theta_{12j}^{[2]} = \beta_{12}^{[2]}, \theta_{13j}^{[2]} = \beta_{13}^{[2]}, \ldots, \theta_{12}^{[n]\cdots nj} = \beta_{12}^{[n]\cdots n}, \quad j = 1, \ldots, N. \tag{4}$$

(To be precise, one additional constraint must be imposed on the parameters in Eq. (2) to identify it, such as fixing one of the β_i values at 0.)

Conjunctive Model Exponential Family Structure

Many useful formal and practical features of conjunctive Rasch kernel stem from their exponential family membership (Andersen, 1980; Lehmann, 1983, 1986). The likelihood for a sample of independent response patterns $\mathbf{u}_1$ through $\mathbf{u}_N$ based on the general Rasch model in Eq. (1) has exponential structure,

$$Pr\{\mathbf{U}_1 = \mathbf{u}_1, \ldots, \mathbf{U}_n = \mathbf{u}_n \mid \Theta_1 = \theta_1, \ldots, \Theta_N = \theta_N; \boldsymbol{\beta}\}$$

$$\propto \exp\Bigg\{\sum_{i=1}^{n}\sum_{j=1}^{N}\theta_{ij}^{[1]}u_{ij} + \sum_{i=1}^{n-1}\sum_{i'=i+1}^{n}\sum_{j=1}^{N}\theta_{ii'j}^{[2]}u_{ij}u_{i'j}$$

$$+ \cdots + \sum_{j=1}^{N}\theta_{1\cdots nj}^{[n]}u_{1j}\cdots u_{nj} - \sum_{i=1}^{n}\beta_i^{[1]}\sum_{j=1}^{N}u_{ij}$$

$$- \sum_{i=1}^{n-1}\sum_{i'=i+1}^{n}\beta_{ii'}^{[2]}\sum_{j=1}^{N}u_{ij}u_{i'j} - \cdots - \beta_{12\cdots n}^{[n]}\sum_{j=1}^{N}u_{1j}\cdots u_{nj}\Bigg\}, \tag{5}$$

and the likelihood based on the conventional Rasch special case in Eq. (2) has exponential structure,

$$Pr\{\mathbf{U}_1 = \mathbf{u}_1, \ldots, \mathbf{U}_N = \mathbf{u}_N \mid \Theta_1 = \theta_1, \ldots, \Theta_N = \theta_N; \boldsymbol{\beta}\}$$

$$\propto \exp\left\{\sum_{j=1}^{N}\theta_j\sum_{i=1}^{n}u_{ij} - \sum_{i=1}^{n}\beta_i\sum_{j=1}^{N}u_{ij}\right\}. \tag{6}$$

The exponential structure in Eq. (5) identifies a linked parameter, sufficient-statistic pair with each exponent term. The maximum likelihood estimate of each parameter is a monotone function of its linked sufficient statistic when all other sufficient statistics are fixed. As a result, special cases of Eq. (5) are easy to interpret. For example, the conventional Rasch model exponential structure in Eq. (6) links each individual's parameter with the number of items passed by that individual, giving individual parameters an ability interpretation. The same structure links each item parameter with the number of individuals passing the item, giving item parameters a difficulty interpretation. Exponential structure will be used to interpret other Rasch conjunctive kernels after reviewing local independence next.

Conjunctive IRT and Local Independence Form

The test theory local independence axiom (Lazarsfeld, 1960; Lord and Novick, 1968) has a formal side and a practical side. Formally, local independence requires test pattern kernels to be products of item response kernels. For example, the conventional Rasch kernel is a locally independent special case of Eq. (1) as the first expression in Eq. (2) shows.

Unlike the conventional Rasch kernel, most other conjunctive Rasch kernels are locally dependent. For example, consider a test made up of t "testlets" (Wainer and Kiely, 1987), with two items in each testlet. One locally dependent kernel for such a test has the form,

$$Pr\{U_{(2\times t)j} = u_{(2\times t)j} \mid (\Theta_j^{[1]}, \Theta_j^{[2]}) = (\theta_j^{[1]}, \theta_j^{[2]}); \beta_{(2\times t)}^{[1]}, \beta_{(t)}^{[2]}\} =$$

$$\prod_{k=1}^{t} \frac{\exp\{(\theta_j^{[1]} - \beta_{1k}^{[1]})u_{1jk} + (\theta_j^{[1]} - \beta_{2k}^{[1]})u_{2jk} + (\theta_j^{[2]} - \beta_{2k}^{[2]})u_{1jk}u_{2jk}\}}{1 + \exp\{\theta_j^{[1]} - \beta_{l1}^{[1]}\} + \exp\{\theta_j^{[1]} - \beta_{2k}^{[1]}\} + \exp\{\theta_j^{[1]} - \beta_{1k}^{[1]} + \theta_j^{[1]} - \beta_{2k}^{[1]} + \theta_j^{[1]} + \theta_j^{[2]} - \beta_k^{[2]}\}}. \tag{7}$$

The test kernel in Eq. (7) indicates that items are locally independent between testlets, because Eq. (7) is a product of its t testlet kernels. Item pairs within testlets are locally dependent, however, because each factor in Eq. (7) is not the product of its two marginal item probabilities. For example, the joint kernel for the first testlet item pair in Eq. (7) is

$$Pr\{(U_{1j1}, U_{2j1}) = (u_{1j1}, u_{2j1}) \mid (\Theta_j^{[1]}, \Theta_j^{[2]}) = (\theta_j^{[1]}, \theta_j^{[2]}); \beta_{11}^{[1]}, \beta_{21}^{[1]}, \beta_1^{[2]}\} =$$

$$\frac{\exp\{(\theta_j^{[1]} - \beta_{11}^{[1]})u_{1j1} + (\theta_j^{[1]} - \beta_{21}^{[1]})u_{2j1} + (\theta_j^{[2]} - \beta_1^{[2]})u_{1j1}u_{2j1}\}}{1 + \exp\{\theta_j^{[1]} - \beta_{11}^{[1]}\} + \exp\{\theta_j^{[1]} - \beta_{21}^{[1]}\} + \exp\{\theta_j^{[1]} - \beta_{11}^{[1]} + \theta_j^{[1]} - \beta_{21}^{[1]} + \theta_j^{[2]} - \beta_1^{[2]}\}}, \tag{8}$$

but it follows from Eq. (7) that its two item kernels are

$$Pr\{U_{1j1} = u_{1j1} \mid (\Theta_j^{[1]}, \Theta_j^{[2]}) = (\theta_j^{[1]}, \theta_j^{[2]}); \beta_{11}^{[1]}, \beta_{21}^{[1]}, \beta_1^{[2]}\} =$$

$$\sum_{u_{2j1}=0}^{1} Pr\{(U_{1j1}, U_{2j1}) = (u_{1j1}, u_{2j1}) \mid (\Theta_j^{[1]}, \Theta_j^{[2]}) = (\theta_j^{[1]}, \theta_j^{[2]}); \beta_{11}^{[1]}, \beta_{21}^{[1]}, \beta_1^{[2]}\} =$$

$$\frac{\exp\{(\theta_j^{[1]} - \beta_{11}^{[1]} u_{1j1}\} + \exp\{(\theta_j^{[1]} - \beta_{11}^{[1]}) u_{1j1} + (\theta_j^{[1]} - \beta_{21}^{[1]}) + (\theta_j^{[2]} - \beta_1^{[2]}) u_{1j1}\}}{1 + \exp\{\theta_j^{[1]} - \beta_{11}^{[1]}\} + \exp\{\theta_j^{[1]} - \beta_{21}^{[1]}\} + \exp\{\theta_j^{[1]} - \beta_{11}^{[1]} + \theta_j^{[1]} - \beta_{21}^{[1]} + \theta_j^{[2]} - \beta_1^{[2]}\}} \tag{9}$$

and

$$Pr\{U_{2j1} = u_{2j1} \mid (\Theta_j^{[1]}, \Theta_j^{[2]}); \beta_{11}^{[1]}, \beta_{21}^{[1]}, \beta_1^{[2]}\} =$$

$$\frac{\exp\{(\theta_j^{[1]} - \beta_{21}^{[1]}) u_{2j1}\} + \exp\{(\theta_j^{[1]} - \beta_{21}^{[1]}) u_{2j1} + (\theta_j^{[1]} - \beta_{11}^{[1]}) + (\theta_j^{[2]} - \beta_1^{[2]}) u_{2j1}\}}{1 + \exp\{\theta_j^{[1]} - \beta_{11}^{[1]}\} + \exp\{\theta_j^{[1]} - \beta_{21}^{[1]}\} + \exp\{\theta_j^{[1]} - \beta_{11}^{[1]} + \theta_j^{[1]} - \beta_{21}^{[1]} + \theta_j^{[2]} - \beta_1^{[2]}\}}, \tag{10}$$

the product of which is distinct from Eq. (8). Thus, the conjunctive kernel in Eq. (7) is formally locally dependent.

Practical Consequences of Local Dependence

The practical side of locally dependent conjunctive models can be seen by examining their conditional probability and exponential family structure. From Eq. (8) and Eq. (10), the conditional probability of passing the second item in testlet 1 once the first item has been taken is,

$$\begin{aligned} & Pr\{U_{2j1} = u_{2j1} \mid U_{1j1} = u_{1j1}; (\Theta_j^{[1]}, \Theta_j^{[2]}) = (\theta_j^{[1]}, \theta_j^{[2]}); \beta_{11}^{[1]}, \beta_{21}^{[1]}, \beta_1^{[2]}\} \\ &= \frac{Pr\{(U_{1j1}, U_{2j1}) = (u_{1j1}, u_{2j1}) \mid (\Theta_j^{[1]}, \Theta_j^{[2]}) = (\theta_j^{[1]}, \theta_j^{[2]}); \beta_{11}^{[1]}, \beta_{21}^{[1]}, \beta_1^{[2]}\}}{Pr\{U_{1j1} = u_{1j1}) \mid (\Theta_j^{[1]}, \Theta_j^{[2]}) = (\theta_j^{[1]}, \theta_j^{[2]}); \beta_{11}^{[1]}, \beta_{21}^{[1]}, \beta_1^{[2]}\}} \\ &= \frac{\exp\{[(\theta_j^{[1]} + \theta_j^{[2]} u_{1j1}) - (\beta_{21}^{[1]} + \beta_1^{[2]} u_{1j1})] u_{2j1}\}}{1 + \exp\{(\theta_j^{[1]} + \theta_j^{[2]} u_{1j1}) - (\beta_{21}^{[1]} + \beta_1^{[2]} u_{1j1})\}}. \end{aligned} \tag{11}$$

Evidently from Eq. (11), U_{2j1} will follow a Rasch model with ability parameter $\theta_j^{[1]}$ and difficulty parameter $\beta_2^{[1]}$ after u_{1j1} has been failed, but it will follow a different Rasch model with ability parameter $(\theta_j^{[1]} + \theta_j^{[2]})$ and difficulty parameter $(\beta_{21}^{[1]} + \beta_1^{[2]})$ after u_{1j1} has been passed. Thus U_{2j1} follows a locally dependent Rasch model, with its ability and difficulty parameters depending on the previous u_{1j1} response.

In practical terms, the structure of Eq. (11) shows that Eq. (7) can model learning during testing. For example, testlet item pairs like those in Eq. (7) can be given in a series of t trials, within which the student is asked to learn during an initial task, the student is next given a reinforcement in keeping with the task response and the student is then given a second task that requires proper comprehension from the first task. In that case, the second-order item parameters $\beta_k^{[2]}$ indicate how students respond to reinforced learning as a group and the second-order person parameters $\theta_j^{[2]}$ indicate how students respond to reinforced learning as individuals.

The conditional probabilities in Eq. (11) for the testlet model in Eq. (7) show that one Rasch model applies if the first item has been passed and another Rasch model applies otherwise. The second-order ability and difficulty parameters in Eq. (11) have similar interpretations to their first-order counterparts in Eq. (11) and in the conventional Rasch model. The second-order difficulty parameter represents the difference between difficulty when the first item is passed and difficulty when the first item is failed, and the second-order ability parameter represents the difference between ability when a first item is passed and ability when a first item is failed.

While its conditional probability structure explains Eq. (7) as a learning model, its exponential family structure justifies it as a learning measurement tool. Its structure based on Eq. (5) is,

$$Pr\{\mathbf{U}_{(2\times t)1} = \mathbf{u}_{(2\times t)1}, \ldots, \mathbf{U}_{(2\times t)N} = \mathbf{u}_{(2\times t)N} \mid$$

$$(\boldsymbol{\Theta}_1^{[1]}, \boldsymbol{\Theta}_1^{[2]}) = (\theta_1^{[1]}, \theta_1^{[2]}), \ldots, (\boldsymbol{\Theta}_t^{[1]}, \boldsymbol{\Theta}_t^{[2]}) = (\theta_t^{[1]}, \theta_t^{[2]}); \beta_{(2\times t)}^{[1]}, \beta_{(t)}^{[2]}\}$$

$$\propto \exp\left\{\sum_{j=1}^{N} \theta_j^{[1]} \sum_{k=1}^{t} (u_{1jk} + u_{2jk}) + \sum_{j=1}^{N} \theta_j^{[2]} \sum_{k=1}^{t} u_{1jk}u_{2jk}\right.$$

$$\left. - \sum_{k=1}^{t} \beta_{1k}^{[1]} \sum_{j=1}^{N} u_{j1k} - \sum_{k=1}^{t} \beta_{2k}^{[1]} \sum_{j=1}^{N} u_{j2k} - \sum_{k=1}^{t} \beta_k^{[2]} \sum_{j=1}^{N} u_{j1k}u_{j2k}\right\}. \tag{12}$$

Thus, the exponential structure in Eq. (12) links each first-order ability parameter $\theta_j^{[1]}$ with the number of items passed by each individual, and it links each first-order difficulty parameter $\beta_{ik}^{[1]}$ with the number of individuals passing the item, just as in the conventional Rasch model. It departs from additive Rasch structure, however, by also linking second-order learning statistics to their corresponding learning parameters.

The testlet item pairs that persons pass are linked to their $\theta_j^{[2]}$ parameters in Eq. (12), giving them a conjunctive learning ability interpretation. Also, among other individuals having the same number-correct scores, higher conjunctive scores indicate the ability to learn through reinforced item passing, and lower conjunctive scores indicate the ability to learn through reinforced item failing. In this way, the conjunctive testlet scores provide extra information about learning during testing that additive item scores cannot.

For example, suppose a test is made up of 20 testlets, each of which involves two comprehension items from a short test paragraph. The test is given by initially presenting the first item in each testlet and receiving the response, next indicating the correct answer to the student and then presenting the second related testlet item. Now consider the subsample of students who get number-correct scores of 20 on the test, that is, students who pass half the test items. Within the subsample, conjunctive scores of 0 through 20 are possible, with a score of 0 indicating students who learn only by failing first testlet items, a score of 20 indicating students who learn only by passing first testlet items and intermediate scores indicating mixed learning styles.

Conjunctive models such as Eq. (7) are useful for ability selection and diagnosis based on number-correct scores, just like the conventional Rasch model. The key difference is that conjunctive models can also measure learning abilities during testing while conventional models cannot. Conjunctive models are especially suitable for concurrent tutoring settings, where learning styles are measured during on-line tutoring and remaining tasks are tailored accordingly.

Related Locally Dependent Models

The testlet model in Eq. (7) is one among many special cases of the CIRT family [Eq. (1)] that have been reviewed elsewhere (Jannarone, 1991). These include Rasch Markov models having items linked into learning chains; pretest-posttest models for assessing learning style after pretest feedback and componential models for assessing individually necessary skills associated with composite tasks. As with the testlet model in Eq. (7), all such CIRT models are distinguished by their nonadditive statistics and justified by their exponential family structure.

Other CIRT models that have been studied include concurrent speed and accuracy (CSA) measurements models (Jannarone, to appear, a) and concurrent information processing (CIP) neural network models (Jannarone, to appear, b). CSA models are based on measuring both item response quickness and correctness, with provisions for reflecting individual differences in cognitive processes. CIP models are designed to produce neurocomputing structures that can learn relationships among measurements, automatically and quickly. All such models rely on nonadditive sufficient statistics within the exponential family that violate local independence.

Returning to the formal side, a variety of CIRT contrasts and connections with traditional test theory have been described elsewhere (Jannarone, 1990, 1991, in press), regarding local independence, sufficient statistic additivity, specific objectivity, item discrimination, dimensionality, item response function form and nonparametric alternatives. Some of these connections will be summarized in the remainder of this section.

Local Independence and Measurement Additivity

A straightforward analysis of Eq. (1) has shown that CIRT special cases are locally independent if and only if they exclude nonadditive sufficient statistics (Jannarone, 1990). This simple result has broad implications once CIRT family generality and its statistically sound (SS) properties and recognized, in terms of both exponential family membership and specific objectivity (Jannarone, in press).

For example, the two-parameter (Birnbaum) model attempts to explain more than the additive Rasch model by including an extra parameter for each item that reflects discrimination power. However, the Birnbaum model falls outside the family of SS models, which poses an interesting question. Can a SS model be constructed that measures differential item discrimination? Interestingly, the answer is that such a model can be found but it must *necessarily* violate local independence. Similar conclusions follow for other extended IRT models that measure differential guessing ability, multivariate latent abilities and the like. Indeed, *any* SS alternative to the Rasch model that extracts extended (i.e., nonadditive) information from binary items *must* violate the local independence axiom (Jannarone, in press).

Thus on the practical side, local independence restricts IRT to settings where people cannot learn during testing. On the formal side, locally independent and SS models are restricted to conventional Rasch models. From both formal and practical viewpoints, therefore, the local independence axiom stands in the way of interesting extensions to test theory and application.

Local Dependence and Dimensionality

Modern IRT has been greatly influenced by factor analysis models, for which a joint normal distribution among latent and observable variables is often assumed (Jöreskog, 1978). Factor analysis models usually also assume that observable variables are uncorrelated if all latent variables are fixed, which with normality implies local independence. Indeed, the existence of a "complete" latent space that can satisfy local independence is a conventional test theory foundation (Lord and Novick, 1968, Sec. 16.3; McDonald, 1981; Yen, 1984).

Given conjunctive family membership, however, latent variables that can account for all local, interitem dependencies may not exist. For example, if a testlet model satisfying Eq. (7) exists with any $\beta_{ii'}^{[2]} \neq \theta_j^{[2]}$, then no equivalent locally independent CIRT counterpart can be constructed. Thus, the traditional notion that conditioning on added dimensions can remove interitem dependencies breaks down in conjunctive IRT, placing it at odds with conventional test theory at the foundation level.

Local Independence and Nonparametrics

Nonparametrics offers a model-free alternative to parametric modeling, which is attractive to some because it avoids making false assumptions.

(Nonparametrics is less attractive to others, because it avoids linking model parameters to sufficient statistics and producing sound alternatives in the process.) When properly conceived, nonparametrics admits useful alternatives that fall outside conventional model families. This subsection will describe one nonparametric approach to test theory that is improperly conceived, because it restricts admissible IRT models to only the locally indepenent variety.

When parametric family membership is not assumed, the local independence assumption is trivial unless other conditions are imposed. For any locally dependent models, Suppes and Zanotti (1981) showed how to construct an equivalent locally independent model, by placing latent variables in one-to-one correspondence with observations. In a similar development, Stout (1990) showed that alternative locally independent and unidimensional models can always explain test scores when items are discrete. However, these alternatives are vacuous as Stout pointed out, because statistical inference is meaningless when only one observation exists per parameter.

To exclude such trivial models from consideration, some authors (Holland, 1981; Holland and Rosenbaum, 1986; Rosenbaum, 1984; Stout, 1987; 1990) developed "nonparametric tests" based on test models that satisfied certain requirements. Unfortunately the requirements they imposed, namely response function (RF) monotonicity and local independence, restricted admissible IRT models to the exclusion of useful parametric models, namely CIRT models. Consequently, the unidimensionality tests that they based on these restrictions are not at all nonparametric.

Understanding the rationale behind imposing the above restrictions is useful, because it clarifies some important distinctions between IRT and CIRT models. Response function monotonicity is appealing because it allows latent variables to be regarded as abilities that increase with item passing probabilities (Holland and Rosenbaum, 1986). Monotonicity along with local independence also guarantee latent trait identifiability in a variety of settings. For example, consider the observable random variable (U_1, U_2) for a two-item test that depends on a single latent trait Θ. Given local independence in this case, a model would not be identifiable if for any $\theta_1 \neq \theta_2$,

$$\begin{aligned}(Pr\{U_1 = 1 \mid \Theta = \theta_1\}, Pr\{U_2 = 1 \mid \Theta = \theta_1\}) \\ = (Pr\{U_1 = 1 \mid \Theta = \theta_2\}, Pr\{U_2 = 1 \mid \Theta = \theta_2\}),\end{aligned} \tag{13}$$

but Eq. (13) would be impossible given RF monotonicity. Thus, besides improving interpretability, monotonicity can help guarantee statistical soundness. Response function monotonicity is restrictive, however, because it excludes useful models from consideration. For example, identifiable CIRT models can be constructed satisfying Eq. (13), much as analysis-of-variance models can be constructed having interactions but no main effects (Jannarone, 1990; Jannarone and Roberts, 1984).

In a related issue, CIRT models illustrate that "nonparametric tests for unidimensionality" (Holland and Rosenbaum, 1986) are misleading. For example, the testlet model in Eq. (7) with the $\theta_j^{[1]} = \theta_j^{[2]}$ is one-dimensional. However, data generated from such a model when the $\theta_j^{[2]} < \beta_k^{[2]}$ would produce negative interitem correlations within testlets, which are considered to be "rather strong evidence that the item responses themselves are not unidimensional" (Holland and Rosenbaum, 1986, p. 1541). Thus, excluding useful models from a restrictive "nonparametric" framework produces misleading conclusions when the framework is applied to them.

Another related issue is Stout's (1990) "essential local independence" requirement, which is satisfied if for each latent trait vector θ,

$$D_n(\theta) \equiv \frac{\sum_{1 \leq i < i' \leq n} Cov(U_i, U_{i'} \mid \Theta = \theta)}{\binom{n}{2}} \to 0 \tag{14}$$

as $n \to \infty$. Stout's definition is misleading in that some special cases of Eq. (1) are "essentially locally independent," but they have measurable and interesting locally dependent properties that prevail asymptotically.

In the testlet model (Eq. (7)) case for example, $Cov(U_i, U_{i'} \mid \Theta = \theta)$ is a positive constant if $i = i'$, a different constant for values of i and i' corresponding to items within testlets and 0 otherwise. Thus, as $n \to \infty$, $D_n(\theta)$ approaches 0, because the denominator of Eq. (10) is of higher order in n than its numerator (2 vs. 1). Stout's conclusion based on Eq. (14) would therefore be that the testlet model in Eq. (7) is "essentially locally independent," which makes no sense in light of its useful locally dependent properties.

The incorrect conclusions that follow when the above results are applied to conjunctive IRT models are worthy of special note, because the above approach is improperly presented as nonparametric. A worthwhile nonparametric approach excludes as few possibilities from consideration as possible, especially those that have clear potential utility. In a broader sense, the same problem holds for the local independence axiom that prevails throughout test theory. The time is at hand for the axiom to be replaced by a more general alternative, now that useful test models have been shown to exist that violate it.

Parameter Estimation

Parameter estimation for binary item conjunctive IRT resembles conventional Rasch model estimation, in that person and item parameters are estimated from person and item sufficient statistics. The soundness and efficiency of conjunctive IRT estimates are also assured by their exponential family membership, just as in the conventional Rasch estimation case.

The simplest person-parameter estimation approach for conjunctive IRT models is to use person sufficient statistics themselves in place of their linked parameters. More efficient schemes are possible for item parameter estimation, but they are much more complicated. Conjunctive Rasch model estimation is more complex than conventional Rasch model estimation, because nonadditive statistic possibilities are restricted when additive statistics values are fixed, and *vice versa*. For example, if a test is made up of five testlets satisfying Eq. (7), person sufficient statistics of the form

$$(s_j^{[1]}, s_j^{[2]}) = \left(\sum_{k=1}^{5} (u_{1jk} + u_{2jk}), \sum_{k=1}^{5} u_{1jk} u_{2jk} \right) \tag{15}$$

have possible $s_j^{[1]}$ values ranging from 0 to 10 and possible $s_j^{[2]}$ values ranging from 0 to 5. However, the range of $s_j^{[2]}$ values is restricted when $s_j^{[1]}$ values are fixed, for example to 0 given that $s_j^{[1]} = 0$, to between 1 and 3 given that $s_j^{[1]} = 6$ and to 4 given that $s_j^{[1]} = 9$. With these and other such restrictions, the end result is that only 21 possible contingencies exist for $(s_j^{[1]}, s_j^{[2]})$ instead of the 66 (11×6) that might be expected, causing $S_j^{[1]}$ to be highly correlated with $S_j^{[2]}$.

Efficient schemes that have been most studied so far are two-stage maximum likelihood estimation (Jannarone, 1987), conditional maximum likelihood estimation (Kelderman and Jannarone, 1989) and "easy Bayes" estimation (Jannarone et al., 1989) for the Rasch Markov model. Besides complexity resulting from additive and nonadditive statistic contingencies, an added source for complexity is the need for iterative procedures such as the Newton-Rapheson algorithm. A second added source for complexity is the need for recursive (elementary symmetric-like) functions to avoid counting all possible test patterns during each iteration.

A third added source for complexity is the need to augment sample data with prior information so that useful estimates can be obtained for all possible contingencies. In the Eq. (7) case involving five testlets, for example, maximum likelihood person parameter estimation is possible for only 6 of the 21 possible $(s_j^{[1]}, s_j^{[2]})$ contingencies, because the other 15 occur at boundary values for one person-statistic when the other person-statistic is fixed. To give one such set of boundary values, $s_j^{[2]}$ values are restricted to between 1 and 3 given that $s_j^{[1]} = 6$, but among these possible contingencies only $(s_j^{[1]}, s_j^{[2]}) = (6, 2)$ admits a maximum likelihood estimate, because $(s_j^{[1]}, s_j^{[2]})$ values of $(6, 1)$ and $(6, 3)$ are conditional boundary values for $s_j^{[2]}$. Such boundary-value contingencies can produce useful "easy Bayes" estimates instead of impossible maximum likelihood estimates, but deriving them is not easy and obtaining them takes iterative convergence time (Jannarone et al., 1990).

Because efficient estimation takes both effort to program and time to converge, the use of simple sufficient statistics in place of efficient parameter estimates is recommended, at least as a basis for initial study. For example, assessing the stepwise correlation between external measurements of interest and $s_j^{[2]}$ values, over and above $s_j^{[1]}$ values, is a natural and simple first step in evaluating the utility of testlet learning measurements. Also, using $s_j^{[2]}$ values instead of efficient $\theta_j^{[2]}$ estimates may be needed in tailored tutoring or testing settings where person estimates must be updated and used concurrently and quickly, before selecting a new task for presentation.

Goodness of Fit

Efficient methods for assessing conjunctive parameters have been developed based on straightforward asymptotic theory (Jannarone, 1986; 1987; Kelderman and Jannarone, 1989), but the use of simple methods based on sufficient statistics is recommended for initial study. For example, second-order testlet parameters are worth estimating only if their linked measurements provide useful predictive power over and above additive sufficient statistics. As in the previous section, the easiest means for utility assessment is through stepwise correlation of second-order sufficient statistics with external measurements, controlling for first-order sufficient statistic correlations.

Less simple methods for assessing goodness of fit have been developed based on consistent conjunctive parameter estimates and multinomial hypothesis testing (Jannarone, 1986). These methods produce asymptotic chi square tests that additive and conjunctive item parameters are zero, which provide global as well as nested assessment of additive Rasch models and their conjunctive extensions. Other asymptotic tests based on maximum likelihood estimates (Jannarone, 1987) and conditional maximum likelihood estimates (Kelderman and Jannarone, 1989) are simple to construct, because CIRT models belong in the exponential family.

Examples

Available empirical results for nonadditive test measurement include simple tests for item cross-product step-wise correlations from personality data (Jannarone and Roberts, 1984), and asymptotically efficient tests of hypotheses that second-order parameters are 0 from educational test data (Jannarone, 1986). Also, Monte Carlo studies have been performed for the Rasch-Markov model, verifying that useful predictability can be obtained from second-order statistics, over and above additive statistical information (Jannarone, 1987).

Results of all such assessments have shown that CIRT models have potential utility over and above additive IRT models. Significantly interacting item counts were found to far exceed chance values in personality data (Jannarone and Roberts, 1984), and significant conjunctive item parameter counts were found to far exceed chance levels in verbal analogies and personality data (Jannarone, 1986).

Simulation studies have also been performed to assess CIRT model utility based on componential item pairs (Jannarone, 1986) and items linked by learning (Jannarone, 1987). Both studies showed that CIRT models produce conjunctive ability estimates with significant predictability over and above additive ability estimates.

Discussion

A natural area for conjunctive IRT application is interactive computer testing and tutoring, where learning performance and task response times can quickly be assessed, reinforcements can quickly be provided and new tasks can quickly be selected accordingly. This area is especially promising now that concurrent information processing procedures are available for automatically learning and responding to input computer measurements as quickly as they arrive (Jannarone, to appear, b). For tailored tutoring and testing applications, this translates to receiving a student's response to an item, measuring its quickness and correctness, quickly updating that student's parameter estimates accordingly and automatically selecting the next task for presentation accordingly.

Bringing IRT into computerized tutoring requires developing entirely new tests that are based on assessing reinforced learning, instead of assessing previously learned aptitude. To the author's knowledge this is an interesting but unexplored field for future IRT study.

As human-computer interaction continues to accelerate its impact on human information processing, a prominent role for IRT in computing technology could bring new vitality to psychometrics. The most promising such role is for concurrent learning assessment during adaptive computerized tutoring. A necessary condition for IRT involvement in this vital new area, however, is that it break away from local independence as a fundamental requirement.

References

Andersen, E.B. (1980). *Discrete Statistical Models with Social Science Applications.* Amsterdam: North Holland.

Andrich, D. (1985). A latent trait model with response dependencies: implications for test construction and analysis. In S.E. Embretson (Ed.), *Test Design: Developments in Psychology and Psychometrics* (pp. 245–275). Orlando, FL: Academic Press.

Bickel, P. and Doksum, K. (1977). *Mathematical Statistics: Basic Ideas and Selected Topics.* San Francisco: Holden-Day.

Embretson, S. (1984). A general latent trait model for item responses. *Psychometrika* **49**, 211–218.

Gibbons, R.D., Bock, R.D., and Hedeker, D.R. (1989). *Conditional Dependence* (Office of Naval Research Final Report No. 89-1). Chicago: University of Chicago.

Holland, P.W. (1981). When are item response models consistent with observed data? *Psychometrika* **46**, 79–92.

Holland, P.W. and Rosenbaum, P.R. (1986). Conditional association and unidimensionality in monotone latent variable models. *Annals of Statistics* **14**, 1523–1543.

Jannarone, R.J. (1986). Conjunctive item response theory kernels. *Psychometrika* **51**, 357–373.

Jannarone, R.J. (1987). *Locally Independent Models for Reflecting Learning Abilities* (Center for Machine Intelligence Report No. 87-67). Columbia, SC: University of South Carolina.

Jannarone, R.J. (1990). *Locally Dependent Cognitive Process Measurement: Contrasts and Connections with Traditional Test Theory* (Center for Machine Intelligence Report No. 90-01). Columbia, SC: University of South Carolina.

Jannarone, R.J. (1991). Conjunctive measurement theory: Cognitive research prospects. In M. Wilson (Ed.), *Objective Measurement: Theory into Practice.* Norwood, NJ: Ablex, 211–236.

Jannarone, R.J. (1994). Local dependence: objectively measurable or objectionably abominable? In M. Wilson (Ed.), *Objective Measurement: Theory into Practice*, Vol. II. Norwood, NJ: Ablex, 211–236.

Jannarone, R.J. (to appear, a). Measuring quickness and correctness concurrently: A conjunctive IRT approach. In M. Wilson (Ed.), *Objective Measurement: Theory into Practice*, Vol. III. Norwood, NJ: Ablex.

Jannarone, R.J. (to appear, b). *Concurrent Information Processing: A Psycho-Statistical Model for Real-Time Neurocomputing.* New York: Van Nostrand Reinhold.

Jannarone, R.J. and Roberts, J.S. (1984). Reflecting interactions in personality scales: Meehl's paradox revisited. *Journal of Personality and Social Psychology* **47**, 621–628.

Jannarone, R.J., Yu, K.F., and Laughlin, J.E. (1990). Easy Bayes estimation for Rasch-type models. *Psychometrika* **55**, 449–460.

Jöreskog, K.G. (1978). Statistical analysis of covariance and correlation matrices. *Psychometrika* **43**, 443–477.

Kelderman, H. and Jannarone, R.J. (1989, April). Conditional maximum likelihood estimation in conjunctive item response models. Paper presented at the meeting of the American Educational Research Association, San Francisco.

Lazarsfeld, P.F. (1960). Latent structure analysis and test theory. In H. Gulliksen and S. Messick (Eds.), *Psychological Scaling: Theory and Applications* (pp. 83–96). New York: McGraw-Hill.

Lehmann, E.L. (1983). *Theory of Point Estimation.* New York: Wiley.

Lehmann, E.L. (1986). *Testing Statistical Hypotheses* (2nd ed.). New York: Wiley.

Lord, F.M. and Novick, M.R. (1968). *Statistical Theories of Mental Test Scores.* Reading, MA: Addison-Wesley.

McDonald, R.P. (1981). The dimensionality of test and items. *British Journal of Mathematical and Statistical Psychology* **34**, 100–117.

Rosenbaum, P.R. (1984). Testing the conditional independence and monotonicity assumptions of item response theory. *Psychometrika* **49**, 425–436.

Rosenbaum, P.R. (1987). Probability inequalities for latent scales. *British Journal of Mathematical and Statistical Psychology* **40**, 157–168.

Spray, J.A. and Ackerman, T.A. (1986, April). The effects of item response dependency on trait or ability dimensionality. Paper presented at the meeting of the Psychometric Society, Toronto.

Stout, W. (1987). A nonparametric approach for assessing latent trait dimensionality. *Psychometrika* **52**, 589–617.

Stout, W. (1990). A nonparametric multidimensional IRT approach with applications to ability estimation. *Psychometrika* **55**, 293–326.

Suppes, P. and Zanotti, M. (1981). When are probabilistic explanations possible? *Synthese* **48**, 191–199.

Wainer, H. and Kiely G. (1987). Item clusters in computerized adaptive testing: A case for tests. *Journal of Educational Measurement* **24**, 185–202.

Yen, W.M. (1984). Effects of local item dependence on the fit and equating performance of the three-parameter logistic model. *Applied Psychological Measurement* **8**, 125–145.

28

Mismatch Models for Test Formats that Permit Partial Information to be Shown

T.P. Hutchinson

Introduction

The conventional IRT models—that is, those for which the probability of examinee j correctly answering item i is $P_i(\theta_j)$, θ being ability and P being an increasing function—make no allowance for the examinee having *partial information* about the question asked. The models are unable to predict what might happen in situations which allow the partial information to be shown. Relations between probabilities of correctness in different formats of test—for example, with different numbers of options to choose from, or permitting a second attempt at items initially answered wrongly—do not fall within their scope.

There are two reasons why the existence of partial information is credible:

1. *Introspection.* Often, one is conscious of having some information relating to the question posed, without being sure of being able to select the correct option.

2. *Experiment.* Among responses chosen with a high degree of confidence, a greater proportion are correct than among those chosen with a low degree of confidence. Second attempts at items initially answered wrongly have a higher-than-chance probability of being correct. And other results of this type.

Much the same can be said concerning perception, e.g., of a faint visual or auditory stimulus. What has been done in that field is to develop *signal detection theory* (SDT). The model to be proposed in this chapter is SDT applied to multiple-choice tests. Just as SDT enables performance in different types of perceptual experiment to be interrelated, so *mismatch theory* enables performance in different formats of ability or achievement test to be interrelated. Over the years, many different formats have been tried at some time or other; among them: (1) varying the number of options; (2)

including some items for which all options are wrong; (3) asking the examinee to accompany the response with a confidence rating; (4) having the examinee mark as many options as are believed to be wrong; and (5) permitting the examinee to make a second attempt at items initially answered wrongly.

More information concerning mismatch theory can be found in Hutchinson (1991). The first publication of the theory was in Hutchinson (1977), with much further development being in Hutchinson (1982).

Presentation of the Models

The Main Ideas

The important features of mismatch theory can be described using a single parameter to represent the ability of the examinee relative to the difficulty of the item. The symbol λ will be used. It is implicit that λ could be more fully written as λ_{ij} (where i labels the item and j labels the examinee); and that it would then be of interest to split λ into item and examinee components, e.g., as $\lambda_{ij} = 1 + \exp(\theta_j - b_i)$.

The central idea is as follows: Each alternative response that is available in a multiple-choice item gives rise within the examinee to a continuously-distributed random variable that reflects how inappropriate the alternative is to the question posed—that is, how much "mismatch" there is between the question and the alternative. The distribution of this random variable, which will be denoted X, is different in the case of the correct option from what it is for the incorrect options. Specifically, the correct answer tends to have a lower value of X than do the incorrect alternatives. The greater the difference between the distributions of X, the easier is the question (or the cleverer is the examinee). Denote the two distributions by F and G, $\Pr(X > x)$ being $F(x)$ for the correct option and $G(x)$ for any incorrect option, where $F < G$. The derivatives $-dF(x)/dx$ and $-dG(x)/dx$ are the respective probability density functions (p.d.f.'s). It is supposed that for each examinee, there is a response threshold T, such that if the mismatch exceeds this for all the alternative options, no choice is made. If at least one alternative gives rise to a value of X less than T, the one with the lowest value of X is selected. Equations for the probabilities of a correct response, of a wrong response, and of omitting the item may readily be obtained. For a given item, ability is measured by how different F and G are. They are chosen so as to jointly contain a single parameter characterizing ability, λ. λ may then be found from the empirical probabilities of correct and wrong responses.

To make any progress, it is necessary to make assumptions about F and G:

1. *Exponential Model.* One possible choice is to say that for the correct alternative, X has an exponential distribution over the range 0 to ∞, with scale parameter 1; and for the incorrect alternatives, X has an exponential distribution with scale parameter λ, with $\lambda \geq 1$. That is, we take $F(x) = \exp(-x)$ and $G(x) = \exp(-x/\lambda)$.

2. *Normal Model.* Another possible choice is to say that X has a normal distribution in both cases, but with different means. That is, $F(x) = 1 - \Phi(x)$ and $G(x) = 1 - \Phi(x - \lambda)$, with $\lambda \geq 0$.

3. *All-or-Nothing Model.* A third possibility is that, for the correct alternative, X has a uniform distribution over the range 0 to 1; and for the distractors, X has a uniform distribution over the range $1 - \lambda^{-1}$ to 1, with $\lambda \geq 1$. The significance of this proposal is that it embodies the conventional idea of all-or-nothing information: if mismatch is less than $1 - \lambda^{-1}$, the option generating it *must* have been the correct one; if mismatch exceeds $1 - \lambda^{-1}$, it carries no information about which sort of option it came from, and the examinee's response is a random guess. (Thus it is appropriate to call this a two-state theory.)

4. *Symmetric Uniform Model.* Take X to have a uniform distribution over the range 0 to 1, or a uniform distribution over the range λ to $1 + \lambda$, with $0 \leq \lambda \leq 1$, for the correct and incorrect options, respectively. This model is almost identical to a model introduced by Garcia-Pérez (1985), who supposes that the truth value of each option is either known (with probability λ) or not known (with probability $1 - \lambda$). That is, there are three possible states:

   a. Known to be correct: This state is entered with probability λ for the correct option.
   b. Status not known: This state is entered with probability $1 - \lambda$ for any option.
   c. Known to be incorrect: This state is entered with probability λ for the incorrect options.

   If no option is in the first state and at least two options are in the second state, then the examinee may (with probability g) guess at random between those options in the second state, or may (with probability $1 - g$) leave the item unanswered.

However, the assumptions about F and G need not be arbitrary, but can be guided by what empirical results are found. For instance, a choice of F and G that enables second-attempt performance to be correctly predicted from first-attempt performance is preferable to a choice that does not. Naturally, mathematical tractability also plays a part in the choice of F and G; the Exponential and All-or-Nothing Models are most convenient in this respect.

An alternative way of viewing this theory is in terms of "association" between options and the questions asked, instead of "mismatch." Association will be the opposite of mismatch, and the examinee will choose the option generating the highest association, rather than the lowest mismatch. There is no compelling reason to prefer either the language of mismatch or that of association.

Application to the Omission of Responses

In what follows, m will be the number of options per item, and c, w, and u will be the probabilities of items being correctly answered, wrongly attempted, and omitted.

Putting the model's assumptions that were described above into mathematical notation,

$$u = F(T)[G(T)]^{m-1}, \tag{1}$$

$$c = \int_{-\infty}^{T} -dF(x)/dx[G(x)]^{m-1}dx. \tag{2}$$

As $w = 1 - u - c$, there are two equations connecting the two unknowns, λ and T, with the two observables, c and w. In words, Eq. (1) says that the probability of not attempting the item is the probability that the mismatches from all options exceed T; and this is obtained by multiplying together the probabilities of the individual mismatches exceeding T, it being assumed these are independent. And Eq. (2) says that to get the probability of answering correctly, we must consider all values less than T of the mismatch from the correct alternative; if this value happens to be x, the mismatches from all incorrect options need to be greater than x if the correct option is to be chosen. Now, the probability that the correct option generated a mismatch between x and $x + dx$ is $(-dF(x)/dx)dx$, the probability that all the other mismatches are greater is $[G(x)]^{m-1}$, and we need to multiply these together and sum over all values of x that are less than T.

Omissions have long been a practical problem in the scoring of tests. One can instruct examinees to attempt all items, and tolerate any error resulting from failure to fully follow this. Or one can use the "correction for guessing" in scoring, and put up with the lack of realism in the random guessing model on which this is based. But it would be better to understand more fully what is happening, and to have a greater variety of actions available in the face of omissions. It is a simple matter to derive the correction for guessing $c - w/(N-1)$ from Eqs. (1) and (2) using the All-or-Nothing Model. If the Exponential Model is assumed instead, the ratio $c/[w/(N-1)]$ is found to be the appropriate measure of ability.

Application to Second-Choice Performance

It is now presumed that all items are attempted and that a second attempt is permitted at items wrongly answered at first. Without loss of generality, X can be taken to have a uniform distribution over the range 0 to 1 in the case of correct options. That is, $-dF/dx$ is 1 for x between 0 and 1 and is 0 elsewhere. Thus all the flexibility of choosing a model is embodied in the choice of $G(x)$. It will be convenient to adopt this formulation now.

It is evident that according to the mismatch theory, the probability that the mismatch takes a value between x and $x + dx$ in the case of the correct option, that exactly k of the wrong options have a higher mismatch, and that exactly $m - 1 - k$ of them have a lower mismatch is

$$\binom{m-1}{k} [G(x)]^k [1 - G(x)]^{m-1-k} dx. \tag{3}$$

Consequently, the probability of making the correct choice at first attempt can be seen to be (on setting $k = m - 1$ and integrating over all possible values of X)

$$c_1 = \int_0^1 [G(x)]^{m-1} dx, \tag{4}$$

and similarly the probability of the correct alternative having the second-lowest mismatch is

$$c_2^* = \int_0^1 (m-1)[G(x)]^{m-2}[1 - G(x)]\, dx. \tag{5}$$

The (conditional) probability of giving the wrong answer when the second choice is made is then $c_2 = c_2^*/(1 - c_1)$.

For some choices of model, the expressions for c_1 and c_2 in terms of λ are simple, and λ can be eliminated from these equations, enabling us to obtain a relationship between c_1 and c_2:

1. If the All-or-Nothing Model is used, $c_2 = 1/(m - 1)$, independent of c_1, is obtained.

2. If the Exponential Model is used, $c_2 = (m - 1)c_1/(m - 2 + c_1)$ is obtained.

What if All Options are Wrong?

Items for which all the options are wrong are, perhaps, not revealing of partial information as such, but the proportion which examinees attempt is a measure of their willingness to answer, and thus helps interpret behavior on normal items.

The most straightforward assumption to make is that the probability distribution of mismatch for all the alternatives listed for any nonsense item is the same as for the incorrect alternatives in the genuine items. Then the probability of leaving a nonsense item unanswered is $[G(T)]^m$. And the probability of answering is $a = 1 - [G(T)]^m$. Once one has made a choice of model, a can be expressed in terms of T; T can be found from responses to conventional items (i.e., from u, c, and w); finally, an equation can be written to predict a from (any two of) u, c, and w.

In the case of the All-or-Nothing Model, a may be found to be

$$\frac{mw}{(m-1)u + mw}. \tag{6}$$

This equation has been given by Ziller (1957). In the case of the Exponential Model, a may be found to be

$$1 - u^{mw/[(m-1)(1-u)]}. \tag{7}$$

"None of the Above"

Suppose that in each item, the final option is "none of the above" (NOTA), and that examinees attempt every item. Let NOTA$^-$ and NOTA$^+$ items be those where NOTA is wrong and correct, respectively. There will be five types of response—for NOTA$^-$ items: correct content option, incorrect content option, and NOTA option; and for NOTA$^+$ items: incorrect content option and NOTA option. Then mismatch theory will suggest that:

$$n_- = F(T)[G(T)]^{m-2}, \tag{8}$$

$$c_- = \int_{-\infty}^{T} \frac{-dF(x)}{dx} [G(x)]^{m-2} dx, \tag{9}$$

$$n_+ = [G(T)]^{m-1}, \tag{10}$$

where n_- is the probability of a NOTA response in a NOTA$^-$ item, c_- is the probability of a correct response in a NOTA$^-$ item, and n_+ is the probability of a NOTA response in a NOTA$^+$ item. (The response threshold T is not necessarily the same as with ordinary items not having the NOTA option.) The probabilities of wrong responses are $w_- = 1 - u_- - c_-$ and $w_+ = 1 - n_+$.

If the Exponential Model holds, it may be shown that the relation

$$\log n_+ = \frac{m-1}{m-2} \cdot \frac{w_-}{c_- + w_-} \cdot \log n_- \tag{11}$$

should hold (see Hutchinson, 1991, Sect. 5.12, which includes a discussion of the paper by Garcia-Pérez and Frary, 1989).

Separate Item and Examinee Parameters

In Hutchinson (1991, Chap. 9), there are some proposals about how λ can be decomposed into separate item and examinee parameters, b_i and θ_j. For example, in the Exponential Model, λ can be anything from 1 to ∞. One might try $\log\log\lambda_{ij} = \theta_j - b_i$, or alternatively $\log(\lambda_{ij} - 1) = \theta_j - b_i$.

This reference also suggests how different wrong options may be allowed for, and the probability of examinee j selecting option k in item i modelled:

1. Take the mismatch distribution to be $G(x; \lambda_{ijk})$ for the jth examinee evaluating the kth option in the ith item. (For compactness of notation, forget about using the symbol F for the distribution for the correct option; let this be one of the G's.)

2. The probability of selecting option k is (if it is assumed that omitting the item is not a possibility, so that the response threshold T can be taken as ∞):

$$\int_{-\infty}^{\infty} \frac{-dG(x; \lambda_{ijk})}{dx} \prod_{l \neq k} G(x; \lambda_{ijl})\, dx. \tag{12}$$

3. When λ is split into option b_{ik} and examinee θ_j components, Eq. (12) (regarded as a function of θ_j) is an option response function (Bock, 1972; this volume). Indeed, a connection may be made between the Exponential Model and the particular equation suggested by Bock (Hutchinson, 1991, Sec. 9.5).

However, no practical trials of splitting λ into b_i and θ_j have yet been performed.

Parameter Estimation

In the empirical studies performed to date (see below), no attempt has been made to split λ into separate examinee and item components. Instead, some expedient like taking a group of items of similar difficulty, and then regarding λ as characteristic of the examinee only, has been adopted. That is, it has not been necessary to fit something like $2n + N$ parameters to a data matrix of size nN (n = number of items, and N = number of examinees); instead, the size of the data matrix has been something like $3N$ (counts of the numbers of items responded to in each of three ways, for each examinee), with the number of parameters being about N.

Consequently, parameter estimation has not been the major technical problem that it is in usual circumstances. It has been satisfactory to take a straightforward likelihood maximization or chi-squared minimization approach, using readily-available software (e.g., that of the Numerical Algorithms Group) to find the optimum. The NAG subroutines require that the user supply a subroutine for calculating the criterion statistic (for example, the log-likelihood) for a given value of the parameter being sought (that is, λ). So all that is needed are formulae for the theoretical probabilities of the different types of response, followed by calculation of the criterion statistic from these theoretical probabilities and the numbers observed in the empirical data.

By way of example, the data might be the number of 5-alternative items answered correctly at first attempt, at second attempt, and in three or more attempts, for each examinee. The relative proportions of these are predicted by Eqs. (4) and (5); naturally, it is necessary to choose the functional form of $G(x)$, and this will have an ability parameter λ.

Occasionally, we may be lucky enough to get an explicit expression for our estimate of λ. Continuing the example of the previous paragraph, suppose we are assuming the All-or-Nothing Model, and using minimum chi-squared as the estimation method. According to the model, the expected number of items in the three categories will be cn, $\frac{1}{4}(1-c)n$, and $\frac{3}{4}(1-c)n$, for any particular examinee whose probability of being correct at first attempt is c (this is what is called c_1 in Eq. (4), and could readily be written in terms of λ). The statistic to be minimized is

$$\frac{(O_1 - cn)^2}{cn} + \frac{(O_2 - \frac{1}{4}(1-c)n)^2}{\frac{1}{4}(1-c)n} + \frac{(O_3 - \frac{3}{4}(1-c)n)^2}{\frac{3}{4}(1-c)n},$$

where the O's are the observed numbers of items in the three categories, for this examinee. Differentiating with respect to c and setting the result equal to 0, the estimated c is found to be the solution of

$$\frac{c^2}{(1-c)^2} = \frac{\frac{3}{4}O_1^2}{3O_2^2 + O_3^2}.$$

As might be expected on commonsense grounds, the resulting estimate is not very different from the simple estimate, O_1/n. For example, if O_1/n is 0.5, and O_2/n is 0.2, and O_3/n is 0.3, then c is estimated by this method to be 0.486.

In the future, methods will need to be developed for estimating examinee and item parameters when λ is split into these. It is not clear whether it would be easy to adapt the methods that have been developed for conventional IRT, or whether new difficulties would be encountered.

Goodness of Fit

As for parameter estimation, the issues with mismatch theory are rather different from those for conventional IRT; since λ is not split into b_i and θ_j, questions about whether this is valid or whether there is interaction between examinee and item have not yet been faced.

A central feature of mismatch theory is that it allows performance in one format of the test to be predicted from performance in another. And it is in evaluating predictions of this type that goodness of fit is assessed.

The goodness of fit question has two sides to it. First, does the theory have *any* success? This can be answered by looking in the data for qualitative features predicted by the theory, and by correlating observed with predicted quantities. Second, is the theory *completely* successful, in the sense that the deviations of the data from the theory can reasonably be ascribed to chance? This can be answered by calculating some statistic like $\Sigma(\text{observed} - \text{expected})^2/\text{expected}$. (Indeed, this may be the criterion that is optimized in parameter estimation, in which case it already has been calculated.)

These two sides to the question will be illustrated in the empirical examples below.

Examples

Second-Choice Performance

If an examinee gets an item wrong and is then permitted a second attempt at it, is the probability of correctly answering it greater than chance? This is an effective contrast between the assumption of all-or-nothing information and theories that incorporate partial information.

Suppose an examinee responds to a 56-item test, each item having five alternatives, and answers 28 correctly at first attempt, leaving 28 to be attempted a second time. Then the All-or-Nothing Model will predict that about 7 items ($28 \times \frac{1}{4}$) will be correctly answered on the second attempt. But the Exponential Model will predict that about 16 items—that is, $28 \times (5-1) \times \frac{1}{2}/(5-2+\frac{1}{2})$—will be correctly answered at second attempt.

In terms of the two aspects of goodness of fit described above, theories incorporating partial information will have some success if c_2 is above $1/(m-1)$ for most examinees; a model will be completely successful if $\Sigma(\text{observed} - \text{expected})^2/\text{expected}$ is close to what it would be expected to be if all deviations of data from the model were chance ones.

These types of analyses were performed in Hutchinson (1991, Chap. 6) [originally, in Hutchinson (1986) and Hutchinson and Barton (1987)]. The data were from answer-until-correct tests of spatial reasoning and of mechanical reasoning, taken by secondary school pupils. In only a few cases were 4 or 5 attempts necessary in 5-alternative items, so the data for each examinee consisted of the numbers of items for which 1, 2, or 3+ attempts were necessary. These observed numbers can be denoted O_1, O_2, O_3. For each of several choices of the model (that is, for each of several choices of $G(x)$), expressions for expected numbers E_1, E_2, E_3 were written (with λ being included as an unknown parameter). The goodness of fit statistic that

TABLE 1. Comparison of the Goodness of Fit of Three Models, Using Three Datasets.

		Model	
Dataset	Exponential	Normal	All-or-Nothing
(1)	453	559	1074
(2)	442	428	803
(3)	370	360	420

was minimized was $\sum_{i=1}^{3}(O_i - E_i)^2/E_i$. To arrive at an overall measure of the goodness of fit of a model, the best (i.e., minimum obtainable) values of this for each examinee were summed over examinees. Models having small totals are obviously preferable to models having larger totals.

Table 1 compares the goodness of fit of the Exponential, Normal, and All-or-Nothing Models using three datasets:

1. 11 five-alternative spatial reasoning items of medium difficulty;
2. 11 five-alternative mechanical reasoning items of medium difficulty;
3. 9 three-alternative mechanical reasoning items of medium difficulty.

As can be seen in the table, one important aspect of the results was that the All-or-Nothing Model was clearly the worst.

Three further features of the data were: There was above-chance performance when making second and subsequent attempts at items initially answered wrongly; this is shown in Table 3.[1] Positive correlation was found between an examinee's probability of success at first attempt and at second attempt, see Table 2. (And there was also a positive correlation between an examinee's probability of success within two attempts and at the third attempt if that was necessary.) Correlations between examinees' abilities estimated from easy, difficult and medium items were rather higher when the abilities were estimated using the Exponential Model than when using the All-or-Nothing Model.

When All Options Are Wrong

As discussed above, an assumption about what $G(x)$ is will imply some particular relation between (on the one hand) the proportions of genuine items answered wrongly and left unanswered, and (on the other hand) the proportion of nonsense items responded to.

The analysis in Hutchinson (1991, Chap. 7) (originally, in Frary and Hutchinson, 1982) was of a test of chemistry that included four nonsense

[1] *Note to Table 3.* The last line gives the guessing probabilities for five-alternative items.

TABLE 2. Correlation Between Examinees' Probabilities of Success at First Attempt and Second Attempt.

Dataset	Correlation
(1)	0.46
(2)	0.33
(3)	0.05

TABLE 3. Conditional Probabilities of Answering Correctly at the qth Attempt, Given that the Previous $q-1$ Attempts Were Wrong.

Dataset	q			
	1	2	3	4
(1)	0.39	0.41	0.39	0.57
(2)	0.49	0.39	0.42	0.58
(3)	0.65	0.66		
$1/(6-n)$	0.25	0.33	0.50	

items having no correct answer. There being so few nonsense items per examinee, the approach taken was as follows. Examinees were grouped into ranges according to their value of Eq. (6); this is their predicted proportion of nonsense items responded to. Then the actual mean proportion responded to by the examinees in each group was found, and the predicted and actual proportions compared. The process was repeated, but with examinees now being grouped according to their value of Eq. (7).

Both Eqs. (6) and (7) enjoyed some degree of success, in the sense that the actual proportions tended to be high in the groups for which the predicted proportions were high, and low in the groups for which the predicted proportions were low. Both Eqs. (6) and (7) were less than perfect, in that they tended to overestimate the proportion of nonsense items that were attempted. See Table 4[2] for quantification of this. Equation (7) was a little more successful than Eq. (6).

Despite the few opportunities each examinee had for responding to nonsense items, an analysis of individual examinees' data was also undertaken: the observed values of a (which could only be 0, $\frac{1}{4}$, $\frac{1}{2}$, $\frac{3}{4}$, or 1) were correlated with the values predicted by Eqs. (6) and (7). The correlations were found to be 0.46 and 0.52, respectively.

[2] *Note to Table 4.* The last line gives the column means.

TABLE 4. Proportions of Nonsense Items Attempted.

Proportion Predicted by Eq. (6)	Actual Mean Response Probability	Proportion Predicted by Eq. (7)	Actual Mean Response Probability
0.90–1.00	0.84	0.90–1.00	0.88
0.80–0.90	0.67	0.80–0.90	0.68
0.70–0.80	0.56	0.70–0.80	0.66
0.60–0.70	0.49	0.69–0.70	0.61
0.50–0.60	0.48	0.50–0.60	0.50
0.00–0.50	0.29	0.40–0.50	0.42
		0.00–0.40	0.30
0.86	0.71	0.80	0.71

Confidence Rating

If examinees are permitted to express their degree of confidence in the response they have selected, it is often found that the higher the level of confidence, the greater the probability of being correct. See Hutchinson (1991, Sec. 5.4) for references.

Similarly, if examinees are persuaded to attempt items they first left unanswered, their performance is typically below their performance on the items they first did attempt, but is above the chance level. See Hutchinson (1991, Sec. 5.5) for references.

Multiple True–False Items

Sometimes an item consists of an introductory statement, together with M further statements, each of which the examinee has to classify as true or false. It ought to be possible to compare performance on a conventional item with that on the equivalent multiple true–false item (which would have 1 true statement and $N - 1$ false ones). Hutchinson (1991, Sec. 5.8) shows that it is indeed possible. (On one set of data published by Kolstad and Kolstad (1989), the Exponential Model was superior to a two-state model. But the comparison is of limited usefulness because the data was aggregated over all examinees and all items.)

Discussion

First, the empirical results that demonstrate partial information are not surprising. Unless one is committed to some strong form of all-or-nothing learning theory, they are qualitatively pretty much as expected. What is surprising is that no way of describing this mathematically has been developed previously—that is, why $c - w/(m-1)$ is well-known as "the" correction for guessing, but not $c/[w/(m-1)]$, and why Eq. (6) was proposed in 1957, but not Eq. (7).

Second, the mismatch model does not tackle the question of why items are answered wrongly—the item characteristics that might explain the b_i, and the characteristics of cognitive development, learning experiences, and personality that might explain the θ_j are not its concern.

Third, notice that there are ideas from cognitive psychology that provide detailed mechanistic accounts of problem-solving; for a review of such models, see Snow and Lohman (1989). Mismatch theory is much more of a broad brush approach than these, while being more explicit about psychological processes than standard IRT is. Since both less abstract and more abstract theories flourish, the mismatch idea falls within the range of what might be useful.

Fourth, as to future research needs, the most urgent line of future development is that of performing a greater number and variety of comparisons of the theoretical predictions with empirical results. Among the formats that ought to be studied are: second attempt permitted (e.g., answer-until-correct), nonsense items, NOTA items, confidence ratings, and multiple true-false items. These are not highly obscure types of test that are impracticable to administer; indeed, there is probably suitable data already in existence that could be confronted with theoretical predictions.

References

Bock, R.D. (1972). Estimating item parameters and latent ability when responses are scored in two or more nominal categories. *Psychometrika* **37**, 29–51.

Frary, R.B. and Hutchinson, T.P. (1982). Willingness to answer multiple-choice questions, as manifested both in genuine and in nonsense items. *Educational and Psychological Measurement* **42**, 815–821.

García-Pérez, M.A. (1985). A finite state theory of performance in multiple-choice tests. In E.E. Roskam and R. Suck (eds.), *Progress in Mathematical Psychology* (Vol. 1, pp. 455–464). Amsterdam: Elsevier.

García-Pérez, M.A. and Frary, R.B. (1989). Testing finite state models of performance in objective tests using items with 'None of the above' as an option. In J.P. Doignon and J.C. Falmagne (eds.), *Mathematical Psychology: Current Developments* (pp. 273–291). Berlin: Springer-Verlag.

Hutchinson, T.P. (1977). On the relevance of signal detection theory to the correction for guessing. *Contemporary Educational Psychology* **2**, 50–54.

Hutchinson, T.P. (1982). Some theories of performance in multiple choice tests, and their implications for variants of the task. *British Journal of Mathematical and Statistical Psychology* **35**, 71–89.

Hutchinson, T.P. (1986). Evidence about partial information from an answer-until-correct administration of a test of spatial reasoning. *Contemporary Educational Psychology* **11**, 264–275.

Hutchinson, T.P. (1991). *Ability, Partial Information, Guessing: Statistical Modelling Applied to Multiple-Choice Tests.* Adelaide: Rumsby Scientific Publishing.

Hutchinson, T.P. and Barton, D.C. (1987). A mechanical reasoning test with answer-until-correct directions confirms a quantitative description of partial information. *Research in Science and Technological Education* **5**, 93–101.

Kolstad, R.K. and Kolstad, R.A. (1989). Strategies used to answer MC test items by examinees in top and bottom quartiles. *Educational Research Quarterly* **13**, 2–5.

Snow, R.E. and Lohman, D.F. (1989). Implications of cognitive psychology for educational measurement. In R.L. Linn (ed.), *Educational Measurement* (3rd ed., pp. 263–331). New York: Macmillan.

Ziller, R.C. (1957). A measurement of the gambling response-set in objective tests. *Psychometrika* **22**, 289–292.

Subject Index

Author Index